Clinical Immunology

CLINICAL

with contributions by

Phil Gold, M.D., PH.D., F.R.C.P.(C)

ASSOCIATE PROFESSOR OF MEDICINE,
MCGILL UNIVERSITY FACULTY OF MEDICINE;
SENIOR RESEARCH ASSOCIATE AND ASSISTANT PHYSICIAN,
DEPARTMENT OF MEDICINE, THE MONTREAL GENERAL HOSPITAL,
MONTREAL, QUEBEC, CANADA

David Hawkins, M.D., F.R.C.P.(C)

ASSISTANT PROFESSOR OF MEDICINE,
MCGILL UNIVERSITY FACULTY OF MEDICINE;
RESEARCH ASSOCIATE AND ASSISTANT PHYSICIAN,
DEPARTMENT OF MEDICINE, THE MONTREAL GENERAL HOSPITAL,
MONTREAL, QUEBEC, CANADA

Joseph Shuster, M.D., PH.D.

ASSISTANT PROFESSOR OF MEDICINE,
MCGILL UNIVERSITY FACULTY OF MEDICINE;
RESEARCH ASSOCIATE AND ASSISTANT PHYSICIAN,
DEPARTMENT OF MEDICINE, THE MONTREAL GENERAL HOSPITAL,
MONTREAL, QUEBEC, CANADA

IMMUNOLOGY

Samuel O. Freedman, M.D., F.R.C.P.(C), F.A.C.P.

PROFESSOR OF MEDICINE, MCGILL UNIVERSITY FACULTY OF MEDICINE;
DIRECTOR, DIVISION OF CLINICAL IMMUNOLOGY AND ALLERGY,
SENIOR RESEARCH ASSOCIATE AND SENIOR PHYSICIAN,
DEPARTMENT OF MEDICINE, THE MONTREAL GENERAL HOSPITAL,
MONTREAL, QUEBEC, CANADA

with 50 illustrations

MEDICAL DEPARTMENT
HARPER & ROW, PUBLISHERS
NEW YORK, EVANSTON, SAN FRANCISCO, LONDON

CLINICAL IMMUNOLOGY

First Edition
Standard Book Number 06-140831-X
LIBRARY OF CONGRESS
CATALOG CARD NUMBER 74-154884

Contents

Preface

Almost every clinical discipline has been influenced by the rapid advances that have taken place in the science of immunology over the past decade. More often than not, however, the practical significance of new developments in immunologic research has remained obscure. The purpose of this book is to bring recent progress in experimental immunology to the bedside in a manner that is both useful and comprehensible. Thus, this volume is written not only for specialists in clinical immunology and allergy, but also for practitioners, teachers, investigators, and postgraduate trainees in the various branches of internal medicine, pediatrics, and surgery. The intention is to provide the reader with an appreciation of the etiology and pathogenesis of common immunologic disorders, as well as with detailed information concerning their clinical manifestations and treatment. In addition, the application of immunologic principles to the prevention of disease is emphasized.

The selection of topics for inclusion in a textbook of this type must be somewhat arbitrary because the scope of clinical immunology is relatively new and ill-defined. Nevertheless, an attempt has been made to stress those disease processes which are encountered most frequently in clinical practice or which illustrate an important immunologic concept. Based on these considerations, the first chapter introduces those immunologic principles that have the greatest relevance to the clinical chapters that follow; it is not intended to be an exhaustive review of basic immunology. Results of animal experimentation are discussed in the first and subsequent chapters only when they are considered essential to the understanding of comparable human disorders. The clinical chapters present a broad viewpoint of immunologic disorders, including immunologic deficiency states, diseases associated with hypergammaglobulinemia and autoantibodies, collagen-vascular and atopic diseases, allergic drug reactions, hypersensitivity to infectious agents, common immunization procedures and the immunologic aspects of transplantation, cancer, rheumatology, dermatology, nephrology, hematology, pulmonary diseases, gastroenterology, ophthalmology, otolaryngology, neurology, endocrinology, and cardiology.

For assistance in the preparation of this volume, I am grateful to a vast number of colleagues, residents, fellows, and medical students. In particular, I must acknowledge my indebtedness to my friends and close associates, Drs. Phil Gold, David Hawkins, and Joseph Shuster, of the Division of Clinical Immunology and Allergy at The Montreal General Hospital. Their outstanding contributions and suggestions, based on their own unique professional backgrounds and special interests, have enriched the text throughout.

Dr. Gold is a Medical Research Associate and Dr. Hawkins and Dr. Shuster are Medical Research Scholars of the Medical Research Council of Canada. We all wish to thank the Medical Research Council of Canada and the National Cancer Institute of Canada for their continued support of our research program in clinical immunology.

For critically reviewing specialized portions of the manuscript, I wish to express my gratitude to the following colleagues at The Montreal General Hospital: Drs. C. F. D. Ackman, Jr., A. J. M. Aguayo, J. H. Burgess, W. Gerstein, C. H. Hollenberg, M. Jabbari, R. A. H. Kinch, D. W. C. Lorenzetti, J. R. Ruedy, and N. B. Whittemore. I also wish to thank the residents and fellows of the Division of Clinical Immunology and Allergy for many valuable suggestions. Among this latter group, I am especially grateful to Dr. Andrej Gutkowski for his assistance in compiling the data for Tables 22-5 and 22-6.

One of my greatest debts is to my devoted secretary, Mrs. Lorraine Habib, who spent hundreds of overtime hours toiling over the numerous revisions of the manuscript. The publisher's staff has been helpful and cooperative at all times, and has contributed in many ways to the final version of this volume.

My wife Norah has spent countless days in revising the text, and she must be given much of the credit for clarity of style and expression. To my wife and my children, David, Daniel, Abraham, and Elizabeth, I can only express my deepest appreciation for their interest and patience while the manuscript was in preparation. Without their constant support and encouragement, this book would not have been possible.

S.O.F.

Montreal, Canada

Clinical Immunology

1

The Biology of the Immune Response

SAMUEL O. FREEDMAN, PHIL GOLD,
DAVID HAWKINS, AND JOSEPH SHUSTER

WHAT IS CLINICAL IMMUNOLOGY?

Immunology as a branch of medical science began in 1796 when Edward Jenner investigated the folk tale that the milk maids of Gloucestershire who had been infected with cowpox were protected from the subsequent development of smallpox. By observation and by experiment, he proved the rumor to be true. It was not until about 100 years later that Landsteiner demonstrated the antigenic differences between human erythrocytes which ultimately led to the delineation of the ABO blood group antigens, and Richet described the phenomena of allergy or hypersensitivity. Each of these three apparently unrelated events contributed significantly to the foundation on which modern immunology is built, since they were all concerned with the reaction of the human host either to substances foreign to the individual or to his own body constituents.

IMMUNITY, ALLERGY, AND HYPERSENSITIVITY

Immune reactions can be beneficial to the host, as exemplified by immunization procedures against infectious diseases, or harmful to the host, as exem-

1

plified by diseases such as allergic asthma, hay fever, or diseases associated with autoantibodies. In either case, the "foreign" substance (antigen) evokes an *immune response* which ultimately results in the synthesis of specifically reactive proteins (antibodies), the production of specifically modified reactive cells, or both. Defined in terms of its most traditional and narrowest meaning, *immunology* is the study of *immunity,* and *immunity* is a state of increased resistance to disease. However, a more modern viewpoint is that immunology is the study of all aspects of the immune response as it affects both man and experimental animals.

The word *allergy,* as originally defined by von Pirquet at the turn of the century, was used to denote a state of altered reactivity which resulted from antigenic exposure, and was harmful to the host. For many years afterward, the terms allergy and *hypersensitivity* were used almost interchangeably to describe a deleterious clinical response to foreign substances, as opposed to the protective effects of immunity. However, the distinction between immunity and allergy or hypersensitivity is somewhat artificial, as the consequences which result from either of these states are by no means mutually exclusive. For example, the common procedure of smallpox vaccination usually results in a high degree of protective immunity, although a small proportion of individuals may also develop a harmful allergic encephalitis (see Chapter 18). In order to avoid semantic confusion, some authors have attempted to restore the word allergy to its original meaning by the introduction of terms such as autoallergic instead of autoimmune, but this suggestion has not yet been widely accepted.

THE CLINICAL IMMUNOLOGIST

The *clinical immunologist* is primarily concerned with: (*1*) the elimination of undesired immune reactions in patients who have a wide variety of disease processes with immunologic features, or in patients undergoing organ transplantation; (*2*) the investigation and management of patients with immune deficiency states; and (*3*) the production of protective immunity in individuals exposed or potentially exposed to infectious diseases. Thus, the clinical immunologist is a process orientated medical specialist rather than an organ or system orientated specialist as is the case with a cardiologist, ophthalmologist, or neurologist.

Ideally, the clinical immunologist should be familiar with both the clinical and laboratory aspects of immunology as they relate to human disease processes. In other words, the role of the clinical immunologist in a modern hospital may be considered as that of a physician-scientist who should be proficient in the clinical evaluation of patients with immunologic diseases, and trained to perform and interpret common laboratory procedures relevant to clinical immunology. (See Chapter 22 for a discussion of laboratory procedures in clinical immunology.)

The range of medical knowledge of the clinical immunologist should be broadly based to include the atopic diseases, collagen-vascular diseases, diseases associated with autoantibodies, immunologic deficiency states, transplantation immunology, cancer immunology, allergic drug reactions, hypersensitivity to infectious agents, immunization procedures, and the immunologic features of rheumatology, dermatology, hematology, pulmonary diseases, nephrology, endocrinology, cardiology, gastroenterology, ophthalmology, and neurology.

In many institutions, the clinical immunologist often fulfills an important research function in addition to his clinical and laboratory responsibilities. In fact, immunology has always been a branch of medical science in which fundamental advances have quickly led to practical applications of outstanding importance. The effective control of poliomyelitis, the prevention of the tragic consequences of hemolytic disease of the newborn, and the continuing progress in organ transplantation are but a few recent examples of the close link between basic research in immunology and the eradication of human disease.

ANTIGENS

IMMUNOGENS AND ANTIGENS

Although the terms immunogen and antigen are frequently used interchangeably, they are not necessarily synonymous. *Immunogenicity* may be defined as the capacity of a substance to initiate a humoral or cell-mediated immune response, whereas *antigenicity* may be defined as the capacity of a substance to bind specifically with the antibody molecules whose formation it has elicited. The word *ligand* has also been employed to describe the latter property of specific binding to antibodies. Employed correctly, the term *immunogen* specifies that a substance acts at the afferent limb of the immune response (see subsequent discussion in this chapter for a description of the afferent and efferent limbs of the immune response). However, unless otherwise stated, the term *antigen* will be used throughout the text to describe substances which have immunogenic capacity, antigenic capacity, or both.

Most conventional antigens possess both immunogenic and antigenic capacities, although in some instances these may not be apparent due to a state of immunologic unresponsiveness (see subsequent discussion in this chapter), or due to genetic inability of the host to synthesize antibodies with certain specificities. The lower limit of molecular weight at which a substance may be an immunogen is probably of the order of 10,000, and thus most immunogens are large molecules such as proteins, polysaccharides, polypeptides, and polynucleotides.

HAPTENS

Low molecular weight substances introduced into the body may bind with tissue or circulating protein constituents in order to enlarge the ultimate molecular size of the immunogenic complex. This concept is best illustrated by studies of antibody production directed against simple chemical materials, such as 2,4-dinitrophenyl (DNP) or 2,4-dinitrofluorobenzene (DNFB), which have molecular weights of no more than a few hundred and are themselves nonimmunogenic. When coupled to large protein molecules, however, the resulting conjugate acquires immunogenic capacity and evokes an antibody response directed primarily against the simple chemical grouping which serves as the antigenic determinant, although some reactivity is also elicited against the carrier molecule. The low molecular weight substances which participate in this type of immune response are called *haptens.*

Each one of the many haptenic groups which may be bound to the carrier-protein serves as a single combining site (univalent site) on the immunogenic conjugate. Since the serologic manifestations of antigen-antibody interaction require multivalency of the antigen (see Chapter 22), a hapten in the absence of a carrier-protein cannot take part in such reactions. However, the hapten is a ligand which is capable of binding to the reactive site on its corresponding antibody. Hence, the action of a hapten is best demonstrated by its ability to inhibit the reaction of its specific antibody with the complete antigen (i.e., the hapten plus the carrier-protein).

It has been clearly demonstrated that the major specificity of the immunogen formed between hapten and carrier-protein is independent of the protein molecule. Thus, antibodies evoked by DNP-bovine serum albumin will also react with DNP-bovine gamma globulin. The reason a carrier-protein is needed for immunogenicity remains unclear. One possible explanation is that a minimal molecular size is necessary for antigen processing to occur in the afferent limb of the immune response.

ALLERGENS

Allergens are a special group of antigens which are innocuous to the majority of the population, but may cause disease when predisposed individuals are exposed to them by inhalation, ingestion, injection, or by contact with the skin surface. Allergens may be very simple compounds (e.g., sulfadiazine) which probably require protein-carriers during the immunogenic phase. Other substances in the allergen class are more complex (e.g., rag-weed pollen), frequently contain both protein and carbohydrate components, and have molecular weights of up to 40,000.

The *atopic diseases,* such as allergic bronchial asthma and hay fever, tend to manifest themselves in individuals with a hereditary predisposition to produce reagins (skin-sensitizing antibodies) on exposure to environmental allergens. There is also evidence to suggest that atopic individuals may have an increased sensitivity to the chemical mediators of allergic reactions such as histamine, acetylcholine, or serotonin (see Chapter 3).

In considering the action of allergens in atopic individuals, the portal of entry is of some importance. Individuals genetically predisposed to the development of atopic disease are usually sensitized by exposure to the allergen by way of the bronchial or gastrointestinal mucosae. Whether a specific form of interaction between the mucosal lining and the allergen is required for this material to enter the body in an immunogenic form is uncertain. Regardless of the mechanism, exposure of an atopic individual to the appropriate allergen results in the formation of specific antibodies of the IgE class of immunoglobulins (reagins, skin-sensitizing antibodies). On the other hand, the administration of the allergen by injection, to either atopic or non-atopic individuals, usually results in the formation of IgG antibodies, IgE antibodies, or both types of antibodies.

MICROBIAL ANTIGENS

The contention that a large proportion of the activity of the immune system is directed against microbial antigens is based on the observation that serum immunoglobulin levels in germ-free animals are usually depressed. The antigenic composition of bacteria, viruses, fungi, and rickettsial organisms is extremely varied and complex. Potent microbial antigens may include such chemically diverse substances as the polysaccharide constituents of the pneumococcal capsule, the largely protein endotoxins of a variety of bacteria, and the primarily lipid antigens of the mycobacterial organisms. The specific antigenic determinant groups which elicit an antibody response following invasion of the body by microorganisms remain virtually unknown. Although there are a number of important exceptions, most of the antibodies formed during microbial invasion serve a protective function in the host.

TISSUE ANTIGENS

Tissue components form a group of highly immunogenic antigens. These substances include a wide variety of proteins, polysaccharides, and lipids

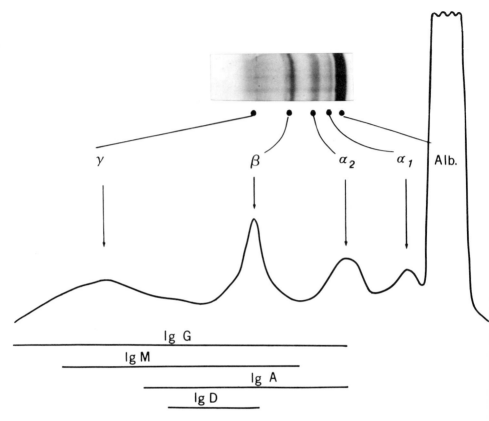

FIG. 1-1. Diagram of electrophoretic distribution of human immunoglobulins.

that are capable of evoking either a humoral or a cell-mediated immune response. Pregnancy, passive immunization with foreign antisera, and blood transfusions are the most common means by which humans are immunized to tissue components. However, the increasing frequency of human organ transplantation has provided a major stimulus for the study of the immune response following exposure to tissue antigens. This latter problem is considered in greater detail in a subsequent section of this chapter and in Chapter 14.

IMMUNOGLOBULIN STRUCTURE AND SYNTHESIS

Serum proteins separated by various electrophoretic techniques were originally designated as albumin, $\alpha 1$, $\alpha 2$, β and γ-globulins. The term *immunoglobulin,* as distinct from the term gamma-globulin, is commonly used in a somewhat broader context to describe serum proteins with antibody characteristics which include the γ-globulins, but extend into the β and α2 range of electrophoretic mobility (Fig. 1-1). In humans, there are at least five major classes of immunoglobulins known as IgG, IgA, IgM, IgD, and IgE.

STRUCTURE OF IMMUNOGLOBULINS

The basic structure of immunoglobulins in all vertebrates capable of humoral antibody synthesis is similar, and consists of four polypeptide chains. In each molecule there are two identical heavy chains and two identical light chains held together by covalent disulfide bonds and by noncovalent hydrophobic bonds (Fig. 1-2). Superimposed upon the prototype four chain structure are differences in size, biologic activity, carbohydrate content, and antigenicity of antibody molecules which vary with each immunoglobulin class (Table 1-1).

The initial structural studies were made on the IgG class of antibody molecules and subsequently extended to other immunoglobulins. The IgG light chains have a molecular weight of 22,500, and are structurally identical to the monomeric units of the Bence-Jones proteins found in the urine or serum of some patients with multiple myeloma (see Chapter 10). On the other hand, the heavy chains of IgG molecules (γ chains) have a molecular weight of 53,000. The observation that antisera prepared in rabbits against isolated light and heavy chains show no cross-reactivity indicates that the two types of chains are antigenically distinct.

Hydrolysis of the IgG molecule with the proteolytic enzymes trypsin, papain, and pepsin produces characteristic products illustrated diagramatically in Figure 1-2. Papain and trypsin attack the heavy chain on the N-terminal (amino terminal) side of the interheavy chain disulfide bonds liberating three fragments: the Fc fragment and two Fab fragments. The Fc fragment is a dimer of the C-terminal (carboxyl terminal) side of the heavy chain, whereas the two Fab fragments are composed of an intact light chain and the N-terminal half of the heavy chain (the Fd fragment) linked to each other by a single disulfide bond. It is the Fab fragment which contains the antibody combining site, and, hence, the IgG immunoglobulin molecule is divalent.

The Fc fragment contains most of the carbohydrate moiety, has a tendency to crystallize, but does not have the capacity to combine with antigen. Nevertheless, this fragment confers important biologic properties on antibody molecules such as the capacities to fix complement, traverse the placenta, combine with rheumatoid factor, or adhere to tissue mast cells. By contrast, the monovalent Fab fragments retain the ability to bind antigen.

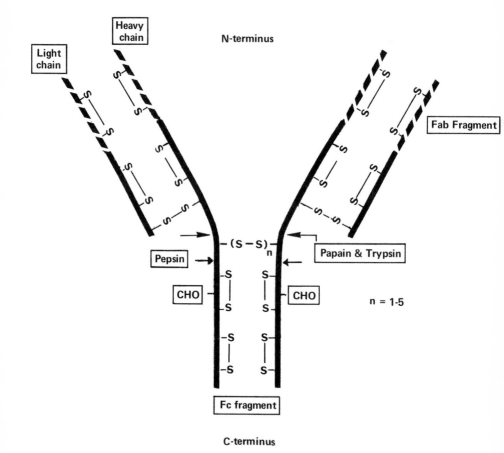

FIG. 1-2. Structure of IgG Immunoglobulins. Electron microscopic studies have demonstrated IgG molecules are "Y" shaped. Solid lines indicate regions of constant amino acid sequences; broken lines indicate variable regions. Note symmetry in structure of molecule. One intrachain disulfide loop recurs for every 110–120 amino acid residues along heavy and light chains; about 60 residues are contained within each loop. From 1–5 interheavy chain disulfide bonds are present in each molecule depending on subclass of heavy chain. Points of cleavage of heavy chains by proteolytic enzymes papain, trypsin, and pepsin, in relation to the interheavy chain disulfide bonds are indicated.

Pepsin, as distinct from papain or trypsin, hydrolyses the immunoglobulin molecule on the C-terminal side of the interheavy chain disulfide bonds, liberating a single bivalent antibody fragment called $F(ab')_2$. The fragment has a molecular weight of 110,000 and remains active as an antibody.

TABLE 1-1. Classes of Human Immunoglobulins

Characteristics	Class				
	IgG	IgA	IgM	IgD	IgE
Molecular weight	150,000	170,000 to 500,000	900,000	200,000	200,000
Heavy chains:					
Class	γ	α	μ	δ	ϵ
Subclasses	γ1, 2, 3, 4	α1, 2	μ1, 2	—	—
Molecular weight	53,000	63,000	75,000	77,000·	75,000
Allotypes	Gm	Am	—	—	—
Light chains:					
Class	κ,λ	κ,λ	κ,λ	κ,λ	κ,λ
Molecular weight	22,500	22,500	22,500	22,500	22,500
Allotypes	Inv	Inv	Inv	Inv	Inv
Molecular formula	$(\kappa_2\gamma_2)$ or $(\lambda_2\gamma_2)$	$(\kappa_2\alpha_2)_n$ or $(\lambda_2\alpha_2)_n$ n = 1,2,3	$(\kappa_2\mu_2)_5$ or $(\lambda_2\mu_2)_5$	$(\kappa_2\delta_2)$ or $(\lambda_2\delta_2)$	$(\kappa_2\epsilon_2)$ or $(\lambda_2\epsilon_2)$
Antigen binding sites	2	2	5–10	2	2
$S_{20, w}$	6.5–7.0	7, 10, 13, 15	18–20	6.2–6.8	8.2
Carbohydrates (%)	2.9	7.5	11.8	14.8	10.7
Serum levels (mg/%)	600–1600	20–500	60–200	0.1–40	0.01–0.9
Synthesis (mg/kg/day)	20–40	3–55	3–17	0.03–1.5	0.2
Catabolism (% IV pool/day)	4–7	14–34	14–25	18–60	89
Complement fixing	+	0	+		0
Skin sensitizing	heterologous species	0	0	0	human reagins
Placental transfer	+	0	0	0	0
Presence in CSF	+	+	0	0	
Exocrine secretion	+	+++	+	±	±

Mild reduction and alkylation of the F(ab')$_2$ fragment splits the interheavy chain disulfide bonds to produce two identical fragments called Fab' which are immunochemically and functionally similar to the monovalent Fab fragments produced by papain and trypsin digestion. Pepsin completely hydrolyses the C-terminal portion of the heavy chain to small peptides, and thus an Fc-like fragment is not produced by this enzyme.

A similar four chain core structure is found in all the other classes of immunoglobulins. Antigenically identical light chains are found in IgG, IgA, IgM, IgD, and IgE immunoglobulins, whereas the heavy chains are antigenically distinctive for each class of immunoglobulins (Fig. 1-3).

The light chains of all classes of immunoglobulins can be divided into 2 antigenic types: kappa (κ) and lambda (λ). Any given normal immunoglobulin molecule contains either two kappa chains or two lambda chains, but never one of each. The antigenic differences between the kappa and lambda chains can be correlated with specific amino acid sequence differences in the C-terminal half of the light chains.

The heavy chains of IgG, IgA, IgM, IgD, and IgE molecules are termed γ- (gamma), α- (alpha), μ- (mu), δ- (delta) and ϵ- (epsilon) chains, respectively. In addition to the structural and antigenic differences between the heavy chains of various immunoglobulin classes (see Table 1-1), antigenic differences within the heavy chains of each major class have also been delineated. Four such subclasses called γ1, γ2, γ3 and γ4 are found in γ chains, and two subclasses have been noted in both α and μ chains. The total serum immunoglobulins of normal individuals contain all of the heavy chain subclasses, but a single immunoglobulin molecule belongs to only one antigenic subclass.

The γ3 molecules are catabolized rapidly, probably due to their susceptibility to the action of proteolytic enzymes, while γ4 molecules are non-complement-fixing and do not attach to heterologous skin. Only γ1 and γ3 molecules are recognized by receptors on the surface of macrophages. The α1 and α2 subclasses are correlated with a structural difference in the type of bonding between the heavy and light chains. In the α2 subclass, the disulfide bond between the heavy and light chains is absent and the chains are held together by noncovalent forces. The two subclasses of μ chains appear to be correlated with the ability to bind Clq, the first component of the complement sequence.

The only structural variation from the four chain prototype of the immunoglobulin molecule is found in the IgM and in the secretory IgA molecules. IgM immunoglobulins or macroglobulins have a molecular weight of 900,000 and appear to be pentamers of the four chain prototype. The five monomeric units of 160,000 which comprise an IgM molecule are joined together by disulfide bonds between the heavy chains.

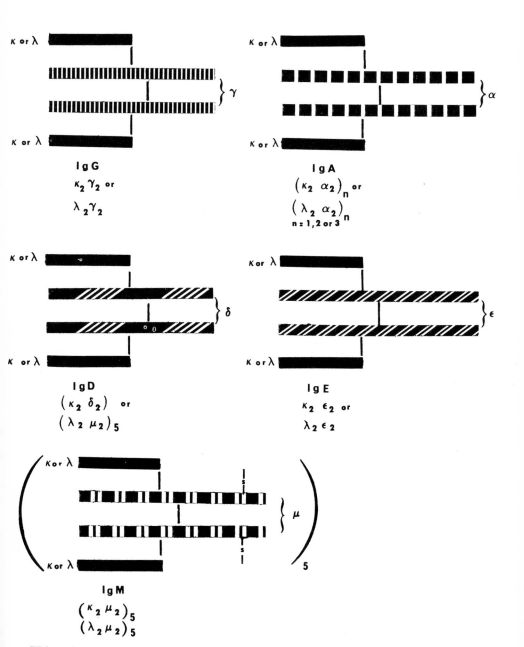

FIG. 1-3. Schematic representation of molecular structures and formulas of the various immunoglobulin classes.

11

Secretory IgA molecules constitute a major immunoglobulin component of exocrine secretions exposed to the external environment such as tears, saliva, gastric juice, small and large bowel secretions, and colostrum. The secretory IgA molecule differs from serum IgA in that it contains an extra antigenic chain, known as the secretory or transport piece, in addition to heavy and light chains similar to those found in serum IgA. Structurally, secretory IgA appears to be a trimolecular complex of 400,000 molecular weight consisting of two monomeric four chain units linked together to the secretory piece by disulfide bonds.

The IgA immunoglobulin moiety in exocrine secretions is synthesized by plasma cells located in submucosal tissues of the exocrine glands. The secretory piece, on the other hand, is synthesized by the columnar epithelial cells and is presumably added to IgA as the IgA molecules pass between the epithelial cells. An alternative hypothesis is that the union between the secretory piece and IgA takes place in the secretions themselves in the lumina of the exocrine glands.

SYNTHESIS OF IMMUNOGLOBULINS

Immunoglobulin molecules are produced according to the laws governing protein synthesis in general. It has been shown that the individual polypeptide chains of immunoglobulin molecules are assembled as a single unit on separate ribosomes. Amino acid residues are bonded into the growing polypeptide chain beginning at the N-terminal side. Subsequently the light and heavy chains are united into a protein molecule with the disulfide bonds contributing to the overall three dimensional arrangement of the chains. The carbohydrate components are attached both during the time when the polypeptide chain is growing as well as after the individual chains have been constituted into a complete molecule.

CHEMICAL BASIS FOR ANTIBODY SPECIFICITY

As noted previously, univalent antibody combining sites are found on the Fab fragment, and both the heavy and light chains of this fragment are required for optimum antigen binding. Recent experimental observations have clearly shown that antibody specificity is determined by the distinctive amino acid sequence of immunoglobulin polypeptide chains. This view is in contrast to the older, instructionist theories of antibody formation in which it was held that immunoglobulin polypeptide chains of common amino acid sequence are somehow folded in response to an antigenic template.

Detailed amino acid sequence studies have been carried out on human and mouse myeloma proteins and on Bence-Jones proteins because these paraproteins provide relatively large quantities of homogeneous immuno-globulins which are the product of a single line (or clone) of neoplastic plasma cells. In these studies it was found that the heavy and light chains contain invariant (constant) and variable sequences of amino acids (Fig. 1-2). The N-terminal half of the light chains and the N-terminal quarter of the heavy chains constitute the variable portions of the polypeptide chains, while the remaining C-terminal portions are relatively invariant for each class of immunoglobulins. Thus, each light chain (κ and λ) and each heavy chain (γ, α, μ, δ, and ϵ) subclass has a distinctive amino acid sequence in the invariant portion of the polypeptide chain. However, small differences in the amino acid sequence in the invariant portion of the chain do exist, and these appear to be genetically determined. The sequence differences in the invariable portions of the heavy or light chains are prob-ably sufficient to account for the diversity of antibody specificities generated in response to various antigens.

THE IMMUNE RESPONSE

Immunologic responses are classically divided into those mediated by hu-moral antibodies and those mediated by cells. In either case, the hallmark of the immune response is its *specificity*. Characteristic of this specificity is the ability of the organism to recognize an antigen as foreign, and to respond by the synthesis of specifically reactive immunoglobulins (humoral antibodies), the production of specifically sensitized lymphocytes (cell-mediated immunity), or both.

Detailed studies on the chemical basis of the recognition process are made extremely difficult by the large number of immunogenic configurations present in almost all antigens. However, it is clear that antibody producing cells must, in some way, be able to distinguish the chemical configuration of antigens which are capable of eliciting an immune response from those which are native to the host. Having once recognized a particular antigen as foreign, subsequent exposure to the same antigen usually results in a secondary response which is more rapid and more extensive than that which occurs on the first encounter. This capacity for *immunologic memory*, like the capacity for *antigen recognition* is fundamental to the specific nature of the immune response.

The complex series of biologic phenomena which constitute the immune response will be considered under the following headings: (*1*) development and organization of the immune system; (*2*) capture and processing of antigens; (*3*) antigen recognition; (*4*) cell-mediated immunity; and (*5*) immunity mediated by humoral antibodies; (*6*) immunologic unresponsiveness; and (7) autoimmunity. The capture, processing, and recognition of antigens is sometimes referred to as the *afferent limb* of the immune response, and the sequence of events which follows antigen recognition is referred to as the *efferent limb* of the immune response.

The concept of the immune response outlined in Figure 1-4 and described in this Section is an operational one based on currently available experimental data obtained largely in animal models. Modifications of these concepts will undoubtedly appear in the future as more becomes known about the immune response in humans.

DEVELOPMENT AND ORGANIZATION OF THE IMMUNE SYSTEM

Both antigen recognition and immunologic memory are associated with the small lymphocytes which are themselves ultimately derived from bone marrow precursors. In addition, the property of *immunologic competence,* or the ability to recognize antigens as foreign and respond to them, is dependent on a unique lymphoid organ—the thymus gland. For example, it has been shown in newborn animals that immunologic competence is markedly impaired by removal of the thymus gland, and is restored by the subsequent reimplantation of thymic tissue. Thus, in order to be fully immunologically competent, an animal must have a normally developed thymus in utero, and the thymus must usually remain intact for several days after birth. It should be emphasized, however, that most of the experiments on the role of the thymus in immunity have been carried out in inbred strains of mice, and their relationship to the immune response in humans has not been defined.

Even in mice, it is not yet established whether the *central lymphoid tissue* (e.g., the thymus) supplies lymphocytes to *peripheral lymphoid tissues* (e.g., spleen and lymph nodes), or merely conditions lymphocytes brought to it from other areas of lymphopoiesis such as the bone marrow and extramedullary sites. There is some experimental evidence that the thymus secretes a hormone which is essential for the normal functioning of the peripheral lymphoid tissues.

Considerable insight into the effect of the thymus gland has been obtained from experiments in the chicken. In this species, neonatal thymectomy prevents the subsequent development of cell-mediated immune reactions such as homograft rejection and delayed type hypersensitivity, as well as the humoral response to certain antigens. By contrast, removal of the bursa of Fabricius in the chicken profoundly impairs the capacity of the animal to produce circulating antibodies but has no effect on cell-mediated immunity. At present, the analogue of the bursa of Fabricius has not been identified in man or other mammals, although both the tonsils and the gut-associated lymphoid tissue have been suggested as possible bursa equivalents.

When considered together, all of these observations have led to the hypothesis that stem cells originating in the bone marrow differentiate to form two distinct lymphocyte populations: the thymic-dependent T-lymphocytes which are responsible for the initiation of cell-mediated immunity, and the thymic-independent (bursa-equivalent) B-lymphocytes which are responsible for the initiation of humoral antibody synthesis (see Fig. 1-4). The T-lymphocytes form the greater part of the circulating pool of small lymphocytes and have a relatively long lifespan, whereas the B-lymphocytes tend to remain in the lymphoid tissues and are relatively short-lived. Furthermore, the T-lymphocytes carry a specific antigen called the θ antigen on their cell surfaces. It has been postulated that the θ antigen is acquired by the T-lymphocytes during their sojourn in the thymus.

CAPTURE AND PROCESSING OF ANTIGENS

The capture of antigens is primarily carried out by two groups of cells: (1) the fixed phagocytes such as the macrophages which line the sinusoids of the liver, spleen, and lymph nodes; and (2) the wandering phagocytes such as the polymorphonuclear leukocytes, monocytes, and histiocytes of the blood and tissue spaces.

The initial phase of phagocytosis involves contact between the antigenic particle and the surface of the phagocytic cell, and it is at this stage that serum opsonins (see Chapter 11) may be of importance in facilitating the entry of antigenic material into the cell. However, it should be emphasized that not all phagocytic cells (e.g., the polymorphonuclear leukocytes) are capable of processing antigen. Furthermore, phagocytosis itself is not necessarily implicated in the immune response to all antigens. It is the interaction between antigen and antigen processing cells or between antigen and antigen reactive cells (see subsequent discussion in this chapter) which appears to be critical for the initiation of the immune response.

A currently popular hypothesis is that the first stage in the immune response to microbial and some macromolecular antigens is the phagocytosis of antigen by macrophages. Once the phagocytic cells have ingested the particulate or macromolecular antigens, these cells usually break down the antigen into immunogenic fragments. Some of the immunogenic fragments may attach to a small molecule of RNA which has no detectable immunogenic properties of its own to form a "superantigen complex." Another and larger form of m-RNA probably does not bind antigen, but seems to have the capacity to be programmed with specific immunologic information. Both forms of specifically altered RNA are apparently able to stimulate

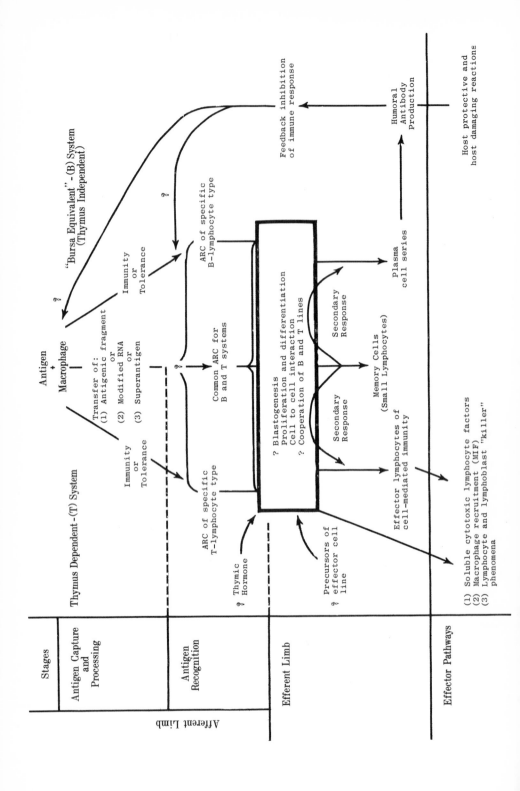

the small lymphocyte which is the next cell in the immune response. There is also evidence to suggest that, under certain circumstances, the immunogenic fragment alone may be released from the antigen processing cell (see Fig. 1-4).

According to another hypothesis, the antigen under certain circumstances is adsorbed onto the surface of the antigen processing cell and never enters the cytoplasmic compartment.

ANTIGEN RECOGNITION

It is likely that both the T-lymphocyte and B-lymphocyte populations contain antigen-reactive cells (ARC, antigen sensitive cells) which are capable of antigen recognition. It is currently believed that the recognition of antigen is mediated by an antibody-like molecule synthesized in the cell and bound to the surface membrane. According to this theory, the specificity of the surface antibody is determined by the genetic programming of the individual lymphocyte, and the combination of the surface antibody with its corresponding antigen serves to initiate the subsequent steps of the immune response.

On contact with antigen the T-lymphocytes enter into a poorly understood series of cellular events which ultimately result in the development of cell-mediated immunity, whereas the B-lymphocytes differentiate, proliferate, and ultimately result in the formation of plasma cells that synthesize humoral antibodies. In vitro studies suggest that both T-lymphocytes and B-lymphocytes are transformed into large blast cells following contact with antigen. On the other hand, it is possible that the blast cells are derived from a common stem cell or stem cell precursor, and that differentiation into specifically modified lymphocytes and plasma cells occurs only after blastogenesis has taken place. The primed antigen reactive cells which provide immunologic memory are also believed to be derived from the long-lived T-lymphocytes (see Fig. 1-4).

To date, there is no evidence to suggest that antigen-reactive cells are able to produce antibodies. Operationally, they are recognized by their ability to stimulate the development of groups of antibody producing cells when injected into immunologically compatible animals. For example, if sensitized cells from an immunized animal are injected intravenously into an irradiated syngeneic recipient, clusters of antibody producing cells can be demonstrated scattered throughout the spleen and lymphoid tissues.

It would appear that individual antigen-reactive cells cannot recognize every antigen, but it is not known at the present time whether they can respond to several antigens or only to one antigen. However, during the

FIG. 1-4. Schematic representation of current hypotheses regarding the sequence of biologic events in the immune response. See text for explanation.

early phases of the immune response, each antigen-reactive cell is probably capable of recruiting numerous uncommitted antibody producing cells as well as proliferating to form additional antigen-reactive cells. The latter cells may be derived from the immunologic memory cells.

CELL-MEDIATED IMMUNITY

Considerable information on the nature of the cell-mediated immune response has been obtained from studies on diverse "model systems" of delayed hypersensitivity such as lymphocyte transformation in culture, the macrophage migration inhibitory factor (M.I.F.), and Lawrence's transfer factor.

Lymphocyte Transformation in Culture

There appears to be a definite, but not absolute, correlation between the capacity of an antigen to induce lymphocyte transformation in culture and the ability of the same antigen to elicit cell-mediated hypersensitivity reactions in the leukocyte donor. If one accepts the previous hypothesis that there are two populations of ARC, then it would be the T-lymphocytes that participate in the phenomena of in vitro lymphocyte transformation.

The addition of a nonspecific mitogenic agent such as phytohemagglutinin (PHA) to human peripheral blood leukocytes in culture causes the majority of the small lymphocytes to enlarge into "blast" cells morphologically similar to the large pyroninophilic cells that arise from small lymphocytes during homograft rejection (see Chapter 14). Some of these transformed cells go on to mitosis, and, like the pyroninophilic cells, are capable of synthesizing new DNA. The addition of specific antigen to peripheral blood cultures obtained from appropriately sensitized human subjects will also induce a similar form of blastogenesis, although a much smaller percentage of cells are affected than with PHA. The degree of blastogenesis is most readily measured in quantitative terms by determining the amount of tritiated thymidine that is incorporated into the DNA synthesized by the cells during transformation.

It is of interest that contact between macrophages and lymphocytes is frequently observed in the cell preparations used for lymphocyte transformation. Furthermore, when phagocytic cells are removed from the cell preparations, there is a diminished response of lymphocytes to antigen. However, the capacity to undergo blastogenesis on antigen stimulation can be restored by the subsequent addition of macrophages or polymorphonuclear leukocytes. These observations would suggest that antigen processing by macrophages is necessary in at least some in vitro situations, but it is still not clear whether antigens may also stimulate T-lymphocytes directly. There is also evidence to suggest that the cells in culture that initially respond to antigen release a blastogenic factor which nonspecifically transforms other T-lymphocytes and thus accelerates the transformation reaction.

Migration Inhibitory Factor (M.I.F.)

If peritoneal exudate cells from guinea pigs are packed into a capillary tube placed horizontally on the floor of a chamber containing culture fluid, the cells tend to migrate fan-wise from the end of the tube after a period of time which ranges from several hours to two days. However, if the peritoneal exudate cells are obtained from animals sensitized to tuberculin or other antigens and the same antigen is added to the culture fluid, there is specific inhibition of migration of macrophages. In the guinea pig, there appears to be an excellent correlation between the degree of macrophage inhibition and the delayed type skin reactivity of the cell donor.

The current opinion is that the interaction of antigen with sensitized T-lymphocytes in the peritoneal exudate leads to the release of a soluble migration inhibitory factor which inhibits the migration of wandering macrophages in tissue culture. If peritoneal exudate cells from a sensitized guinea pig are mixed with those from a normal guinea pig, the M.I.F. exerts its effect on all the macrophages in the preparation. Thus, under these experimental conditions, the release of M.I.F. appears to be a specific phenomenon, but its action appears to be partly nonspecific.

Lawrence's Transfer Factor

Delayed type cutaneous hypersensitivity to tuberculin, streptococcal proteins, and other antigens can be successfully transferred in man by means of either whole peripheral blood leukocytes or leukocyte extracts. For example, a leukocyte extract obtained from a positive skin reactor to tuberculin, and injected into a tuberculin-negative recipient at one skin site, will result in the development of a delayed type skin reaction when the recipient is subsequently challenged intradermally with tuberculin at another site. The leukocyte transfer factor of Lawrence is soluble, of low molecular weight, and withstands treatment with proteases and nucleases. Immune responses mediated by humoral antibodies cannot be transferred in this manner.

The mode of action of transfer factor in inducing cell-mediated hyper-sensitivity is poorly understood. However, its effect on human recipients appears to be one of active sensitization since the hypersensitivity it induces may persist for weeks or months. At present it appears more likely that "transfer factor" is a sensitizer acting on the T-lymphocytes of the recipient, rather than an effector of cell-mediated immune responses.

Other Soluble Lymphocyte Factors

Other soluble factors released from sensitized lymphocytes may: (1) kill target cells (lymphocytotoxic factor); (2) cause inhibition of growth of target cells in tissue culture; (3) increase vascular permeability in the skin of experimental animals; and (4) promote chemotaxis of mononuclear cells.

Cell-Mediated Hypersensitivity in Humans

By extrapolation from the experimental data discussed in the preceding sections, it is possible to form a working hypothesis concerning the possible mechanisms of cell-mediated hypersensitivity in humans (see Fig. 1-4). The term *delayed type hypersensitivity* which has been used for many years to describe the clinical manifestations of cell-mediated immunity is somewhat confusing. Although the skin response to intradermal testing is delayed compared to skin reactions mediated by humoral antibodies, the clinical manifestations of delayed hypersensitivity often appear sooner following antigenic stimulation than the clinical manifestations of hypersensitivity mediated by humoral antibodies.

The best available theory to explain the development of cell-mediated immunity is that the T-lymphocytes migrate through the tissues in relatively large numbers, thus permitting their sensitization or restimulation by antigen localized in the tissues. The contact between antigen and ARC may possibly result in lymphocyte transformation in vivo, but this hypothesis remains to be established by direct observation. The significance of antigen processing by macrophages or the role of blastogenic factor in inducing the postulated in vivo transformation of lymphocytes in humans is also unknown at the present time. Current evidence would suggest that the specifically sensitized lymphocyte behaves as a "killer-cell," and its cytotoxic action on graft target cells is probably effected by the direct release of C8 and C9 from the lymphocyte. (The actions of the complement components are discussed in a subsequent section of this chapter.)

In addition, it is possible that the release of soluble factors from sensitized lymphocytes leads to some of the other tissue changes considered to be characteristic of delayed type hypersensitivity. For instance, the accumulation of mononuclear leukocytes and the vascular changes which occur at the site of the familiar tuberculin reaction may be mediated in part by soluble lymphocyte factors. The effect of M.I.F. in vivo might be to immobilize randomly wandering macrophages at the site of interaction between antigen and sensitized T-lymphocytes. The exact role of macrophages in this situation is obscure, but it has been postulated that they may have a cytotoxic action of their own on target cells. On the other hand, it is possible that the macrophages which accumulate locally merely serve as scavengers that phagocytose previously damaged cells.

IMMUNITY MEDIATED BY HUMORAL ANTIBODIES

Humoral Antibody Formation

The mechanism whereby antigen-reactive B-lymphocytes lead to the development of the antibody forming cells of the plasmacyte cell line is not yet clear. In particular, it is not known whether macrophages are directly involved in the primary antibody response or not. In addition, there is conclusive evidence from animal experiments that in certain situations there is direct "cooperation" between T-lymphocytes and B-lymphocytes in the process of humoral antibody synthesis. It has been suggested that antigen bound to the surface of the T-lymphocyte provides a higher local concentration of antigen during cell-to-cell contact with the B-lymphocyte than would be possible if the antigen were uniformly dispersed throughout the body fluids (see Fig. 1-4). This phenomenon occurs primarily within the lymph node.

After a latent period of 4–24 hours, antibody producing cells of the plasmacyte series appear, proliferate, and begin to produce antibody. The level of serum antibody over the next few days rises exponentially in direct proportion to the number of antibody producing cells. However, as the immune response continues, the recruitment of new antibody producing cells declines, possibly due to an inhibitory effect of circulating antibodies. The existence of this form of *feed-back inhibition* is based on the observation that small amounts of IgG antibody tend to depress the immune response to the corresponding antigen. In fact, this is probably the mechanism whereby Rh sensitization is suppressed by the administration of small quantities of anti-Rh_0(D) antibody (see Chapter 9). Thus, as the result of depletion of antigen and failure to recruit new antibody producing cells, antibody synthesis gradually declines and antibody titers fall.

Many investigators feel that the first type of antibody to appear in response to primary antigenic stimulation belongs to the IgM class of immunoglobulins, although this phenomenon may be related to the method of antibody detection. After continued antigenic exposure or re-exposure to the same antigen, the IgM antibodies are usually replaced by IgG in much larger amounts. Thus, the primary antibody response is characterized by a relatively low titer of antibodies which are primarily IgM, whereas the secondary response is characterized by a much higher titer of antibodies which are primarily IgG. It is conceivable that the late IgG response may inhibit the synthesis of IgM antibody through a negative feed-back mechanism similar to that discussed in the preceding paragraph.

The induction of antibody formation following exposure to antigen may therefore be considered as the culmination of a series of cellular events that eventually results in a cell secreting antibodies specific for the original antigen. A heterogeneous group of antibody molecules with different amino acid sequences in the variable region of the polypeptide chain is produced by the organism, although a single cell is usually capable of producing antibodies of only a single immunoglobulin class with a single antigenic specificity.

As noted in the section in this chapter on the synthesis of antibodies, current experimental evidence favors selective rather than instructive theories of antibody formation. The clonal selection theory, as originally proposed, stated that the capacity of a cell to form a specific antibody was restricted for genetic reasons. In other words, a given cell (cell line or clone) was capable of producing antibody against only one antigen, and thus only a limited number of specifically committed cells would proliferate on contact with that antigen. The elaboration of large quantities of homogeneous immunoglobulins from a single line of neoplastic plasma cells provides an example of this form of clonal proliferation.

It has subsequently been shown that under certain experimental circumstances, a single cell may produce more than one type of antigen specific molecule. Nevertheless, current opinion still holds that some form of selective process forms the basis of the humoral antibody response to antigenic stimulation. A selective theory of antibody formation implies that in a given individual there exists all the necessary information to specify antigen combining sites on structurally diverse antibody molecules. The observed variations in the amino acid sequence at various portions of the N-terminal regions of both the heavy and light chains are sufficient to account for the wide variety of antibody specificities which can be generated by humans or experimental animals.

In recent years, there has been considerable speculation concerning the genetic factors that are responsible for clonal responses and antibody diversity. One view holds that during the evolution of the species, point mutation and selection results in coding being stored for a large variety of individual antibody specificities in the germ-line of genes. Several other hypotheses are based on the somatic mutation and recombination of a few immunoglobulin coding genes. However, neither the germ-line nor the somatic mutation theories proposed to date completely explain the amino acid sequence data that is currently available.

Protective Effects of Humoral Antibodies

In considering the biologic significance of humoral antibodies, it should be remembered that one of the most important functions of the immunologic system is the removal or neutralization of potentially noxious substances such as bacteria, bacterial toxins, viruses, fungi, or immune complexes. In general, humoral antibodies formed against particulate antigens have a protective function that leads to the ultimate destruction of the inciting agent. The consequences of deficient humoral antibody production in terms of increased susceptibility to infection are discussed in Chapters 10 and 11, while the significance of humoral antibodies in the prevention, treatment, and diagnosis of infectious diseases is discussed in Chapter 21.

Adverse Effects of Antigen-Antibody Interactions

Immune reactions mediated by humoral antibodies can be harmful to the organism in a number of ways. The distinction between the various mechanisms is somewhat artificial since a single clinical syndrome may be the result of several mechanisms, or a single type of antibody may act in several ways. Nevertheless, there are at least three distinct pathways by which antibodies may initiate tissue damage: (1) homocytotropic, (2) cytotoxic (cytolytic); and (3) immune-complex. It should be emphasized that it is not the antibodies themselves which are harmful to the organism. Instead, it is the sequence of events which follows antigen-antibody interaction that results in the tissue damage to be described in this and subsequent sections of this chapter.

Homocytotropic Mechanism. In humans, the IgE class of immunoglobulins appears to have the unique property of adhering to tissue mast cells or peripheral blood leukocytes, presumably because of a specific polypeptide configuration on the Fc portion of its heavy chain. Because IgE (reaginic) antibodies become fixed to the cells of target organs they are often referred to as homocytotropic antibodies. However, the homocytotropic antibodies have no immunologic specificity for the affected cells. Thus, it is believed that the homocytotropic type of immune reaction is initiated by an allergen reacting with tissue cells passively sensitized by IgE produced elsewhere in the body. The antigen-antibody reaction which takes place at the cell surface, through a sequence of events which is poorly understood, ultimately results in the release of chemical mediators such as histamine and serotonin from mast cells, and in the release of slow-reacting substance (SRS) from polymorphonuclear leukocytes.

The homocytotropic mechanism is manifested clinically in humans by the atopic diseases such as bronchial asthma, hay fever, and some forms of urticaria, as well as by anaphylactic reactions similar to those which occur in experimental animals.

The presence of reagins in the sera of an atopic patient was first described in 1921. In this classic experiment, Prausnitz passively sensitized an area of his own skin to fish by the intradermal injection of serum from an allergic patient named Küstner. The sensitized skin site developed a wheal and flare reaction on rechallenge with an extract of fish. Since then, the Prausnitz-Küstner passive transfer experiment has been repeated by many investigators with numerous allergens such as animal danders, pollens, and foreign sera. However, it is only within the last few years that reaginic antibodies have been shown to be largely, if not entirely, associated with the IgE class of immunoglobulins (see Chapter 3).

Cytotoxic (Cytolytic) Mechanism.   In contrast to the homocytotropic type of mechanism, cytolytic antibodies bind to cells because their specific antigen is located at the cell surface. The antigen may be an intrinsic component of the tissue cells, as in hemolytic disease of the newborn due to Rh incompatibility, or it may be an antigen or hapten which has become intimately associated with blood cells, as in penicillin-induced hemolytic anemia. Thus, the pathogenetic immunoglobulins bind to the tissue cells by means of antigen-specific configurations on their Fab portions rather than by means of the non-antigen-specific binding postulated for homocytotropic antibodies. The cytolytic antibodies almost always belong to the IgG class of immunoglobulins with the important exception of IgM cold hemagglutinins.

The coating of cells by cytolytic antibodies renders them more susceptible to intravascular and extravascular destruction (see Chapter 9 for a detailed discussion of the fate of antibody coated blood cells). Unlike the homocytotropic mechanism, complement components are involved in the sequence of events which leads to most forms of immune cytolysis.

In humans, the cytotoxic mechanism is most commonly manifested by blood transfusion reactions, hemolytic disease of the newborn, autoimmune hemolytic anemias, immunologic leukopenia, immunologic thrombocytopenia, and, perhaps, by certain aspects of homograft rejection.

The "anti-tissue" mechanism of immune injury is really a variant of the cytotoxic mechanism except that the antibodies are directed against a fixed tissue instead of cells. An example of anti-tissue antibodies are the anti-GBM antibodies found in Goodpasture's syndrome (see Chapter 6).

Immune Complex Mechanism.   In man and experimental animals, insoluble antigen-antibody complexes, as well as large soluble complexes, are usually cleared from the circulation and tissue spaces by the cells of the reticuloendothelial system, and are thus rendered harmless. However, if soluble immune complexes of intermediate size are formed in moderate antigen excess (see Chapter 22), they are not removed from the circulation. Immune complexes which are not cleared tend to localize in organs such as the kidney which filter large quantities of blood, or in vessels whose permeability is abnormally increased. In addition, the uptake of immune complexes by phagocytic cells in the tissues may trigger a localized inflammatory reaction.

The antibodies responsible for immune complex disease in humans belong to the IgG or IgM class of immunoglobulins. The mechanisms whereby immune complexes produce tissue damage through the activation of the complement system and other mediators of immune injury will be discussed in a subsequent section of this chapter.

Examples of immune complex disease in animals are the *Arthus reaction* and experimental serum sickness. A typical Arthus reaction occurs when one immune reactant (e.g., antigen) is injected intravascularly, and the other (e.g., antibody) is injected extravascularly, usually in the skin. The two reactants diffuse and meet in the vessel wall where immune complexes in precipitate form are produced. A sequence of events is thereby initiated which results in a severe inflammatory reaction and eventually culminates in a necrotizing vasculitis. Thus, the Arthus reaction takes place primarily in the tissues and not in the circulation.

By contrast, in experimental serum sickness, the antigen must remain in the circulation until antibodies appear. Pathogenetic immune complexes in antigen excess are formed at the stage when large amounts of antigen are still present in the circulation, but humoral antibody synthesis is just beginning. It has been demonstrated that the soluble antigen-antibody complexes so produced localize in the kidney, aorta, and other large vessels. These immune complexes initiate a process which results in tissue injury.

Tissue damage in humans due to circulating antigen-antibody complexes is best illustrated by systemic lupus erythematosus, some types of acute glomerulonephritis, certain hypersensitivity diseases of the lung parenchyma (see Chapter 4), and some features of human serum sickness. Some tissues, particularly the formed elements of the blood, are not damaged as a direct consequence of the immune complex mechanism, but are indirectly injured as "innocent bystanders" (see Chapter 9).

IMMUNOLOGIC UNRESPONSIVENESS

Neonatal Tolerance

The original concept that the immune system was developed in order to protect the host from invasion by foreign antigenic material implied that the body was capable of distinguishing "self" from "nonself." The failure of the individual to produce antibodies against his own circulating and tissue proteins, or *natural immunologic tolerance,* was thought to be completely under the control of genetic mechanisms.

In 1945, however, these concepts were challenged by the demonstration that there was a lack of immunologic reactivity between dizygotic cattle twins who had shared the same placenta during fetal life. This observation indicated that immunologic unresponsiveness might well be an acquired state, caused by exposure of the immunologic system to tissue antigens during fetal life. Eight years later, a classic series of experiments revealed that mice inoculated during fetal life with cells from an unrelated donor would, in later life, accept skin grafts from the same donor or animals genetically identical to that donor.

It was subsequently demonstrated that the phenomenon of *acquired immunologic tolerance* could be induced in a variety of fowl and rodents during the neonatal period by the administration of relatively small quantities of viruses, bacteria, carbohydrates, proteins, synthetic polypeptides, haptens, erythrocytes, and transplantation antigens. There is a marked species variation in the ease with which neonatal animals develop acquired immunologic tolerance. Newborn mice, rabbits, and chickens are relatively susceptible to the development of this state, whereas sheep, guinea pigs, and humans are extremely resistant.

It has been shown that acquired immunologic tolerance is exquisitely specific. For instance, chickens rendered tolerant to the erythrocytes of one turkey were still able to produce antibodies against the erythrocytes of another individual turkey. Furthermore, rabbits made tolerant to bovine serum albumin during neonatal life showed no tolerance to the albumins of other mammalian species or to bovine serum albumin coupled to diazonium derivatives of arsanilic and sulfonilic acids.

Recovery from tolerance occurs spontaneously in the absence of continued administration of antigen. The only apparent exceptions to this general statement are: (*1*) tolerance produced by antigens such as pneumococcal polysaccharides and poly-D-amino acids which are poorly metabolized; and (*2*) tolerance produced by viable cells. In both of these situations, there is a source of continuous endogenous antigenic stimulation which serves to maintain the state of tolerance. The recovery from tolerance is usually gradual, extending over periods of weeks to years, and is frequently incomplete. On the other hand, indefinite prolongation of the tolerant state can be achieved by the administration of relatively small doses of antigen during adult life.

During recovery from tolerance to a complex mixture of antigens, the immune response to some antigens may return while tolerance to others persists. It is even possible that antibody production may be limited to one antigenic group out of many possible ones on a protein molecule. This phenomenon is referred to as *split tolerance*. Other variations of the tolerant state include forms of *partial tolerance* or *immune deviation*. Under these circumstances a restriction of the immunologic response is observed which may extend to the absolute amount of antibody produced, or to the immunoglobulin class of the antibody being synthesized.

Adult Tolerance

Although it was originally believed that acquired immunologic tolerance as described above could be induced only during perinatal life, it had been noted previously that poorly metabolized antigens such as pneumococcal polysaccharides, given in large quantity, were able to induce a state of immunologic unresponsiveness in mature animals. Furthermore, when a sufficiently high dose of material is administered, a comparable state of unresponsiveness can be achieved with a variety of antigenic materials regardless of the manner in which they are metabolized. The phenomenon of the induction of immunologic unresponsiveness in adults is known as *immunologic paralysis*. Neonatal immunologic tolerance and adult immunologic paralysis may be grouped together under the general term of *immunologic unresponsiveness*.

Because a much higher concentration of antigen per unit body weight is required to induce immunologic paralysis as compared to neonatal tolerance, it was originally felt that the mechanisms underlying the development of these two conditions were quite different. However, once immunologic unresponsiveness is achieved, either by small quantities of antigen in the neonatal animal or with much greater quantities of antigen in the adult animal, the same maintenance dose is required in order to maintain the unresponsive state. Moreover, immunologic unresponsiveness can be achieved in adult animals with smaller doses of antigen if they are administered at a time when general immunologic responsiveness is partially impaired by radiation, cytotoxic drug therapy, thymectomy, thoracic duct drainage, or the administration of antilymphocytic serum.

More recent studies have demonstrated that immunologic unresponsiveness in adults may be produced in a dosage range below that required for the induction of an immune response. This state is termed *low-zone paralysis,* and is most easily achieved in mice with antigens that are only weakly immunogenic such as certain components of bovine γ-globulin and poly-D-amino acids. Immunosuppression tends to increase the likelihood of low-zone paralysis, whereas the administration of antigen in adjuvants impairs its development.

Thus, it would appear that the initial administration of antigen may lead to a state of either immunity or paralysis depending upon the immunogenicity of the antigen and the dose administered. If the antigen is weakly immunogenic, low-zone paralysis is achieved with antigen concentrations less than that required for the production of immunity. If the antigen is highly immunogenic, unresponsiveness to the antigen can only be obtained with high concentrations of antigen to produce a state of *high-zone paralysis*.

Cellular Basis for Immunologic Unresponsiveness

The observations regarding low-zone paralysis in adults suggest that the mechanisms underlying acquired immunologic tolerance and immunologic paralysis are probably identical. Essential to an understanding of immunologic unresponsiveness is a clear distinction between (*1*) central failure of the immune response caused by an alteration in the properties of immunologically competent cells; and (*2*) peripheral failure of the immune response caused by interference with antigen access to antigen-reactive cells (ARC) or by masking of the antibody subsequently produced by excessive quantities of antigen. The most significant studies in this area demonstrated an abrogation of immunologic unresponsiveness by the transfer of immunologically competent cells from a genetically identical normal donor. Since the transferred cells were able to respond in a normal fashion in the previously tolerant host, immunologic unresponsiveness would appear to be due to a central failure of immunologically competent cells.

It has been clearly shown that the macrophage functions normally in its handling of antigen in the tolerant animal, and evidence currently available suggests that acquired immunologic tolerance is brought about by interference with the ARC of the lymphoid series, or their precursors.

It has been proposed that neonatal tolerance is a high-zone paralysis phenomenon most easily induced by the action of an antigen upon an ARC precursor. At birth, few ARC are present in the peripheral lymphoid tissues, but these are rapidly generated via stem cells and precursors in the neonatal period. Thus, very low levels of antigen administered during the first weeks of life, in rodents at least, are capable of interacting with ARC precursors as they are generated, and either destroy or suppress the ARC with regard to the specific antigen administered.

In the adult, however, a relatively large ARC population is available for interaction with any given antigen. Moreover, these cells are apparently very heterogeneous with respect to the dose of antigen which may induce either immunity or paralysis. In the case of moderately immunogenic antigens, very small doses may induce low-zone paralysis in a majority of the

ARC population, but they probably initiate an immune response on the part of the more sensitive cells in the group. Larger doses of antigen stimulate an immune response in the majority of the ARC, with a few very sensitive and a few very resistant cells developing high-zone and low-zone paralysis, respectively. Under these circumstances, which prevail for most common antigens, immunologic unresponsiveness in the adult can only be achieved by high-zone paralysis after the administration of extremely large quantities of antigen.

A somewhat different situation is observed when less immunogenic antigens are administered to adult animals. Under these circumstances it is possible to achieve a low-zone paralysis in the entire ARC population without reaching a concentration of antigen which will trigger an immune response in even the most sensitive members of this group. Thus, because of the weak immunogenicity of the antigen involved, an apparently homogeneous response is obtained despite the heterogeneity of the cell population.

The manner in which recovery from immunologic unresponsiveness occurs remains unclear. At present, it appears probable that the ARC which have reacted with antigen under inhibitory conditions become differentially susceptible to cell death, and thus there is a temporary hiatus in the production of a particular ARC line. Recovery from tolerance or paralysis must then require the gradual replenishment of specific ARC from a precursor or stem cell population. In certain rodents, it appears that the thymus is essential for this type of repopulation to occur. With the advent of a freshly populated specific ARC line, alterations in the antigen-ARC interaction may then favor stimulation rather than inhibition. Thus, there is subsequent development of an immune response instead of immunologic unresponsiveness.

AUTOIMMUNITY

The mechanisms of immunologic unresponsiveness afford the body tissues a large measure of protection against an immune system developed for the destruction or elimination of antigenically foreign substances. Nevertheless, a number of well established clinical syndromes exist in which the self-recognition process apparently fails, and the immune response is directed against autologous antigens.

The autoantibodies which appear in these disease states demonstrate different degrees of specificity with respect to both tissue and species. Tissue-specific autoantibodies include those which react against erythrocyte stromal antigens, platelets, antihemophilic globulin, thyroid tissue, and γ-globulin (rheumatoid factor). Autoantibodies without tissue specificity include antinuclear, antinucleoprotein, anti-DNA, and anticytoplasmic antibodies. Autoantibodies directed against the formed elements of the blood can undoubtedly induce disease by causing the destruction and removal of these cells from the circulation. However, it is far less certain whether other types of autoantibodies play pathogenic roles.

Most studies of autoantibodies in both humans and animals have concentrated on the reactivity of humoral constituents. However, it should be remembered that the cell-mediated immune response is far more efficient in terms of tissue destruction. Since humoral antibodies have been shown, under appropriate circumstances, to prevent cell-mediated tissue damage, it is conceivable that they may have a protective rather than a destructive function.

There is presently no indication whether the autoantibodies detected in human disease represent a primary manifestation of the disease itself or a secondary event stimulated by an underlying, but unrelated, abnormality. In either event, the mechanisms which may be responsible for the abrogation of natural immunologic tolerance are worthy of consideration. Four general mechanisms have been proposed in the pathogenesis of auto-antibody production: (1) alterations in the structure or distribution of antigens; (2) formation of cross-reactive antibodies following exposure to extrinsic antigens; (3) release of sequestered antigens; and (4) abnormalities of immunologic responsiveness.

Alterations in the Structure or Distribution of Antigens

The interaction of normal body constituents with a variety of exogenous agents may lead to a modification in antigenic structure. Possibly inciting agents include microorganisms, radiation, thermal changes, and chemicals or drugs. In general, any form of tissue destruction may be associated with antigenic alteration. A drastic antigenic change is unlikely to result in the formation of autoantibodies which cross-react with normal body constituents, and is therefore relatively harmless. More subtle, nongenetic, molecular modifications, such as those induced on cell surfaces by certain viral infection or by drugs, are more likely to evoke an immune response in which the autoantibodies cross-react with native constituents and may result in tissue damage. The autoantibody production may be a temporary phenomenon, extending only for that period of time during which the agent is present. It is, however, possible that exposure to the modified material may result in a permanent loss of tolerance to the native component.

Chronic autoantibody production might also be elicited by a permanent change in the structure of native components. For example, some viral infections, irradiation, and mutagenic drugs are capable of altering the genetic information of cells which, in turn, may result in the synthesis of abnormal macromolecules.

Cross-Reactive Antigens

The fortuitous antigenic similarity between constituents of infecting micro-organisms and components of the body might, during chronic infection, lead to a persistent state of autoantibody production.

Sequestered Antigens

Since continued exposure of the immune system to antigen is necessary for the maintenance of immunologic unresponsiveness, tolerance may be lost to "sequestered" antigens that are not accessible to the blood and lymphatic circulation. Tissue damage leading to exposure of the sequestered components, with or without molecular modification, might then be associated with autoantibody production since these products would no longer be looked upon as "self." Moreover, a vicious cycle might develop in which autoantibody production leading to tissue destruction might further augment the autoantibody response.

Abnormalities of Immunologic Unresponsiveness

Multiple autoantibodies are detected in certain disease states. Unless a general mechanism is postulated which could alter numerous tissue constituents simultaneously, the events leading to autoantibody production might be more easily explained on the basis of an alteration of the immune apparatus. Although no evidence for this type of mechanism has been demonstrated, a number of possibilities have been put forward: (1) the ARC might become resistant to antigen-induced tolerance; (2) an ARC accumulation might occur on the basis of either increased production or decreased destruction and thus lead to a heightened immune response; (3) the ARC might become hyperresponsive to certain autologous antigens; and (4) macrophage function might become abnormal leading to increased cellular processing and the production of highly immunogenic "superantigen complexes" by combination with RNA. The first three possibilities noted above may be grouped together as the "forbidden clone" theory of auto-antibody formation.

MEDIATION OF IMMUNOLOGIC TISSUE INJURY

In considering the mechanisms of immunologic tissue injury, it should be remembered that one of the most important functions of the immunologic system is the removal or neutralization of potentially noxious agents such as microorganisms and foreign antigens. The inflammatory reaction which often forms part of the immune response to these agents not infrequently results in inadvertent damage to the host and, on occasion, may be primarily directed against the host. In this context, it is worth emphasizing again that antibodies, even when combined with their corresponding antigens, are seldom the final effectors or mediators of adverse immunologic reactions.

In many immune disorders, more than one inflammatory mediator contributes to tissue damage, and frequently both cells and humoral factors are involved. Furthermore, many of the mediation systems, of both cellular and humoral origin, may be activated by nonimmunologic means. Examples of this latter phenomenon include the codeine-induced release of histamine from mast cells in certain individuals, and the increase in vascular permeability which occurs in hereditary angioedema (see Chapter 5).

In the ensuing discussion, the consideration of each system as an isolated mediator is somewhat artificial. The final inflammatory process is usually the result of a complex interaction of cells (e.g., mast cells, polymorphonuclear leukocytes, platelets, monocytes, and lymphocytes) and humoral factors such as the complement, coagulation, kinin, and fibrinolytic systems.

COMPLEMENT SYSTEM

Biochemistry of the Complement System

The complement system consists of 11 distinct serum proteins which react with each other to produce a variety of biologic effects. The system is comparable in some ways to the coagulation mechanism, particularly in the interaction of components in a "cascade" type of sequence. The ultimate effect of this interaction is damage to a cell membrane that results in cytolysis. However, intermediate steps in the activation sequence generate products which have biologic effects. Examples of this "biologic fallout" include the production of chemotactic factors and anaphylatoxins.

The classic complement sequence leading to membrane damage (usually of the red blood cell membrane) is depicted schematically in Figure 1-5. The symbol S is used to denote a cell surface antigen against which an antibody, designated by the symbol A, is directed. Complement components associated with enzyme activity are indicated by a bar above the numerals or letters used for their designation. For the sake of simplicity, inactivated components have not been shown in the diagram. The cleavage of some components into sub-fragments is indicated by small letters such as 2a, 3b, etc.

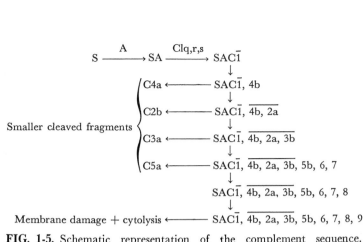

FIG. 1-5. Schematic representation of the complement sequence. S = cell surface antigen; A = antibody; complement components associated with enzyme activity indicated by bar above numerals and letters used for their designation; cleavage of components into subfragments indicated by small letters. (Adapted from Müller-Eberhard, H. J. *Ann. Rev. Biochem. 38*:389, 1969.)

Activation of the complement sequence begins when antibody with complement-fixing capacity combines with its specific antigen. The C1 complex attaches to the Fc fragment of the antibody through binding sites on its C1q subunit, presumably as the result of a configurational change in the Fc fragment of the immunoglobulin molecule. Through the action of C1r, C1s is activated to form C1 esterase (activated C1), and, thus, C1 functions as a three unit complex.

Activated C1 in turn activates C4 and C2 to form an enzyme, C3 convertase (C4b, 2a) which splits C3 into two fragments. The smaller fragment, C3a, possesses anaphylatoxic and chemotactic activity, whereas the larger fragment, C3b, is bound to the cell surface and permits the next three components to interact. C5, like C3, is split into two fragments: C5a, which also possesses chemotactic and anaphylatoxic activity, and C5b, which binds to the cell. C5b, C6, and C7 act as a functional trimolecular complex which has chemotactic activity for polymorphonuclear leukocytes and permits binding of the last two components, C8 and C9. It is these last two components of the complement sequence which act in concert to produce membrane damage and ultimately cytolysis.

In general, fragmentation of complement components results in the formation of: (*1*) a smaller molecule which is unable to participate further in the complement sequence but frequently possesses biologic activity; and (*2*) a larger fragment (e.g., C3b or C5b) which is capable of entering the cytolytic sequence. In addition to cleavage of C3 and C5, there is evidence for the occurrence of a similar cleavage of C4 and C2. Although

33

biologic effects have not been definitely attributed to smaller fragments of these components, it has been suggested recently that fragments of C2 and C4 may provide complement derived kinin-like peptides. Furthermore, C4 which has been acted on by C1 esterase may be capable of releasing serotonin.

Activation of the complement sequence can occur in the absence of bound antibody, but the cytolytic efficiency of the process is greatly enhanced when it is triggered by an antigen-antibody reaction.

Biologic Effects of the Complement System

A number of complement dependent reactions that have been described in vitro are listed in Table 1-2. There is considerable evidence that a number of these in vitro reactions have their in vivo counterparts, particularly in experimental immunologic diseases such as experimental vasculitis, nephrotoxic nephritis, and serum sickness arteritis. Furthermore, it seems reasonable to assume that most of these reactions may also have a protective function in the host, particularly as a defense against invasion by microorganisms.

TABLE 1-2. Complement Dependent Biologic Reactions
in Vitro

Reaction	Major complement components
Immune cytolysis	C1–9
Bactericidal reaction	C1–9
Immune adherence	C3,4
Immune conglutination	C3
Anaphylatoxin production	C3a, C5a
Leukocyte chemotaxis	C5, 6, 7; C3a; C5a
Phagocytosis	Probably several
Complement dependent non-cytotoxic histamine release	C1–C5?
Clot lysis	C3,C4
Kinin-like activity	C2, C4?

Immune Cytolysis.   A number of cell types such as red blood cells and mast cells are susceptible to immune cytolysis. The complement dependent immune hemolysis which is observed in a number of human isoimmune and autoimmune hemolytic anemias provides a good example of this type of reaction (see Chapter 9). Immune cytolysis generally requires the participation of the entire sequence of complement components.

Bactericidal Reaction. Complement may attack the bacterial cell wall in a manner similar to that described for other cell membranes and cause destruction of the bacteria. This phenomenon is particularly common in Gram-negative organisms where the cell wall is more susceptible to complement-induced damage. In addition, complement may aid in the destruction of bacteria by enhancing phagocytosis and by promoting chemotaxis of phagocytic cells such as polymorphonuclear leukocytes.

Immune Adherence. The binding of complement to antigen-antibody complexes confers on them the property of adhering to nonsensitized cells such as erythrocytes, leukocytes, and platelets. This adherence, particularly to leukocytes, probably promotes phagocytosis and accounts, at least in part, for the ability of complement to act as an opsonin. Should the antigen by a microorganism, the phenomenon of immune adherence would promote the adherence of phagocytic cells and the removal of the offending organism. Immune adherence appears to be a function of both C3 and C4, but either one can produce the phenomenon independently of the other.

Conglutination and Immune Conglutination. When C3 is bound to cells it undergoes a configurational change that permits the formation of a true autoantibody, *immunoconglutinin,* directed against the bound molecule. In addition, a nonantibody protein, known as conglutinin, which appears to have specificity for bound C3 has been found in bovine serum. Immunoconglutinin is presumed to enhance resistance to infection, perhaps by promoting phagocytosis of particles which have fixed antibody and complement. However, its true significance in human disease is as yet unclear.

Anaphylatoxin Production. It has been known for many years that when immune precipitates are reacted with fresh serum, a substance is generated which can induce a syndrome similar to anaphylactic shock. As noted in the section on the complement sequence, at least two molecular species, C3a and C5a, have now been identified which have the properties ascribed to anaphylatoxin, i.e., smooth muscle contraction and increase in vascular permeability. Both molecules are capable of liberating histamine from mast cells, and their anaphylatoxic properties can probably be explained in part by their mastocytolytic (histamine releasing) effect. Anaphylatoxin also appears to act directly on blood vessels.

C3a can also be produced by a number of proteolytic enzymes which act independently of the complement sequence. Thus, this biologically active fragment can be generated by nonimmunologic mechanisms. In addition to its anaphylatoxic properties, C3a is chemotactic for polymorphonuclear leukocytes, but the chemotactic and anaphylatoxic properties probably reside on different portions of the C3a molecule. The inflammatory enhancing properties of C3a are evident. Histamine release leads to enhanced vascular permeability, while the chemotaxis of polymorphonuclear leukocytes brings cells which contain a number of proteolytic enzymes and vascular permeability factors to the site of inflammation.

Like C3a, C5a may be generated by mechanisms other than through the usual complement sequence. For instance, the action of trypsin on C5 will result in the formation of the anaphylatoxin, C5a. Of interest is the fact that both molecular species of anaphylatoxin, C3a and C5a, are positively charged molecules and bear a certain resemblance to a mastocytolytic factor which is present in the polymorphonuclear leukocyte granules of some species.

Leukocyte Chemotaxis.   It is a well established fact that factors derived from the complement system can promote directional migration of polymophonuclear leukocytes in vitro. Three distinct species of complement-derived chemotactic factors have been described, one of high molecular weight and two of low molecular weight. The former consists of a complex of C5, C6, and C7 in an activated state. This complex is generated by the action of the preceding complement components, and has a molecular weight which exceeds 200,000. The low molecular weight (less than 15,000) chemotactic fragments are C3a and C5a. Two esterases associated with polymorphonuclear leukocytes are the final effectors of the chemotactic activity of the C5, 6, 7 complex. One esterase exists in an activated form and the other is apparently activated by the C5, 6, 7 complex itself. The chemotactic factors derived from complement are the best defined, but it is also known that chemotactic factors of low molecular weight are elaborated by some species of bacteria. Recent studies suggest that C5a may be a more significant anaphylatoxic and chemotactic factor than C3a.

Phagocytosis.   A number of complement properties such as immune adherence, immunoconglutination, and chemotaxis serve to enhance phagocytosis. In addition to providing a protective mechanism for the disposal of bacteria and immune complexes, the phagocytic process leads to the release of bioactive substances from polymorphonuclear leukocytes. The bioactive substances, in turn, are capable of inflicting tissue injury on the host.

Complement Dependent Noncytotoxic Histamine Release.   A mechanism of histamine release from mast cells which is distinct from the homocytotropic or reagin mediated mechanism and is also distinct from the cytolytic mechanism has been described in nonhuman species. This process is dependent on the complement sequence through C5, but the exact mechanism is unknown.

Clot Lysis.   Inhibition of clot lysis in vitro has been observed with the use of specific antisera to C3 and C4. The results of this experiment suggest that complement may play an important role in clot lysis, although the mechanism is not understood. The ability of bound C3 to adhere to platelets may be related to this phenomenon.

Regulation of the Complement System

Because of the potent biologic effects of the complement system, it is essential that regulatory mechanisms exist to prevent inappropriate activation of the sequence. Certain regulatory mechanisms are intrinsic to the system such as: (1) rapid decay of certain components; (2) loss of binding capacity; and (3) dissociation of components leading to loss of enzyme activity. In addition, there are a number of extrinsic inhibitors of the complement system. The best defined is the serum inhibitor of C1 esterase (activated C1) which, when deficient, leads to a disease state in humans known as hereditary angioedema (see Chapter 5). A number of other inhibitors or inactivators of complement components have been found including those directed against native C4, cell-bound C3, and cell-bound C6. Recently an 11S α2-globulin has been detected in human serum which inactivates the two anaphylatoxic fragments, C3a and C5a.

POLYMORPHONUCLEAR LEUKOCYTES (PMN'S)

The polymorphonuclear leukocytes (PMN) is an important mediator of immunologic tissue injury in a number of experimental immunologic diseases and has recently been implicated in similar disease processes in humans. Its role as an effector of tissue damage is intimately related to the complement system. As noted in the previous section, chemotactic factors generated from complement can promote directional migration of PMN's and bound C3 or C4 can cause adherence of PMN's at the sites of immunologic reactions.

PMN's in Experimental Immunologic Disease

In the Arthus phenomenon, serum sickness arteritis, and nephrotoxic nephritis, the infiltration of PMN's into the site of the immunologic reaction is associated with functional and structural changes in the target organ. Prior depletion of these cells either eliminates or greatly reduces the degree of tissue injury. In most immunologic diseases studied it appears that a prerequisite for involvement of the PMN is an antibody which is capable of fixing complement. Thus a pathway of mediation has been delineated which involves the union of antigen and antibody, the fixation of complement, the generation of complement-derived chemotactic factors, and the accumulation of PMN's (see Fig. 1-6). Although this mediation system is of proven importance in a number of experimental diseases and probably in many human disorders, it is certainly not the sole pathway involved in tissue damage.

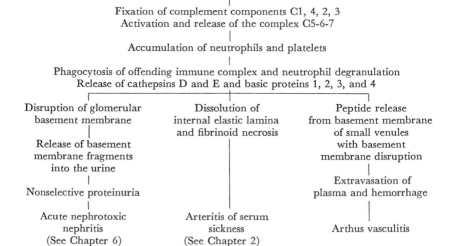

FIG. 1-6. Suggested mechanism for the production of various types of experimental immunologic tissue injury. (Adapted from Cochrane, C. G. Immunologic tissue injury mediated by neutrophilic leukocytes. *Advances Immun.* 9:97, 1968.)

Many immunologic lesions begin in the walls of blood vessels or in the glomeruli, and it is these structures which appear to be the primary targets against which the leukocyte attack is directed. The PMN contains a number of substances, predominantly in its lysosomal granules, which are capable of altering vascular structures. PMN factors which have been found to be of significance in immunologic tissue injury include: (*1*) proteolytic enzymes (acid proteases or cathepsins) which are capable of hydrolyzing glomerular basement membrane in vitro; (*2*) a number of permeability factors which are capable of increasing vascular permeability; (*3*) a permeability factor with mastocytolytic (histamine releasing) properties; and (*4*) an elastase and a collagenase.

In addition, under certain experimental conditions, PMN's have been shown to be a source of other inflammatory mediators such as slow-reacting substance (SRS-A), kininases, and kininogenases (see section which follows on the kinin system). PMN's also appear to be capable of converting prothrombin to thrombin. This latter property may, in part, account for the frequent accumulation of fibrin at the sites of immunologic tissue injury.

PMN's in Human Immunologic Disease

Most of the work on the role of complement and the PMN in immunologic tissue injury has been done, of necessity, in experimental animals where depletion of these substances can be readily accomplished. The evidence for their role in human immunologic diseases is more circumstantial and, in the case of the PMN, depends largely on morphologic observations. As in the experimental lesions, PMN's are frequently found infiltrating the site of an immunologic reaction where complement has been fixed. For example, accumulation of PMN's may be seen in the glomerular lesions associated with acute poststreptococcal nephritis, anaphylactoid purpura, and Goodpasture's syndrome, as well as in the vasculitides associated with rheumatoid arthritis, systemic lupus erythematosus, anaphylactoid purpura, or mixed cryoglobulinemia.

It is conceivable that a number of anti-inflammatory agents, useful in the treatment of immunologic diseases, exert their beneficial role, in part, through their action on the PMN. The corticosteroids, chloroquine, and salicylates are all lysosomal stabilizers, and, thus, might retard the release of inflammatory products from the PMN. Furthermore, a number of widely used anti-rheumatic agents such as the corticosteroids, chloroquine, colchicine, and indomethacin, appear to inhibit the chemotactic activity of the PMN.

KININ SYSTEM

The kinins are a group of extremely potent vasoactive peptides which are split off from plasma precursors known as kininogens (Fig. 1-7). Several vasoactive peptides may be derived from these $\alpha2$-globulins depending on the nature of the enzyme which acts upon them, but the major ones are lysl-bradykinin (a decapeptide) and bradykinin (a nonapeptide). The most important of the proteolytic enzymes which are capable of cleaving kinins from kininogens are the kallikreins. Several different kallikreins have been described and these, in turn, can be activated by a number of other enzymes.

At least one such pathway involves the sequential activation of Hageman factor (coagulation Factor XII), another proteolytic enzyme known as PF/dil, and a plasma kallikrein (Fig. 1-7). It is currently thought that this constitutes the major pathway for the activation of plasma kinins.

Hageman factor → Activated Hageman factor

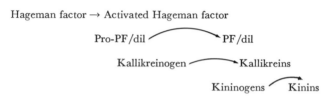

FIG. 1-7. Suggested pathway for the activation of plasma kinins.

As with other potent bioactive systems of this type whose inadvertent activation might lead to undesirable consequences, a number of inhibitors exist which minimize this eventuality. For example, the kinins themselves are rapidly destroyed in plasma by kininases. In addition, kallikrein can be inhibited by a material obtained from beef organs which has been used therapeutically under the name of Trasylol. Whether a comparable substance exists in humans is not known. Lastly, the inhibitor of C1 esterase also inhibits plasma kallikrein and PF/dil (see Chapter 5).

Despite extensive study of these vasoactive peptides for a number of years, the significance of the kinins in physiologic control systems and in pathologic states in man is uncertain. However, it is well established that kinins can produce many of the signs of inflammation. When injected locally they cause pain and an increase in vascular permeability. Their effect on smooth muscle is variable, but generally they tend to produce contraction of nonvascular smooth muscle and relaxation of vascular smooth muscle. This latter property renders them potent hypotensive agents.

Since kinins produce most of the signs of acute inflammation, it is in inflammatory conditions that they are most likely implicated. Kinin concentrations are increased at sites of tissue injury and are released from kininogens by the enzymes of inflammatory cells such as polymorphonuclear leukocytes. This latter reaction appears to require the presence of Hageman factor (Factor XII). In support of this hypothesis is the observation that a number of anti-inflammatory agents such as corticosteroids and salicylates inhibit the release of kinins.

Evidence that kinins might be significant mediators in allergic disease is largely circumstantial thus far, but the following observations are of interest: (1) antigen-antibody complexes are capable of inducing kinin release; (2) increased levels of kinins have been identified in the blood of a number of animal species during anaphylactic reactions; (3) kinins are capable of inducing bronchoconstriction in the guinea pig; (4) kinins cause bronchoconstriction when administered to asthmatic patients by aerosol in doses which do not produce any change in normal subjects; and (5) increased levels of kinins have been demonstrated in the blood of patients with asthmatic attacks and in the nasal secretions of patients with allergic rhinitis.

SLOW-REACTING SUBSTANCE OF ANAPHYLAXIS (SRS-A)

The lack of effectiveness of antihistamines in the treatment of human bronchial asthma has led to the suggestion that chemical mediators other than histamine might be involved in its pathogenesis (see Chapter 3). At least one such substance has been identified in animals and has been implicated as a mediator in human bronchial asthma. This substance, known as slow-reacting substance (SRS-A), can be distinguished from other mediators of inflammation by: (1) its ability to contract guinea pig ileum and human bronchial smooth muscle in the presence of antihistamines; (2) its ability to contract guinea pig ileum made refractory to the action of histamine; and (3) the absence of any effect on rat uterus. The fact that SRS-A is not destroyed by proteolytic enzymes would suggest that it is not protein in nature, but it may be an acid lipid.

When challenged in vitro with specific antigen, SRS-A is released from lung tissue obtained from sensitized guinea pigs as well as from lung tissue obtained from patients with extrinsic bronchial asthma. SRS-A is also capable of producing an increase in cutaneous vascular permeability.

Recent studies in the rat have shown that a distinct immunologic pathway exists for the release of SRS-A which is quite different from that involved in the release of histamine. The release of histamine may be effected by either homocytotropic antibody or antibody associated with the IgGa class of rat immunoglobulin, whereas SRS-A is released by the latter immunoglobulin only. Furthermore, the mast cell appears to be the major source of histamine, while the polymorphonuclear leukocyte is the major source of SRS-A.

Of considerable interest is the fact that these two pathways can be selectively inhibited by different pharmacologic agents. SRS-A release can be blocked by a piperazine analogue, diethylcarbamazine, which does not block histamine release. On the other hand, disodium cromoglycate inhibits histamine release but has no effect on the release of SRS-A. The therapeutic potential of these two agents in human allergic disorders has not yet been fully explored (see Chapter 3).

SEROTONIN

The role of serotonin in human allergic and immunologic disorders is not known. However, like SRS-A, it has been suggested as a mediator of immunologic injury in situations where histamine alone does not appear to account for all the observed phenomena. Of particular interest is the association of wheezing with the increased levels of circulating serotonin found in the carcinoid syndrome. On the other hand, the intravenous injection of serotonin in man does not consistently produce bronchoconstriction, whereas the administration of aerosolized serotonin to asthmatic subjects does produce bronchoconstriction. In this context, it may be of significance that the serotonin content of the human lung is negligible.

Serotonin has rather complex effects on other types of smooth muscle, particularly in the vascular system. In man, serotonin appears to constrict the larger arteries and veins, and to dilate the smaller blood vessels. When injected locally it is capable of producing pain. These latter two properties suggest that it may produce some of the features of the inflammatory process.

There is evidence in several other species that serotonin may play an important role in immunologic tissue injury. In the rabbit, the release of vasoactive amines, including serotonin, from platelets during serum sickness is responsible for the transient increase in vascular permeability which permits the localization of circulating immune complexes. Anaphylaxis in the mouse can be inhibited by a serotonin antagonist, d-lysergic acid diethylamide (LSD). However, it should be noted that the mouse lung contains relatively large amounts of serotonin compared to the human lung. In man, the bulk of serotonin is contained in the gastrointestinal mucosa, while smaller amounts occur in blood platelets. Since platelets participate in some immunologic reactions (see subsequent discussion in this chapter), it is conceivable that serotonin may contribute to certain forms of human immunologic tissue injury.

HISTAMINE

Histamine appears to play a key role in many human immunologic disorders, particularly of the atopic variety. Its actions have been extensively studied, and, compared to those of other mediators, are relatively well defined. When injected locally it produces the well known triple response which consists of: (1) primary, local dilatation of small vessels; (2) widespread arteriolar dilatation mediated through local axon reflexes; and (3) local increased vascular permeability. In addition to these vascular effects, histamine causes contraction of smooth muscle, especially in the gastrointestinal tract and bronchioles.

The major source of histamine in the body is the mast cell which contains histamine and heparin within its granules, but does not appear to contain any other vasoactive amines. Mast cells are widely distributed in human tissues such as the skin, gastrointestinal tract, and lung. In some tissues, histamine may be formed through the action of histidine decarboxylase, but this mechanism probably does not account for most of the histamine produced in the body.

A number of mechanisms for the release of histamine from the mast cell have been described in animal species, particularly the rat. One mechanism involves homocytotropic antibody which fixes to the rat mast cell without involvement of the complement system. On subsequent challenge with specific antigen, histamine is released from the mast cell in the absence of cytolysis. A second mechanism is cytolytic and requires the presence of anti-rat mast cell antibodies as well as the entire complement sequence. A third mechanism has also been described in which a different type of antibody is directed against rat immunoglobulin on the surface of the mast cell. Complement components C1–5 are essential for histamine release in this latter system which is noncytolytic and has been termed immune-aggregate-induced complement-dependent histamine release.

In addition to these mechanisms which involve antibody directly, a number of other substances are liberated during immunologic reactions which are capable of causing mastocytolysis with histamine release. As noted in previous sections of this chapter, these latter substances include the anaphylatoxins (C3a and C5a), and a low molecular weight protein obtained from PMN's. Finally, certain drugs, such as codeine, may induce release of histamine from mast cells by entirely non-immunologic means.

PLATELETS

Platelets may contribute to immunologic tissue injury by virtue of their ability to respond to antigen-antibody complexes or to γ-globulin bound to the surfaces of cells. Phagocytosis of antigen-antibody complexes by platelets leads to release of bioactive substances while exposure to bound γ-globulin, immune complexes, or damaged vascular walls induces platelet aggregation and the release of inflammatory mediators. The enzyme adenosinediphosphate (ADP) is also released by aggregated platelets and this substance induces further platelet aggregation and release of bioactive substances.

The platelet contains histamine, serotinin, and a vascular permeability factor which does not appear to be a kinin, anaphylatoxin, or SRS-A.

Detailed experimental studies in vitro have demonstrated several mechanisms of antibody-mediated release from vasoactive amines from the rabbit platelet. In some instances release is dependent on complement and may be enhanced by PMN's, or the phenomenon of immune adherence may trigger platelet aggregation around immune complexes. Once aggregated, the platelet can participate in the process of blood coagulation. It is of interest that antigen-antibody complexes may also activate Hageman factor and thus initiate coagulation independently of the platelets.

Many of the in vivo studies on the platelet in immunologic tissue injury have been done in the serum sickness model in the rabbit. There it was found that the initiation of vascular lesions required the release of vasoactive amines from platelets, while the more advanced and destructive lesions were dependent on complement and PMN's.

Infusion of antigen into a sensitized animal or of preformed antigen-antibody complexes into a normal animal produces a rapid fall in platelet count, acceleration of blood coagulation, and obstruction of the pulmonary vessels by thrombi. Frequently these animals develop peripheral vasodilatation, acute shock, and death. However, if platelet aggregation is inhibited by drugs such as sulfinpyrazone or salicylates, shock and death do not occur. This finding suggests that platelet aggregation may be involved in some of the systemic reactions associated with antigen-antibody complexes.

In the generalized Shwartzman reaction in animals (see subsequent discussion in this chapter), the deposition of fibrin in the golmeruli and bilateral renal cortical necrosis can be prevented by drugs which inhibit endotoxin-induced platelet aggregation. In humans, it has been found that administration of an antiplatelet aggregator such as phenylbutazone is capable of reversing the disturbance in renal function associated with hyperacute renal homograft rejection (see Chapter 14).

Thus, the platelet may contribute to immunologic tissue injury through: (1) release of vasoactive amines and permeability factors; (2) release of coagulation factors which lead to localized or generalized fibrin deposition; and (3) formation of platelet aggregates with plugging of vessels.

COAGULATION SYSTEM

A rather complex interrelationship exists between the coagulation, fibrinolytic, kinin and complement systems. Antigen-antibody complexes can trigger coagulation through activation of both Hageman factor (Factor XII) and platelets, and may also convert plasminogen to plasmin. Hageman factor, in turn, can activate kinins and may act directly on plasminogen to form plasmin. Subsequently, plasmin may activate complement (C1 and C3) and kinins with the release of anaphylatoxins, chemotactic substances, and substances which increase vascular permeability (see preceding sections in this chapter).

In addition, the conversion of fibrinogen to fibrin results in the formation of a potent vasoconstrictor peptide which might contribute to renal ischemia in some forms of immunologic renal injury. Another factor of possible significance is that PMN's, which are attracted to sites of injury by complement-derived chemotactic factors, have procoagulant activities. Thus, the coagulation and fibrinolytic systems may be readily activated in a number of ways once antigen-antibody complexing has occurred. Several examples serve to illustrate the relationship between coagulation, fibrinolytic systems, and immunologic tissue injury.

In nephrotoxic nephritis and several human nephritides, fibrin can be identified by immunofluorescence in the damaged glomeruli where it may contribute to subacute and chronic changes. Treatment of acute nephritic animals with anticoagulants greatly modifies the lesion and appears to prevent glomerular obliteration and crescent formation. Reversal of severe renal impairment has been observed in patients with acute glomerulonephritis who were treated with high doses of heparin (see Chapter 6). In humans, fibrinogen fragments have been detected in the urine of patients during allograft rejection. There is evidence that plasmin is activated in the kidneys of these patients and may contribute to renal damage (see Chapter 14).

SANARELLI-SHWARTZMAN PHENOMENON

Although it is not usually initiated by antigen-antibody interaction, the Sanarelli-Shwartzman phenomenon (Shwartzman reaction) provides yet another example of the complex relationship between the coagulation system and immunologic phenomena. Furthermore, its participation in acute disease processes of immunologic interest has long been suspected.

In experimental animals, a *local Shwartzman reaction* is produced most readily by the intradermal injection of bacterial endotoxin followed several hours later by the intravenous injection of the same or a different bacterial endotovin. The second intravenous injection results in a hemorrhagic necrotic lesion at the site of the first injection. The *generalized Shwartzman reaction* is produced by giving both injections intravenously. Under these latter experimental conditions, the predominant lesion is bilateral cortical necrosis of the kidneys due to extensive vascular obstruction caused by platelet, polymorphonuclear leukocyte, and fibrin thrombi. Thus, the ultimate effects of the generalized Shwartzman reaction are increased intravascular coagulation and, possibly, a consumptive coagulopathy.

It is not yet established whether there is a significant immunologic component to the Sanarelli-Shwartzman phenomenon. However, it is conceivable that vasoactive substances released by bacterial endotoxins may have a nonspecific effect in enhancing the functional consequences of immunologic reactions. The best example of this hypothetical synergistic interaction between immune responses and the generalized Shwartzman reaction is provided by some patients with hyperacute rejection of renal homografts (see Chapter 14).

IMMUNOGENETICS

The term immunogenetics may be defined as the study of the interaction between the disciplines of immunology and genetics. Two major areas are included in this field: (1) the genetic mechanisms involved in the control of immune response (e.g., the capacity of inbred strains of mice to produce antibodies to certain synthetic polypeptides is a genetically determined trait), and (2) the application of immunologic methods to the recognition of individual antigenic differences within a species (alloantigens) for genetic study. The discussion in this section will be limited to a consideration of alloantigenic differences that can be demonstrated between serum immunoglobulins (allotypes) and between antigens on the surfaces of cells (e.g., blood group, histocompatibility, leukocyte, and platelet antigens).

In discussing genetic differences between individuals it is important to distinguish between the meanings of the words genotype and phenotype. The term *genotype* refers to the genetic constitution of the individual, whereas the word *phenotype* refers to the outward expression from which the observer may make deductions about the genotype.

GENETIC POLYMORPHISM (ALLOTYPES) OF IMMUNOGLOBULINS

Antigenic differences between similar immunoglobulin classes in individuals within a species form the basis for demonstrating the genetic *polymorphism* (variation) of human immunoglobulins. These antigenic differences (*allotypes*) are inherited as autosomal codominant genetic traits and form a system of genetic markers similar in many ways to the blood group antigens.

Two major allotypic systems, Gm and Inv, have been described in humans. The three Inv allotypes are found on the kappa light chains of all immunoglobulin classes, whereas the Gm factors are found only on the heavy chains (γ chains) of IgG molecules. Preliminary reports have described antigenic polymorphism among heavy chains (α chains) of IgA molecules, but allotypic systems for the heavy chains of the other immunoglobulin classes have not yet been defined.

TABLE 1-3. Gm and Inv Allotypes
in Humans

Nomenclature	
Numerical	Alphabetical
Gm(1)	Gm(a)
Gm(2)	Gm(x)
Gm(3)	Gm(b²)* or (bʷ)
Gm(4)	Gm(f)*
Gm(5)	Gm(b¹)*
Gm(6)	Gm(c³)
Gm(7)	Gm(r)
Gm(8)	Gm(e)
Gm(9)	Gm(p)
Gm(10)	Gm(bᵅ)*
Gm(11)	Gm(bᵝ) or (b⁰)
Gm(12)	Gm(bᵞ)*
Gm(13)	Gm(b³)*
Gm(14)	Gm(b⁴)
Gm(15)	Gm(s)
Gm(16)	Gm(t)
Gm(17)	Gm(z)
Gm(20)	—
Gm(21)	Gm(g)
Gm(22)	Gm(y)
Gm(23)	Gm(n)
Gm(24)	Gm(c⁵)
Inv(1)	Inv(l)
Inv(2)	Inv(a)
Inv(3)	Inv(b)

* Gm(b²) and Gm(f) are probably
identical. Similarly Gm(b¹) probably
corresponds to Gm(bᵞ), and Gm(bᵅ)
probably corresponds to Gm(b³).

The Gm system is composed of approximately 20 distinct antigenic determinants which have been described according to a numerical and an
alphabetical nomenclature (see Table 1-3). In this text the alphabetical
nomenclature will be used throughout. The serum Gm phenotype is the
sum of the individual phenotypes present on individual antibody molecules.
Investigations employing myeloma proteins have shown that the Gm factors

thus far described are specifically associated with $\gamma 1$, $\gamma 2$, and $\gamma 3$ heavy chains, but not with $\gamma 4$ heavy chains (Table 1-4). Furthermore, it has been demonstrated in family and population studies that the Gm factors are inherited in linked genetic units (gene complexes) or in combinations called phenogroups.

TABLE 1-4. Molecular Localization and Segregation of the Gm Factors Among the Heavy Chain Subclasses

IgG subclass nomenclature		Associated Gm factors and heavy chain localization	
New	Old	Fc fragment	Fd fragment
$\gamma G1$, IgG1	γ_{2b}, We	a, y, x, 20	z, f
$\gamma G2$, IgG2	γ_{2a}, Ne, Cr	n	none
$\gamma G3$, IgG3	γ_{2c}, Vi, Zu	b^0, b^1, b^3, b^4, b^5, s, t, c^3, c^5	none
$\gamma G4$, IgG4	γ_{2d}, Ge	none	none

The phenogroups or gene complexes which are characteristic of various populations are summarized in Table 1-5. In the table, the phenogroups are arranged in a vertical fashion according to the subgroup of the γ chain with which a Gm factor is associated. For example, in Caucasians, a common homozygous gene complex or phenotype is Gm ($a^+z^+g^+$). This is made up of Gm (a^+) and Gm (z) found on the same $\gamma 1$ heavy chain, and Gm (g) found on the $\gamma 3$ heavy chain. The allotypes of the $\gamma 2$ and $\gamma 4$ molecules that would complete the gene complex have not yet been described.

From Table 1-5, it is apparent that although different Gm factors are present on different molecules, certain Gm factors are always inherited together as a genetic unit. Thus, if a homozygous Gm ($a^+z^+g^+$) male marries a homozygous female with the phenotype Gm ($y^+f^+b^+n^+$), the offspring will always be heterozygous and will have the phenotype Gm ($a^+z^+g^+y^+f^+b^+n^+$), having inherited a complete gene complex from each parent. These facts, as well as the demonstration that crossing over of Gm factors has sometimes been observed in myeloma proteins or in the immunoglobulins of rare families, have led to the suggestion that the synthesis of heavy chains is controlled by four closely linked autosomal loci. Also documented in Table 1-5 is the fact that certain Gm factors (e.g., Gm (c), (s), and (t)) are indigenous to certain populations. Thus, this system can be useful in anthropological studies.

TABLE 1-5. Gene Complexes of Different Social Groups Arranged According to the Subgroup of Heavy Chain Involved

Heavy chain subclass	Caucasian				Negroid				Mongoloid			
γG_1	x										x	a
	a	a	y	y	a	a	a	a	a	a	a	y
	z	z	f	f	z	z	z	z	z	z	z	f
γG_3	g	g	b^0	b^0	b^0	b^0	b^0	b^0	b^0	g	g	b^0
			b^1	b^1	b^1	b^1	b^1	s	st			b^1
			b^4	b^4	b^4		b^4					b^4
			b^5	b^5	b^5	c^5	b^5	b^5	b^5			b^5
			b^3	b^3	b^3	c^3	c^3	b^3	b^3			b^3
γG_2		n										n

From Litwin, S.D., and Kunkel, H.G. *J. Exp. Med. 125:*847, 1967.

The chemical basis for Gm specificity has been extensively studied. For example, tryptic peptide maps of isolated heavy chains of IgG serum or myeloma proteins have demonstrated a characteristic association of specific peptides with certain Gm phenotypes. All Gm (a⁺) molecules contain a unique peptide called the "a" peptide, whereas all Gm (a⁻) molecules contain another unique peptide called the "non-a" peptide. Phylogenetic studies of these peptides showed that individual allotypic differences arose from point mutations in genes coding for immunoglobulins.

HUMAN BLOOD GROUPS

In 1900, Landsteiner first demonstrated the alloantigenic differences on human erythrocytes which ultimately led to the delineation of the ABO blood group antigens. Since then an extensive number of alloantigens have been discovered that can conveniently be divided into blood group systems based on patterns of inheritance (see Table 1-6). Generally speaking, the blood group antigens are dominantly inherited Mendelian traits, but in some instances the interaction of two gene products results in the expression of a different phenotype. From a clinical point of view (see Chapter 9), the blood group antigens which are of major importance in transfusion practice are the ABO, Rh, and Kell systems.

TABLE 1-6. Erythrocyte Antigens in Man*

System	Number of antigens†	Major antigens
ABO-H	4	A, A_1, B, H‡(O)
MN	29	M, N, S, s
P	4	P_1, P(Tj^a), Luke‡
Rh	30	Rh1(D,Rh_o), Rh2(C,rh^1), Rh3(E,rh^{11}), Rh4(c,hr^1), Rh5(e,hr^{11}), Rh6(f,ce,hr), Rh7(Ce,rh_i), Rh8(C^w,rh^{w1}), Rh9(C^x,rh^x), Rh10(V,ce^s,hr^v), Rh11(E^w,rh^{w2}), Rh12(G,rh^G), Rh20(VS,e^s), Rh22(CE), Rh23(D^{Wiel}), Rh24(E^T), Rh25(LW)‡, Rh27(cE)
Lutheran	4	Lu^a, Lu^b
Kell	9	K1(k), K2(k)
Lewis	5	Le^a, Le^b
Duffy	2	Fy^a, Fy^b
Kidd	3	Jk^a, Jk^b
Diego	2	Di^a, Di^b
Cartwright	2	Yt^a, Yt^b
I	4	I, i
Xg	1	Xg^a
Dombrock	1	Do^a
Cs	1	Cs^a
Wright	1	Wr^a
Sciana	2	Sm, Bu^a
DBG	4	Ho, Ot, DBG
Gerbich	2	Ge, Yussel

* The following high incidence antigens are not associated with any blood group system: At^a, Co^a, Gy^a, Lan, Vel.

† Number of antigens described by July, 1968.

‡ Genetically independent part of the system.

ABO Blood Group System

The ABO blood group antigens are distributed in a wide variety of cells and tissues such as erythrocytes, leukocytes, lymphocytes, platelets, epidermal cells, capillary endothelium, spleen sinusoids, various bodily secretions, and gut epithelium, as well as in certain plants and bacteria. Natural isoantibodies to ABO blood group antigens, usually IgM in type, are present in normal human sera. In any given individual these antibodies are directed against the ABO antigens which are not present in the erythrocytes of the donor whose serum is being tested (Table 1-7). These isoantibodies (isoagglutinins) presumably arise as the result of antigenic stimulation from colonic microorganisms containing ABO-like surface antigens.

TABLE 1-7. ABO System

Phenotype	Genotype	Antigens	Natural isoantibodies		
			Anti-A	Anti-A$_1$	Anti-B
A$_1$	A$_1$O, A$_1$A$_1$, A$_1$A$_2$	A, A$_1$	0	0	+
A$_2$	A$_2$A$_2$, A$_2$O	A	0	±	+
B	BB, BO	B	+	+	0
A$_1$B	A$_1$B	A, A$_1$, B	0	0	0
A$_2$B	A$_2$B	AB	0	±	0
O	OO	H	+	+	+

The existence of the A$_1$ and A$_2$ subgroups of the A antigen is of importance in blood typing since cells of subgroup A$_2$ react weakly in vitro with anti-A antisera, and thus more care is needed to detect this antigen. Furthermore, the sera of A$_2$B individuals may contain natural Anti-A$_1$ isoantibodies that are not easily detected by routine methods (see Chapter 9).

Lewis Substances

The Lewis system is defined by two major antigens, Le^a and Le^b, which are actually soluble substances present in the serum and in secretions such as the saliva. The erythrocytes acquire the Lewis phenotype by absorbing Lewis substances from the serum.

Genetics and Chemical Nature of the ABO and Lewis Blood Group Antigens

Four independent but closely interrelated gene systems, ABO, Hh, LeLe, and SeSe, determine the synthesis of five blood group specificities: A, B, H, Le^a, and Le^b (Table 1-8). The secretor (Se) gene determines the capacity of the individual to secrete A, B, and H antigens, and the Lewis phenotype is closely related to the secretor status of the individual. For

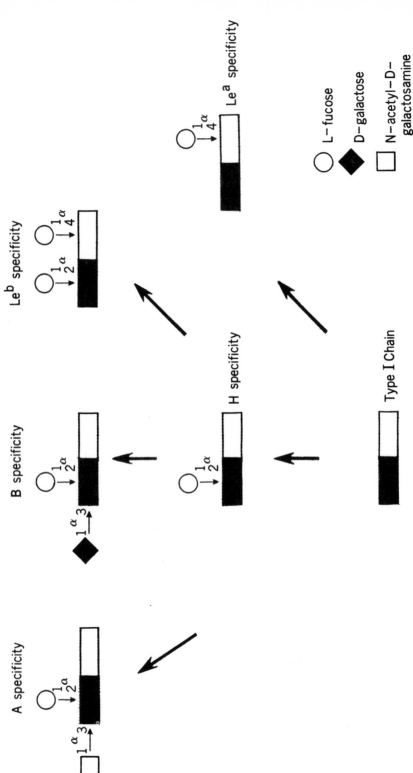

FIG. 1-8. The symbol ▭ represents the two sugars at the non-reducing terminal end of the type 1 precursor chain of the ABO and Lewis blood group antigens. Dark area represents a D-galactose residue attached *via* a β(1 = 3) linkage to adjacent N-acetyl-D-glucosamine (light area). In type 2 chains, these same sugars are joined by a β(1 = 4) linkage. Numbers and letters of Greek alphabet refer to bonds between sugar residues.

example, a person who is a nonsecretor (genotype sese) is of the Lewis type Le^a, but those who secrete blood group substances (genotype Sese or SeSe) are of the Le^b phenotype. There is no Le^b gene, but the Le^b determinant is the product of the combined action of the H and Le genes. In addition, there is no such entity as the O antigen since the erythrocytes of group O individuals contain H substance on their surfaces. However, the term group O erythrocytes is still retained for historic reasons.

TABLE 1-8. Relationship Between Genotype, Erythrocyte Phenotype and Antigenic Specificities Detectable in Secretions

Probable gene combination	Antigens detectable on red cells			Specificities detectable in secretions		
	ABH	Le^a	Le^b	ABH	Le^a	Le^b
ABO, H, Se, Le	+++	−	++	+++	+	++
ABO, H, sese, Le	+++	+++	−	−	+++	−
ABO, H, Se, lele	+++	−	−	+++	−	−
ABO, H, sese, lele	+++	−	−	−	−	−
ABO, hh, Le(Se or sese)	−	+++	−	−	+++	−
ABO, hh, lele(Se or sese)	−	−	−	−	−	−

From Watkins, W. M. *Science 152:* 172, 1966.

Both the ABH and Lewis antigens are carbohydrates linked to a peptide backbone (Fig. 1-8). Antigenic specificity is determined by the mode of linkage of four sugars, D-galactose, L-fucose, N-acetyl-D-galactosamine, and N-acetyl-D-glucosamine, to two types of backbone precursor structures (type 1 and type 2 chains). The two precursor chains differ in the mode of linkage of galactose and N-acetyl-glucosamine, but both cross-react with pneumococcal type XIV polysaccharide. The ABH and Le genes regulate the synthesis of specific glycosyl transferases which, in turn, are responsible for the mode of linkage of the sugars to the type 1 and type 2 chains.

For example, the conversion of precursor substances to H substance under the influence of the H gene occurs upon addition of L-fucose via an $\alpha(1–2)$ linkage to D-galactose. H substance, in turn, is the precursor of the Le^b, A, and B antigens. The A and B genes elaborate glycosyl transferases which add N-acetyl-D-galactosamine and D-galactose, respectively, to the H substance, and thus determine the A and B antigenic specificities. The Lewis gene directs the addition of fucose to C-4 of N-acetyl-D-galactosamine of type 1 chains to form the Le^a determinant.

Rh Blood Group System

At present at least 27 distinct antigenic determinants have been described for the Rh blood group system, and three different types of nomenclature have been developed for their designation (Table 1-6). Unlike the ABO system, very little is known of the chemical nature of the Rh antigens.

From a clinical point of view the Rh1 (Rh$_0$,D) antigen is of major importance because it is highly antigenic and is involved in the production of most cases of Rh hemolytic disease of the newborn. Despite the obvious complexity of the Rh system, considerable insight into the genetic relationships between the Rh antigens has been gained by the application of Fisher's hypothesis. According to this hypothesis, there are three genes at closely linked loci which have two possible alleles, C or c, D or d, and E or e, at each locus. Thus, the Rh gene complex can be assembled in eight different ways, CDe, cde, cDE, cDe, cdE, Cde, CDE, and CdE. Over the years, this experimental model has served as a basis for the large amount of research effort that has taken place in this area.

LEUKOCYTE OR TRANSPLANTATION ANTIGENS

Although antigenic polymorphisms specific to leukocytes probably exist, the term leukocyte antigens is usually employed to designate tissue transplantation antigens that are detected by tests which utilize white blood cell preparations (see Chapter 14). The determinants of these antigens are most likely protein components of the lipoglycoprotein molecules which are associated with both the surface and intracellular membranes.

In man, there are a number of genetically determined histocompatibility loci, but the synthesis of transplantation antigens primarily responsible for graft rejection is directed by a single, major genetic grouping referred to as the HL-A locus. The HL-A locus occurs in autosomal chromosomes and consists of at least two, and possibly as many as five, closely linked gene clusters or subloci. The various alleles of the HL-A system can code information for the synthesis of at least eight major, and an even greater number of minor, transplantation antigens. The inheritance of human transplantation antigens is expressed in a codominant fashion.

Unfortunately, no standard nomenclature has as yet been established for these constituents. Moreover, duplication of experiments in different laboratories, as well as difficulties in obtaining completely monospecific antisera, has given rise to a redundant and somewhat confusing terminology

TABLE 1-9. Nomenclature Equivalents of HL-A Specificities Described by Different Investigators

| WHO Nomenclature | Investigators | | | | | | | | | | | Frequency (%) |
	Amos	Bat-chelor	Ceppel-lini	Daus-set	Engel-friet	Kiss-meyer	Payne and Bodmer	van Rood	Shul-man	Tera-saki	Walford	
HL-A 1	19	1	8	11	4	LA1	LA1	LA1		1	Lc-1	21–40
HL-A 2 (Mac)	1	5	9	1	2	LA2	LA2	8a	B1	2	LC-2	36–61
HL-A 3	4		10	12		LA3	LA3	LA3	Hill	8	Lc-3	26–37
HL-A 5	12	25	5	5	7	MH	4d			6	Slaughter	4–24
HL-A 7	2		20	10	3	7C	4c	7c		11	Lc-8	14–40
HL-A 8	56	2	7	8	1	7D	SLA4	7d		5	Lc-7	14–29
HL-A 9	Stewart	3	12	16		LA4				4	Lc-11	19–29
HL-A 10			13	17						12	Lc-20	19–31
HL-A 11			26	21						13	Lc-20	?
HL-A 12	15		11	4		T12	4a			9	Lc-26	23–39
HL-A 13			21			HN				26		?

which will eventually require international agreement for clarification (Table 1-9).

Family studies have revealed that the ten most common combinations of alleles at the HL-A subloci occur with the relatively low frequencies of 3–14 per cent. Nevertheless, distinct groups of antigens almost invariably appear together. Thus, although much less well defined, the situation is comparable to the allotypic groupings seen within the Gm system of the IgG immunoglobulins (see Chapter 14 for a more complete discussion of transplantation antigens).

PLATELET ANTIGENS

To a large extent, the most potent platelet antigens are transplantation antigens which are shared with other tissues. There are, however, a number of immunogenic platelet constituents specific for this cell type (Table 1-10). Platelet antigens, in general, have been implicated in a number of clinical conditions including thrombocytopenic purpura, sensitization to allografts, and problems of alloimmunization with secondary effects on "self" constituents (see Chapter 9).

TABLE 1-10. Distribution of Human Platelet Antigens

Name	Population frequency (%)
$Zw^a(Pl^{A1})$	98
Zw^b	26
Ko^a	15
Ko^b	99
Pl^{E1}	99
Pl^{E2}	5

SUGGESTED READING LIST

Antigens

1. Sela, M. Antigenicity: some molecular aspects. *Science 166:*1365, 1969.

Immunoglobulin Structure and Synthesis

1. Cohen, S., and Milstein, C. Structure and biological properties of immunoglobulins. *Advances Immun.* 7:1, 1967.

2. Edelman, G. M., and Gall, W. E. The antibody problem. *Ann. Rev. Biochem.* *38:*415, 1969.

The Immune Response

1. Dresser, D. W., and Mitchison, N. A. The mechanism of immunologic paralysis. *Advances Immun. 8:*129, 1968.

2. Holborrow, E. J. Cellular immune faculties. Competence and memory. *Lancet 1:*995, 1967.

3. Holborrow, E. J. The immunological capability of small lymphocytes. *Lancet 1:*1049, 1967.

4. Janeway, C. A. Progress in immunology. Syndromes of diminished resistance to infection. *Pediatrics 72:*885, 1968.

5. Lichtenstein, L. M., and Norman, P. S. Human allergic reactions. *Amer. J. Med. 46:*163, 1969.

6. Parker, C. W., and Varva, J. D. Immunosuppression. *Progr. Hemat. 6:*1, 1969.

7. Roitt, I. M., Greaves, M. F., Torrigiani, G., Brostoff, J., and Playfair, J. H. L. The cellular basis of immunological responses. A synthesis of some current views. *Lancet 2:*367, 1969.

8. Schwartz, R. S. Therapeutic strategy in clinical immunology. *New Eng. J. Med. 280:*367, 1969.

9. Uhr, J. W., and Möller, G. Regulatory effect of antibody on the immune response. *Advances Immun. 8:*81, 1968.

Mediation of Immunologic Tissue Injury

1. Cochrane, C. G. Immunologic tissue injury mediated by neutrophilic leukocytes. *Advances Immun. 9:*97, 1968.

2. Kellermeyer, R. W., and Graham, R. C., Jr. Kinins-possible physiologic and pathologic roles in man. *New Eng. J. Med. 279:*754, 1968.

3. Macfarlane, R. G. (Ed.) A discussion on triggered enzyme systems in blood plasma. *Proc. Roy. Soc. 173:*257, 1969.

4. Müller-Eberhard, H. J. Complement. *Ann. Rev. Biochem. 38:*389, 1969.

5. Mustard, J. F., Evans, G., Packham, M. A., and Nishizawa, E. E. "The Platelet in Intravascular Immunologic Reactions," in *Cellular and Humoral Mechanisms in Anaphylaxis and Allergy,* ed. by Movat, H. Z. Basel, S. Karger, 1969, p. 151.

6. Orange, R. P., and Austen, K. F. "Slow Reacting Substance of Anaphylaxis in the Rat," in *Cellular and Humoral Mechanisms in Anaphylaxis and Allergy,* ed. by Movat, H. Z. Basel, S. Karger, 1969, p. 196.

Immunogenetics

1. Bach, F. H. Transplantation: pairing of donor and recipient. *Science* *168*:1170, 1970.

2. Giblett, E. R. *Genetic Markers in Human Blood.* Oxford, Blackwell, 1969.

3. Litwin, S. D., and Kunkel, H. G. The genetic control of γ-globulin heavy chains. *J. Exp. Med. 125*:847, 1967.

4. Marcus, D. N. ABO and Lewis blood group system. *New Eng. J. Med. 28*:993, 1969.

2

Human Anaphylaxis
and Serum Sickness

SAMUEL O. FREEDMAN

ANAPHYLAXIS

Anaphylaxis is an acute, severe, and sometimes fatal reaction, occurring within seconds or minutes after exposure to an allergenic agent to which an individual is specifically hypersensitive. The clinical syndrome closely resembles systemic anaphylaxis in the guinea pig, and may be considered as the human counterpart of experimental anaphylaxis. At present, the bulk of the available evidence suggests that human anaphylaxis is an immunologic reaction primarily mediated by homocytotropic antibodies belonging to the IgE class of immunoglobulins (reagins).

Before considering the etiology, pathophysiology, immunology, and clinical manifestations of human anaphylaxis, a brief description of experimental anaphylaxis may contribute to the understanding of the anaphylactic process in humans. If a soluble antigen is injected intravenously into an animal previously immunized with the same antigen, an explosive generalized response often occurs within 2 to 3 minutes. The nature of this response varies considerably between species: e.g., in *guinea pigs* the principal manifestations of systemic anaphylaxis consist of respiratory distress, bronchiolar constriction, and acute emphysema; in *rabbits* the principal manifestations are obstruction of pulmonary capillaries with leukocyte-platelet thrombi (see Chapter 1), and right-sided heart failure with passive congestion of the liver and intestines; in *dogs* the principal manifestations are hepatic engorgement and hemorrhage in the intestines and lungs. Depending on the conditions of the experiment, systemic anaphylaxis may terminate in the rapid death of the animal, or may be a transient phenomenon lasting from 30 to 60 minutes.

In the guinea pig, antibodies which correspond to human antibodies of the IgG immunoglobulin class can be separated electrophoretically into two sub-classes, γ1 and γ2. It is the antibodies of the γ1 sub-class which have homocytotropic properties analogous to human IgE, and have an affinity for guinea pig mast cells in the target organs.[32] Various pharmacologically active agents such as histamine, kinins, and SRS-A have been implicated as chemical mediators in systemic anaphylaxis in the guinea pig (see Chapter 1).

In addition to the homocytotropic mechanism briefly described above, at least two other immunologic mechanisms may be operative in guinea pig anaphylaxis. For example, a single intravenous injection of a relatively large quantity of soluble antigen-antibody complexes may evoke fatal anaphylactic shock. It is postulated that this *immune-complex* type of anaphylaxis leads to the formation of anaphylatoxins which, in turn, release histamine from mast cells (see Chapter 1). Furthermore, *cytotoxic* mechanisms may play a role in the anaphylaxis which occurs when guinea pigs are injected with rabbit antibodies to Forssman antigen, a natural constituent of all guinea pig cell membranes.

Passive cutaneous anaphylaxis (PCA) is a special form of anaphylaxis which is frequently utilized, instead of systemic anaphylaxis, for evaluating the capacity of antisera to elicit anaphylactic responses in homologous and heterologous species.[20a] In order to perform the PCA reaction, the antiserum is first injected intracutaneously in the test animal. After a latent period of several hours, the corresponding antigen is mixed with an appropriate dye and is injected intravenously. An accumulation of dye at the site of the original intradermal injection of antibody is considered to constitute a positive test. The principal advantages of this technique are its simplicity, its economy of reagents, and its suitability for semi-quantitative determinations.

Temporary protection against fatal anaphylaxis in guinea pigs can often be achieved by the repeated injection of small amounts of antigen at frequent intervals. This process of desensitization is believed to be dependent on the neutralization of the antibodies responsible for the anaphylactic response.

ETIOLOGY

The great majority of anaphylactic reactions occur as the result of: (*1*) the injection of therapeutic or diagnostic agents; (*2*) the ingestion of a drug (see Chapter 20) or food; or (*3*) accidentally following an insect sting (see Table 2-1). Some of the causes of anaphylaxis are discussed in more detail below.

TABLE 2-1. Common Causes of Human Anaphylaxis

Foreign proteins
    1. Insect stings (bee, wasp, yellow jacket, hornet)
    2. Foreign serums (tetanus antitoxin, antilymphocyte serum)
    3. Biological extracts (pollen extracts, insulin, chymotrypsin, heparin, relaxin)
    4. Vaccines (diphtheria toxoid, typhus, influenza)
    5. Parasites (hydatid cyst)
    6. Foods (isolated case reports)

Non-protein drugs
    1. Penicillin and its homologues
    2. Procaine hydrochloride and its homologues
    3. Organic iodides
    4. Sodium dehydrocholate
    5. Mercurials
    6. Acetylsalicylic acid
    7. Thiamine hydrochloride
    8. Vancomycin
    9. Dextran
    10. Sulfobromphthalein
    11. Nitrofurantoin
    12. Tetracycline and its homologues
    13. Diphenhydramine hydrochloride
    14. Thiopental
    15. Triphenylmethane
    16. Probenecid

Insect Stings

Severe and fatal reactions to stings from insects of the order *Hymenoptera* (honey bee, wasp, yellow jacket, and hornet) have been recognized for many years. Because the clinical features of many of these reactions are similar to anaphylaxis and antibodies to insect antigens are detected in the sera of affected individuals, the role of hypersensitivity in their pathogenesis is generally accepted. However, it has been demonstrated that most *Hymenoptera* venoms contain varying quantities of histamine, serotonin, acetylcholine, and kinins. It is conceivable that these pharmacologically active substances may account for some of the manifestations of severe reactions to insect stings, and may be entirely responsible for some of the milder reactions such as transient urticaria or local tissue edema.

Foreign Serums

Horse serum is now a much less frequent cause of anaphylaxis in North America and Western Europe than formerly because human antitetanus immunoglobulin rather than equine antitoxin is readily available for passive immunization against tetanus (see Chapter 21). On the other hand, if antilymphocyte serum becomes widely used in organ transplantation (see Chapter 14) or in the treatment of "autoimmune" disorders, there may be a marked increase in the prevalence of anaphylactic reactions due to foreign serums.

Biologic Extracts

Extracts from animal or plant sources are usually impure and frequently contain numerous high molecular weight contaminants in addition to pharmacologically active components of potential allergenicity. Well documented anaphylactic reactions have been reported following the administration of pollen extracts, insulin, posterior pituitary extract, ACTH, chymotrypsin, heparin, and relaxin.

Vaccines

Human anaphylaxis has been described following the injection of diphtheria toxoid, typhus vaccine, and influenza virus vaccine. Many virus vaccines are prepared on chick embryos, although in recent years there has been a trend towards the use of other culture media. The reported cases of anaphylactic reactions to virus vaccines have been attributed to extreme egg sensitivity. In addition, bacterial or viral vaccines and toxoids contain numerous allergenic constituents including antibiotic agents and protein contaminants derived from the culture media.

Parasites

In Echinococcus disease, surgical or accidental rupture of an intra-abdominal hydatid cyst may result in the typical manifestations of anaphylactic shock. The acute symptoms are believed to occur as the result of the release of fluid containing highly antigenic protein into the peritoneal cavity, but mechanical or surgical shock may sometimes constitute a contributory factor.

Foods

Case reports of anaphylactic reactions to ingested foods have appeared sporadically, but their true incidence is difficult to evaluate because similar symptoms may occur on a toxic basis. For example, poisoning caused by staphylococcal toxins in spoiled food may be confused with anaphylactic shock. In addition, foods such as mushrooms, shellfish, and certain species of fish may contain chemical poisons which, on occasion, produce a clinical picture similar to anaphylaxis. Nevertheless, it is well established that clinical anaphylaxis may be induced by intradermal testing with potent food allergens such as nuts, fish, eggs, and shellfish. This latter observation would suggest an immunologic basis for the infrequent occurrence of true anaphylactic sensitivity to ingested food allergens. It has been suggested that certain instances of unexpected sudden death in infants (cot death) may be due to anaphylactic sensitivity to cow's milk[21] (see Chapter 16). However, this hypothesis has yet to be fully substantiated.

Human Seminal Fluid

Anaphylactic shock has been reported following coitus in a woman sensitized to the glycoprotein constituents of her husband's seminal fluid.[13]

Drugs

Concomitant with the introduction of thousands of new pharmaceutical products during the past 25 years, numerous case reports of anaphylactic reactions to nonprotein drugs have appeared in the literature. These reports are often difficult to evaluate because the pharmacologic properties of the suspected drug may, in some individuals, closely mimic the clinical features of anaphylaxis. However, true anaphylactic reactions substantiated by positive skin tests, characteristic autopsy findings, or multiple case reports appear to have taken place with the drugs listed in Table 2-1.[27]

At the present time, penicillin and its homologues are probably the most frequent causes of severe anaphylactic reactions in humans. The prevalence of allergic reactions to penicillin is approximately 1 per cent in veneral disease clinics and in other large scale treatment programs such as the prophylaxis of rheumatic fever in military recruits.[30] The incidence of acute anaphylactic reactions to penicillin appears to range between 10 and 40 per 100,000 injections, while the risk of a fatal anaphylactic reaction is approximately 2 in 100,000.[16]

Shock Reactions to Human Normal Immunoglobulin

Shock reactions have been described following the administration of human normal immunoglobulin (IgG) to patients with hypogammaglobulinemia (see Chapter 11). Most of these reactions are probably not the result of antigen-antibody interactions. Instead, they appear to be associated either with the presence of biologically active aggregates of IgG which release histamine or with other pharmacologic mediators from human cells.[23]

PATHOPHYSIOLOGY

The autopsy findings in human anaphylaxis vary considerably among subjects.[17] The most common features are acute pulmonary emphysema, acute pulmonary edema, and edema of the entire upper respiratory tract including the hypopharynx, epiglottis, and trachea. The pulmonary changes at necropsy may be interpreted as reflecting the existence of acute bronchospasm in the living state. Edema of the pharynx would appear to be unique to man as it is not found in experimental anaphylaxis. In some patients, especially those who had symptoms of vascular collapse only, there may be no abnormal findings at autopsy.

There is no available data on the pharmacology of anaphylaxis in man because the reaction takes place so swiftly and unexpectedly. However, it is unlikely that all of the symptoms can be accounted for by postulating a massive release of histamine as the result of antigen-antibody interaction.[10] Histamine is capable of producing urticaria, local tissue edema, and drop in blood pressure in humans, but not profound bronchospasm. It has been suggested that the bronchospasm which occurs in human anaphylaxis may be due to slow-reacting substance (SRS-A), and that the vascular reactions may be due to plasma kinins released during the acute reaction.[2]

It is also possible that hypotension may, in some instances, be the result of varying degrees of heart block which is known to occur in fatal animal anaphylaxis. Serial electrocardiograms recorded in nonfatal cases of human anaphylaxis showed evidence of arrhythmias and right-sided chamber enlargement during the acute phase, as well as ischemic changes evolving over a period of several days.[4] The selective chamber enlargement is probably related to severe bronchospasm, but it is not known whether the myocardial damage is related to acute changes in the coronary arteries, hypotension, or drugs used in the therapy of anaphylaxis. None of the subjects studied had pre-existing heart disease, and the electrocardiographic changes reverted to normal after recovery. Myocardial changes are not demonstrable at autopsy, presumably because of the rapidity of death.

Detailed hemodynamic studies of patients in acute anaphylactic shock revealed that shock was primarily due to a marked reduction in plasma volume related to a loss of fluid from the intravascular compartment.[15] Peripheral vascular resistance was increased rather than decreased, indicating that hypotension in human anaphylaxis cannot be explained by arteriolar vasodilation. Improvement in shock in the patients studied was brought about only by the infusion of large volumes of fluid. Adrenergic vasoconstrictor drugs were ineffectual and probably added to the workload of the heart by increasing peripheral arterial resistance.

Similarly, focal neurologic changes in nonfatal human anaphylaxis may result from acute changes in cerebral vessels or may be the result of prolonged hypotension. Cerebral edema, intraventricular hemorrhage, and diffuse petechiae in the central nervous system have been described at necropsy in patients dying from anaphylactic reactions to insect stings. However, it is difficult to generalize from the findings in insect sting anaphylaxis, because *Hymenoptera* venoms contain neurotoxins which may induce almost identical changes in susceptible individuals.

IMMUNOLOGY

Whether reagins or antibodies which enter into conventional serologic reactions mediate systemic anaphylaxis in man is not yet completely understood. It is known that, in humans, reagins take part in the pathogenesis of asthma and urticaria, both of which have their counterparts in systemic anaphylaxis. Furthermore, whenever suitable skin test antigens exist, reagins can be demonstrated by direct and passive transfer skin testing in individuals recovering from anaphylaxis. It is also of significance that anaphylactic shock may occur in atopic patients receiving their first injection of pollen extract for skin testing or hyposensitization purposes. Thus an initial sensitizing injection of antigen does not appear to be a necessary prerequisite for anaphylaxis in humans as it is in animals.

On the other hand, antibodies capable of inducing passive cutaneous anaphylaxis (PCA) in the guinea pig have been demonstrated in the sera of patients recovering from insect sting anaphylaxis,[28] whereas human reagins are not capable of producing PCA reactions in the guinea pig. Antibodies which participate in hemagglutination reactions have been detected in the sera of patients recovering from anaphylaxis due to penicillin[31] and horse serum,[24] as well as in patients allergic to ragweed who have received no hyposensitization therapy.[12] An investigation of a single case of nonfatal human anaphylaxis due to horse serum is of considerable immunologic interest.[24] Both reagins and hemagglutinins were present at the time of the reaction, but precipitins did not appear until one week after recovery.

On the basis of these observations, it may be concluded that the weight of evidence suggests that human anaphylaxis is primarily mediated by reagins. Precipitins do not appear until several days after the reaction has taken place, and there is no experimental model that would implicate hemagglutinins. However, the possibility that precipitins may exist during the early stages of anaphylaxis at levels too low to be detected by currently available methods cannot be excluded completely. Thus, it is conceivable that the formation of soluble antigen-antibody complexes during the course of human anaphylaxis may result in the release of anaphylatoxins secondary to activation of the complement sequence (see Chapter 1). Anaphylatoxins are known to be capable of releasing histamine from mast cells, and may thus account for the urticaria, tissue edema, and shock which are characteristic of many cases of human anaphylaxis. It is also possible that cytotoxic mechanisms may account for some of the anaphylactic components of acute hemolytic transfusion reactions in man (see Chapter 9).

CLINICAL MANIFESTATIONS

The clinical manifestations of generalized anaphylaxis in man may affect the skin, the upper and lower respiratory tract, the gastrointestinal tract, and the cardiovascular system.[2] Not every patient will have involvement of all systems.

When they occur, cutaneous manifestations are usually the first to appear. A few seconds or minutes after the injection or ingestion of the allergenic substance, the patient may complain of generalized pruritus often most pronounced over the face, upper chest, palms, axillae, and groin. If pruritus occurs, it is usually followed by diffuse erythema and generalized urticaria. Respiratory symptoms may consist of tightness or pain in the chest, dry cough, laryngeal stridor, wheezing, dyspnea, and cyanosis. Spasm of gastrointestinal smooth muscle is usually indicated by vomiting, severe abdominal cramps, and diarrhea which is occasionally bloody. Female patients, who recover, occasionally describe their abdominal pain as being similar to menstrual cramps or to the pain of childbirth, suggesting that contraction of uterine smooth muscle may also take place.

Vascular collapse with profound hypotension and circulatory failure may be the sole manifestation of human anaphylaxis or may follow cutaneous, respiratory, or gastrointestinal symptoms. In fatal cases, the interval between administration of the causative agent and death varies from 15 to

120 minutes.[17] Death is usually the result of asphyxia or peripheral circulatory failure.

DIAGNOSIS

In the acute emergency situation, the diagnosis must be made solely on clinical grounds.[3] Serologic methods are time consuming and, furthermore, titers of reagins, hemagglutinins, and antibodies which participate in the PCA reaction do not correlate well enough with clinical findings to be of value in predicting potential anaphylactic reactors.

The major conditions to be considered in the differential diagnosis are vasodepressor syncope and cardiac arrest. Neither of these conditions is characterized by urticaria, bronchospasm, or gastrointestinal symptoms, but they may be confused with anaphylaxis manifested by vasomotor collapse only. On examination, the patient with vasodepressor syncope will show marked pallor, sweating, and hypotension similar to that seen in anaphylactic shock. However, syncopal attacks will invariably terminate spontaneously in about 30 seconds if the patient is allowed to be flat. Sudden cardiac arrest is characterized by gasping, irregular respirations, no pulse or blood pressure, and widely dilated pupils. Complete cessation of respiration may occur within 20 to 30 seconds of the onset of symptoms.

A knowledge of the drugs or biologic agents known to cause human anaphylaxis (see Table 2-1) is also very helpful in establishing the diagnosis.

TREATMENT

The single most effective agent in combating human anaphylaxis is epinephrine. It antagonizes edema of the respiratory mucous membranes and antagonizes constriction of the bronchial musculature. As a result, many of the pathophysiologic consequences of human anaphylaxis are reversed by epinephrine. The action of antihistamines is slower and weaker than epinephrine, and this class of drugs has no significant effect on bronchoconstriction. Corticosteroids have little place in the treatment of acute anaphylaxis because of the delayed onset of their therapeutic effect, but they may provide additional symptomatic relief during the recovery period.

At the first sign of systemic anaphylaxis the patient should be placed flat on his back with his feet elevated to combat shock. If the patient has severe bronchospasm or laryngeal stridor, his head should be temporarily elevated and then lowered again when the respiratory symptoms have disappeared. If a subcutaneous or intramuscular injection has been given in the arm, a tourniquet should be placed proximal to the injection site to slow further systemic absorption of the drug.

Following these measures, the patient should be given 0.5 ml of 1:1000 aqueous epinephrine subcutaneously. Unless there is profound shock from the outset, intravenous epinephrine should be avoided because of its tendency to cause cardiac arryhthmias in anaphylaxis. If considered to be necessary, intravenous epinephrine may be administered by diluting 0.2 ml of 1:1000 aqueous epinephrine in 5 ml of isotonic saline and injecting it slowly over 2 to 3 minutes. Chlorpheniramine maleate, 10 mg, may be given intravenously at the same time as the first dose of epinephrine.

Most patients will respond quickly to this relatively simple treatment. Should recovery not occur within 5 minutes after the initial injection of epinephrine, an additional 0.3 ml of 1:1000 aqueous epinephrine should be given every 5 minutes until the desired effect is obtained, or until marked tachycardia and excitability prevent further administration of the drug.

The nature of further treatment will depend on the subsequent clinical course of the reaction. Refractory hypotension which persists despite the administration of epinephrine is an absolute indication for the prompt and rapid administration of large volumes of plasma or plasma substitutes. Vasopressor agents are of little value in maintaining blood pressure in acute anaphylaxis.[15]

Hypoxia manifested by increasing cyanosis constitutes a life-threatening emergency. If epinephrine fails to relieve bronchial obstruction, aminophylline, 500 mg, should be injected intravenously. Persistent laryngeal edema may require emergency tracheostomy and assisted respiration. As respiratory failure inevitably leads to cardiac arrest, external cardiac massage may be indicated in extreme situations.

SERUM SICKNESS SYNDROME

Classic serum sickness caused by the injection of foreign serum into humans is considerably less common than it was 20 to 30 years ago. Widespread immunization programs, the development of potent antibiotic agents, and the increasing use of human antitetanus immunoglobulin have all contributed to the declining incidence of this syndrome. On the other hand, serum sickness-like reactions due to nonprotein drugs, especially penicillin, remain a problem of considerable magnitude (see Table 2-2). Furthermore, the use of antilymphocyte serum as an immunosuppressive agent will undoubtedly result in a significant increase in the number of cases of serum sickness over the next several years.

Experimental serum sickness has been studied most extensively in the

TABLE 2-2. Common Causes of Human Serum Sickness

Foreign proteins
1. Horse serum (tetanus antitoxin, antisera in rabies,
   botulism, gas gangrene, and snake bites)
2. ACTH
3. Bee venom

Nonprotein drugs
1. Penicillin
2. Sulfonamides
3. Hydantoin compounds
4. Piperazine citrate.

---

rabbit.[7a] In this species, animals immunized with a heterologous protein, such as bovine serum albumin (BSA) develop cardiovascular, joint, and kidney lesions 7 to 14 days after the initial injection of antigen. The latent period is sufficient to allow the synthesis of antibodies to occur while circulating antigen persists at detectable levels. If ^{131}I-labeled BSA is used as the antigen, it is noted that the level of free antigen declines rapidly at precisely the time that symptoms become apparent. During this same period of antigen disappearance soluble antigen-antibody complexes can be detected in the serum, and the level of serum complement is depressed because it is fixed by the antigen-antibody complexes. In addition to these observations, it has been shown that the glomerulonephritis associated with experimental serum sickness is of the "immune-complex" type; i.e., host antibody, host complement, and antigen are demonstrable by immunofluorescence along the outer side of the glomerular basement membrane (GBM) in a granular, discrete pattern (see Chapter 6). From this data, it is possible to conclude that the manifestations of serum sickness in rabbits are primarily mediated by soluble immune complexes (see Chapter 1).

ETIOLOGY

Horse Serum

Horse serum contains multiple antigenic components located in either the γ-globulin or β-globulin fractions, or both.[26] In general, the frequency and severity of serum sickness varies directly with the volume of horse serum administered and the purity of the preparation. If 100 ml of unpurified horse serum is given, approximately 90 per cent of recipients will develop serum sickness; whereas, if 10 ml is given, only 10 per cent will develop the disease.[19]

In former years, large quantities of unpurified horse serum were administered in the treatment of pneumococcal pneumonia and diphtheria, and in the prophylaxis of tetanus. There was a high incidence of adverse reactions. Since the advent of the antibiotic era, horse serum is no longer used in treatment of pneumococcal pneumonia or diphtheria. Furthermore, tetanus antitoxin has been purified and concentrated so that many antigenic components which have no antibody activity are removed and the volume of serum injected is greatly reduced.

Despite these precautions, the incidence of serum sickness in a random series of patients given prophylactic tetanus antitoxin of equine origin was 2.5 per cent.[20] Human antitetanus immunoglobulin and active immunization have now largely supplanted equine antitoxin in the prevention of tetanus, but horse serum is still occasionally used in the prophylaxis and treatment of rabies, gas gangrene, botulism, and snake bites (see Chapter 21). The incidence of serum sickness following antirabies serum is higher than with tetanus antitoxin, occurring in about 15 per cent of cases.[18] The higher proportion of serum sickness reactions reported with antirabies serum may be attributed to the fact that it is more difficult to purify and concentrate without destroying antibody activity.

Other Foreign Proteins

Reactions which are clinically identical to classic serum sickness have been reported occasionally with foreign proteins such as ACTH and bee venom.

Drugs

Serum sickness-like reactions which occur following the administration of nonprotein drugs are now more prevalent than those due to foreign proteins. Oral and parenteral penicillin and its homologues are by far the most common etiologic agents in this category,[8] but well documented serum-sickness-like reactions have also been described following orally administered sulfonamides, hydantoin drugs, and piperazine citrate (see Chapter 20).

Whether one uses the term serum sickness to describe these reactions becomes a question of semantics. It is perhaps unfortunate that a syndrome which can be initiated by a variety of antigens was first described following the administration of foreign serum. There is probably no fundamental immunologic difference between human serum sickness due to horse serum and that which occurs following the administration of penicillin or sulfonamides.

PATHOLOGY

Uncomplicated serum sickness is a transient, self-limited disease which is almost never fatal. The only autopsy reports are those of patients whose drug-induced serum sickness syndrome progressed to polyarteritis nodosa,[22] or who died of intercurrent disease. Typical lesions of acute glomerulonephritis were described in three patients who developed fatal serum sickness following the infusion of unusually large quantities of unpurified anticancer serum of equine origin.[7] This latter finding once again illustrates the importance of dosage in the pathogenesis of serum sickness due to horse serum. However, it must be emphasized that these autopsy reports represent exceptionally severe manifestations of serum sickness occurring under unusual circumstances. There is no knowledge of the pathologic findings in the common variety of transient human serum sickness syndrome.

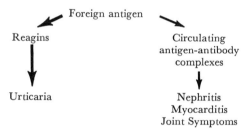

FIG. 2-1. Schematic representation of possible immunologic mechanisms in human serum sickness.

IMMUNOLOGY

As with anaphylaxis, there is much more known about the immunologic mechanisms of serum sickness in animals than in man. Currently available evidence suggests that the urticarial lesions of human serum sickness are mediated by reagins (IgE, homocytotropic antibodies), whereas the lesions of the heart, kidneys, and joints are probably mediated by soluble antigen-antibody complexes analogous to those found in experimental serum sickness[6] (see Fig. 2-1). However, it should be emphasized that the vascular lesions of the heart, kidneys, and arteries which are so prominent in experimental serum sickness appear to be of considerably less significance in its human counterpart. On the other hand, serum sickness differs from other reagin-mediated diseases such as asthma and hay fever in that a hereditary predisposition seems much less important, particularly if large volumes of foreign serum are administered.

If the antibody response is studied in patients who develop serum sickness due to horse serum, it is found that precipitins, hemagglutinins, and antibodies demonstrable by the PCA reaction in guinea pigs may be detected in the sera of some, but not all, patients with the characteristic clinical findings.[25] The pathogenetic significance of these antibodies has not been established. By contrast, reagins are demonstrable by direct or passive transfer skin tests in almost every case of human serum sickness.

Heterophile antibodies which could be absorbed out with guinea pig tissue were frequently found in patients with serum sickness in the days when large doses of native horse serum were given, but they are rarely detected in serum sickness today. The occasional demonstration of free light chains in the serum,[29] peripheral blood plasmacytosis, and polyclonal hypergammaglobulinemia[14] provides indirect evidence of increased antibody production in serum sickness.

The immunopathogenesis of the peripheral neuritis in serum sickness remains obscure. It has been postulated that the involved nerves are compressed by perineural edema analogous to urticaria because the skin and nervous tissue share a common ectodermal origin. On the other hand, serum neuritis may be due to a vasculitis of the vasa nervorum, or even the result of a direct toxic action of serum on peripheral nerves. Because the swelling of lymphoid tissue tends to be most pronounced in the lymph nodes draining the area of injection, it may be reasoned that the lymphadenopathy and occasional splenomegaly which occurs in serum sickness reflects increased antibody production.

CLINICAL MANIFESTATIONS

The characteristic clinical picture consists of urticaria, fever, arthralgias, lymphadenopathy, and, less commonly, peripheral neuritis. The usual incubation period between the administration of the causative agent and the onset of symptoms varies from 6 days to 3 weeks. However, in certain individuals where there are low residual titers of antibodies following previous exposure, an "accelerated" reaction may occur with the onset in 1 to 5 days.

Generalized swelling of the lymph nodes is often the first sign of serum sickness and may occasionally be accompanied by splenomegaly. Fever ranging from 100° to 104° F. is almost always present. The cutaneous eruption is urticarial in about 90 per cent of cases, but may occasionally consist solely of erythema, purpura, morbilliform rash, or erythema multiforme. Some clinicians hesitate to make the diagnosis in the absence of cutaneous manifestations, but skin eruptions may be absent in 3 per cent of otherwise typical cases of serum sickness. A local reaction of erythema and edema often appears at the site of injection 1 to 3 days before the onset of generalized skin manifestations. Angioedema of the face and extremities is occasionally present.

Pain and stiffness of the joints occurs in about 50 per cent of patients with serum sickness. In the more severe cases, the affected joints are swollen, hot, and tender, with effusion into the synovial spaces. The joint fluid, if aspirated, contains large numbers of polymorphonuclear leukocytes. The large and medium joints are most frequently involved.

The urticaria, fever, and arthralgias appear at about the same time and may disappear within 2 or 3 days, or may persist for several weeks. For reasons which are not well understood, protracted urticaria may follow serum sickness syndrome due to penicillin.

A small number of patients develop a peripheral neuritis. The cervical portion of the brachial plexus (C5-C6) is most frequently involved, with the shoulder girdle, arm, and hand affected in decreasing order of frequency. The neurologic manifestations are occasionally generalized and result in a clinical picture indistinguishable from idiopathic polyneuritis (see Chapter 18). In former years, when large volumes of horse serum were commonly administered, there were occasional reports of optic neuritis, retinal edema with hemorrhage, and iritis occurring during the course of serum sickness. These optic manifestations are rarely encountered at the present time.

The laboratory findings in the serum sickness syndrome are not characteristic. The hemogram may or may not reveal the presence of leukopenia with a decrease in polymorphonuclear leukocytes, an eosinophilia, and an elevated erythrocyte sedimentation rate. Plasmacytosis occurs occasionally in serum sickness, making it one of the few human diseases in which plasma cells are found in the peripheral blood. Albumin and nyaline casts may be detected in the urine in some of the more severe cases, suggesting the presence of renal lesions similar to those found in experimental serum sickness. Electrocardiographic findings suggestive of myocardial infarction or severe coronary insufficiency during the course of serum sickness have been described in individuals with no previous history of coronary artery disease.[5]

DIAGNOSIS

The clinical picture of serum sickness is characteristic, and usually presents little difficulty in differential diagnosis. However, if a patient has been given both penicillin and tetanus antitoxin following injury, the etiology of a subsequent episode of serum sickness may be in doubt. Involvement of the temporomandibular joint in serum sickness may occasionally be misdiagnosed as tetanus. Similarly, serum sickness following penicillin given for a streptococcal pharyngitis may be confused with rheumatic fever, particularly if the skin eruption consists of erythema multiforme rather than urticaria. There is no laboratory procedure which will firmly establish the diagnosis of serum sickness.

TREATMENT

Milder cases usually respond well to hydroxyzine, 25 mg, four times daily, for pruritus, and salicylates for joint pain and fever. More severe attacks may require short courses of prednisone, 20 to 40 mg daily, in divided doses. As serum sickness is usually a self-limited disease, there should be little hesitancy in prescribing systemic corticosteroids in otherwise healthy individuals.

PREVENTION OF ANAPHYLAXIS AND SERUM SICKNESS

HORSE SERUM

If the administration of horse serum is contemplated, some attempt must be made to determine whether the patient is hypersensitive to it. Both reagins and hemagglutinins are usually present prior to the onset of symptoms and thus may be of prognostic significance. The subsequent development of serum sickness shows a definite correlation with the titer of hemagglutinins,[1] but the test procedure is time consuming and technically demanding. It is therefore of limited value in an emergency situation.

In most instances, reliance must be placed on the history and the results of the immediate type intradermal skin test. Intradermal testing is usually carried out with 0.025 ml of horse serum in a dilution of 1:100. If this test is negative, it should be repeated at a dilution of 1:10 to exclude horse serum sensitivity. Any patient who has a history of rhinitis or asthma due to horse dander, or a previous history of serum sickness due to horse serum, should be presumed sensitive to horse serum even if the intradermal test is negative. If the patient is considered to be sensitive to horse serum, it may be necessary to attempt desensitization as there is no conclusive evidence that treatment with antihistamines or corticosteroids will prevent anaphylaxis. However, massive corticosteroid therapy may suppress the manifestations of serum sickness.

A tentative schedule for desensitization to horse serum is outlined in Table 2-3. It should be recognized that this procedure is potentially hazardous, and is less likely to succeed where there is a history of atopic sensitivity to horse dander.

TABLE 2-3. Tentative Schedule for Horse Serum Desensitization (Doses given subcutaneously every 20 minutes. Total dose 1 ml)

Dilution of antiserum	Amount injected (ml)
1:100	0.2
	0.4
	0.7
	1.0
1:10	0.2
	0.4
	0.7
	1.0
Undiluted	0.1
	0.2
	0.3
	0.4

PENICILLIN

At present, there is no rapid and reliable method for predicting penicillin sensitivity (see Chapter 20). Penicillin, or one of its homologues, is rarely the only available life-saving drug, except perhaps in certain cases of subacute bacterial endocarditis. Whenever there is any suspicion of a previous adverse reaction to penicillin, it would be prudent to choose a different class of antibiotic. However, if a specific bactericidal effect is considered essential, the incidence of anaphylactic reactions to penicillin can be markedly reduced by prescribing oral rather than parenteral penicillin. Therapeutically satisfactory blood levels can be rapidly achieved with most oral penicillin preparations.

The management of patients with proved subacute bacterial endocarditis who are known to be, or suspected of being, penicillin sensitive occasionally presents a therapeutic dilemma of major proportions. It is in this situation that skin testing with both penicilloylpolylysine and crystalline potassium penicillin G may be of assistance (see Chapter 20). If either of these tests is positive, or if there is a convincing history of penicillin hypersensitivity, intravenous penicillin should be administered only after careful weighing of the anticipated risk of an anaphylactic reaction against the anticipated risk of withholding a bactericidal drug. Under these circumstances, desensitization to penicillin is feasible,[11] but should be carried out with full recognition of the potential hazards. A tentative desensitization schedule for penicillin is outlined in Table 2-4. It is not clear in the case of penicillin whether this procedure achieves desensitization in the immunologic sense, results in the production of IgG "blocking" antibodies which have a protective effect, or merely demonstrates that the patient is no longer hypersensitive.[9]

TABLE 2-4. Tentative Schedule for Penicillin Desensitization (Doses of crystalline penicillin G given subcutaneously every 20 minutes)

Concentration (units/ml)	Amount injected (ml)
1,000	0.05
	0.1
	0.2
	0.4
	0.7
10,000	0.15
	0.2
	0.4
	0.7
100,000	0.15
	0.2
	0.4
	0.7
1,000,000	0.15
	0.2
	0.4
	0.7
	1.0*

* To be followed immediately by continuous therapy with intravenous crystalline penicillin G.

As with horse serum, prophylactic coverage with conventional doses of corticosteroids probably does not prevent anaphylaxis, but will suppress serum sickness.

REFERENCES

1. Arbesman, C. E., Kantor, S. Z., Rose, N. R., and Witebsky, E. Serum sickness: Serologic studies following prophylactic tetanus antitoxin. *J. Allergy 31:*257, 1960.

2. Austen, K. F. Systemic anaphylaxis in man. *J.A.M.A. 192:*116, 1965.

3. Booth, B., and Patterson, R. Anaphylaxis: A consideration in the differential diagnosis of shock. *J. Allergy 42:*364, 1968.

4. Booth, B., and Patterson, R. Electrocardiographic abnormalities during human anaphylaxis. *J. Allergy 43:*159, 1969.

5. Catalano, T. C. Myocardial infarction after serum sickness from tetanus antitoxin. *J.A.M.A 188:*1154, 1964.

6. Christian, C. L. Immune-complex disease. *New Eng. J. Med. 280:*878, 1969.

7. De la Pava, S., Nigogosyian, G., and Pickren, J. W. Fatal glomerulonephritis after receiving horse anticancer serum. *Arch. Intern. Med. 109:*391, 1962.

7a. Dixon, F. J. The role of antigen-antibody complexes in disease. *Harvey Lect. 58:*21, 1963.

8. Fellner, M. J., and Baer, R. L. Immunologic studies in patients with serum sickness-like reactions following penicillin therapy. *J. Invest. Derm. 48:*384, 1967.

9. Fellner, M. J., Van Hecke, E., Rozan, M., and Baer, R. L. Mechanisms of clinical desensitization in urticarial hypersensitivity to penicillin. *J. Allergy 45:*55, 1970.

10. Frick, O. L. Mediators of atopic and anaphylactic reactions. *Pediat. Clin. N. Amer. 16:*95, 1969.

11. Green, G. R., Peters, G. A., and Geraci, J. E. Treatment of bacterial endocarditis in patients with penicillin hypersensitivity. *Ann. Intern. Med. 67:*235, 1967.

12. Gyenes, L., and Sehon, A. H. The nature and properties of antibodies in sera of allergic individuals. A review. *Int. Arch. Allerg. 18:*330, 1961.

13. Halpern, B. N., Ky, T., and Robert, B. Clinical and immunological study of an exceptional case of reaginic type sensitization to human seminal fluid. *Immunology 12:*247, 1967.

14. Han, T., Chawla, P. L., and Sokal, J. E. Sulfapyridine-induced serum-sickness-like syndrome associated with plasmacytosis, lymphocytosis, and multiclonal gamma-globulinopathy. *New Eng. J. Med. 280:*547, 1969.

15. Hanashiro, P. K., and Weil, M. H. Anaphylactic shock in man: Report of two cases with detailed hemodynamic and metabolic studies. *Arch. Intern. Med. 119:*129, 1967.

16. Idsøe, O., Guthe, T., Willcox, R. R., and de Weck, A. L. Nature and extent of penicillin side-reactions with particular reference to fatalities from anaphylactic shock. *Bull. WHO 38:*159, 1968.

17. James, L. P, Jr., and Austen, K. F. Fatal systemic anaphylaxis in man. *New Eng. J. Med. 270:*597, 1964.

18. Karliner, J. S., and Belaval, G. S. Incidence of reactions following antirabies serum: Study of 526 Cases. *J.A.M.A. 193:*359, 1965.

19. Mackenzie, G. M., and Hanger, F. M. Serum disease and serum accidents. *J.A.M.A. 94:*260, 1930.

20. Moynihan, N. H. Serum sickness and local reactions in tetanus prophylaxis. *Lancet 2:*264, 1955.

20a. Ovary, Z., Benacerraf, B., and Bloch, K. J. Properties of guinea pig 7S antibodies. II. Identification of antibodies involved in passive cutaneous and systemic anaphylaxis. *J. Exp. Med. 117:*951, 1963.

21. Parish, W. E., Richards, C. B., France, N. E., and Coombs, R. R. A. Further investigations on the hypothesis that some cases of cot-death are due to a modified anaphylactic reaction to cow's milk. *Int. Arch. Allerg. 24:*215, 1964.

22. Rich, A. R. The role of hypersensitivity in periarteritis nodosa. As indicated by seven cases developing during serum sickness and sulfonamide therapy. *Bull. Johns Hopkins Hosp. 71:*123, 1942.

23. Richerson, H. B., and Seebohm, P. M. Anaphylactoid reaction to human gamma globulin. *Arch. Intern. Med. 117:*568, 1966.

24. Reisman, R. E., Arbesman, C. E., and Rose, N. R. Anaphylactoid reaction following an intradermal test of tetanus antitoxin. *Ann. Intern. Med. 59:*883, 1963.

25. Reisman, R. E., Rose, N. R., Witebsky, E., and Arbesman, C. E. Serum sickness. II. Demonstration and characteristics of antibodies. *J. Allerg. 32:*531, 1961.

26. Rose, N. R., Reisman, R. E., Witebsky, E., and Arbesman, C. E. Serum sickness. III. Characterization of antigens. *J. Allergy. 33:*250, 1962.

27. Samter, M., and Berryman, G. H. Drug allergy. *Ann. Rev. Pharmacol. 4:*265, 1964.

28. Schwartz, H. J., and Kahn, B.: Hymenoptera sensitivity. II. The role of atopy in the detection of clinical hypersensitivity. *J. Allerg. 45:*87, 1970.

29. Vaughan, J. H., Barnett, E. V., and Leadley, P. J. Serum sickness. Evidence in man of antigen-antibody complexes and free light chains in the circulation during the acute reaction. *Ann. Intern. Med. 67:*597, 1967.

30. van Arsdel, P. P., Jr. The risk of penicillin reactions. *Ann. Intern. Med. 69:*1071, 1968.

31. Voss, H. E., Redmond, A. P., and Levine, B. B. Clinical detection of the potential allergic reactor to penicillin by immunologic tests. *J.A.M.A. 196:*679, 1966.

32. Zvaifler, N. J., and Robinson, J. O. Rabbit homocytotropic antibody. A unique rabbit immunoglobulin analogous to human IgE. *J. Exp. Med. 130:*907, 1969.

3

Clinical Immunology of the Nose and Bronchi (Allergic Rhinitis and Bronchial Asthma)

SAMUEL O. FREEDMAN

Allergic rhinitis is a reaction of the nasal mucosa manifested by edema, hypersecretion of mucus, and pruritus. It is frequently, but not invariably, accompanied by allergic conjunctivitis. Bronchial asthma, on the other hand, is a reaction of the bronchial mucosa and bronchial smooth muscle characterized by edema of the mucosa, hypersecretion of mucus, and smooth muscle contraction. Clinically, there are two types of bronchial asthma: (1) extrinsic asthma initiated by external allergens and mediated by well defined immunologic mechanisms; and (2) intrinsic asthma due to essentially unknown causes. Although the distinction between extrinsic and intrinsic asthma is a useful one, it should be noted that the allergic and nonallergic forms of bronchial asthma are not mutually exclusive. In fact, they frequently coexist in the same individual.

79

Allergic rhinitis and bronchial asthma will be considered together as they often share a common etiologic, genetic, and immunologic background.

ETIOLOGY AND PATHOGENESIS

Because the clinical syndrome known as bronchial asthma probably represents a spectrum of disease entities rather than a single disorder, the different pathogenetic mechanisms which may be operative in any individual patient will be reviewed below. It is more than likely that similar mechanisms exist for allergic rhinitis, but they are less well defined.

GENETIC PREDISPOSITION

Respiratory allergy usually occurs in individuals with a genetic predisposition to the development of atopic diseases. Most surveys have placed the incidence of atopy in the immediate relatives of asthmatic patients at between 60 and 70 per cent.[32] However, the mode of inheritance has not been established with certainty.

EXTRINSIC ALLERGENS

Inhaled allergens are a much more common cause of extrinsic bronchial asthma and rhinitis than food, as might be expected from their portal of entry through the respiratory tract. Traditionally, the inhalant allergens are divided into seasonal allergens such as ragweed pollen, tree pollens, grass pollens, and mold spores, and perennial allergens such as house dust, feathers, and animal danders. Certain occupational allergens may be of importance in industrial or agricultural communities. Included in this category are the fine dusts which emanate from flour, cottonseed, flaxseed, castor bean, coffee bean, and grain.

From the foregoing discussion, it is apparent that most of the agents which provoke symptoms of respiratory allergy in susceptible individuals are chemically complex substances derived from plant or animal sources. The nature of the allergenic constituents of these substances is, for the most part, poorly understood, but they have been tentatively identified in certain isolated instances. For instance, there is evidence to suggest that chlorogenic acid, a simple phenolic compound of low molecular weight, may be an allergenic component of green coffee bean.[11] Similarly, the recent demonstration of direct and passive transfer intradermal tests to platinum salts in a patient who developed violent asthma on exposure to these simple chemicals is of interest in understanding the immunogenicity of allergens in atopic diseases.[10] These low molecular weight allergens may act as haptens by combining with body constituents to form allergenic conjugates. On the other hand, it is conceivable that the allergen alters or "denatures" body proteins to the point where they are foreign to the atopic host.

ROLE OF INFECTION

The role of bacteria or other microorganisms in the pathogenesis of allergic rhinitis and asthma is much more difficult to assess, despite the common clinical observation that acute episodes of intrinsic asthma may be provoked by respiratory infection. The major support for the concept of bacterial allergy rests on two pieces of indirect evidence. The first is the observation, familiar to clinical allergists who use bacterial vaccines, that the subcutaneous injection of relatively small amounts of bacterial vaccine will occasionally precipitate an attack of severe asthma within 6 to 12 hours of administration. Secondly, it has been demonstrated that the inhalation of an aerosol containing an extract of *Neisseria catarrhalis,* a normal respiratory organism, will initiate immediate airways obstruction in patients with intrinsic asthma, but not in normal controls.[12] However, reagins to bacteria or bacterial products have never been consistently demonstrated in intrinsic asthma, and it is quite possible that the relationship between asthma and infection is nonimmunologic.

INCREASED SENSITIVITY TO CHEMICAL MEDIATORS

It has been demonstrated that minute quantities of inhaled histamine or methacholine, in doses which are harmless for normal individuals, will produce severe bronchoconstriction in most asthmatic subjects.[17] It has also been shown that repeated injections of polyvalent influenza virus vaccine will enhance the bronchoconstrictor response aerosolized methacholine in subjects with bronchial asthma, but will have no such effect in nonatopic individuals.[23] These studies suggest that the increased sensitivity of the asthmatic subject to the chemical mediators of allergic reactions may be accentuated by common respiratory pathogens.

β-ADRENERGIC THEORY OF BRONCHIAL ASTHMA

It has been observed in animals that blockade of β-adrenergic receptors leads to an increased response to the pharmacologic mediators of antigen-antibody reactions such as histamine, acetylcholine, and serotonin. In humans, partial blockade of β-adrenergic receptors by propanolol has been found to increase the asthmatic response of atopic subjects to ragweed pollen.[24] These observations have led to the tentative hypothesis that there is a partial anatomic deficiency or physiologic blockade of β-receptors in the bronchial glands, smooth muscles, or mucosal blood vessels of asthmatic patients.[27] Since stimulation of β-receptors normally dilates the airway, their deficiency would allow an unopposed constrictor effect mediated by α-adrenergic receptors or by parasympathetic vagus fibers.

MECHANICAL IRRITANTS

The mechanical or irritating properties of inhaled substances must also be considered in the pathogenesis of bronchial asthma and rhinitis. Even normal individuals will respond to the inhalation of inert dusts by a sudden increase in airway resistance. The asthmatic subject, like the patient with rhinitis, is often peculiarly susceptible to sudden exacerbations of their disease induced by nonspecific irritants such as perfumes, soap powders, cigarette smoke, cold air, gasoline fumes, and fresh paint.

EMOTIONAL FACTORS

Some authorities feel that psychologic factors are frequent primary causes of bronchial asthma or rhinitis, whereas others contend that the psychologic changes which occur in some patients are either unrelated or secondary to the underlying disease process. It is well known that emotional stress may frequently provoke an attack of bronchial asthma or rhinitis in an individual already susceptible to these diseases, but it is unlikely that psychodynamic mechanisms are of primary importance in the majority of patients.

PATHOLOGY

ALLERGIC RHINITIS

In pathologic sections of the nasal mucosa of patients with allergic rhinitis, there is hyperplasia of the mucous glands of the surface epithelium, eosinophilic infiltration in the submucosa, and changes in the intensity of staining in the ground substance.

BRONCHIAL ASTHMA

In patients who have died of uncomplicated asthma, the lungs are pale and distended at necropsy. Thick, viscid mucus plugs are seen in the medium and small-sized bronchi, and there is visible thickening of the walls of the larger bronchi. The characteristic features of the microscopic examination are marked thickening and hyalinization of the basement membranes of the bronchial mucosa, and an increase in the number of goblet cells and eosinophils in the subepithelium. In many patients, mast cells in the subepithelial connective tissue are degranulated and decreased in number.[28] The bronchial lumina frequently contain eosinophils, mucin, and shed epithelial cells. The exact significance of the increase in thickness of the basement membrane or the profuse shedding of ciliated epithelial cells which occurs in many asthmatics is not understood.

IMMUNOLOGY

REAGINS

There appears to be little doubt that allergic rhinitis and extrinsic bronchial asthma are mediated by reagins (IgE, homocytotropic antibodies). When there is a good clinical history of respiratory allergy to inhalant substances, direct or passive transfer skin testing usually provides convincing evidence for the presence of cell-fixed and circulating reagins to the suspected allergen. Human serum containing reagins has been shown to produce in vitro sensitization of normal monkey ileum[15] and normal human appendix,[4] as demonstrated by muscle contraction on exposure to antigen. Furthermore, it has been demonstrated that monkeys will develop asthma on antigenic challenge following the intravenous infusion of human serum containing high titers of reagins.[25]

There is now convincing evidence that reaginic activity is largely, if not entirely, associated with the IgE class of immunoglobulins[13] (see Chapter 1). Minute amounts of IgE (0.160 μg/ml) are present in the sera of normal individuals, but the sera of atopic patients may contain up to six times the amount of IgE found in normal subjects. The serum levels of IgE are significantly increased in approximately 65 per cent of patients with extrinsic asthma, whereas they are increased in only 5 per cent of patients with intrinsic asthma.[14] The latter observation would tend to confirm the impression that intrinsic asthma is not mediated by reagins.

It has been postulated that the combination of cell-bound homocytotropic antibody with its specific allergen induces a conformational change in the Fc region of the antibody molecule. One of the consequences of this structural change is the initiation of a reaction at the surface of the mast cell which leads to the activation of a series of enzymes responsible for the release of histamine, 5-hydroxytryptamine, and other chemical mediators of allergic inflammation. The ability of human cells to bind IgE immunoglobulins has been studied indirectly by measuring histamine release from leukocytes treated with human sera containing reaginic antibodies.[22a] The available evidence from this in vitro system would suggest that the release of histamine is triggered by a reaction on the cell surface between IgE and allergen. Furthermore, there appears to be little doubt that the peripheral blood basophil is the major source of cellular histamine liberated under these experimental conditions.

Immunofluorescent studies with anti-IgE antisera provided evidence that the major sites of IgE production in the human are localized in the plasma cells and germinal centers of the tonsils and adenoids, as well as in the plasma cells of the bronchial and peritoneal lymph nodes, the respiratory mucosa, and the gastrointestinal mucosa.[13] The results of the studies on the distribution of IgE-producing cells suggest that IgE antibodies may be formed locally in the respiratory and gastrointestinal tracts, and may account for the fact that many reagin-mediated allergic manifestations occur predominantly in these organs.

Some of the highest levels of serum IgE have been reported in patients with parasitic infections, particularly those with *Ascaris* infestations.[14] This finding is of particular interest with respect to a single report of a 90 per cent incidence of infection with *Ascaris lumbricoides, Strongyloides stercoralis,* and *Necator americanus* in a group of 200 patients with bronchial asthma living in a temperate climate.[31]

BLOCKING ANTIBODIES

Blocking antibodies, associated with the IgG class of immunoglobulins, appear during the course of hyposensitization therapy with pollen extracts, and may be present in trace amounts in patients who have never received hyposensitization injections.[26] There is little convincing evidence that blocking antibodies are directly responsible for clinical improvement, as there is no correlation between titers of blocking antibodies and decrease in symptoms. It appears more likely that blocking antibodies influence the course of pollen asthma and hay fever by increasing the patient's ability to receive injections of pollen extract without adverse reactions. Protracted hyposensitization therapy is in turn associated with a decrease in the titer of reagins.[6] The mechanism of reduction in reagin titer is not understood, but it has been suggested that hyposensitization therapy may induce a state comparable to immunologic tolerance.[5]

OTHER ANTIBODIES

Hemagglutinins, antibodies which bind ^{131}I-labelled antigen, and precipitins directed against pollen allergens have all been detected in the sera of atopic patients. Their significance, if any, in the pathogenesis of allergic rhinitis and bronchial asthma has not been established.

CELL-MEDIATED IMMUNITY

It has also been shown that there is evidence for the existence of cell-mediated hypersensitivity to pollen extracts, as determined by delayed type skin reactions, lymphocyte transformation in vitro, and inhibition of leukocyte migration in patients with seasonal allergic rhinitis.[7a] However, the pathogenetic significance of cell-mediated immunity in allergic rhinitis and bronchial asthma requires further elucidation at present.

CHEMICAL MEDIATORS IN BRONCHIAL ASTHMA

In bronchial asthma, there is a complex relationship between antigen-antibody interaction, the autonomic nervous system, and the release of chemical mediators of allergic inflammation. It was demonstrated about 20 years ago that bronchial smooth muscle obtained during surgery from a patient with extrinsic asthma contracted when exposed to antigen in a water bath. More recent experiments have provided evidence that human asthmatic lung tissue will release both histamine and slow-reacting substance (SRS-A) when perfused in vitro with specific antigen.[29] However, SRS-A appears to be a more likely chemical mediator of human asthma than histamine. This supposition is supported by the observation that bronchial ring preparations from asthmatic patients contract in vitro when challenged with allergen in the presence of an antihistaminic agent. Currently available experimental evidence indicates that IgE antibodies are responsible for the release of histamine and SRS-A from human lungs.

PATHOPHYSIOLOGY

ALLERGIC RHINITIS

Allergic rhinitis is characterized by vasodilation and increased permeability of blood vessels in the nasal mucosa secondary to the liberation of histamine and other pharmacologically active mediators of allergic inflammation. Essentially similar functional changes occur in the nasal mucosae of many individuals in whom there is no demonstrable allergic mechanism. The term vasomotor rhinitis is used to describe this syndrome which, in susceptible individuals, may be markedly aggravated by a number of nonspecific factors such as strong odors, intense emotion, pregnancy, or sudden changes in temperature or humidity. The pathophysiologic mechanisms responsible for nonallergic or vasomotor rhinitis have not been extensively investigated.

BRONCHIAL ASTHMA

The functional consequences of bronchial asthma cannot be explained solely by constriction of bronchial smooth muscle secondary to the release of chemical mediators. Mucosal edema and the formation of thick tenacious mucus plugs in small bronchioles are, at least, of equal importance in producing airway obstruction.

Because uncomplicated bronchial asthma is an episodic disease, pulmonary function studies will vary greatly depending upon whether the patient is in remission, is having moderately severe symptoms, or is in status asthmaticus. The principal functional abnormalities take place as the result of bronchial obstruction occurring in the absence of significant changes in the lung parenchyma. Clinically detectable bronchospasm is usually reflected in low values for the maximum breathing capacity (MBC), forced expiratory volume (FEV) over a measured period of time, and maximum mid-expiratory flow rate. Inhalation of a bronchodilator drug often produces a dramatic reversal of abnormal ventilatory function in asthmatic patients.

Blood gases are usually normal except during severe attacks of asthma. In this situation, pulmonary segments or lobules become obstructed to the point that there is a significant decrease in ventilation in relation to perfusion. The result may be marked arterial hypoxia with pO_2 values of 45 to 55 mg Hg in the absence of CO_2 retention.[19] Hypercarbia seldom occurs, except as a terminal event, because the asthmatic patient tends to hyperventilate and "blow off" the extra CO_2. Marked CO_2 retention with pCO_2 values of 80 to 90 mm Hg in patients with bronchial asthma uncomplicated by pulmonary emphysema is usually a sign of impending death due to massive airway obstruction.[20]

Studies with radioactive xenon have demonstrated that there may be marked differences in pulmonary ventilation among various zones of the lung, even when the asthma is in remission.[1] This finding would suggest considerable independence of bronchial function in the various portions of the lung.

CLINICAL MANIFESTATIONS

PREVALENCE

Allergic rhinitis and bronchial asthma are common diseases in North America, particularly in areas where ragweed pollen is prevalent. Epidemiologic studies have indicated that seasonal allergic rhinitis occurs in

4 to 15 per cent of individuals at some time in their lives, depending on the diagnostic criteria employed. The available figures for bronchial asthma suggest a prevalence of 3 to 4 per cent.[2] The mortality rate from bronchial asthma is almost impossible to estimate because diagnostic criteria for the reporting of respiratory diseases vary widely between different institutions and between different countries. However, an annual death rate of 3 per 100,000 population would seem a reasonable estimate from the available data. Bronchial asthma is thus a common disorder and accounts for considerable medical, social, and economic disability in its chronic form.

ALLERGIC RHINITIS

During the acute stage, allergic rhinitis is usually manifested by paroxysms of sneezing, profuse watery nasal discharge, nasal obstruction, and itching of the nares, soft palate, and anterior aspect of the neck. In some patients, itching, burning, or tearing eyes, and swollen eyelids may be the predominant clinical features. Systemic symptoms of marked lassitude and fatigue are not uncommon during the course of acute allergic rhinitis.

Chronic rhinitis, on the other hand, is usually characterized by protracted nasal obstruction without many of the acute features outlined above. In children, the persistent nasal pruritus which often accompanies chronic allergic rhinitis may lead to frequent rubbing of the nose and sniffing—the so-called "allergic salute." Patients with chronic allergic rhinitis of long duration may ultimately develop nasal polyps, which further increases their nasal obstruction.

On examination, the nasal mucosa may be boggy and congested with a pale gray or bluish cast. However, in some acute cases, or in chronic cases with superimposed infection, the nasal mucosa may be normal or even reddened in appearance. Nasal polyps are usually visible as smooth, glistening, grayish-white protrusions within the nasal cavities.

A small number of patients, particularly children, may develop serous otitis as a complication of chronic allergic rhinitis. There is no evidence that serous otitis is a primary allergic phenomenon, but it probably occurs secondarily as the result of obstruction of the Eustachian tubes.

BRONCHIAL ASTHMA

The cardinal manifestations of asthma are wheezing respirations, episodes of acute dyspnea, and protracted cough which may, or may not, be productive of thick tenacious sputum. These symptoms may occur in paroxysms with completely symptom-free periods between, or there may be almost chronic low-grade asthma with periodic exacerbations and remissions. In severe acute asthma, there may be visible cyanosis, and the patient often sits upright with his shoulders leaning slightly forward. Protracted asthma may lead to a constant dull pain across the anterior chest which is probably related to spasm of the thoracic muscles.

Examination of the chest usually reveals a normal percussion note. During the acute attack, numerous sibilant and sonorous rhonchi are heard throughout the chest and are often present in inspiration as well as in expiration. The expiratory phase of respiration is frequently prolonged. Breath sounds or adventitious sounds may be completely absent over one area of the lung if a mucus plug has completely occluded a large segment.

In patients over 40 years of age, a common triad of signs and symptoms is the occurrence of nasal polyps, intrinsic asthma, and peripheral blood eosinophilia, often accompanied by aspirin disease (see Chapter 20).

DIAGNOSIS

Routine Laboratory Tests

A nasal smear for eosinophils is sometimes helpful in confirming the diagnosis of allergic rhinitis. However, the value of this procedure is greatly limited by the fact that many patients with chronic rhinitis do not produce sufficient nasal secretions for an adequate smear. In chronic allergic rhinitis, sinus x-rays may reveal thickening or polypoid changes in the mucous membranes lining the paranasal sinuses.

Unfortunately, there are no laboratory procedures which will, in themselves, establish the diagnosis of bronchial asthma. A radiograph of the chest, taken during the acute phase, may demonstrate overdistension of the lungs and lowering of the diaphragms. Microscopic examination of the sputum may reveal the presence of eosinophils, Charcot-Leyden crystals, or Curschmann's spirals. The characteristic prism-shaped Charcot-Leyden crystals represent crystallized proteins extruded from eosinophils in the lower respiratory tract, whereas Curschmann's spirals probably represent casts of small bronchioles. Peripheral blood eosinophilia is more common in chronic intrinsic bronchial asthma than in acute extrinsic asthma.

As noted in the previous discussion of the pathophysiology of asthma, reversible airway obstruction is the characteristic finding in respiratory function studies. Relatively simple measurements of ventilatory function such as the vital capacity (VC) and the forced expiratory volume over a measured period of time ($FEV_{1.0}$) can be carried out by any physician in his office. If the total vital capacity is relatively normal, reversion of $FEV_{1.0}$ to normal values following inhalation of a bronchodilator aerosol or during a period of remission is strongly suggestive of a diagnosis of uncomplicated bronchial asthma.

Skin Tests

Intradermal or scratch tests with pollens, molds, or animal danders are often useful in confirming an etiologic diagnosis suspected on the basis of the history. However, they do not, in themselves, establish allergy as a cause of the patient's symptoms. Many atopic patients will show positive skin tests to inhalant allergens without evidence of clinical sensitivity. Furthermore, certain inhalant allergens such as house dust, feathers, wool, silk, and stinging insects are often potentially irritating to normal skin. In this connection, it is significant that approximately 10 per cent of normal, nonatopic individuals will demonstrate skin reactivity to one or more common respiratory allergens. It has been suggested that household mites may be the major allergenic constituent of house dust.[30] It is therefore conceivable that skin tests with mite extracts may lead to a more precise diagnosis of house dust allergy than is possible with the crude, heterogeneous extracts of house dust currently available.[18]

Intradermal or scratch testing with food allergens shows even less correlation with clinical symptoms, presumably because food substances are broken down in the digestive tract to degradation products of unknown allergenic potentiality. Intradermal testing with egg white, nuts, fish, or shellfish may provoke severe constitutional reactions in patients with extreme clinical sensitivity, and should therefore be avoided when the history is obviously diagnostic.

It is rarely necessary to perform a large number of skin tests as a routine or screening procedure in the investigation of patients with allergic rhinitis or bronchial asthma. A list of common allergens suitable for testing in most patients is presented in Table 3-1. Other allergens may be added as suggested by the history.

Elimination Diets

Respiratory allergy due to food allergens usually manifests itself in the form of acute symptoms appearing within one hour of food ingestion. It is rarely possible, by any means, to implicate foods in the pathogenesis of chronic allergic rhinitis or chronic bronchial asthma in adults. In the experience of many clinical allergists, elimination diets in adults are not helpful in establishing foods as a cause of chronic respiratory allergy. Extensive dietary trials suffer from the double disadvantage of extreme inconve-

TABLE 3-1. Suggested List of Allergens* for Intradermal Testing in Respiratory Allergy

House dust conc.	Dog dander 100	Cat dander 100
Grasses 100†	Wool 1000	Trees 1000†
Alternaria 1000†	Horse dander 100	Hormodendrum 1000†
Feathers 1000	Ragweed 100	Saline control

* Standardized in protein nitrogen units per milliliter.

† Selection of grasses, trees and molds will depend on geographic location. (For further details, see Sheldon, J. M., Lovell, R. G., and Mathews, K. P. *A Manual of Clinical Allergy*, Philadelphia, Saunders, 1967, pp. 326–436.)

nience for even the most cooperative patient, and lack of reproducibility. Furthermore, well controlled studies, carried out on a double-blind basis, have failed to provide convincing evidence of improvement following withdrawal of suspected food allergens in chronic bronchial asthma.[33] The subject of alimentary and gastrointestinal allergy, particularly as applied to children, is more fully discussed in Chapter 16.

In Vitro Tests

Recently, a radioimmunoassay[34] and a modification of the indirect Coombs' test[7] have been developed for the detection of IgE antibodies against inhalant allergens. The results of studies on the clinical applications of these procedures are awaited with interest.

DIFFERENTIAL DIAGNOSIS

ALLERGIC RHINITIS

Acute allergic rhinitis due to seasonal pollens or due to intermittent exposure to perennial inhalant allergens usually presents little difficulty in differential diagnosis. However, the distinction between chronic nonseasonal allergic rhinitis, vasomotor rhinitis, and infective rhinitis may present certain problems.

In general, chronic allergic rhinitis is associated with a family or personal history of atopic diseases, positive intradermal or scratch tests, and a definite historic correlation between symptoms and exposure to the suspected allergen. Vasomotor rhinitis is usually distinguished by a clinical picture similar to chronic allergic rhinitis, but there is no atopic background and no laboratory or clinical evidence for extrinsic allergic factors. Infective rhinitis is characterized by thick, purulent nasal secretions, the isolation of pathogens on nasal culture, and associated sinus infection. However, it should be remembered that infection commonly occurs as a complication of both acute and chronic allergic rhinitis. The presence of enlarged adenoids must be excluded as a cause of chronic nasal obstruction in children. The administration of Rauwolfia compounds or contraceptive medication may occasionally produce symptoms of chronic nasal congestion in adults.

BRONCHIAL ASTHMA

As is the case with allergic rhinitis, there is usually no difficulty in diagnosing acute episodic asthma due to extrinsic agents. It is chronic intrinsic bronchial asthma which is most frequently confused with chronic bronchitis or cardiac asthma. In favor of a diagnosis of bronchial asthma is a history of attacks of acute airway obstruction occurring, at least on some occasions, at rest. An atopic background, correlation of symptoms with environmental allergens, positive skin tests, peripheral blood eosinophilia, and demonstrated reversible airway obstruction all tend to confirm the diagnosis.

On the other hand, patients whose airway obstruction is entirely due to chronic bronchitis and pulmonary emphysema usually experience dyspnea only on exertion, and, except in advanced cases, are usually quite comfortable at rest. Respiratory function tests characteristic of pulmonary emphysema such as the demonstration of diffuse airway obstruction, reduced diffusing capacity, and an increased pulmonary compliance are very useful in establishing the diagnosis of this condition. Bronchial asthma and pulmonary emphysema may coexist in the same patient, and both may be aggravated by respiratory infection.

The term "cardiac asthma" has been used for many years to describe episodes of left ventricular failure in which the physical signs of bronchial obstruction are almost indistinguishable from those encountered in bronchial asthma. The majority of patients who develop bronchospasm as the major manifestation in pulmonary edema usually have a history of coexisting bronchial asthma or chronic bronchitis in addition to the usual signs and symptoms of heart disease. Therefore, the term "cardiac asthma" is, in a sense, a misnomer as the syndrome occurs primarily in patients with pre-existing bronchial disease.

Other pulmonary and systemic diseases which should be considered in the differential diagnosis of bronchial asthma are summarized in Table 3-2.

TABLE 3-2. Differential Diagnosis of Bronchial Asthma

Chronic Bronchitis

Pulmonary Emphysema

Hereditary α-antitrypsin Deficiency

Left Ventricular Failure ("cardiac asthma")

Diseases of the Lung Parenchyma with Immunologic Features
Collagen-vascular diseases, allergic alveolitis, pulmonary infiltration with eosin-ophilia, fibrosing alveolitis

Mechanical Irritation
Nitrogen dioxide (silo-filler's disease), sulfur dioxide, alkyd resins, toluene di-isocyanate

Localized Bronchial Obstruction
Foreign bodies, bronchial adenoma or carcinoma, metastatic neoplasms, tuber-culosis, enlarged hilar or mediastinal lymph nodes, vascular anomalies, substernal thyroid

Pediatric Lung Diseases
Mucoviscoidosis, bronchiolitis, croup, whooping cough, congenital anomalies of trachea, larynx, or great vessels

---

TREATMENT

From the preceding discussion, it is apparent that not all individuals with bronchial asthma or allergic rhinitis can be successfully treated by the removal of specific allergens or by hyposensitization therapy. The treatment of chronic respiratory allergy is frequently a frustrating experience for both the physician and the patient because no single therapeutic measure is likely to produce dramatic and permanent relief of symptoms. Successful management, in most cases, requires constant and meticulous attention to the correction or suppression of multiple etiologic factors.

AVOIDANCE OF ALLERGENS

Where applicable, the removal of allergens from the patient's environment or the removal of the patient from his environment constitutes the simplest and most effective form of treatment, provided such environmental manipulation can be carried out without excessive economic or psychologic disturbance to the patient. Certain common perennial allergens such as animal danders, feathers, and wool can usually be removed from the patient's environment with relative ease if the patient is sufficiently motivated. On the other hand, it is rarely possible to eliminate all traces of house dust or seasonal pollen allergens from the patient's immediate surroundings. Removal of the patient from the environment is occasionally indicated in respiratory allergy caused by occupational allergens, but the patient should not be advised to change occupations unless the diagnosis is firmly established and all other treatment measures have failed.

DRUG THERAPY

Drug therapy is frequently effective as the sole method of treatment in allergic rhinitis or bronchial asthma, provided that satisfactory relief can be achieved without unpleasant or deleterious side-effects.

Allergic Rhinitis

Most patients with allergic rhinitis will show some degree of beneficial response to an orally administered antihistamine such as chlorpheniramine, 4 to 8 mg, four times daily or to an orally administered nasal decongestant such as ephedrine, 15 mg, three times daily. A useful combination of drugs consists of the antihistamine tripolidine, 2.5 mg, and pseudoephedrine, 60 mg (Actifed). The excessive use of topical nasal decongestants should be discouraged in chronic allergic rhinitis, as the inevitable result is secondary irritation of the nasal mucosae or rebound congestion.

Bronchial Asthma

Antihistamines are of limited value in the treatment of bronchial asthma because other chemical mediators such as SRS-A seem to be of primary importance in its pathogenesis. The recent introduction of disodium cromoglycate represents a new pharmacologic approach to the treatment of asthma. This drug is not an antagonist of histamine or SRS-A, but appears to act by inhibiting the release of histamine from sensitized cells at the earliest stages of antigen-antibody interaction.[22] Since the drug is poorly absorbed by mouth, it must be administered as a powder inhalation either alone or in combination with isoproterenol. Preliminary clinical trials suggest that disodium cromoglycate is a mildly effective drug in the prophylaxis of bronchial asthma, and not infrequently reduces the requirement for corticosteroid drugs in patients with refractory symptoms.[3] The best clinical responses were obtained, as might be expected, in patients with a strong allergic component to their asthma. Diethylcarbamazine citrate inhibits the release of SRS-A in experimental animals, and has been shown to be effective in the treatment of a limited number of patients with bronchospasm associated with the P.I.E. syndrome (see Chapter 4). Preliminary clinical trials suggest that this drug is of little or no value in the management of bronchial asthma.

The major form of drug therapy in bronchial asthma consists of drugs which reverse the functional consequences of allergic inflammation in human bronchi. Adrenergic drugs which stimulate α-receptor sites act by reducing mucosal blood flow and by reducing mucus secretion, whereas the β-stimulating drugs act by relaxing the bronchial musculature. Epinephrine, ephedrine, and related compounds are widely used in the treatment of bronchial asthma because they possess both α- and β-stimulating activity. Isoproterenol is a more powerful β-stimulant than epinephrine, but has no effect on α-receptor sites. Typical adult dosages are: ephedrine 30 to 60 mg, four times daily by mouth for chronic asthma; aqueous epinephrine, 0.5 ml of 1:1000 solution, subcutaneously for acute asthma; or isoproterenol, 0.5% solution, by aerosol inhalation for asthma of moderate severity. The excessive or repeated use of nebulized isoproterenol preparations may occasionally lead to the development of severe paradoxical airway resistance.[12a] The cause of this refractory state is unknown.

Theophylline compounds have no direct effect on either α- or β-receptors, but are widely used for their relaxing effect on the bronchial musculature. Typical adult dosage forms are: choline theophylline, 100 to 200 mg, four times daily by mouth, or aminophylline suppositories, 250 to 500 mg, at bedtime for chronic bronchial asthma; and aminophylline, 250 to 500 mg, intravenously for acute asthma. Tablets or capsules containing various combinations of ephedrine, theophylline derivatives, and barbiturates have long enjoyed widespread popularity in the treatment of bronchial asthma. The most serious side-effect of theophylline compounds is the toxicity which occasionally occurs in infants and children as the result of overdosage. Typical signs and symptoms consist of central nervous system stimulation, convulsions, vomiting, and dehydration.

Corticosteroids often produce dramatic relief of symptoms in bronchial asthma by blocking or suppressing the allergic inflammatory response, but their well documented side-effects makes their protracted use hazardous in most individuals. Nevertheless, there is an occasional patient in whom the emotional, social, and economic incapacity resulting from uncontrolled chronic bronchial asthma may be more damaging than the anticipated side-effects of prolonged steroid therapy with all its attendant risks. In addition, this class of drugs may be lifesaving in severe status asthmaticus. Common adult dosage forms are prednisone, 10 to 40 mg, daily in divided doses by mouth for chronic asthma; and hydrocortisone sodium succinate, 100 mg, intravenously every 6 hours in severe acute asthma. Where possible, the occurrence of steroid-induced side-effects may be diminished by administering the drug for several days or weeks when the patient's asthma is particularly severe, and then discontinuing during relatively symptom-free periods.

Intercurrent infection should be treated promptly with appropriate antibiotics selected on the basis of bacteriologic sensitivity studies. Intermittent positive-pressure breathing accompanied by adequate humidification is a useful ancilliary measure when there are copious amounts of thick tenacious sputum. This procedure simultaneously moistens inspissated mucus secretions, distributes bronchodilator medication evenly through the bronchial tree, and reinflates atelectatic lobules. On the other hand, the excessive use of intermittent positive-pressure breathing may only serve to irritate sensitive bronchi in patients with bronchospasm as the predominant feature of their illness. Mild sedation for the apprehensive patient, the cautious administration of oxygen, and adequate hydration all have their place as general supportive measures. The oral administration of iodides (e.g., saturated solution of potassium iodide, 10 drops t.i.d.) may sometimes provide additional relief through its expectorant action.

The presence of cyanosis, drowsiness, or an arterial CO_2 tension greater than 80 mm Hg in bronchial asthma uncomplicated by pulmonary emphysema constitutes a grave emergency. The patient should be moved without delay to an intensive care unit if one is available. Under these circumstances, endotracheal intubation, the use of muscle relaxants, and assisted respiration may be necessary as life-saving procedures.

HYPOSENSITIZATION THERAPY

If allergic rhinitis or extrinsic bronchial asthma cannot be controlled by environmental manipulation or simple medication, hyposensitization therapy may be considered. However, it should be emphasized that this form of treatment is both inconvenient and expensive for the patient, and its value is not unequivocally established. Hyposensitization injections are unnecessary in the majority of patients with allergic rhinitis or bronchial asthma, but, when given, the best results are usually obtained with pollen allergens. Double-blind studies have demonstrated the clinical effectiveness of perennial hyposensitization therapy with aqueous pollen extracts in the treatment of ragweed hayfever.[16] Similar double-blind studies demonstrated that the best results can be anticipated with relatively high doses of ragweed pollen extract close to the patient's tolerance level.[9]

Aqueous pollen extracts may be administered according to preseasonal (see Table 3-3) or perennial dosage schedules. With the preseasonal method, treatment is usually begun 3 to 4 months before the onset of the pollen season. Weekly injections of increasing strength are given according to the patient's tolerance until the beginning of the pollen season and are then discontinued until the following spring. With the perennial method, the highest dose of extract reached just prior to the pollen season is maintained throughout the year at monthly intervals. Comparable results are obtained with both types of schedules, but the perennial method in which the patient receives 12 to 15 evenly spaced injections throughout the year is usually more convenient for both the patient and physician. Hyposensitization injections with seasonal pollen allergens should be continued until the patient has experienced two consecutive symptom-free pollen seasons. Two to four years of continuous therapy is usually required before this stage is reached in the treatment program. If there is a reappearance of hay fever or asthma after cessation of hyposensitization therapy, treatment can be resumed the following year.

The introduction of the repository form of hyposensitization therapy in which a water-in-oil emulsion of a pollen extract is injected as a single dose several weeks prior to the pollen season has provoked considerable controversy among clinical allergists during the past ten years. Well controlled double blind studies have failed to demonstrate the effectiveness of this form of injection therapy.[21] At the time of this writing, its use in the United States is limited by government regulation to qualified clinical investigators.

The results of hyposensitization therapy with other inhalant allergens have not been investigated by the double-blind method. A two-year double-blind study on the clinical effectiveness of hyposensitization therapy with bacterial vaccines in children with infectious asthma showed no significant difference between the treated and control groups.[8] Nevertheless, many experienced clinical allergists recommend hyposensitization therapy with perennial inhalant allergens, molds, or bacterial vaccines in refractory cases of respiratory allergy.

In the writer's own clinic, the following criteria must be met before a trial of hyposensitization therapy with aqueous pollen extracts is recommended: (1) symptoms severe enough to cause significant physical, economic, or psychological incapacity; (2) demonstrated failure of simple symptomatic medication; and (3) impossibility of allergen avoidance during the pollen season. Hyposensitization therapy with house dust, bacterial vaccines, or molds is recommended for a trial period of 6 months only in those patients whose symptoms are uncontrolled by other treatment methods.

There is no evidence that injection treatment of seasonal allergic rhinitis will prevent or modify the later development of seasonal bronchial asthma.[2] Therefore, hyposensitization injections should be recommended on their

TABLE 3-3. Typical Schedules for Preseasonal Hyposensitization Therapy with Aqueous Pollen Extracts*

Dose Number	Weak† (p.n.u.)‖	Standard‡ (p.n.u.)	Accelerated§ (p.n.u.)
1	5	10	20
2	10	20	40
3	20	40	80
4	35	75	150
5	50	125	300
6	70	200	600
7	100	300	900
8	150	500	1250
9	200	700	1750
10	300	1000	2500
11	400	1500	3250
12	600	2000	4000
13	800	2500	5000
14	1000		

* Should be modified if there is any tendency for reactions to occur.

† Recommended for all patients beginning hyposensitization therapy, patients with pollen asthma, or patients with a previous history of constitutional reactions.

‡ Recommended for patients who have tolerated hyposensitization therapy in the preceding year without constitutional or severe local reactions.

§ Recommended for patients who have tolerated hyposensitization therapy for several years without constitutional or severe local reactions and who show evidence of decrease in the size of the intradermal skin reaction to the allergen.

‖ Protein nitrogen units.

own merit for the alleviation of otherwise uncontrollable hay fever, and not as a form of preventive medicine.

REFERENCES

1. Bentivoglio, L. G., Beerel, F., Bryan, A. C., Stewart, P. B., Rose, B., and Bates, D. V. Regional pulmonary function studies with xenon[133] in patients with bronchial asthma. *J. Clin. Invest.* 42:1193, 1963.

2. Broder, I., Barlow, P. P., and Horton, R. J. M. The epidemiology of asthma and hay fever in a total community, Tecumseh, Michigan. I. Description of study and general findings. *J. Allerg. 33*:513, 1962.

3. Chai, H., Molk, L., and Middleton, E., Jr. Disodium cromoglycate in bronchial asthma. *Ann. Int. Med. 71*:1212, 1969.

4. Chopra, S. L., Kovacs, B. A., Rose, B., and Goodfriend, L. Detection of human reagins by Shulz-Dale technique using human appendix. *Intern. Arch. Allerg. 29*:393, 1966.

5. Claman, H. N. Does injection therapy produce tolerence or immunity? *J. Allerg. 35*:371, 1964.

6. Connell, J. T., and Sherman, W. B. Changes in skin-sensitizing antibody titer after injections of aqueous pollen extract. *J. Allerg. 43*:22, 1969.

7. Coombs, R. R. A., Hunter, A., Jonas, W. E., Bennich, H., Johansson, S. G. O., and Panzani, R. Detection of IgE (IgND) specific antibody (probably reagin) to castor-bean allergen by the red-cell-linked antigen-antiglobulin reaction. *Lancet 1*:1115, 1968.

7a. Editorial. Cell-mediated immunity in hay fever. *Lancet 1*:27, 1970.

8. Fontana, V. J., Salanitro, A. S., Wolfe, H. I., and Moreno, F. Bacterial vaccine and infectious asthma. *J.A.M.A. 193*:123, 1965.

9. Franklin, W., and Lowell, F. C. Comparison of two dosage levels of ragweed extract in the treatment of pollenosis. *J.A.M.A. 201*:915, 1967.

10. Freedman, S. O., and Krupey, J. Respiratory allergy caused by platinum salts. *J. Allerg. 42*:233, 1968.

11. Freedman, S. O., Krupey, J., and Sehon, A. H. Chlorogenic acid: An allergen in green coffee bean. *Nature 192*:241, 1961.

12. Hampton, S. F., Johnson, M. C., and Galakatos, E. Studies of bacterial hypersensitivity in asthma I: The preparation of antigens of *Neisseria Catarrhalis,* the induction of asthma by aerosols, the performance of skin and passive transfer tests. *J. Allerg. 34*:63, 1963.

12a. Inman, W. H. W., and Adelstein, A. M. Rise and fall of asthma mortality in England and Wales in relation to use or pressurized aerosols. *Lancet 2*:179, 1969.

13. Ishizaka, K., and Ishizaka, T. Biological function of γE antibodies and mechanisms of reaginic hypersensitivity. *Clin. Exp. Immunol. 6*:25, 1970.

14. Johansson, S. G. O., Bennich, H., Berg, T., and Hogman, C. Some factors influencing the serum IgE levels in atopic diseases. *Clin. Exp. Immunol. 6*:43, 1970.

15. Kobayashi, S., Girard, J. P., and Arbesman, C. E. Demonstration of human reagin in monkey tissues. III. In-vitro passive sensitization of monkey ileum with sera of atopic patients. Physiologic and enhancing experiments. *J. Allerg. 40*:26, 1967.

16. Lowell, F. C., and Franklin, W. A double-blind study of the effectiveness of injection therapy in ragweed hay fever. *New Eng. J. Med. 273*:675, 1965.

17. Makino, S. Clinical significance of bronchial sensitivity to acetylcholine and histamine in bronchial asthma. *J. Allerg. 38*:127, 1966.

18. Maunsell, K., Wraith, D. G., and Cunnington, A. M. Mites and house-dust allergy in bronchial asthma. *Lancet 1*:1267, 1968.

19. McFadden, E. R., Jr., and Lyons, H. A. Arterial-blood gas tension in asthma. *New Eng. J. Med. 278*:1029, 1968.

20. Miyamoto, T., Mizuno, K., and Furuya, K. Arterial blood gases in bronchial asthma. *J. Allerg. 45*:248, 1970.

21. Norman, P. S., Winkenwerder, W. L., and D'Lugoff, B. C. D. Controlled evaluations of repository therapy in ragweed hay fever. *J. Allerg. 39*:82, 1967.

22. Orange, R. P., and Austen, K. F. Guest editorial—Prospects in asthma therapy: Disodium cromoglycate and diethylcarbamazine. *New Eng. J. Med. 279*:1055, 1968.

22a. Osler, A. G. Immunology of reaginic allergy: *In vitro* studies. *Clin. Exp. Immunol. 6*:13, 1970.

23. Ouellette, J. J., and Reed, C. E. Increased response of asthmatic subjects to methacholine after influenza vaccine. *J. Allerg. 36*:588, 1965.

24. Ouellette, J. J., and Reed, C. E. The effect of partial beta-adrenergic blockade on the bronchial response of hay fever subjects to ragweed aerosol. *J. Allerg. 39*:160, 1967.

25. Patterson, R., Miyamoto, T., Reynolds, L., and Pruznansky, J. J. Comparative studies of two models of allergic respiratory disease. *Intern. Arch. Allerg. 32*:31, 1967.

26. Perelmutter, L., Lea, D. J., Freedman, S. O., and Sehon, A. H. Demonstration of precipitating antibodies in sera of ragweed-allergic individuals by the agar-gel technique. *Intern. Arch. Allerg. 20*:355, 1962.

27. Reed, C. E. Beta-adrenergic blockade, bronchial asthma and atopy. *J. Allerg. 42*:238, 1968.

28. Salvato, G. Some histologic changes in chronic bronchitis and asthma. *Thorax 23*:168, 1968.

29. Sheard, P., Killingback, P. G., and Blair, A. M. J. N. Antigen induced release of histamine and SRS-A from human lung passively sensitized with reaginic serum. *Nature 216*:283, 1967.

30. Spieksma, F. Th. M. Biological aspects of the house dust mite (*Dermatophagoides pteronyssinus*) in relation to house dust atopy. *Clin. Exp. Immunol. 6*:61, 1970.

31. Tullis, D. C. H. Bronchial asthma associated with intestinal parasites. *New Eng. J. Med. 282*:370, 1970.

32. Van Arsdel, P. P., Jr., and Motulsky, A. G. Frequency and hereditability of asthma and allergic rhinitis in college students. *Acta Genet. (Basel) 9*:101, 1959.

33. Van Metre, T. E., Jr., Anderson, A. S., Barnard, J. H., Bernstein, I. L., Chafee, F. H., Crawford, L. V., and Wittig, H. J. The effects on chronic asthma of a rigid elimination diet. *J. Allerg. 41*:195, 1968.

34. Wide, L., Bennich, H., and Johannson, S. G. O. Diagnosis of allergy by an in-vitro test for allergen antibodies. *Lancet 2*:1105, 1967.

4

Clinical Immunology of the Lung Parenchyma

SAMUEL O. FREEDMAN

A number of pulmonary diseases with immunologic features affect the lung parenchyma rather than the bronchial tree. Although there is sometimes considerable clinical overlap between these disorders and bronchial asthma, they differ in that the primary immunologic response takes place in the alveoli or interstitial tissues of the lung instead of in the bronchial mucosa.

ALLERGIC ALVEOLITIS (HYPERSENSITIVITY PNEUMONITIS)

DISEASES CAUSED BY THERMOPHILIC ACTINOMYCETES

Traditionally, farmer's lung, bagassosis, and mushroom worker's disease have been considered as separate disease entities. However, recent evidence would suggest that they are all due to a pulmonary hypersensitivity response to the fungal spores of the thermophilic actinomycetes (see Table 4-1).

100

TABLE 4-1. Allergic Alveolitis

Disease	Suspected antigens
Farmer's lung	Thermophilic actinomycetes
Mushroom worker's lung	Thermophilic actinomycetes
Bagassosis	Thermophilic actinomycetes
Malt worker's disease	*Aspergillus clavatus*
Bird breeder's disease	Avian proteins
Maple bark disease	*Cryptostroma corticale*
Wood worker's disease	Sawdust from oak, mahogany, cedar, and redwood
Inhaled vegetable dusts	Dust from sisal, hemp, paprika, cotton, kapok, palm kernels, cork, thatched roofs
Inhaled organic antigens	Emanations from wheat weevils (*Sitophilus granarius*), pituitary snuff, smallpox scabs, and proteolytic enzymes from *Bacillus subtilis*

In addition, the clinical and laboratory findings are remarkably similar in each of these conditions. Therefore, the diseases caused by thermophilic actinomycetes will be considered together rather than separately.

Pathology

Examination of biopsy specimens in both farmer's lung and bagassosis typically show evidence of focal granulomatous inflammation which takes place predominantly within the walls of the alveoli, but may involve the interstitial tissues as well. Chronic cases may progress to interstitial pulmonary fibrosis.

Immunology and Pathogenesis

Farmer's Lung. Farmer's lung is an occupational disease of agricultural workers who are exposed to moldy hay or silage. The pathogenesis of this disease is of considerable interest because the sera of most patients contain precipitins against extracts of moldy hay.[12] Further studies have provided evidence that the principal antigenic component of moldy hay responsible for precipitin formation is derived from fungi such as *Micropolyspora faeni* and *Thermoactinomyces vulgaris*.[17] These thermophilic actinomycetes thrive at temperatures of 40° to 60° C which are reached when hay is stored with too high a moisture content. The spores of the actinomycetes are about 1 μ in diameter and are therefore capable of deep penetration into the lung parenchyma.

Precipitin reactions against the antigens of *M. faeni* were obtained in the sera of 87 per cent of patients with farmer's lung, but were also found in 18 per cent of farmers exposed to moldy hay without signs of clinical disease.[17] Additional evidence for the participation of *M. faeni* in the pathogenesis of this condition comes from a report of the isolation of the organism from a lung biopsy specimen obtained from a patient with farmer's lung.[28] On the other hand, reagins against moldy hay antigens or fungal antigens cannot be demonstrated in patients with farmer's lung.

The question then arises as to whether the disease is caused by mycotic infection of the lung or whether it represents a hypersensitivity response to fungal antigens. At the time of writing, there has been no reported evidence for fungal growth or proliferation in biopsy specimens. Furthermore, the disease can be reproduced experimentally in susceptible patients by the inhalation of aerosolized extracts of moldy hay.[2] The mechanism of the hypersensitivity response in farmer's lung remains to be established. It has been suggested that the precipitins demonstrated in this disease may form antigen-antibody complexes which are injurious to lung tissue in a manner analogous to the Arthus reaction.

Fog fever, a pulmonary disease of cattle, constitutes an interesting animal model for farmer's lung. The disease has been attributed to the inhalation of moldy hay antigens by the animals and precipitins against thermophilic actinomycetes have been detected in the sera of affected cattle.

Mushroom Worker's Lung.   Mushroom worker's lung is probably identical to farmer's lung. At certain stages in their life cycle, domestic mushrooms are grown on compost which is subjected to temperatures of 55° to 60° C and 100 per cent humidity. Workers in the mushroom industry occasionally develop an acute pulmonary illness similar to farmer's lung. Precipitins to *M. faeni* and *T. vulgaris* have been demonstrated in the sera of some of these patients.[19]

Bagassosis.   Bagassosis, a respiratory disease which affects workers who handle sugar cane fibers (bagasse) has many clinical and immunologic features similar to those seen in farmer's lung. Immunologic studies revealed the presence of precipitins against a crude extract of bagasse in the sera of 98 per cent of patients with bagassosis.[20] On the other hand, precipitins were also detected in 95 per cent of apparently healthy workers chronically exposed to bagasse. Further studies of the antigenic components of crude bagasse have demonstrated well defined precipitin bands against *T. vulgaris* in the sera of over 50 per cent of patients with bagassosis. Reagins to extracts of crude bagasse or fungal antigens are occasionally present in patients with bagassosis. The comments made previously regarding the pathogenetic significance of precipitins in farmer's lung are probably equally valid for bagassosis.

Clinical Manifestations

The clinical picture in the pulmonary diseases attributed to thermophilic actinomycetes is primarily that of an interstitial pneumonitis. The onset of symtoms may take place acutely within 5 to 6 hours after exposure to the etiologic agent, or may develop insidiously over a period of several days.

The acute syndrome is characterized by cough, fever, chills, dyspnea, and occasional hemoptysis, all of which usually clear over a period of several days. Auscultation of the chest usually reveals the presence of scattered inspiratory crepitations. Clinical evidence of airway obstruction is not common, but may be a prominent feature in the early or acute phases of the disease process. In those individuals where the onset is slower, there may be progressive development of dyspnea, cough, and cyanosis over a period of several weeks. Repeated exposure may eventually lead to diffuse interstitial pulmonary fibrosis with symptoms of severe chronic exertional dyspnea.

Chest radiographs may show a "ground glass" appearance, or fine reticulation with granular mottling during the acute or subacute phases. Respiratory function studies are comparable to those seen in most forms of pulmonary infiltrative disease. The lung volumes are reduced due to decreased pulmonary compliance and there is a reduction in the pulmonary diffusing capacity. There is little or no evidence of significant airway obstruction, except in the occasional patient during the acute phase. The arterial oxygen tension often falls abruptly during exercise due to an uneven distribution of perfusion and ventilation, but is usually normal or slightly decreased at rest.

Treatment

The most important principle of management in farmer's lung, mushroom worker's disease, or bagassosis is to remove the patient from all further contact with thermophilic actinomycetes. Spontaneous recovery is the general rule, but the adminstration of corticosteroids (e.g., prednisone, 40 mg, daily in divided doses) may be of benefit in the treatment of severe acute symptoms. Concomitant or superimposed infection with pathogenic bacteria should be treated with appropriate antibiotics.

MALT WORKER'S DISEASE

A form of allergic alveolitis clinically similar to farmer's lung has been described in Scottish distillery workers exposed to malt.[6] The causative agent has now been identified as the fungus *Aspergillus clavatus* on the basis of sputum cultures and provocative inhalation tests. Precipitins against *A. clavatus* were found in approximately 25 per cent of symptomatic subjects, but were also detected in malt workers without clinical evidence of pulmonary disease.

BIRD BREEDER'S DISEASE

A pulmonary disease process similar to that seen in farmer's lung and bagassosis occasionally occurs in individuals chronically exposed to pigeons, budgerigars, or related domestic birds. The acute phase is characterized by symptoms of chills, fever, cough, and dyspnea. Radiographic and respiratory function studies are typical of an acute interstitial pneumonitis.[23] The syndrome can be reproduced in susceptible pigeon breeders by provocative inhalation challenge with aerosolized extracts of pigeon droppings, pigeon feather dust, and sterile pigeon serum.

Immunologic studies demonstrated that: (*1*) the sera of all individuals with pigeon breeder's disease contained high titers of precipitins to pigeon antigens; and (*2*) an Arthus type of skin reactivity to pigeon antigens was found in all patients.[9] There was, however, no evidence of reaginic or delayed type hypersensitivity to these antigens.

The pneumonitis associated with hen litter would appear to be a condition closely related to bird breeder's disease.

MAPLE BARK DISEASE

Maple bark disease is a rare form of pneumonitis occurring in paper mill workers exposed to sawdust. Patients with this disorder were found to have both immediate and slower developing skin-test reactions to an extract of the fungus *Cryptostroma corticale* isolated from maple bark. In addition, precipitins against *C. corticale* have been demonstrated in their sera.[8]

WOOD WORKER'S LUNG

An etiologically different form of allergic alveolitis has been reported in woodworkers exposed to the sawdust from oak, mahogany, cedar, and redwood.[23a] Immediate and delayed type skin reactions, precipitins, and positive provocative inhalation tests to the specific wood dust have been documented in a small number of patients.

VEGETABLE DUSTS

A variety of vegetable dusts such as those from sisal, cotton (byssinosis), cork (suberosis), hemp, paprika, and thatched roofs in New Guinea have been reported to cause acute respiratory symptoms on occupational exposure. Circulating precipitins to cotton, kapok, coffee, sisal, hemp, palm kernels, and extracts of thatched roofs have been demonstrated in the sera of workers exposed to these substances. However, as in the case with other occupational lung diseases with immunologic features, the significance of these antibodies in the pathogenesis of the disease is not yet clear.

OTHER ORGANIC ANTIGENS

Similar forms of hypersensitivity pneumonitis have been reported occasionally in individuals exposed to the wheat weevil (mill worker's asthma), pituitary snuff, smallpox scabs, and proteolytic enzymes derived from *Bacillus subtilis* used in the detergent industry.[10]

PULMONARY INFILTRATION WITH EOSINOPHILIA

In 1932, Loeffler described a syndrome of transient pulmonary infiltrations, associated with peripheral blood eosinophilia, cough, sputum, and malaise, which cleared spontaneously within 1 or 2 weeks. The term Loeffler's syndrome, if it has any application whatsoever in the light of modern concepts, should be restricted to this benign, self-limited condition which is not associated with any other underlying disease process. Following Loeffler's original description, however, it soon became apparent that a number of other conditions with a less favorable prognosis and a more protracted course occasionally presented with similar clinical features.[5] Hence, the term pulmonary infiltration with eosinophilia (P.I.E. syndrome) was introduced to describe this general category of diseases.

ETIOLOGY

The common causes of P.I.E. syndrome are listed in Table 4-2. Collagen-vascular diseases such as polyarteritis nodosa or rheumatoid arthritis are among the most frequent of the underlying disease processes. In addition, typical clinical and laboratory features of P.I.E. syndrome may occur as a transient phenomenon during the course of severe protracted bronchial asthma. Allergic reactions to such diverse drugs as penicillin, sulfonamides, para-aminosalicylic acid, hydralazine, nitrofurantoin,[10c] mephenesin carbonate and nickel in association with dermatitis may occasionally initiate the P.I.E. syndrome.

TABLE 4-2. Causes of Pulmonary Infiltration with Eosinophilia (P.I.E. Syndrome)

Collagen-vascular diseases
Bronchial asthma
Drug reactions
Bronchopulmonary aspergillosis
Tropical eosinophilia (filarial infestation of the lung)
Other parasitic infestations
Idiopathic

In the past decade, there has been considerable interest in the possible role of pulmonary hypersensitivity to the fungus *Aspergillus fumigatus* in the pathogenesis of some cases of P.I.E. syndrome. It is postulated that a pulmonary hypersensitivity reaction is initiated as the result of infection with the spores of this fungus.[17]

P.I.E. syndrome may also occur as the result of direct invasion of the lung by a number of parasites such as ascaris, schistosomes, lung flukes, hookworms, Echinococcus, Strongyloides, and cheese mites. In addition, invasion of organs other than the lung by *Trichinella spiralis, Entameba histolytica,* whipworms, *Toxocara canis,* liver flukes, and beef tapeworm may induce a similar clinical picture by presumed hypersensitivity mechanisms. Tropical eosinophilia, a related disease which occurs in the Near and Far East, is probably due to pulmonary infiltration with microfilariae.

PATHOLOGY

The gross and microscopic lesions in P.I.E. syndrome show great variability, depending upon the underlying cause. A typical finding on microscopic examination of a lung biopsy specimen consists of focal patches of massive cellular exudates consisting primarily of eosinophilic leukocytes. These patches also contain variable proportions of histiocytes, lymphocytes, and plasma cells. The cellular exudate is present in the alveoli as well as in the interstitial spaces.[7] At times, the lesions may be focal and have a granulomatous appearance.

IMMUNOLOGY AND PATHOGENESIS

The pathogenesis of bronchopulmonary aspergillosis and tropical eosino-philia has been investigated to a greater extent than any of the other causes of pulmonary eosinophilia. The immunologic features of other disorders associated with the P.I.E. syndrome are less well defined.

Bronchopulmonary Aspergillosis

The immunologic response to pulmonary infection with *Aspergillus fumigatus* may be divided into three main patterns, although there is considerable overlap between these groupings.[17]

Group I.   Some atopic patients develop typical symptoms of allergic rhinitis and asthma similar to those described for other extrinsic allergens (see Chapter 3). This first group of patients has immediate-type skin reactions on direct intradermal testing with extracts of *A. fumigatus,* and reagins against *A. fumigatus* can be demonstrated in their sera by passive transfer testing. About 10 per cent of patients in this category have detectable precipitins to *A. fumigatus* in their sera.

Group II.   A second category of patients may develop transient P.I.E. syndrome during the course of otherwise typical bronchial asthma of varying etiology, duration, and severity. Approximately 90 per cent of these patients have both reagins and precipitins to *A. fumigatus* in their sera, and show immediate wheal and flare reactions as well as Arthus type skin reactions to protein antigens of *A. fumigatus* (Fig. 4-1). Both the immediate and Arthus types of skin reactivity to *A. fumigatus* have been passively transferred to the skin of a rhesus monkey using serum from a patient with bronchopulmonary aspergillosis.[10a] In addition, a rhesus monkey given an intravenous infusion of human aspergillosis serum, and subsequently challenged with aspergillus antigen, developed pulmonary lesions similar to human bronchopulmonary aspergillosis.

It has been postulated that the precipitins demonstrated in this form of bronchopulmonary aspergillosis may form antigen-antibody complexes which are injurious to lung tissue in a manner analogous to the Arthus reaction. In addition, direct infection of the lower respiratory tract by *A. fumigatus* and reagin-mediated obstructive airway disease are of un-doubted pathogenetic significance. Bronchopulmonary aspergillosis occurring during the course of chronic asthma is not uncommon in England, but is reported to be relatively infrequent on the eastern seaboard of the United States.[1]

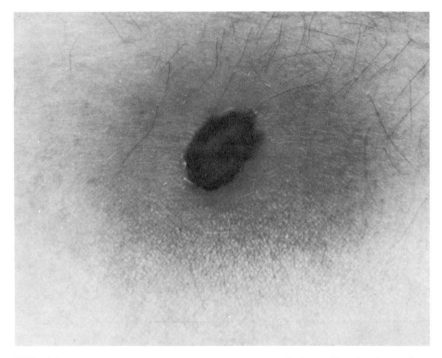

FIG. 4-1. Arthus type skin reaction to an extract of *Aspergillus fumigatus* in a patient with bronchopulmonary aspergillosis.

Group III. The third category of patients in this group presents with the signs and symptoms of pulmonary mycetoma due to *Aspergillus* infection of damaged areas of the lung. The lesions, which are almost always secondary to other chronic cavitary pulmonary diseases such as bronchiectasis, carcinoma, lung abscess, or tuberculosis, are usually not associated with P.I.E. syndrome or other allergic manifestations. Precipitins to *A. fumigatus* are almost always present, but there are no positive skin tests unless there is coexisting P.I.E. syndrome or bronchial asthma. Positive sputum cultures for *A. fumigatus* may be obtained if the aspergilloma communicates with a bronchus.

Tropical Eosinophilia

There is now fairly convincing evidence that tropical eosinophilia is the result of a hypersensitivity response in the lung to microfilariae of an unknown species. In filariasis, the adult worms live in various parts of the human body, and the females give birth to elongate embryos (150 μ to

350 μ) known as microfilariae. The microfilariae migrate through the blood stream to various parts of the body, and hence are able to penetrate the lung parenchyma by virtue of their motility rather than their small size. The geographic distribution of tropical eosinophilia, which is almost entirely restricted to the Near and Far East, is identical to that of filariasis. Furthermore, 90 per cent of patients with the disease show positive filarial complement fixation tests in dilutions of 1:10 or greater, and a similar number show positive skin reactions with filarial antigens. Histologic examination of biopsy specimens obtained at the time of open lung biopsy demonstrated degenerating microfilariae in focal eosinophilic granulomata.[7] However, no microfilariae have ever been demonstrated in the peripheral blood of patients with tropical eosinophilia, nor has the definitive host, vector, or filarial species been established.

There have been occasional reports of mites recovered from the sputum of patients with tropical eosinophilia. Although these organisms probably represent contaminants, their possible role in the pathogenesis of the disease cannot be completely excluded.

CLINICAL MANIFESTATIONS

The commonest symptoms of P.I.E. syndrome are cough, fever, hemoptysis, and dyspnea. Asthmatic manifestations are more likely to occur in those patients with preexisting bronchial asthma or when the underlying process is polyarteritis nodosa. Many patients with the syndrome experience diffuse nonspecific chest pain, which is not related to respiration, on the side of the lesion. Other patients with marked radiographic changes and pronounced peripheral blood eosinophilia may experience only mild symptoms, or none at all.

Depending on the etiology, examination of the chest may reveal auscultatory evidence of severe bronchial obstruction, with sibilant and sonorous inspiratory and expiratory rhonchi heard throughout both lung fields. Persistent basilar crepitations may be present where there is massive pulmonary involvement. Eosinophilic pleural effusions occasionally occur during the course of the P.I.E. syndrome.[4] These effusions contain large numbers of eosinophils, are almost always unilateral, and are frequently hemorrhagic.

Characteristic radiographic changes consist of fleeting, ill-defined, homogenous or mottled densities which are nonsegmental in distribution. There may also be an increase in hilar markings with streaking into the bases. More constant and protracted lesions may occur particularly in those cases associated with pulmonary aspergillosis or collagen-vascular diseases. Respiratory function studies in P.I.E. syndrome are essentially similar to those found in other forms of pulmonary infiltrative disease.

Tropical eosinophilia can usually be distinguished from other causes of P.I.E. syndrome by its characteristic geographic distribution, the male to female ratio of 7:1, and the presence of an absolute eosinophil count of 4000 or greater in 90 per cent of cases. The eosinophil counts tend to be more moderate in P.I.E. syndrome due to other causes.

Eosinophilic granuloma of the lung, one of the histiocytoses-X, represents another cause of pulmonary eosinophilia. The disease is usually mild and self-limited, but may occasionally progress to severe lung destruction.

Eosinophilic pleural effusions which are not associated with P.I.E. syndrome may occasionally occur in association with pulmonary neoplasms, pulmonary infarction, chest trauma, hemothorax, and subdiaphragmatic infection.

TREATMENT

Transient episodes of P.I.E. syndrome of less than 2 weeks duration rarely require specific treatment unless the patient is in severe discomfort. Persistence of the disease for more than 2 weeks maybe considered as an indication for treatment with corticosteroids such as prednisone, 10 to 40 mg, daily in divided doses. However, it should be noted that P.I.E. syndrome secondary to polyarteritis nodosa frequently pursues a progressive course despite corticosteroid therapy. Preliminary evidence suggests that aerosolized amphotericin B may be of value in the treatment of allergic bronchopulmonary aspergillosis.

Tropical eosinophilia due to pulmonary infiltration with microfilariae usually responds dramatically to treatment with the antiparasitic agent diethylcarbamazine, given orally in doses of 8 to 12 mg/kg of body weight in divided doses for 1 week.

FIBROSING ALVEOLITIS (DIFFUSE INTERSTITIAL PULMONARY FIBROSIS)

The term fibrosing alveolitis[22] will be used to describe parenchymal lung diseases of varied etiology characterized by cellular thickening of alveolar walls with a tendency to fibrosis (see Table 4-3). Diffuse interstitial pulmonary fibrosis and the Hamman-Rich syndrome are terms which have also been applied to the same general category of disease processes. An altered immune response has been suggested as a possible factor in the pathogenesis of fibrosing alveolitis because of its frequent association with multiple autoantibodies, hypergammaglobulinemia, and systemic collagen-vascular disease.

TABLE 4-3. Causes of Fibrosing Alveolitis

With immunologic features
Collagen-vascular diseases (rheumatoid arthritis,
progressive systemic sclerosis Sjögren's syndrome
systemic lupus erythematosus, polymyositis)
Familial (associated with hypergammaglobulinemia)
Drug reactions (busulfan)
Idiopathic (associated with hypergammaglobulin-
emia or autoantibodies)

Without immunologic features
Desquamative interstitial pneumonia
Pulmonary muscular hyperplasia
Chronic pulmonary venous obstruction
Carcinoma of the lung
Tuberous sclerosis
Neurofibromatosis

PATHOLOGY

Lung biopsy or necropsy specimens demonstrate the essential morphologic features of fibrosing alveolitis in varying degrees, depending upon the underlying etiology and the duration and severity of disease. Cellular thickening and fibrosis of alveolar walls is most pronounced in those cases associated with collagen-vascular diseases (Fig. 4-2). Other pathologic features may include the presence of other forms of cellular or fibrinous exudate in the alveolar spaces, hyaline membrane formation, and hyperplasia of lymphoid follicles. Chronic fibrosis may lead to gross and microscopic anatomic changes such as honeycombing of the lungs, apparent excess of smooth muscle, and hyperplasia of the bronchiolar epithelium lining residual air spaces.

ETIOLOGY AND PATHOGENESIS

Fibrosing alveolitis may occur as an isolated event, or in association with some other systemic disease process. Most prominent among the latter are the collagen-vascular diseases such as rheumatoid arthritis,[21] progressive systemic sclerosis, Sjögren's syndrome, systemic lupus erythematosus, and polymyositis.

The possible importance of silica dust in the production of the pulmonary fibrosis associated with collagen-vascular diseases was first suggested by

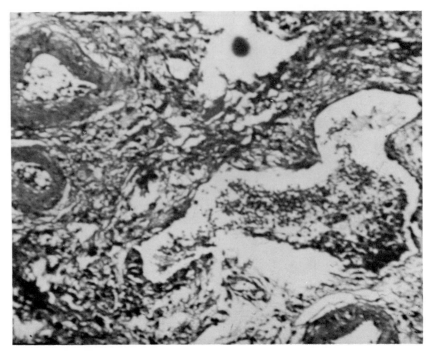

FIG. 4-2. Lung biopsy from a patient with idiopathic fibrosing alveolitis, positive RA test, and diffuse hypergammaglobulinemia. There is marked thickening and fibrosis of alveolar walls with complete destruction of the normal architecture of the lung parenchyma.

studies in Welsh coal miners with rheumatoid arthritis. Subsequent investigators have described in detail the exaggerated fibrotic response (Caplan's syndrome) which occurs in this group of patients. The nodular fibrotic pulmonary lesions can, in many instances, be distinguished both radiologically and pathologically from silicosis which occurs in individuals without rheumatoid arthritis.[13] Similarly, an unusually high incidence of patients with the pulmonary manifestations of progressive systemic sclerosis have a history of prolonged exposure to silica dust.[18] Thus, it may be postulated that the combination of extrinsic agents capable of penetrating the lung parenchyma and an altered state of immunologic reactivity may initiate the process of fibrosing alveolitis in certain patients with preexisting collagen-vascular diseases (see Chapter 8).

Fibrosing alveolitis has also been described as a genetically determined disease transmitted as an autosomal dominant trait.[24a] However, the reported familial occurrence does not exclude possible immunologic associations, since the affected members of some of the families studied also had evidence of hypergammaglobulinemia, monoclonal gammaglobulinopathies, and peripheral blood eosinophilia.[3] Furthermore, there was a high incidence of autoimmune disorders in the asymptomatic relatives of patients with familial pulmonary fibrosis.

Typical lesions of fibrosing alveolitis have been reported to occur following busulfan treatment for leukemia.

Fibrosing alveolitis has also been described in association with nonimmunologic disorders such as desquamative interstitial pneumonia, pulmonary muscular hyperplasia, chronic pulmonary venous obstruction, peripheral carcinoma of the lung, tuberous sclerosis, and neurofibromatosis.[29]

IMMUNOLOGY

Increased values for one or more immunoglobulins were found in 40 per cent of patients with fibrosing alveolitis, regardless of etiology.[11] In another study, positive tests for rheumatoid factor were obtained with the sera of approximately 50 per cent of patients including those without joint manifestations.[26] It has been suggested that pulmonary involvement in patients with high titer rheumatoid factor or abnormal immunoglobulins might be due to the desposition of antigen-antibody complexes or macromolecules in pulmonary capillaries leading to secondary ischemia and fibrosis.[25]

Positive serologic tests for antinuclear factor are found in about 30 per cent of patients with fibrosing alveolitis. Of these, at least one-half have idiopathic pulmonary disease without overt evidence of systemic lupus erythmatosus or other collagen-vascular diseases. The presence of IgM in the alveolar septae was recently demonstrated by immunofluorescent methods in a lung biopsy obtained from a patient with serum IgM antinuclear factor and idiopathic pulmonary fibrosis.[16] This observation would suggest that deposition of immunoglobulins in the lung parenchyma may be of importance in the pathogenesis of fibrosing alveolitis.

CLINICAL MANIFESTATIONS

Severe, progressive, exertional dyspnea is the most common presenting symptom and may become incapacitating in patients with advanced disease. In addition, symptoms of nonproductive cough, weight loss, fatigue, and increased susceptibility to upper respiratory infection occur in most patients with fibrosing alveolitis. Hemoptysis is found less frequently, but may occur in the occasional patient.

On auscultation of the chest, the most common finding consists of crackling rales heard at the lung bases bilaterally. The rales of fibrosing alveolitis are very characteristic in that they are high pitched and occur late in inspiration. Diffuse rhonchi are occasionally present, but are not usually as high pitched as those heard in bronchial asthma. Finger clubbing, visible cyanosis, and cor pulmonale with signs of congestive heart failure are frequently seen in patients with advanced or terminal disease. The usual cause of death is respiratory or cardiac failure precipitated by respiratory infection.

Chest radiographs vary considerably, depending on the etiology and severity of the underlying disease process. The chest film may appear normal, there may be reticular and nodular mottling involving the entire lung bilaterally, or there may be a honeycomb appearance to the lungs. Radiographically, the lower lung fields are usually involved to the greatest extent (Fig. 4-3). Respiratory function studies are similar to those described for other forms of pulmonary infiltrative disease.

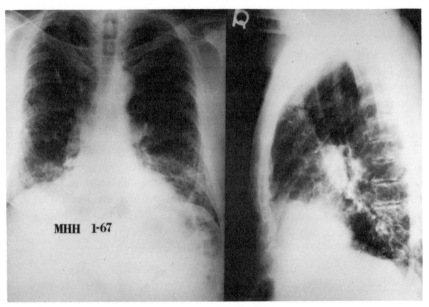

FIG. 4-3. Chest x-ray from same patient as Figure 4-2. The characteristic fibrotic changes are best seen at the lung bases.

TREATMENT

The only effective form of specific treatment is with corticosteroids. Oral prednisone, 10 to 40 mg, daily, may be prescribed in divided doses. Patients with fibrosing alveolitis show a variable response to corticosteroid therapy, and there is no documented evidence that this form of treatment slows the progression of the disease or alters the prognosis. However, dramatic temporary relief of incapacitating symptoms may be achieved in some patients. The prognosis is extremely variable, ranging from a relatively benign chronic condition to a disabling, rapidly fatal illness.

COLLAGEN-VASCULAR DISEASES

In addition to their association with infiltrative pulmonary diseases such as P.I.E. syndrome and fibrosing alveolitis, the collagen-vascular disorders may produce parenchymal lung damage by other mechanisms. The vascular and granulomatous abnormalities of the lung which occur in Goodpasture's syndrome, polyarteritis nodosa, systemic lupus erythematosus, and Wegener's granulomatosis are described in Chapters 6 and 8.

PULMONARY TUBERCULOSIS

The immunologic response of the human host to infection with *Mycobacterium tuberculosis* is of unquestioned importance in the pathogenesis of pulmonary tuberculosis. However, despite approximately 50 years of detailed study, the relationship between hypersensitivity and acquired resistance to tuberculosis remains obscure.[14]

About 3 weeks after the initial infection with *M. tuberculosis,* there is evidence in humans of both immediate and delayed type hypersensitivity to the organism (see Chapter 21). There is considerable clinical evidence to suggest that delayed hypersensitivity is closely associated with resistance to tuberculosis, and is of more significance in this respect than is the presence of circulating antibodies. However, it is not clear from the available data whether delayed hypersensitivity is an integral part of acquired resistance to tuberculosis or is merely a concomitant phenomenon. Similarly, the mechanisms of tissue damage attributable to delayed hypersensitivity are poorly understood.

Epidemiologic data derived from well controlled studies of heavily exposed individuals would indicate that tuberculin negative subjects developed active pulmonary tuberculosis in direct proportion to the degree of exposure, whereas tuberculin reactors enjoyed a relative protection from development of the disease.[24] Agammaglobulinemic individuals, who produce no detectable humoral antibodies, but who are capable of developing delayed type hypersensitivity, demonstrate the same degree of resistance to tuberculous infection as normal individuals. Conversely, patients with immunologic deficiency syndromes who have a normal capacity to produce circulating antibodies, but are deficient in delayed hypersensitivity, are often unusually susceptible to tuberculosis (see Chapters 11 and 12).

OPPORTUNISTIC PULMONARY INFECTIONS

The term opportunistic is frequently used to describe infections that adapt themselves to unique circumstances favoring their development.[15] In the lung, the clinical picture may be extremely complex because opportunistic infections usually occur as a result of the interaction between a variety of unusual organisms and a decrease in host resistance due to underlying disease. The conditions which are known to predispose an individual to opportunistic infections, and the organisms most commonly responsible for them, are listed in Table 4-4. It will be noted that almost all of the predisposing causes are associated with a diminished immunologic response. By definition, many of the common bacterial infections that show increased virulence due to alteration in host resistance are opportunistic, but these will be excluded from the present discussion.

Pneumocystitis, cytomegalovirus infection, nocardiosis, aspergillosis, candidiasis, and mucormycosis are probably the most important forms of opportunistic pulmonary infections. Because pulmonary infections caused by cytomegalovirus and *Pneumocystis carinii* have certain unusual features they will be described briefly below.

CYTOMEGALOVIRUS INFECTION

Cytomegalovirus is a DNA virus of the herpes group which morphologically indistinguishable from herpes simplex and varicella. Clinically, the disease appears in three major forms: (*1*) an overwhelming congenital or neonatal infection; (*2*) an inapparent infection, especially of the salivary glands; and (*3*) a secondary infection in patients with debilitating diseases, in patients with immunologic deficiency states, or in patients receiving immunosuppressive drugs. The characteristic features of extensive neonatal infection include hepatosplenomegaly, jaundice, thrombocytopenic purpura, periventricular calcification, mental retardation, microcephaly, chorioretinitis (see Chapter 17), and optic atrophy. In the secondary forms of the disease, cytomegalovirus pneumonia is usually the predominant clinical manifestation of infection.

The definitive diagnosis is made by the isolation of the virus in tissue culture or by serologic tests. There is no known specific treatment.

TABLE 4-4. Opportunistic Pulmonary Infections

Predisposing Conditions
  With immunologic features
    Leukemia and lymphoproliferative disorders
      (Chapter 12)
    Malignancy (Chapter 13)
    Collagen-vascular diseases (Chapter 8)
    Immunologic deficiency states (Chapter 11)
    Neutropenia, aplastic anemia, splenectomy
      (Chapter 9)
    Immunosuppressive agents (corticosteroids, aza-
      thioprine, cancer chemotherapeutic drugs,
      radiation therapy)
  Without immunologic features
    Diabetes mellitus
    Cushing's disease
    Alveolar proteinosis
    Antibiotic therapy

Types of Infections
  Fungal
    Histoplasmosis
    Coccidiomycosis
    Blastomycosis
    Actinomycosis
    Nocardiosis
    Cryptococcosis
    Candidiasis
    Mucormycosis
    Aspergillosis
    Other phycomycoses
  Viral
    Cytomegalovirus infection
  Protozoal
    Pneumocystis carinii pneumonia

PNEUMOCYSTIS CARINII PNEUMONIA

The precise taxonomic classification of *Pneumocystis carinii* is still in doubt, but the organism is widely believed to be a protozoa.[27] *P. carinii* pneumonia occurs most commonly in debilitated newborn infants, in patients with immunologic deficiency states, in patients with malignant diseases, and in patients receiving immunosuppressive drugs.[10b] Clinically, the disease is often characterized by an unusual degree of cyanosis and tachypnea in the absence of significant auscultatory findings in the lung. A diffuse bilateral, rapidly progressive interstitial pneumonitis is the most common finding on chest x-ray.

The diagnosis is made by the histologic demonstration of the organisms in the sputum, in secretions obtained by tracheal lavage, or in tissues obtained by lung biopsy. *P. carinii* organisms have not yet been successfully established in tissue culture. Preliminary reports suggest that pentamidine isethionate in a single daily intramuscular injection of 4 mg/kg constitutes an effective form of treatment for *P. carinii* infection.

REFERENCES

1. Agbanyani, B. F., Norman, P. S., and Winkenwerder, W. L. The incidence of allergic aspergillosis in chronic asthma. *J. Allerg. 40:*319, 1967.

2. Barbee, R. A., Dickie, H. A., and Rankin, J. Pathogenicity of specific glycopeptide antigen in farmer's lung. *Proc. Soc. Exper. Biol. Med. 118:*546, 1965.

3. Bonnani, P. P., Frymoyer, J. W., and Jacox, R. F. A family study of idiopathic pulmonary fibrosis. A possible dysproteinemic and genetically determined disease. *Amer. J. Med. 39:*411, 1965.

4. Bower, G. Eosinophilic pleural effusion: A condition with multiple causes. *Amer. Rev. Resp. Dis. 95:*746, 1967.

5. Carrington, C. B., Addington, W. W., Goff, A. M., Madoff, I. M., Marks, A., Schwaber, J. R., and Gaensler, E. A. Chronic eosinophilic pneumonia. *New Eng. J. Med. 280:*787, 1969.

6. Channell, S., Blyth, W., Lloyd, M., Weir, D. M., Amos, W. M. G., Littlewood, A. P., Riddle, H. F. V., and Grant, I. W. B. Allergic alveolitis in maltworkers. A clinical, mycological, and immunological study. *Quart. J. Med. 38:*351, 1969.

7. Danaraj, T. J., Pacheo, G., Shanmugartum, K., and Beaver, P. C. The etiology and pathology of eosinophilic lung. *Amer. J. Trop. Med. 15:*183, 1966.

8. Emanuel, D. A., Wenzel, F. J., and Lawton, B. R. Pneumonitis due to cryptostroma corticale (maple-bark disease). *New Eng. J. Med. 274:*1413, 1966.

9. Fink, J. N., Sosman, A. J., Barboriak, J. J., Schlueter, D. P., and Holmes, R. A. Pigeon breeders' disease. A clinical study of a hypersensitivity pneumonitis. *Ann. Intern. Med. 68:*1205, 1968.

10. Flindt, M. L. H. Pulmonary disease due to inhalation of derivatives of *Bacillus subtilis* containing proteolytic enzyme. *Lancet 1:*1177, 1969.

10a. Golbert, T. M., and Patterson, R. Pulmonary allergic aspergillosis. *Ann Intern. Med., 72:*395, 1970.

10b. Goodell, B., Jacobs, J. B., Powell, R. D., and De Vita, V. T. *Pneumocystis carinii:* The spectrum of diffuse interstitial pneumonia in patients with neoplastic diseases. *Ann. Intern. Med. 72:*337, 1970.

10c. Hailey, F. J., Glascock, H. W. Jr., and Hewitt, W. F. Pleuropneumonic reactions to nitrofurantoin. *New Eng. J. Med. 281:*1087, 1969.

11. Hobbs, J. R., and Turner-Warwick, M. Assay of circulating immunoglobulins in patients with fibrosing alveolitis. *Clin. Exp. Immun. 2:*645, 1967.

12. Kobayashi, M., Stahmann, M. A., Rankin, J., and Dickie, H. A. Antigens in moldy hay as the cause of farmer's lung. *Proc. Soc. Exp. Biol. Med. 113:*472, 1963.

13. Lendars, D. C., and Davies, D. Rheumatoid pneumoconioses. A study in colliery populations in the east midlands coalfield. *Thorax 22:*525, 1967.

14. Mackaness, G. B. The relationship of delayed hypersensitivity to acquired cellular resistance. *Brit. Med. Bull. 23:*52, 1967.

15. Murray, J. F., Haegelin, H. F., Hewitt, W. L., Latta, H., McVickar, D., Rasmussen, A. F., Jr., and Rigler, L. G. Opportunistic pulmonary infections. *Ann. Intern. Med. 65:*566, 1966.

16. Nigaya, H., Buckley, E. C., III, Sieker, H. O. Positive antinuclear factor in patients with unexplained pulmonary fibrosis. *Ann. Intern. Med. 70:*1135, 1969.

17. Pepys, J. Pulmonary hypersensitivity disease due to inhaled organic antigens. *Ann. Intern. Med. 64:*943, 1966.

18. Rodnan, G. P., Benedek, T. G., Medsger, T. A., Jr., and Cammarata, R. J. The association of progressive systemic sclerosis (Scleroderma) with coal miner's pneumoconiosis and other forms of silicosis. *Ann. Intern. Med. 66:*323, 1967.

19. Sakula, A. Mushroom-worker's lung. *Brit. Med. J. 3:*691, 1967.

20. Salvaggio, J. E., Buechner, H. A., Seabury, J. H., and Arquembourg, P. Bagassosis: I. Precipitins against extracts of crude bagasse in the serum of patients. *Ann. Intern. Med. 64:*748, 1966.

21. Scadding, J. G. The lungs in rheumatoid arthritis. *Proc. Roy. Soc. Med. 62:*227, 1969.

22. Scadding, J. G., and Hinson, K. F. W. Diffuse fibrosing alveolitis (diffuse interstitial fibrosis of the lungs): Correlation of histology at biopsy with prognosis. *Thorax 22:*291, 1967.

23. Schlueter, D. P., Fink, J. N., and Sosman, A. J. Pulmonary function in pigeon breeders' disease. A hypersensitivity pneumonitis. *Ann. Intern. Med. 70:*457, 1969.

23a. Sosman, A. J., Schlueter, D. P., Fink, J. N., and Barboriak, J. J. Hypersensitivity to wood dust. *New Eng. J. Med. 281:*977, 1969.

24. Stead, W. W. Pathogenesis of the first episode of pulmonary tuberculosis in man. *Amer. Rev. Resp. Dis. 95:*729, 1967.

24a. Swaye, P., Van Ordstrand, H. S., McCormack, L. J., and Wolpaw, S. E. Familial Hamman-Rich syndrome. Report of eight cases. *Dis. Chest 55:*7, 1969.

25. Tomasi, T. B., Jr., Fudenberg, H. H., and Finby, N. Possible relationship of rheumatoid factor and pulmonary disease. *Amer. J. Med. 33*:243, 1962.

26. Turner-Warwick, M., and Doniach, D. Auto-antibody studies in interstitial pulmonary fibrosis. *Brit. Med. J. 1*:886, 1965.

27. Vogel, C. L., Cohen, M. H., Powell, R. D., Jr., and DeVita, V. T. *Pneumocystis Carinii* pneumonia. *Ann. Intern. Med. 68*:97, 1968.

28. Wenzel, F. J., Emanuel, D. A., Lawton, B. R., and Magnin, G. E. Isolation of the causative agent of farmer's lung. *Ann. Allerg. 22*:533, 1964.

29. Ziskind, M. M., Weill, H., and George, R. B. Diffuse pulmonary diseases. *Amer. J. Med. Sci. 254*:95, 1967.

5

Clinical Immunology of the Skin

SAMUEL O. FREEDMAN

ALLERGIC CONTACT DERMATITIS

Allergic contact dermatitis (ACD) probably provides the best example of an immunologic reaction producing disease of the human skin. The causative agent or contact allergen is usually a small molecular weight compound such as a drug, dye, plant oleoresin, plastic, or industrial chemical. In a previously sensitized individual, acute dermatitis commonly occurs within 48 hours at the site of exposure to the contact allergen. Unlike atopic dermatitis, the tendency to develop ACD does not appear to depend on an inherited predisposition.

PATHOLOGY

Biopsy specimens from patients with ACD demonstrate no specific morphologic features different from those found in other allergic dermatoses. In the acute phase, the epidermis shows spongiosis followed by intraepidermal vesiculation. In the more chronic stages, there may be varying degrees of hyperkeratosis and irregular epidermal thickening. Nonspecific inflammatory

121

changes, often accompanied by mononuclear infiltration, are seen in the dermis.

IMMUNOLOGY

It is generally agreed that ACD is a manifestation of cell-mediated hypersensitivity in the epidermis, immunologically similar to the tuberculin reaction which takes place in the dermis. Immunochemical studies in animals and man indicate that the most potent cutaneous sensitizers are small molecules which combine readily with proteins, but do not significantly alter the internal structure of the carrier protein. On the other hand, compounds such as nitric acid and sulfuric acid may act as primary irritants, but are poor sensitizers. The exact mechanism by which small molecules induce cell-mediated cutaneous hypersensitivity is not completely understood. However, several experimental observations are of interest in this connection.

In animals, painting of the skin with a small molecular weight compound such as 2,4 dinitrochlorobenzene will consistently result in an eczematous response on subsequent cutaneous exposure to 2,4 dinitrochlorobenzene. However, if the small molecule, without conjugation to a carrier protein, is injected intravenously or intramuscularly, no cutaneous sensitization will occur. Guinea pig experiments also suggest that intact lymphatic pathways between the skin and regional lymph nodes are essential for the development of contact hypersensitivity. It thus seems reasonable to postulate the following steps in the process of allergic contact sensitization: (1) the small molecular weight allergen conjugates with epidermal proteins at the site of application; (2) the conjugate is transported via lymphatic pathways to regional lymph nodes; (3) the regional lymph nodes produce specifically modified lymphocytes (see Chapter 1); and (4) the specifically modified lymphocytes return to the epidermis to result in a hypersensitivity reaction on subsequent challenge with the original contact allergen.

In humans, attempts to passively transfer contact type hypersensitivity to low molecular weight allergens by means of leukocytes obtained from sensitized donors have been generally unsuccessful in contrast to the results obtained with tuberculin hypersensitivity. The only apparent exception to this general rule is the observation that cutaneous hypersensitivity to procaine, in which there is a strong dermal component, can be passively transferred with relative ease by peripheral blood leukocytes.[10] Agammaglobulinemic individuals retain their capacity to develop ACD, but this capacity is frequently absent or diminished in patients with immunologic deficiency states which are associated with a decrease in the cell-mediated immune response (see Chapters 11 and 12). ACD cannot be passively transferred with serum.

CLINICAL MANIFESTATIONS

The clinical manifestations vary, depending upon the stage of the disease process, the site of the lesion, and the possible coexistence of other cutaneous diseases. The acute phase is usually characterized by vesiculation, exudation of fluid, and localized edema of the skin. In the more chronic stages, eczematization, scaling, crusting, and lichenification predominate. Some patients tend to lose their cutaneous hypersensitivity to a given contact allergen after a period of years for no obvious reason.

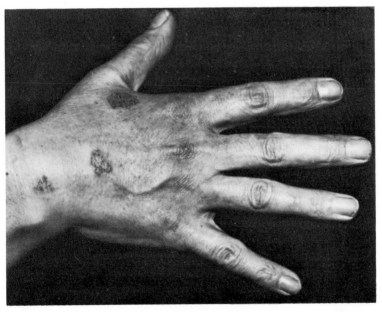

FIG. 5-1. Allergic contact dermatitis in a nurse following the accidental spillage of three drops of streptomycin solution on the dorsum of the hand.

Contact dermatitis can usually be distinguished from other dermatoses with similar clinical features (e.g., atopic dermatitis, nummular eczema, solar dermatitis, and fungal diseases with eczematization) by its tendency to appear in localized areas, and by the history of suspected contact (Fig. 5-1). The face, neck, dorsal aspects of the hands and feet, and lateral aspects of the arms and legs are most commonly affected, whereas the palms, soles, and hairy areas of the body are usually free of lesions. Primary irritant contact dermatitis, particularly of the occupational variety, may, at times, be impossible to distinguish clinically from ACD. Primary irritant dermatitis often appears within 1 to 2 hours after contact rather than after 48 hours, and prior exposure to the causative agent is not required. However, the differential diagnosis depends ultimately on a thorough familiarity with known primary skin irritants such as soaps, mineral oils, solvents, and numerous industrial chemicals.[4]

ACD may occasionally coexist with other dermatologic disorders, either as the result of the application of topical medication or because the contact allergen is more easily absorbed through the diseased skin surface. In this situation, the clinical diagnosis of ACD may be extraordinarily difficult.

DIAGNOSIS

Once the clinical diagnosis of ACD is established or suspected, an attempt should be made in most cases to determine the specific cause of the dermatitis in order to avoid a possible recurrence. The successful detection of a specific contact allergen usually demands a thorough knowledge of: (1) the technique and numerous pitfalls associated with the use of the patch test as a diagnostic procedure; (2) the substances which most commonly cause contact dermatitis; and (3) the characteristic locations of dermatitis caused by common contact allergens.

The patch test is the standard procedure for the diagnosis of ACD. This method involves deliberate reproduction of the disease on a miniature scale by applying the suspected contact allergen to the skin for a period of up to 48 hours.[26]

Although the method is simple in principle, there are many potential fallacies in the interpretation of patch tests. Once generalized eczematous sensitivity is established, the skin threshold for irritation may become so low that normally nonirritating concentrations of some substances may exert a primary irritant effect, thereby producing false-positive patch tests. Furthermore, it has been repeatedly observed that many contact allergens may evoke positive patch tests in individuals who have never had ACD. This type of reaction is thought to reflect a state of latent or potential contact allergy. Another problem in the interpretation of patch tests is cross-sensitivity between chemically related allergens.

False-negative reactions, on the other hand, tend to occur following the administration of systemic corticosteroids which suppress cell-mediated hypersensitivity. Patch testing should not be performed until systemic corticosteroids or ACTH have been withdrawn for a period of at least 3 weeks. Antihistamines exert no significant effect on patch test reactions.

It has been suggested that intradermal testing with water-soluble contact allergens, scarification procedures, or the use of dimethylsulfoxide may increase the sensitivity of epidermal reactions to contact allergens by increasing penetration. The same objective can probably be achieved by a slight increase in concentration of solutions used for patch testing.

Patch testing practices vary somewhat between North America and European centers. In North America, selective testing with suspected contact allergens is the rule, whereas in Europe a large battery of screening tests is frequently employed. In the author's clinic, a small series of screening tests is occasionally employed in those patients where the suspected allergen is not obvious from the history. A short list of common contact allergens, sources of contact, and recommended patch testing concentrations is presented in Table 5-1. The risk of inducing sensitization to a contact allergen in a patient who has not been previously exposed is negligible with a single patch test at the recommented concentration.

The location of ACD may be of considerable assistance in establishing a specific etiologic diagnosis. For example, ACD due to nickel or chromium may occur under watchbands, necklaces, garter belts, bracelets or buckles, or on exposure to chrome tanned leather. Rubber dermatitis may occur under foundation garments, elastic hose, or the box toes of shoes which contain rubber compounds. ACD due to industrial chemicals may occur on the exposed areas of the body. ACD due to topical medications or cosmetics usually occurs at the sites of application. The linear distribution on the exposed areas of the body and the history of a picnic or walk in the woods is so characteristic of poison ivy dermatitis that patch testing is rarely necessary for confirmation. Poison ivy dermatitis differs from most other forms of ACD in that the majority of the population are susceptible to the disorder after sufficient exposure. A recent investigation of occupational ACD in forest workers demonstrated that the affected workers had positive patch tests to *Frullania,* a genus of liverworts. The allergenic component of the *Frullania* oleoresins was identified as a sesquiterpene lactone of low molecular weight, and preliminany data would suggest that the presence of a carbon-carbon double bond conjugated to the lactone group is essential for allergenicity.[16]

TREATMENT

Removal of the patient from all further contact with the suspected contact allergen is a self-evident, but sometimes neglected, first principle of treatment. Removal of the allergen may also present a somewhat difficult economic problem in occupational dermatoses where the patient's means of earning a living may depend on his handling substances to which he has become sensitized. Under these circumstances, well designed protective clothing is much more likely to provide adequate protection against sensitizing agents than one of the numerous barrier creams currently available.

TABLE 5-1. Common Contact Allergens*

Contact allergen	Suggested concentration for patch testing	Possible sources of contact
Potassium dichromate	0.5 % in water	Chromium compounds in jewelry, watches, chrome tanned leather, cement, etc
Nickel sulfate†	5 % in water	Nickel compounds in jewelry, watches, clasps, garter belts, earrings, stainless steel, white gold, etc
Formaldehyde	5 % in water	Fabrics, facial tissue, nail hardeners
p-Phenylendiamine	2 % in petrolatum	Black, brown, and blue dyes for hair, furs and textiles
Mercaptobenzothiazole	1 % in petrolatum	Rubber (box toes of shoes may contain rubber)
Tetramethylthiuram disulfide	5 % in petrolatum	Rubber
Balsam of Peru	25 % in petrolatum	Ingredient of tincture of benzoin (frequently applied under adhesive tape)
Neomycin sulfate	20 % in petrolatum	Topical antibiotic
Iodochlorhydroxyquin	Vioform ointment (as is)	Topical antiseptic
Thiomersol (Merthiolate)	1 % in water	Topical antiseptic
Tripelennamine	Pyribenzamine ointment (as is)	Topical antihistamine
Methapyriline	Histadyl ointment (as is)	Topical antihistamine
Benzocaine	10 % in petrolatum	Topical anesthetic
Dibucaine	Nupercainal ointment (as is)	Topical anesthetic
Cyclomethycaine	Surfacaine ointment (as is)	Topical anesthetic

* Cosmetics, topical medications, and industrial contactants to which the patient is specifically exposed must also be considered in addition to the allergens listed above.

† Cobalt frequently cross-reacts with nickel, but does not appear to be an important allergen in itself.

In the acute phases of ACD, cool saline compresses combined with a topical steroid lotion constitute the most effective form of treatment. Lotions are much easier to apply to weeping lesions than ointments or creams. In the subacute or chronic phases, a cream or ointment containing one of the fluorinated hydrocortisones (e.g., triamcinolone, betamethasone, or fluocino-lone) is the treatment of choice. Systemic corticosteroids may occasionally be justified in the management of an acute, isolated episode of ACD, such as that due to poison ivy.

Desensitization to posion ivy oleoresin is not a widely accepted procedure because of lack of agreement as to its effectiveness. In addition, unpleasant and occasionally serious side-effects such as generalized dermatitis, pruritus ani, or nephrotic syndrome may follow such treatment. Occasional attempts to desensitize patients with other common contact allergens such as potassium dichromate have not been successful.

PHOTOSENSITIVITY DERMATITIS

Dermatitis which occurs only after exposure to strong sunlight may follow the topical or systemic administration of certain drugs. Two basic mechanisms, phototoxic and photoallergic reactions, appear to be responsible for most cases of photosensitivity induced by drugs.[1]

ETIOLOGY AND PATHOGENESIS

In *phototoxic* drug reactions, the presence of the drug renders the skin more sensitive to light, producing an exaggerated form of sunburn. The assumption is that light with a wavelength in the ultraviolet range (280 to 400 mμ) activates the drug (photoactivation) to a level where sufficient energy is liberated to damage the surrounding skin. The absorption spectrum required to produce this type of reaction is specific for each drug and is not related to the sunburn spectrum of the normal human skin. The reaction is thus nonimmunologic in nature and, like primary irritant contact dermatitis, will occur in almost all persons even in the absence of previous exposure to the drug. Common examples of drugs that may induce a phototoxic dermatitis are presented in Table 5-2.

Conversely, *photoallergic* drug reactions occur in only a small percentage of the exposed population, require an induction period, and are probably dependent on immunologic mechanisms. It is postulated that the drug is converted in the skin to a new allergenic hapten through the action of absorbed light. The newly formed allergenic compound then induces a state of cell-mediated hypersensitivity similar to that found in allergic contact dermatitis. Because the mechanism is immunologic rather than toxic, a much lower drug concentration is required for a photoallergic drug reaction

TABLE 5-2. Common Causes of Photosensitivity Dermatitis

Probable phototoxic mechanism
Coal tar derivatives (topical)
Sulfonamides (systemic)
Demethylchlortetracycline (systemic)
Furocoumarins (used topically to treat vitiligo)

Probable photoallergic mechanism
Sulfonamides (systemic)
Sulfonamide derivatives (e.g., thiazides, chlorpropamide, tolbutamide)
Phenothiazines
Sun screen agents (e.g., digalloyl trioleate, aminobenzoic acid)
Artificial sweeteners (e.g., calcium cyclamate)
Phytophotodermatitis (e.g., wild parsnip, gas plant, fig trees)

---

as compared to a phototoxic drug reaction. Examples of the classes of drugs which will produce a photoallergic dermatitis are listed in Table 5-2.

A less common variety of photosensitivity dermatitis is phytophotodermatitis secondary to contact with plants of the families Umbelliferae, Rutaceae, and Moraceae (Table 5-2).[29] Despite the dependence of the syndrome on exposure to sunlight, it is frequently confused with poison ivy dermatitis.

Some drugs may act by both photoallergic and phototoxic mechanisms or may induce both photosensitivity dermatitis and allergic contact dermatitis. Cross-reactive photoallergic reactions can occur between chemically related drugs such as the sulfonamides, oral hypoglycemic agents, and oral diuretics. Photosensitivity may also be associated with porphyria, pellagra, and systemic lupus erythematosus.

CLINICAL MANIFESTATIONS

Clinically, the lesions of photosensitivity dermatitis characteristically involve the areas of the body most frequently exposed to sunlight (face, V-area of the neck, arms, legs, and hands). In its milder forms, the dermatitis consists of an exaggerated erythema response. In more severe cases, there may also be edema, vesiculation, and bullae. An occasional clinical problem is that of the "persistent light reactor." These patients display persistent eruptions on exposure to sunlight for many months after their last known contact with the photosensitizing agent.

DIAGNOSIS

A definitive diagnosis of photoallergic dermatitis can be made by photopatch testing. The test is performed by first applying a conventional patch test with a suspected contact allergen or by administering a suspected systemic allergen by mouth. Forty-eight hours later, the skin is exposed to ultraviolet light of a wave length based on the known action spectrum of the drug for 1 to 5 minutes. As sources of monochromatic light are not readily available in most clinics, precise testing in photosensitivity dermatitis remains a research procedure. In the majority of instances, the diagnosis can be made on the history of exposure to light, the use of photosensitizing drugs, and the patient's response to drug withdrawal.

TREATMENT

Treatment consists of withdrawal of the sensitizing drug, avoidance of strong sunlight for a short period, and topical therapy similar to that described for ACD.

ID REACTIONS

It has been suggested that secondary eczematous eruptions (or id reactions) may occur as the result of hypersensitivity to microbial antigens present in primary sites remote from the eczematous lesions. The commonest examples of this type of reaction are the generalized eczema which occasionally occurs over the face, trunk, and arms in individuals with chronic infected varicose ulcers, or the lesions which occur on the palms of the hands in patients with fungal infections elsewhere in the body. Unfortunately, after many years of investigation, there is very little experimental evidence to support the concept of secondary cutaneous hypersensitivity to microorganisms.

ATOPIC DERMATITIS

The importance of immunologic mechanisms in atopic dermatitis is much less well-defined than in allergic contact dermatitis or photosensitivity dermatitis. Traditionally, the term atopic dermatitis has been used to describe a characteristic form of eczematous skin eruption which is frequently associated with other allergic diseases such as asthma and hay fever. This relationship does not necessarily mean that the lesions of atopic dermatitis are directly dependent on immunologic mechanisms.

There is some disagreement regarding terminology in atopic dermatitis. In this section, the characteristic exudative eczematous process which occurs in infants will be referred to as infantile atopic dermatitis, whereas the dry, lichenified, flexural lesions which occur in older children or adults will be referred to as adult atopic dermatitis. In Europe, the term prurigo Besnier is frequently used to describe atopic dermatitis.

PATHOLOGY

There are no characteristic features which distinguish biopsy specimens obtained from patients with atopic dermatitis from other allergic dermatoses. Light microscopy in the acute phase usually reveals intraepithelial vesicles (spongiosis), vascular dilatation in the dermis, and perivascular infiltration with inflammatory cells. The findings in more chronic lesions include hyperkeratosis of the epidermis, acanthosis, and suprapapillary epidermal thickening. Electron microscopic studies often reveal the presence of lysosomes in the stratum granulosum of atopic skin, and it has been suggested that these lysosomes may have an autodigestive function of pathogenetic significance.

PATHOPHYSIOLOGY

The nature of the defect in atopic dermatitis has given rise to considerable speculation over the years. Much attention has been paid to the cutaneous vascular supply, and a number of vascular abnormalities have been described in atopic dermatitis.[33]

In normal individuals, the usual response to firm stroking of the skin with a blunt instrument is a red line followed by a wheal and flare response. In patients with atopic dermatitis, however, the red line is often replaced by a white line surrounded by an area of blanching. This abnormal response of white dermographism is not specific for atopic dermatitis and may be observed in other dermatoses.

Another paradoxical vascular response that occurs in about 50 per cent of atopic patients is the delayed blanch phenomenon.[17] This phenomenon takes place following the intradermal injection of acetylcholine or methacholine, and consists of a spreading area of white reaction that begins 5 to 30 minutes after the injection and lasts for 10 to 60 minutes. Normally, the intradermal injection of acetylcholine produces vasodilation.

The possible role of catecholamines in the pathogenesis of atopic dermatitis has also been the subject of considerable investigation. Decreased levels of circulating plasma norepinephrine were demonstrated in a small number of patients with atopic dermatitis. In addition, when ^{14}C-labelled norepinephrine was injected intravenously into patients with acute atopic dermatitis, these patients were found to store more of the labelled norepinephrine in the affected areas of skin than normal controls or patients with other dermatoses.[28] These findings have led to the hypothesis that patients with atopic dermatitis have a tendency to bind norepinephrine excessively in the skin.

IMMUNOLOGY

At present, there is little evidence to suggest that reagins or other antibodies are directly responsible for the lesions of atopic dermatitis.[27] Unquestionably, the majority of patients have a personal or family history of asthma and hay fever, and many have numerous positive skin tests of the immediate type. However, the only proven cutaneous reaction between an allergen and reagins is a wheal and flare response of the type found in patients with extrinsic bronchial asthma and allergic rhinitis. The positive skin tests in atopic dermatitis never become eczematous, suggesting that there is no direct cause and effect relationship between the allergen which produces the wheal and flare reaction and the characteristic lesions of atopic dermatitis. Patch testing with suspected inhalant or food allergens is almost always negative in patients with atopic dermatitis.

It is a common observation that the ingestion of certain foods by a small percentage of infants with atopic dermatitis will consistently result in an exacerbation of skin lesions due to mechanisms which are poorly understood. It has been the experience of most allergists and dermatologists that removal of suspected food allergens from the patient's diet rarely produces improvement in atopic dermatitis, except in the minority of cases where the etiologic importance of foods is immediately obvious from the history.

On the other hand, there are a few pieces of indirect evidence to suggest that immunologic abnormalities may occur in association with atopic dermatitis. Extracts of normal skin were reported to induce blast cell transformation in the cultured lymphocytes of patients with infantile atopic dermatitis, but not in the lymphocytes of normal individuals.[32] In addition, it has been demonstrated that serum IgG levels are higher[5] and serum complement levels are lower[14] in patients with active atopic dermatitis than in patients with other forms of eczema. These latter changes may simply reflect the chronic skin infections which are often present in association with atopic dermatitis. It is also of interest that there is an unusual frequency of atopic dermatitis, in the absence of demonstrable wheal and erythema allergy, among boys with the sex-linked form of primary agammaglobulinemia, and in infants with the Wiskott-Aldrich syndrome (see Chapter 11).

CLINICAL MANIFESTATIONS

Natural History

The prevalence of atopic dermatitis in children under the age of 5 years has been estimated to be about 3 per cent. Approximately 60 per cent of children with atopic dermatitis have a family history of asthma and hay fever, and 50 per cent have other allergic manifestations at some time in their lives.[31] Contrary to a widely held viewpoint, atopic dermatitis frequently persists into adult life or may even appear for the first time in the adult years. A retrospective survey revealed that only 40 per cent of patients with mild lesions and 29 per cent of patients with severe lesions in infancy were completely free of atopic dermatitis at the age of 20 years.[22]

Signs and Symptoms

The lesions of atopic dermatitis are usually sufficiently characteristic in appearance and distribution to cause little difficulty in differential diagnosis. However, the clinical picture varies considerably with age.

In infants (2 to 24 months), the lesions tend to be vesicular, exudative, and crusted. Infantile atopic dermatitis is most common on the scalp and cheeks, but in more severe cases there may be scattered patches over the trunk and extremities or a generalized eruption which covers the entire body. In the childhood phase (2 to 12 years), the lesions tend to be drier, more lichenified and confined primarily to the antecubital fossae, the popliteal fossae, the wrists, ankles, and flexures of the buttocks. In adolescents and adults, the tendency to intense pruritus and dry, thickened, lichenified lesions in the flexural areas is even more pronounced. There may also be involvement of the face, neck, hands, and feet in adults.

The incidence of several congenital anomalies is significantly higher in children with atopic eczema than in normal children. For instance, vitiligo, spotty hyperpigmentation of the skin, or mongolian folds of the eyelids are not infrequently seen in association with chronic atopic dermatitis. Ocular cataracts and keratoconus (degeneration of the cornea with bulging in the presence of normal intraocular pressure) also occur more commonly in patients with atopic dermatitis than in normal individuals in the same age group.

Differential Diagnosis

It is often difficult to differentiate between seborrheic dermatitis in the infant and the infantile form of atopic dermatitis. Many infants who develop "cradle cap" or acute exudative eczema localized to the scalp subsequently develop typical atopic dermatitis in later years. The two conditions, as they occur in infancy, are indistinguishable on microscopic examination of biopsy specimens. In older children and adults, seborrheic dermatitis is quite different in its manifestations from atopic dermatitis.

Infantile atopic dermatitis must also be differentiated from several rare, but serious, eczematous processes which occur in infancy (see Table 5-3). Leiner's disease (erythroderma desquamativum) occurs in the first few weeks of life and is characterized by a generalized scaling dermatitis, minimal itching, and severe protracted diarrhea. Ritter's disease (dermatitis exfoliativa neonatorum) is a form of exfoliative dermatitis which usually develops within the first 2 weeks of life. It has recently been shown that the injection of Group 2 coagulase-positive staphylococci, isolated from infants with Ritter's disease, produced exfoliation in newborn mice.[15b] An eczematous eruption, clinically indistinguishable from atopic dermatitis, may also appear during the course of Letterer-Siwe's disease or phenylketonuria. Atopic erythrodermia is probably not a separate entity, but represents a severe form of generalized infantile atopic dermatitis with secondary infection.

TABLE 5-3. Differential Diagnosis of In-fantile Atopic Dermatitis

Seborrheic dermatitis
Leiner's disease
Ritter's disease
Wiskott-Aldrich syndrome
Sex-linked form of primary agammaglobulinemia
Phenylketonuria
Letterer-Siwe's disease

TREATMENT

Most patients are seen for the first time in infancy or early childhood. At the time of the first interview, it is our practice to give the parents a careful and detailed explanation to the effect that atopic dermatitis is basically an inherited defect of the skin which usually responds very well to topical therapy. In this way, it is usually possible to avoid the behavioral and feeding problems which are the inevitable result of excessive dietary restrictions based on misconceptions regarding etiology.

The first choice in topical therapy is one of the fluorinated hydrocortisones (fluocinolone, betamethasone, flurandrenolone, or triamcinolone) in a water soluble base applied three times daily until the skin appears normal. For weeping or exudative lesions, wet saline dressings applied several times daily at room temperature constitute the most effective form of treatment. Care should be taken to avoid maceration of the skin caused by protracted application of moist dressings. When the lesions are thick and lichenified, one of the coal tar preparations may be necessary to achieve complete clearing of the skin. Crude coal tar, 1%, in Lassar's paste or cold cream is probably the most satisfactory. However, most patients prefer one of the more refined, but less effective proprietary coal tar preparations. The patient should be warned that coal tar derivatives may sensitize the skin to strong sunlight.

Hydroxyzine, 5 to 25 mg, four times daily, is often helpful in reducing the inevitable pruritus which is directly responsible for the cycle of scratching, excoriation, and flaring of lesions. Hydroxyzine also has a mild sedative effect. If secondary infection is present, one of the quinolone antiseptics (iodochlorhydroxyquin, 3%; diiodohydroxyquin, 1%; or chlorquinaldol, 3%) may be combined with the corticosteroid preparation. The antibiotics neomycin and bacitracin are equally effective in combating secondary infection, but are less acceptable because of their potential sensitizing properties. Occlusive dressings in combination with corticosteroid creams are tolerated poorly by most patients with atopic dermatitis and are rarely used.

The skin of patients with atopic dermatitis is easily irritated by a number of nonspecific factors such as excessive sweating in hot weather, chapping of the skin in cold weather, wool and nylon fabrics, detergents and strong soaps, too frequent bathing, and emotional stress. A careful history will often determine which of these secondary factors are most important in a particular patient. Smallpox vaccination should be avoided in all patients with active atopic dermatitis because of the danger of generalized vaccinia (see Chapter 21).

The use of systemic corticosteroids should be considered only when: (1) all other measures have failed; and (2) the patient is so incapacitated by his atopic dermatitis that he must spend weeks in hospital, or is unable to attend school or carry on with his regular occupation. Under these circumstances, it is sometimes possible to keep the patient relatively free of dermatitis on relatively small doses of prednisone (e.g., 5 to 10 mg daily) combined with a full regimen of topical therapy. Systemic corticosteroids are especially contraindicated in children as, even in small doses,

they tend to suppress growth if continued over a period of years. Nevertheless, they may occasionally be recommended as a last resort in children
with severe atopic dermatitis when repeated or continuous hospitalization
is probably more harmful to the patient and his family than small doses
of systemic corticosteroids.

URTICARIAL DISEASES

Urticaria is a localized or generalized cutaneous eruption consisting of
sharply circumscribed, elevated areas of edema of the skin. If the swelling
is more extensive and involves the subcutaneous tissues as well as the skin,
the term angioedema is used to describe an essentially similar pathophysiologic process. In the older literature the word angioneurotic edema is frequently employed instead of angioedema. However, as there is little evidence
at present for a primary neurogenic mechanism in most individuals with
angioedema, the name angioneurotic edema should be abandoned. Current
evidence would suggest that identical urticarial skin lesions may be produced
by a wide variety of immunologic and nonimmunologic causes.

In considering both the prevalence and pathogenesis of urticarial lesions,
a sharp distinction must be made between acute and chronic urticaria.
All urticaria, of course, begins as acute urticaria. Its prevalence in the
general population has been estimated at 10 to 25 per cent. Chronic urticaria, on the other hand, may be arbitrarily defined as recurrent urticarial
skin lesions and/or angioedema lasting more than 8 weeks. No reliable
figures are available concerning the epidemiology or natural history of
chronic urticaria because patients are rarely hospitalized for this condition
and there is negligible mortality. However, there is sufficient data available
to conclude that chronic urticaria occurs more commonly in individuals
with a personal or family history of asthma and hay fever and that it
is rare in children under the age of 5 years.

ETIOLOGY

Allergic reactions to foods, drugs, insects, and physical agents as well as
psychologic stress account for a large proportion of isolated episodes of
acute urticaria. The causative factor in acute urticaria is usually quite
obvious to the patient, medical attention is seldom sought, and there is
rarely any need for detailed investigation.

In chronic urticaria, however, there is considerable disagreement as to
the actual percentage of cases in which definite etiologic factors are un-

equivocally established. In one large series of patients with chronic urticaria, no specific cause was found in 70 per cent of patients, 22 per cent were classified as psychogenic, and in only 8 per cent were allergic or physical factors thought to be of significance.[11] Nevertheless, the possible causes of chronic urticaria are reviewed below in some detail because removal of specific causative factors constitutes the simplest and most effective form of treatment of this annoying and troublesome affliction (see Table 5-4).

TABLE 5-4. Causes of Chronic Urticarial Lesions

Idiopathic (90 per cent of cases)
Drugs
Foods
Infection
Physical allergy
    Heat, cold, sunlight, effort
Dermographism
Urticaria pigmentosa
Inhalant allergens
Systemic diseases
    Collagen-vascular diseases, infectious mononucleosis, serum hepatitis, Hodgkin's disease, cancer, and amyloidosis

Drugs

Urticaria as a manifestation of drug allergy may occur as an isolated symptom or as part of the serum sickness syndrome (see Chapter 2). Urticaria due to drugs may result either from an antigen-antibody reaction or from drug-induced histamine release. Commonly used drugs which induce non-immunologic histamine release in man or experimental animals include the opium alkaloids (especially codeine), d-tubocurare, polymyxin B, thiamine, and sodium dehydrocholate. The most common causes of drug-induced allergic urticaria include: penicillin and its derivatives, tetracycline and its derivatives, the phenothiazine derivatives, and the sulfonamides (including chemically related drugs such as chlorothiazide, acetazolamide and tolbutamide). Although it is generally assumed that many drugs, such as those listed above, produce urticaria on an allergic basis, the immunologic mechanisms are poorly understood.

Two of the commonest causes of drug-induced urticaria, acetylsalicylic acid and penicillin, present special problems which make the role of allergy difficult to assess in individual cases. It has been observed that approximately one-third of patients with chronic urticaria will note aggravation of their symptoms following the use of aspirin; the aggravation is proportional to the dosage. One suggested mechanism for this nonimmunologic type of response is that aspirin and related compounds may increase the sensitivity of peripheral chemoreceptors to the chemical mediators of allergic reactions[24] (see Chapter 20). The significance of trace amounts of penicillin in dairy products as a cause of persistent urticaria is equally difficult to evaluate because of the paucity of well controlled studies in this area.

Foods

Certain foods which are commonly associated with *acute* urticaria, such as shellfish, strawberries, and citrus fruits, contain potent histamine liberating substances which may contribute considerably to the development of urticaria in some individuals. The importance of foods in the etiology of *chronic* urticaria has probably been greatly overemphasized over the years by patients and physicians alike.

Infection

Urticaria may occur during the course of parasitic infections, presumably as the result of an allergic reaction to foreign proteins. This form of urticaria is seen most commonly in helminthic infections such as ascariasis, hookworm infection, strongyloidiasis, filariasis, echinococcocis, and schistosomiasis, but may also occur less commonly with protozoan infections such as malaria, giardiasis, amebiasis, trichomoniasis. Parasitic diseases are relatively uncommon in temperate climates, and thus represent an infrequent cause of chronic urticaria in North America and Europe.

Chronic urticaria has been attributed to foci of bacterial infection, but the evidence for this hypothesis is less well substantiated than for parasitic diseases.

Physical Allergy

Urticaria secondary to cold, light, heat, and effort are well documented but uncommon entities.

Cold urticaria typically occurs following a sudden drop in air temperature, immersion of the extremities in cold water, or the handling of cold objects. Occasional cases of drowning due to histamine shock after diving into cold water have been reported in patients known to be susceptible to cold urticaria. Cold urticaria may occur as an idiopathic or familial phenomenon, or may be associated with underlying disease processes such as cryoglobulinemia, cryofibrinogenemia, paroxysmal cold hemoglobinuria, or the presence of cold hemagglutinins (see Chapter 9).

Whealing on exposure to sunlight (solar urticaria) is one of the rarer forms of dermatologic reactions to light. The lesions occur over the exposed areas of the body and are triggered in any individual patient by ultraviolet light of a specific wave length (action spectrum). The majority of patients are sensitive to light at wave lengths of about 300 mμ, but action spectra between 400 to 500 mμ are found in a significant number of patients. Solar urticaria is usually idiopathic, but may occasionally be associated with porphyria.

Generalized urticaria provoked by heat and effort (cholinergic urticaria) is characterized by the appearance of minute (1 to 3 mm) wheals surrounded by a disproportionately large flare. The lesions tend to appear immediately following exposure to heat, exercise, strong emotion, or bathing in hot water. This form of urticaria is almost always associated with sweating, and can be reproduced by the intradermal injection of cholinergic drugs. Conversely, no lesions will appear over sympathectomized areas where there is a complete absence of sweating. However, the etiologic role of cholinergic substances in the pathogenesis of this form of urticaria is by no means unequivocally established. Localized heat urticaria is a rare syndrome in which the topical application of heat produces a localized wheal, but there are no symptoms after physical exertion or the intradermal injection of cholinergic drugs.[7]

Dermographism

Dermographism consists of an immediate wheal and flare reaction following light stroking of the skin.[9] Clinically, lesions may occur in pressure areas, along the belt line, or beneath tight undergarments. Dermographism is an occasional feature of chronic urticaria due to other causes, but more frequently appears as an isolated, idiopathic condition. For reasons which are not well understood, acute urticarial penicillin reactions may be followed by dermographism which persists for months or years after the acute episode.

Pressure urticaria differs from dermographism in that the lesions appear only after sustained heavy pressure and only after a latent period of several hours. Typically, the patient develops massive swelling of the feet after walking for several miles, or swelling of the hands after carrying a heavy weight. Pressure urticaria must also be differentiated from hereditary angioedema.

Urticaria Pigmentosa

Urticaria pigmentosa is an infrequent disease characterized by infiltration of the dermis with mast cells. Stroking of the typical reddish-brown, flat papules produces localized urticaria due to histamine release. The condition is usually a mild disorder of children which disappears at puberty in 70 per cent of patients. However, in some children, and in most adults with the disease, there may be infiltration of the spleen, lymph nodes, liver, and bones with mast cells (systemic mastocytosis) in addition to cutaneous involvement. Some patients with systemic mastocytosis may experience flushing, hypotensive episodes, headaches, or asthma due to generalized release of histamine and serotonin.

Inhalant Allergens

Potent inhalant allergens such as pollens, animal danders, or the odor of cooked fish may occasionally produce urticaria, even in the absence of respiratory symptoms.

Other Diseases

Chronic urticaria sometimes occurs during the course of other systemic diseases such as systemic lupus erythematosus or other collagen-vascular diseases, infectious mononucleosis, serum hepatitis, Hodgkin's disease, cancer, and amyloidosis.

PATHOPHYSIOLOGY

Much attention has been focussed in recent years on the role of chemical mediators in the pathogenesis of urticaria.[30] The localized vasodilatation, increased capillary permeability, and pruritus that characterize urticaria can all be reproduced by the intradermal injection of histamine. Furthermore, there is experimental evidence to suggest that histamine is released in some forms of urticaria. In many patients with cold urticaria, an increase in plasma histamine concentration is found in venous blood returning from limbs exposed to the cold.[15a] It has also been reported that the average level of blood histamine is slightly elevated in patients with chronic urticaria.[21] The average value of histamine in biopsies of urticarial wheals is lower than in normal skin, and an accentuated reaction to histamine iontophoresis is observed in patients with chronic urticaria.

Despite the demonstrated significance of histamine, many other chemical mediators are known to produce dilatation of small blood vessels and increased capillary permeability. The importance of substances such as acetylcholine, serotonin, kinins, and proteases in the pathogenesis of human urticaria remains to be established. None of the postulated chemical mediators except histamine are capable of producing the intense pruritus that is usually a prominent symptom in human urticaria. On the other hand, the duration of action of histamine is considered to be too short to explain all of the clinical manifestations of urticaria and angioedema.

IMMUNOLOGY

The reagin-mediated release of chemical mediators is the probable mechanism underlying acute urticaria which is clearly due to specific extrinsic allergens such as certain drugs or foods. The role of immunologic factors in other forms of acute or chronic urticaria is less well established. It is conceivable that antigen-antibody interaction may result in the release of anaphylatoxin secondary to activation of the complement sequence (see Chapter 1). Anaphylatoxins are known to be capable of releasing histamine from mast cells and thereby may be responsible for changes in capillary permeability.

In one patient with cold urticaria and cryoglobulinemia, it was shown that the cryoglobulin was exclusively kappa type IgG, the cold urticaria could be passively transferred to normal recipients by means of the isolated cold precipitable IgG, and there was a drop in complement levels in the patient's serum after the production of cold urticaria.[6] Solar urticaria has, on occasion, been passively transferred by serum to normal recipients. Another interesting, but unexplained finding is the association of chronic urticaria, chronic infection, and significantly depressed levels of IgG, IgA, and IgM in infants and children.[5]

CLINICAL MANIFESTATIONS

The cutaneous lesions of urticaria and angioedema are sufficiently distinctive to rarely present a problem in differential diagnosis.

The typical urticarial wheal consists of elevated red or whitish papules, macules, or patches of varying size and shape on an erythematous base. The lesions produced by scabies or biting insects usually have a characteristic distribution, but may occasionally be confused with urticaria. Angioedema, particularly of the face, should be distinguished from myxedema, nephrotic syndrome, superior vena cava syndrome, and trichiniasis. Idiopathic edema of the eyelids, particularly on arising, is a relatively common symptom in women over the age of 40 years. No underlying immunologic, endocrine, or metabolic abnormality is found in the majority of patients with angioedema limited to the eyelids.

DIAGNOSIS

Because most cases of urticaria and angioedema are idiopathic in nature, special diagnostic procedures are unnecessary unless the history or examination suggests one of the specific causes discussed in the section on etiology.

Allergy skin tests are sometimes helpful in confirming that acute urticaria is due to food or insect allergens. In most patients, skin tests should be limited to allergens which appear to have an historic relationship to acute symptoms.

The diagnosis of *"cholinergic"* urticaria may be supported by an intradermal test with 0.05 ml of methacholine (1:5000). A positive reaction consists of a flare greater than 20 mm with or without satellite wheals. *Cold* urticaria may be demonstrated by placing an ice cube on the skin for 5 minutes followed by warming of the site. Unless a source of monochromatic light is available, the diagnosis of *solar* urticaria is most easily confirmed by exposing the skin to the unfiltered rays from a Kromayer mercury arc lamp for 1 to 2 minutes. If no localized urticaria results, then a further test may be performed by 10 to 15 minutes' exposure to rays from the Kromayer lamp filtered through plate glass.

The diagnosis of *urticaria pigmentosa* is made by biopsy of the suspected skin lesions. Special stains such as Giemsa or toluidine blue are required to demonstrate the characteristic histologic features. A typical biopsy specimen shows infiltration of the upper half of the dermis with mast cells containing numerous cytoplasmic granules. The granules are a source of histamine, serotonin, and possibly other chemical mediators liberated in this condition.

TREATMENT

About 90 per cent of patients will obtain some relief of symptoms with antihistamine medication. In most cases of acute or chronic urticaria due to any cause, therapy may be initiated with chlorpheniramine, 4 to 8 mg, four times daily. If no relief is obtained, hydroxyzine, 10 to 25 mg, four times daily, or cyproheptadine, 4 mg, three times daily may prove to be more effective. Hydroxyzine is more potent than chlorpheniramine in suppressing experimentally induced histamine wheals in humans. Cyproheptadine possesses both antihistamine and antiserotonin activity, but there is no definite evidence that its antiserotonin properties are responsible for suppression of urticaria.

Corticosteroids have a very unpredictable effect in both acute and chronic urticaria. There is, therefore, little justification for their use when less hazardous drugs are almost always beneficial. Aqueous epinephrine (0.5 ml of 1:1000 solution) given subcutaneously will often produce dramatic, but temporary, relief of the manifestations of acute urticaria.

Drugs and foods known to produce acute urticaria should, of course, be avoided. On the other hand, elimination diets have been demonstrated to be of no value in 75 per cent of cases of chronic urticaria and only slightly helpful in 19 per cent.[11]

Avoidance of excessive exposure to light, heat, or sudden drop in temperature is an essential part of the treatment of urticaria due to physical allergy. A sunscreen cream such as one of the commercial preparations containing titanium dioxide and menthyl anthranilate is occasionally helpful in reducing the severity of solar urticaria.

Most cases of "cholinergic urticaria" can be managed successfully with antihistamine drugs as outlined above. The occasional patient with refractory symptoms may respond to propantheline bromide, 15 mg, three times daily.

HEREDITARY ANGIOEDEMA

Hereditary angioedema (HAE) is a rare familial disease characterized by recurrent episodes of acute edema of the skin, upper respiratory tract, and gastrointestinal tract. There has been considerable interest in this condition in recent years because an inherited biochemical defect has been demonstrated as the cause.[20]

PATHOPHYSIOLOGY

The nature of the biochemical defect in HAE is related to the absence or functional deficiency of the normal α_2-globulin inhibitor of C1 esterase (see Chapter 1). The same α_2-globulin (α_2 neuraminoglycoprotein) also appears to inhibit plasma permeability factors such as PF/dil, kallikrein and plasmins, as well as other complement components. In addition, it has been shown that this deficiency, through mechanisms which are not yet completely understood, leads to the release of a small polypeptide molecule that increases cutaneous vascular permeability.[8]

The mechanism by which a deficiency of the natural inhibitor of C1 esterase leads to the manifestations of hereditary angioedema has led to considerable speculation.[22a] It has been shown that the intradermal injection of activated C1 esterase (in the form of purified C1s) will produce localized, self-limited angioedema in normal individuals, and will reproduce an attack of angioedema in genetically predisposed individuals. Furthermore, it has been established that acute attacks of HAE are associated with the appearance of activated C1 esterase (C1s) in the patient's blood. It is also possible that the unopposed action of substances such as PF/dil, kallikrein, and plasmins may play an important role in the pathogenesis of HAE.

The laboratory diagnosis of hereditary angioedema requires the demonstration of a functional deficiency of C1 esterase inhibitor in the patient's serum.[23] The detection of decreased levels of C2 or C4, the natural substrates of C1 esterase, constitutes a reliable and relatively simple screening test for HAE. In the absence of C1 esterase inhibitor, the unopposed action of C1 esterase on C2 or C4 diminishes their serum concentrations (see Chapter 1). The levels of C2 and C4 in patients with HAE are lower than normal in asymptomatic periods and tend to drop to even lower levels during acute attacks.

CLINICAL MANIFESTATIONS

In typical patients, HAE has its onset in early adolescence, persists through adult life, and, if the patient survives, becomes less severe after the age of 45 years. There appears to be no relationship between other allergic disorders and HAE.

Clinically, HAE is readily distinguished from other urticarial diseases by its inheritance as an autosomal dominant trait (Fig. 5-2), the absence of urticaria and pruritus, and the frequent association between trauma and localized attacks of edema. Characteristically, local edema may occur on the extremities or face several hours after minor trauma and usually disappears within 24 to 48 hours (Fig. 5-3). Apparently spontaneous episodes of edema of the tongue, soft palate, or larynx may constitute a life-threatening emergency. Involvement of the gastrointestinal tract is common and may produce symptoms of nausea, vomiting, diarrhea, and colic. Unless the correct diagnosis is recognized, many patients with HAE undergo unnecessary abdominal surgery.

The most serious aspect of the disease is the frequent occurrence of laryngeal edema of sufficient severity to result in death from asphyxiation. Dental surgery is particularly hazardous in patients with HAE. It has been estimated that approximately 20 per cent of patients with HAE die from acute upper respiratory obstruction, usually before the age of 30. In this respect, HAE differs from ordinary benign nonfamilial angioedema in which there is a negligible mortality due to respiratory obstruction.

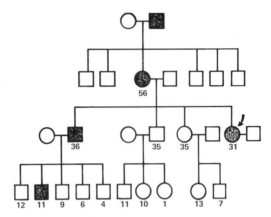

FIG. 5-2. Pedigree of the T. family indicating members with clinical symptoms of hereditary angioedema. Patient whose hand is shown in Figure 5-3 is indicated by **arrow**. In interpreting findings in the fourth generation, it should be noted that symptoms usually do not appear until adolescence.

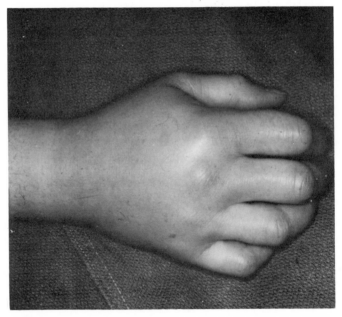

FIG. 5-3. Characteristic edema of the hand following minor trauma in a female patient with hereditary angioedema. Episode occurred 12 hours after patient had used scissors to cut a thick piece of carpet.

TREATMENT

The treatment of HAE is difficult to assess because of its episodic nature. Methyltestosterone, in doses of 5 to 10 mg daily, is occasionally useful in reducing the frequency and severity of acute episodes, but its mode of action is not understood. Abdominal pain may be severe enough to require parenteral meperidine for relief. Acute laryngeal edema may respond to subcutaneous epinephrine. However, if rapid improvement does not occur, immediate tracheostomy and assisted respiration is indicated as a life-saving procedure. Antihistamines and corticosteroids are of questionable value in HAE.

BULLOUS DERMATOSES

In recent years, there has been a certain amount of evidence to implicate immunologic factors in the pathogenesis of dermatoses characterized by bullous or vesicular lesions. A bulla (or bleb) may be defined as an elevation of the epidermis, beneath which there is an accumulation of serum, plasma, or blood. A vesicle is similar to a bulla, but is smaller in size. A number of apparently unrelated dermatologic conditions with immunologic features are characterized by the formation of bullae or vesicles which may occur either singly or in groups.

PEMPHIGUS AND BULLOUS PEMPHIGOID

By means of an indirect immunofluorescent technique, it has been shown that the sera of approximately two-thirds of patients with pemphigus vulgaris contain an antibody which localizes in the intercellular areas of stratified squamous epithelium.[19] The areas of immunofluorescent staining correspond to the intraepithelial bullae which are considered to be the hallmark of pemphigus vulgaris. There appears to be good correlation between the level of antibodies and the severity of the disease. A possible clue to the significance of autoantibodies in pemphigus and other bullous dermatoses is provided by animal experiments in which antiepithelial antibodies were shown to facilitate acantholysis.[12] The process of acantholysis (separation of individual cells from the epidermis and their subsequent isolation within the fluid of a bulla or vesicle) is an important pathologic feature of most of the bullous dermatoses.

By contrast, antibodies localized to the epithelial basement membrane are detected by the indirect immunofluorescence technique in the sera of approximately two-thirds of patients with bullous pemphigoid. No anti-bodies of either the intraepithelial or basement membrane type are found in the sera of patients with dermatitis herpetiformis, erythema multiforme, or other bullous skin diseases.[2] Thus, immunofluorescent studies may be extremely helpful in distinguishing pemphigus vulgaris, which is associated with a high fatality rate, from the more benign lesions of bullous pemphigoid. Furthermore, bullous pemphigoid is frequently difficult to distinguish from dermatitis herpetiformis or erythema multiforme on clinical grounds or by classic histologic methods, and it is likely that immunofluorescent serologic tests will prove to be of considerable value in their differential diagnosis (see Table 5-5).

TABLE 5-5. Patterns of Immunofluorescent Staining in Bullous Dermatoses

	Intra-epithelial	Epithelial basement membrane	Epidermal nuclei
Pemphigus vulgaris	+	−	−
Bullous pemphigoid	−	+	−
Dermatitis herpetiformis	−	−	−
Erythema multiforme bullosum	−	−	−
Pemphigus erythematosus	+	−	+

Pemphigus erythmatosus (Sennear-Usher syndrome) has clinical and pathologic features suggestive of both pemphigus vulgaris and systemic lupus erythematosus. The impression was confirmed by indirect immunofluorescence studies in which there was staining of both intraepithelial substance and epidermal nuclei (antinuclear antibodies)[14a] (see Chapter 8).

DERMATITIS HERPETIFORMIS

The lesions of dermatitis herpetiformis consist of groups of pruritic vesicles or bullae distributed symmetrically over the scapular regions, buttocks, or extremities. Collections of eosinophils are frequently, but not invariably, found within the vesicles. Decreased levels of serum IgA have been reported in this disease.[15]

ERYTHEMA MULTIFORME AND STEVENS-JOHNSON SYNDROME

Erythema multiforme is a polymorphous skin eruption characterized by the appearance of concentric erythematous rings known as target or iris lesions. There is frequent occurrence of bullae (erythema multiforme bullosum) during the course of the disease. The mucous membranes may be involved as well as the skin. Stevens-Johnson syndrome is considered to be a more severe variant of erythema multiforme bullosum. It is characterized by fever, malaise, arthralgias, and bullous eruptions which may involve the skin, mucous membranes, and genitourinary tract. Toxic epidermal necrolysis is another severe variant of erythema multiforme bullosum in which the patient's skin appears as if it had been severely scalded. The etiology of erythema multiforme and its variants remains obscure, but hypersensitivity reactions to viruses or drugs have been frequently suggested as possible causes.

There is little doubt as to the direct cause and effect relationship between viral infection and the vesicular lesions of variola, varicella, herpes simplex, and herpes zoster. In the case of erythema multiforme, a more indirect relationship has been postulated. Herpes simplex virus has been isolated from throat swabbings in patients with erythema multiforme and there is frequently a rise in antibody titer to herpes virus. Hypersensitivity to herpes virus as a cause of erythema multiforme is also suggested by the observation that the local vesiculobullous lesions can be reproduced by the intradermal injection of antigen prepared from killed herpes simplex organisms.[25] *Mycoplasma pneumonia* has been isolated from blister fluid in severe cases of erythema multiforme, and titers of complement-fixing antibodies to *M. pneumonia* were elevated in the same individuals. Erythema multiforme also occurs in association with acute histoplasmosis.

Long-acting sulfonamides have been suspected as an etiologic agent in Stevens-Johnson syndrome, but this widely held impression was not confirmed in a detailed retrospective study.[3] The importance of other anti-infective drugs in the pathogenesis of erythema multiforme is even more difficult to assess because it is usually impossible to decide whether the lesions appeared as a result of an alleged infection or as the result of a drug used to treat the infection.

ERYTHEMA NODOSUM

The lesions of erythema nodosum consist of multiple, painful subcutaneous nodules which occur mainly on the anterior aspects of the lower part of the leg. Less commonly, there may be similar lesions on the arms, trunk, or face. Swelling of the legs and ankles as the result of lymphatic obstruction is a frequent complication, and the disease is usually associated with fever, arthralgia, and malaise. Microscopic examination of typical lesions reveals swelling and fragmentation of collagen fibers in the lower layers of the dermis, evidence of vasculitis, and infiltration with giant cells of the foreign body type. The etiology is unknown, but has been attributed to hypersensitivity reactions to infective agents or drugs.

There is no direct immunologic evidence to link erythema nodosum with any specific causative agent. However, the disease is frequently seen in association with a number of systemic disease states, suggesting a possible relationship. At the present time, one of the more commonly reported syndromes is that of erythema nodosum, diffuse arthralgias, fever, and bilateral hilar lymphadenopathy occurring during the early stages of sarcoidosis. Other relatively common associations include acute histoplasmosis, coccidioidomycosis, lymphogranuloma venereum, ulcerative colitis, and leukemia. In the older literature, tuberculosis and streptococcal infections are mentioned frequently as possible causes. As is the case with erythema multiforme, alleged allergic reactions to drugs are extremely difficult to evaluate as etiologic factors.

PAPULAR MUCINOSIS (LICHEN MYXOMATOSUS)

Papular mucinosis (lichen myxomatosus) is a relatively uncommon condition. It has been described as generalized localized myxedema. The typical papular lesions usually occur in rows on the extremities or on the face, and are characterized by deposits of mucin in the cutis. The observation that the skin becomes hardened and fibrotic in some patients with papular mucinosis has led to the suggestion that the disease is a variant of scleroderma.

The sera of some, but not all, patients with papular mucinosis contains an abnormal γ-globulin which appears to be characteristic of the disease.[13] The specific protein (PM protein) is closely related to myeloma proteins in that it is homogeneous in electrophoretic mobility and homogeneous with respect to light chain antigenic groups. However, the benign clinical course of papular mucinosis is quite different from multiple myeloma with cutaneous involvement (see Chapter 10). The sera of patients with scleroderma-like lesions are more likely to contain the PM protein than are the sera of patients with predominantly papular skin lesions.

VITILIGO

An interesting association between vitiligo and a tendency to increased autoantibody formation has been reported.[4a] In a series of 80 patients there was a significantly increased incidence of autoantibodies directed against thyroid cytoplasm, thyroglobulin, gastric parietal cells, and adrenal cytoplasm as compared to control subjects. There is also a clinical association between vitiligo and thyroiditis, pernicious anemia, and diabetes mellitus. The precise significance of these findings in relation to the pathogenesis of vitiligo is not understood at present.

REFERENCES

1. Baer, R. L., and Harber, L. C. Photosensitivity induced by drugs. *J.A.M.A.* *192:*989, 1965.

2. Beutner, E. H., Rhodes, E. L., and Holborrow, E. J. Autoimmunity in chronic bullous skin diseases. Immunofluorescent demonstration of three types of antibody to skin in sera of patients with pemphigus, bullous pemphigoid and in other human sera. *Clin. Exp. Immun. 2:*141, 1967.

3. Bianchine, J. R., Macaraeg, P. V. J., Lasagna, L., Azaroff, D. L., Brunk, S. F., Huidberg, E. F., and Owen, J. A. Drugs as etiologic factors in Stevens-Johnson syndrome. *Amer. J. Med. 44:*390, 1968.

4. Birmingham, D. J. Skin hygiene and dermatitis in industry. *Arch. Environ. Health (Chicago) 10:*653, 1965.

4a. Brostoff, J., Bor, S., and Feiwel, M. Autoantibodies in patients with vitiligo. *Lancet 2:*177, 1969.

5. Buckley, R. H., and Dees, S. C. Serum immunoglobulins. III. Abnormalities associated with chronic urticaria in children. *J. Allerg. 40:*294, 1967.

6. Constanzi, J. J., Coltman, C. A., Jr., and Donaldson, V. H. Activation of complement by a monoclonal cryoglobulin associated with cold urticaria. *J. Lab. Clin. Med. 74:*902, 1969.

7. Delorme, P. Localized Heat Urticaria. *J. Allerg. 43:*284, 1969.

8. Donaldson, V. H., Ratnoff, O. D., DaSilva, W. D., and Rosen, F. S. Permeability-increasing activity in hereditary angioneurotic edema plasma. II. Mechanism of formation and partial characterization. *J. Clin. Invest. 48:*642, 1969.

9. Ebken, R. K., Bauschard, F. A., and Levine, M. I. Dermographism: Its definition, demonstration and prevalence. *J. Allerg. 41:*338, 1968.

10. Freedman, S. O., and Fish, A. J. The passive cellular transfer of delayed type hypersensitivity to intradermal procaine. *J. Invest. Derm. 38:*363, 1963.

11. Green, G. R., Koelsche, G. A., and Kierland, R. R. Etiology and pathogenesis of chronic urticaria. *Ann. Allerg. 23:*30, 1965.

12. Inderbitzen, T. H., and Grob, P. J. Destruction of epithelial cells in-vivo by antiepithelial antibodies. *J. Invest. Derm. 49:*642, 1967.

13. James, K., Fudenberg, H. H., Epstein, W. L., and Shuster, J. Studies on a unique diagnostic serum globulin in papular mucinosis (lichen myxedematosus). *Clin. Exp. Immun., 2:*153, 1967.

14. Kaufman, H. S., Frick, O. L., and Fink, D. Serum complement (β_{1C}) in young children with atopic dermatitis. *J. Allerg. 42:1*, 1968.

14a. Kay, D. M., and Tuffanelli, D. L. Immunofluorescent techniques in clinical diagnosis of cutaneous disease. *Ann. Intern. Med. 71:753*, 1969.

15. Kjartansson, S., Fusaro, R. M., and Peterson, W. C., Jr. Dermatitis herpetiformis and herpes gestationis. Analysis of A and M serum proteins by immunoelectrophoresis. *J. Invest. Derm. 46:480*, 1966.

15a. Mathews, K. P., and Pan, P. M. Postexercise hyperhistaminemia, dermographia and wheezing. *Ann. Intern. Med. 72:241*, 1970.

15b. Melish, M. E. and Glasgow, L. A. The staphylococcal scalded skin syndrome. Development of an experimental model. *New Eng. J. Med. 282:1114*, 1970.

16. Mitchell, J. C., Fritig, B., Singh, B., and Towers, G. H. N. Allergic contact dermatitis from *Frullania* and *Compositae*. The role of sesquiterpene lactones. *J. Invest. Derm. 54:233*, 1970.

17. Olive, J. T., Jr., O'Connell, E. J., Winkelman, R. K., and Logan, G. B. Delayed blanch phenomenon in children. Reevaluation of 5-year-old children originally tested as newborns. *J. Invest. Derm. 54:546*, 1970.

18. Palacios, J. J., and Blaylock, W. K. The response of lymphocytes in tissue culture to normal and diseased skin extracts. *J. Invest. Derm. 49:214*, 1967.

19. Peck, S. M., Osserman, K. E., Weiner, L. B., Lefkovits, A., and Osserman, R. S. Studies in bullous diseases. Immunofluorescent serologic tests. *New Eng. J. Med. 279:951*, 1968.

20. Pickering, R. J., Gewurz, H., Kelly, J. R., and Good, R. A. The complement system in hereditary angioneurotic oedema—A new perspective. *Clin. Exp. Immun. 3:423*, 1968.

21. Prasad, D. N., Gambhir, S. S., Singh, G., Bhattacharya, S. K., and Das, S. K. Histamine skin sensitivity and blood histamine in patients with urticaria. *Int. Arch. Allergy. 31:230*, 1967.

21a. Rosen, F. S., and Austen, K. F.: The "neurotic edema" (hereditary angioedema). *New Eng. J. Med. 280:1356*, 1969.

22. Roth, H. L., and Kierland, R. R. The natural history of atopic dermatitis. A 20 year follow-up study. *Arch. Derm. (Chicago) 89:209*, 1964.

23. Ruddy, S., and Austen, K. F. Stoichiometric assay for fourth component of complement in whole human serum using EAC'1a^{gp} and functionally pure human second component. *J. Immunol. 99:1162*, 1967.

24. Samter, M., and Beers, R. F., Jr. Intolerance to aspirin: Clinical studies and consideration of its pathogenesis. *Ann. Intern. Med. 68:975*, 1968.

25. Shelley, W. B. Herpes simplex virus as a cause of erythema multiforme. *J.A.M.A. 201:153*, 1967.

26. Shelley, W. B. The patch test. *J.A.M.A. 5:200*, 1967.

27. Solomon, L. M., and Beerman, H. Atopic dermatitis. *Amer. J. Med. Sci. 252:478*, 1966.

28. Solomon, L. M., and Nadler, N. J. Radioautography of nor-adrenaline—¹⁴C in atopic dermatitis. *Canad. Med. Ass. J. 96:*1147, 1967.

29. Sommer, R. G., and Jillson, O. T. Phytophotodermatitis (solar dermatitis from plants). Gas plant and wild parsnip. *New Eng. J. Med. 276:*1485, 1967.

30. Thompson, J. S. Urticaria and angioedema. *Ann. Intern. Med. 69:*361, 1968.

31. Torsney, P., and Blumstein, G. I. Atopic dermatitis and congenital defects, disease and mortality. *Ann. Allerg. 25:*93, 1967.

32. Varelzidis, A., Wilson, A. B., Meara, R. H., and Turk, J. L. Immunoglobulin levels in atopic eczema. *Brit. Med. J., 2:*295, 1966.

33. Winkelman, R. K. Nonallergic factors in atopic dermatitis. *J. Allerg. 37:*29, 1966.

6

Clinical Immunology of the Kidney

DAVID HAWKINS

There is little doubt that immunologic factors play an important role in the production of many human renal diseases. For several years immunologic renal disease has been studied intensively in experimental animal models and through these studies has come an understanding of the immunopathogenetic mechanisms capable of producing renal injury.

EXPERIMENTAL IMMUNOLOGIC RENAL DISEASE

It has been found that experimental immunologic renal disease can be produced in one of two ways. In one model the animal is induced to make or is injected with antibody (Ab) that reacts with its own glomerular basement membrane (GBM), while in the other model the host antibody reacts with a nonglomerular antigen (Ag) which may be either endogenous or exogenous in origin.[4] In the first or "anti-GBM type" of immunologic renal disease the antibody is specifically localized along the glomerular basement membrane, whereas in the second or "immune complex type" the circulating antibody non-GBM antigen complexes are passively trapped or

152

filtered out by the glomerulus. Some of the characteristics of these two immunopathogenetic processes are summarized and compared in Table 6-1.

TABLE 6-1. Characteristics of the Two Immunopathogenetic Types of Glomerulonephritis

Anti-GBM type	Immune-complex type
Antibody directed against host glomerular basement membrane	Antibody directed against endogenous or exogenous nonglomerular antigens
Host Ab and C† found in linear, smooth continuous pattern by immunofluorescence along GBM	Immune reactants (Ag,* host Ab, and C†) found by immunofluorescence in lumpy, granular, discontinuous distribution along GBM
Linear subendothelial deposits or a subendothelial clear space may be found by electron microscopy along GBM	Electron dense lumpy deposits seen subepithelially along GBM by electron microscopy
Anti-GBM antibody may be found in circulation, more readily after total nephrectomy	Immune complexes, Ag, or occasionally Ab may be found in circulation
Masugi or nephrotoxic nephritis and experimental allergic glomerulonephritis are models of this type	Experimental models include serum sickness nephritis in rabbits and Heymann's nephritis or autologous immune complex disease in rats
Goodpasture's syndrome is prototype of human examples	Human diseases include SLE nephritis and nephrotic syndrome with quartan malaria

* Not yet specifically identified in many cases presumed due to immune complexes.
† Complement.

"ANTI-GBM TYPE" GLOMERULONEPHRITIS

The "anti-GBM type" of nephritis was first produced in animals by the administration of antisera to their own GBM which had been produced in a heterologous species (e.g., sheep anti-rabbit GBM). This disease is called nephrotoxic or Masugi nephritis. Subsequently, it was found that immunization of animals with heterologous, homologous or even autologous GBM antigens could result in nephritis.

This experimental allergic glomerulonephritis is characterized by the deposition of host antibody and often complement in a smooth, continuous, linear pattern along the GBM where they are readily demonstrable by immunofluorescent techniques (Fig. 6-1). Occasionally, the immune reactants may also be identified by electron microscopy as a linear subendothelial electron dense deposit or they may produce a subendothelial "clear" space.

The antibody can be eluted from the kidney and shown to have anti-GBM specificity, and the disease can be transferred to normal homologous recipients by serum.[28] Anti-GBM antibody is found in quantity in the circulation of nephritic animals much more readily after total nephrectomy, i.e., after removal of the large antigen pool.

"IMMUNE COMPLEX TYPE" GLOMERULONEPHRITIS

The first experimental model of the "immune-complex type" to be studied in depth was serum sickness nephritis in rabbits. Animals immunized with a heterologous protein antigen (Ag), such as bovine serum albumin, make antibodies against it which complex with the antigen in the circulation. The circulating soluble immune-complexes may then be trapped in the glomerulus and initiate tissue damage. Not all such complexes are pathogenic. For example, extremely small ones tend to remain in the circulation, whereas the largest are rapidly removed by the reticuloendothelial system. The intermediate complexes, large but still soluble, appear to be the most "toxic." The highest incidence of serum sickness nephritis is associated with a less than optimal antibody response.

In this process the immune reactants (i.e., host antibody, host complement, and the antigen), are demonstrable by immunofluorescence along the outer (epithelial) side of the GBM in a lumpy, granular, discrete, discontinuous pattern which is generally readily distinguishable from that seen in the "anti-GBM type" (Fig. 6-1). Furthermore, the immune deposits are often detectable by electron microscopy as discrete electron dense masses lying subepithelially along the GBM.

Experimentally, the most extensively studied disease of the "immune-complex type" is Heymann's nephritis in rats.[8] Immunization of rats with a nephritogenic antigen derived from homologous renal tubular cells results in formation of nonglomerular antigen-antibody complexes which are trapped in the glomerulus. However, the antibody also combines with small amounts of autologous antigen present in the circulation. It is these latter

---

FIG. 6-1. Photomicrographs of renal biopsies stained with fluorescent anti-human IgG. Biopsies on the *left* demonstrate low (*A*) and high (*B*) power views of linear fluorescence along the GBM indicative of anti-GBM antibodies. (From Lerner, R. A., Glassock, R. J., and Dixon, F. J. *J. Exper. Med. 126:*989, 1967.) Biopsies on the *right* (*C* and *D*) display a discontinuous, lumpy, fluorescent pattern along the GBM indicative of immune complex deposition. (Courtesy Dr. Keith Drummond, Montreal Children's Hospital.)

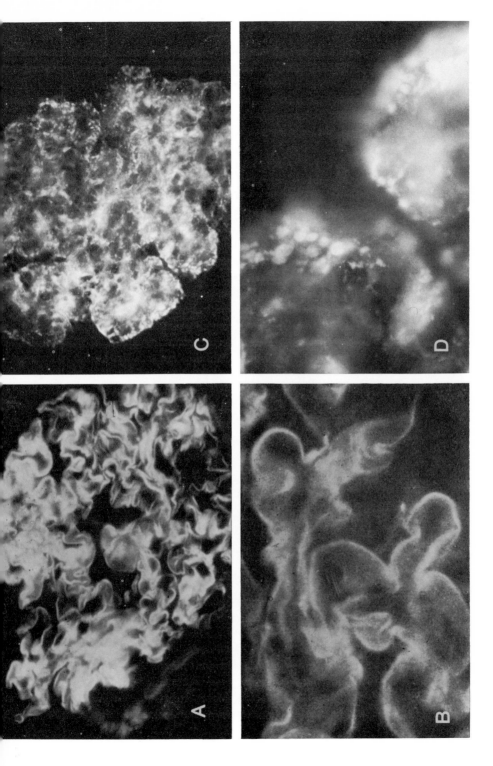

complexes which deposit in the kidney over several weeks and produce a membranous nephritis. Even though the initial stimulus is not autologous, the ultimate disease results from autologous immune complexes and may reasonably be called autoimmune.

MECHANISMS OF RENAL INJURY

In both types of experimental glomerulonephritis, the deposition of immune reactants in the glomerulus initiates a series of reactions which culminate in renal injury. These reactions frequently involve the fixation of host complement by antigen-antibody combination and the subsequent at attraction of polymorphonuclear leukocytes (PMN's) by complement-derived chemotactic factors. The PMN's contain various proteolytic enzymes and permeability factors which are capable of altering the GBM.[11] These pathogenetic pathways are depicted schematically in Figure 6-2.

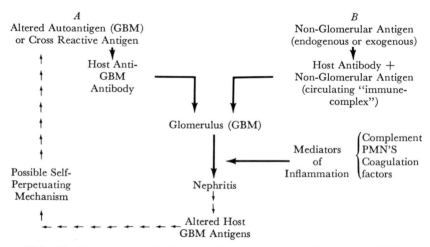

FIG. 6-2. Postulated mechanisms for the pathogenesis of glomerulonephritis.

The complement-PMN pathway is undoubtedly not the sole system for the mediation of immunologic tissue injury. However, its role has been clearly established in certain types of experimental nephritis and strongly implicated in certain human nephritides where complement is demonstrable by immunofluorescence and PMN's are seen lying adjacent to the GBM. The role of humoral factors, such as the kinin system, has not been elucidated.

Similarly the contribution of the coagulation mechanism to the pathogenesis of glomerulonephritis is uncertain. While they may or may not contribute to the acute injury, the coagulation factors may well be important in the production of subacute and chronic changes that lead to glomerular obliteration and renal failure. Fibrinogen derivatives are frequently identified in biopsy material by fluorescent antibody staining in acute poststreptococcal glomerulonephritis as well as in several other human nephritides.

There is in vitro evidence for cell-mediated hypersensitivity to GBM antigens in some patients with glomerulonephritis. However it has not been demonstrated that the sensitized cells are of importance in the pathogenesis of this disorder.

CORRELATION WITH HUMAN RENAL DISEASE

In most patients with nephritis, evidence for an immunologic process rests on the demonstration of immune reactants in the kidney by immunofluorescence and occasionally by electron microscopy. Certain other features, when present, support the concept of an immunologic mechanism, although the evidence they provide is more indirect. These latter features include: (1) the demonstration of a lag period between antigen exposure and the onset of overt clinical disease, (2) the lowering of serum complement levels, and (3) the pattern of light chain distribution in the deposited immunoglobulins. The finding that the light chain type distribution in the glomerular deposits does not reflect the serum light chain pattern suggests that the deposited immunoglobulin may be specific antibody.[12] Ideally, both the antibody and the antigen should be eluted from the diseased kidney and identified, but this is seldom feasible.

Because the immunologic evidence is generally indirect and because few patients have been studied in detail, the relatively neat pathogenetic classification of experimental immunologic renal disease cannot, as yet, be applied satisfactorily to human nephropathies. Nevertheless, a tentative classification is outlined in Table 6-2.

ACUTE GLOMERULONEPHRITIS

POSTSTREPTOCOCCAL GLOMERULONEPHRITIS

Etiology

Acute glomerulonephritis often follows acute Group A β-hemolytic streptococcal infections of the upper respiratory tract or skin. In contrast to the fairly constant attack rate in acute rheumatic fever, the rate in nephritis varies greatly from almost negligible to over one-third of the patients infected. This unusual variation in the incidence of acute glomerulonephritis

TABLE 6-2. Classification of Immunologic Renal Disease

Immune-Complex Type
　Systemic lupus erythematosus
　Nephrotic syndrome with quartan malaria
　Acute poststreptococcal glomerulonephritis
　Subacute and chronic glomerulonephritis (some cases)
　Membranous glomerulonephritis
　Associated with bacteremia (e.g., infected ventriculo-
　　atrial shunt, subacute bacterial endocarditis)
　Cryoglobulinemia, mixed type
　Serum sickness nephritis
　Post-transplantation nephritis (some cases)
　Nephrotic syndrome in syphilis
　D-penicillamine nephropathy

Anti-GBM Type
　Goodpasture's syndrome
　Subacute and chronic glomerulonephritis (some cases)
　Post-transplantation nephritis (some cases)

Mechanism Unknown (Possibly Immunologic)
　Congenital, familial nephrotic syndrome
　Cyclical nephrotic syndrome of pregnancy
　Hypersensitivity nephrotic disease (e.g., insect stings,
　　drugs)
　Anaphylactoid purpura
　Other collagen-vascular diseases (e.g., polyarteritis)
　Amyloidosis
　Multiple myeloma
　Toxemia of pregnancy
　Nephritis in infectious mononucleosis
　Renal vein thrombosis

---

was partially clarified by the demonstration that certain types of Group A β-hemolytic streptococci are "nephritogenic." The typing system is based on differences in a cellular antigen called M-protein. For example, M-types 12, 4, 25, and 49 ("Red Lake") are commonly involved, whereas M-types 1, 3, and 6 are less frequent offenders. Even so, infection with nephritogenic types does not always result in acute glomerulonephritis, and while this may be due to strain differences, it is also possible that differences in host response may play a significant role.

In some patients, organisms other than hemolytic streptococci have been implicated in the etiology of acute glomerulonephritis. These include pneumococcus, staphylococcus, nonhemolytic streptococci and viruses. The evidence which suggests that infectious agents other than β-hemolytic streptococci may cause acute glomerulonephritis will be discussed in the section on nonstreptoccal glomerulonephritis.

Immunopathology

Light microscopy of the kidney during the acute stage shows increased glomerular cellularity due to both fixed and circulating cells. The latter are predominantly polymorphonuclear leukocytes (PMN's) which may be found both within the capillary loops and between the capillary loops in the mesangial region. Endothelial swelling added to the PMN infiltration tends to obliterate the glomerular loops, giving an overall bloodless appearance. The disease is characteristically diffuse, although all glomeruli are not necessarily affected to the same extent. In addition to the proliferative changes there may be varied amounts of exudation. With healing, all these changes regress, although some may persist for as long as 2 years.

There appears to be reasonable evidence for considering acute post-streptococcal nephritis to be an immune-complex disease, although the manner in which certain nephritogenic streptococci initiate the process is unclear. In the majority of patients, fluorescent antibody studies show immunoglobulin and complement in a predominantly discontinuous granular fashion along the basement membrane, and ultrastructural studies demonstrate electron dense deposits along the epithelial side of the basement membrane. Furthermore, the demonstration by ferritin labelled antibody of streptococcal components in the same areas where immunoglobulin and complement were localized has lent further support to the concept of an immune-complex mechanism in the pathogenesis of *sporadic* poststreptococcal glomerulonephritis.[1] On the other hand, recent studies of *epidemic* acute poststreptococcal glomerulonephritis revealed a large number of patients with a focal discontinuous deposition of C3 alone.[7a]

It has also been shown that fluorescent-labelled IgG from the sera of patients with acute glomerulonephritis and from many normal persons will stain the glomerular basement membrane and mesangial areas in early acute glomerulonephritis. On the other hand, no such reaction is found when kidney tissue from other forms of renal disease or from normal subjects is used. The immunofluorescent binding of human IgG is abolished by prior absorption with cell membrane preparations derived from nephritogenic β-hemolytic streptococci, but not by the antigens of other bacteria. It appears that the streptococcal cell plasma membrane is largely responsible for blocking the immunofluorescent reaction.[27] However, other investigators have suggested that a cell wall component is the critical nephritogenic antigen.[1] In either case, the results strongly suggest that streptococcal antigens are present in the glomeruli of patients with acute poststreptococcal glomerulonephritis.

Despite the considerable evidence favoring an immune-complex process due to antibody and streptococcal antigen deposition, some investigators feel that the streptococcus may be antigenically related to human glomerular basement membrane, and infection may lead to the formation of a cross-reacting antibody which specifically localizes in the glomerulus. For instance, there is immunochemical evidence that certain fractions from type 12 nephritogenic streptococci have an antigenic relationship to human glomeruli. Other workers have suggested that the streptococcus may so alter glomerular basement membrane as to render it autoantigenic. However, if anti-GBM autoantibodies or autoantibodies cross-reactive with GBM were involved in the pathogenesis of acute poststreptococcal glomerulonephritis, a continuous, linear deposition of γ-globulin should be demonstrable along the GBM. Such a distribution is not seen in most patients with this disease.

Unfortunately, it has not been possible to develop an entirely satisfactory experimental model of acute poststreptococcal glomerulonephritis, presumably because β-hemolytic streptococcal infections do not occur naturally in most animal species. However, an experimental nephritis has been induced in rats with a strain of streptococcus which is nephritogenic for humans.[16] The disease seems to be due to immune complex deposition in the glomeruli, and the immunoglobulin in the complex shows a specificity for M protein.

Clinical Immunology

The most useful diagnostic procedures of an immunologic nature are those which provide evidence of recent streptococcal infection, and those which indicate that antigen-antibody interaction has occurred.

Antibodies appear early to the "extracellular" antigens of the streptococcus, e.g., antistreptolysin O (ASO) (see Chapter 21). The titer of antibodies to "extracellular" antigens bears no relationship to the possibility of glomerulonephritis, but may have prognostic significance. The highest ASO titers are often found in patients whose renal lesions eventually heal completely.[6] Antibiotics administered during the infection may considerably diminish the antibody response to extracellular antigens without affecting the subsequent course of the glomerulonephritis. Thus, a normal ASO titer is valid evidence against prior streptococcal infection only when antibiotics have not been administered.

Antibodies to the type specific M proteins, which are "cellular" antigens, develop more slowly than those directed against "extracellular" antigens, and tend to be much longer lasting. Presumably, they help confer type-specific immunity which prevents reinfection with the same nephritogenic strain, and may account for the rarity of second attacks of acute glomeruloneph- ritis. Penicillin will suppress the antibody response to M antigen, but the course of therapy must be prolonged and intense to completely prevent antibody production.

A particularly useful determination is that of serum complement. The complement is almost invariably depressed during the acute phase of glomerulonephritis and rises to normal levels with recovery. This depression is reflected in both total hemolytic complement activity (CH_{50}) and in decreased C3 levels. During the acute nephritic phase, the lowered comple- ment level probably reflects its activation in an antigen-antibody interaction. In some cases, there appears to be a prolonged and disproportionate depres- sion of serum C3 levels. It has been suggested that other mechanisms, such as impaired synthesis of C3 or inactivation of C3 by a lytic factor present in nephritic sera, may be responsible.[25] Immunoconglutinin, an antibody to hidden antigenic determinants of C3 and C4 (see Chapter 1), is also elevated in acute glomerulonephritis.

In the light of the current opinion that antikidney antibodies are not involved in the pathogenesis of acute poststreptococcal glomerulonephritis, their significance is unclear. They have been detected by a variety of tech- niques in the sera of some patients with glomerulonephritis. In most in- stances, the test antigen consisted of a crude extract of kidney. The nature of the antigens has not been determined, nor has any relationship been established between the presence of antikidney antibodies and the patho- genesis of acute poststreptococcal glomerulonephritis.

Clinical Manifestations

Proteinuria, hematuria, edema, hypertension, and azotemia are the cardinal clinical features. However, the picture may vary greatly from one of severe illness to one detectable only by abnormal urinary findings or renal morpho- logic changes.

Other characteristic signs and symptoms may consist of mild fever, malaise, headache, puffiness around the eyes and face, and tenderness in the area of the costovertebral angle. Urinary abnormalities include gross and microscopic hematuria, proteinuria, as well as hyaline, granular, and red cell casts. The latter are considered highly indicative of an acute glomerulonephritic process. With impaired renal function, there may be a decrease in the glomerular filtration rate (GFR) and an elevation of the blood urea nitrogen (BUN) and creatinine. The erythrocyte sedimentation rate is increased and a mild normocytic anemia, in part due to fluid retention, may be detected.

The disease generally appears 1 to 2 weeks after the inciting infection, but some patients show microscopic hematuria during the acute infection itself.

Complete clinical recovery within 3 to 4 weeks is the most common outcome. However, there is an acute mortality of 1 to 2 per cent, mainly due to complications. These include hypertensive encephalopathy, congestive heart failure, overwhelming infection, and severe glomerular damage with persistent anuria. The latter is a particularly ominous sign. The nephrotic syndrome may occur early in the acute phase of glomerulonephritis, but does not have the same serious prognostic significance as that which appears months or years after the initial episode.

Diagnosis

The clinical features described above, when superimposed on a picture of recent hemolytic streptococcal infection, provide strong evidence for a diagnosis of acute poststreptococcal glomerulonephritis. The microscopic demonstration of immune reactants and subepithelial deposits in the glomeruli, as well as decreased levels of serum complement, add weight to the diagnosis. It is important to remember, however, that similar clinical features may be seen in a variety of other disorders such as anaphylactoid purpura, systemic lupus erythematosus, Goodpasture's syndrome. and other forms of nonstreptococcal glomerulonephritis.

Natural History

The natural history, course, and prognosis of acute poststreptococcal glomerulonephritis are the subjects of considerable disagreement. The problem has arisen in part because diagnostic criteria are not clearly defined, and because many patients are first seen with subacute or chronic nephritis in whom no history of preceding acute nephritis can be obtained. The wider use of renal biopsy has improved the situation; now the clinical history and postmortem material are no longer the sole sources of information. Despite the fact that acute glomerulonephritis is commonly considered to be a disease of children and young adults, it is now being recognized with increasing frequency in the older age groups.

No evidence of chronic renal disease was found clinically or morphologically in 100 per cent of patients 10 years after the Red Lake epidemic of acute poststreptococcal glomerulonephritis.[22] However, other studies in the pediatric age group indicate that approximately 50 per cent of patients have histopathologic evidence of nonhealing after 2 years.[6] In another series of predominantly adult cases, all of whom were biopsied, there were 6 full recoveries, 5 deaths, and 14 patients with continued evidence of disease from several months to 5 years later. Thus, the generally excellent prognosis based on the Red Lake epidemic may have to be modified, particularly for adult populations.

Those who fail to recover may: (1) proceed directly into a rapidly progressive subacute phase with death in 6 to 18 months; (2) show slow but persistent disease proceeding to chronic nephritis; or (3) appear clinically well but present years later with chronic renal insufficiency. It is assumed that the last group of patients have a prolonged latent phase without overt clinical symptoms.

Acute glomerulonephritis, detected by renal biopsy, may occur in the absence of urinary abnormalities, or in patients who show only a subclinical renal response to streptococcal infection.[10] These observations suggest that clinical and urinary findings may be misleading insofar as the diagnosis of acute glomerulonephritis is concerned, and that renal biopsy may be the only way to establish the correct diagnosis. A subclinical renal response to streptococcal infection does not necessarily ensure a favorable prognosis; some patients develop worsening histologic pictures over a period of 12 to 18 months.

Prophylaxis and Treatment

A reduction in the community-wide prevalence of nephritogenic streptococcal infections produces a reduction in the incidence of acute glomerulonephritis. Penicillin is effective in producing such a reduction, although prompt eradication of the organism may not always prevent the disease. The use of streptococcal vaccines is still an unproven experimental procedure, but has obvious theoretic usefulness should it be possible to develop effective vaccines against selected nephritogenic strains.

Once acute glomerulonephritis has occured, there is no therapeutic measure known which will consistently alter the glomerular inflammatory process or produce more rapid healing. Therefore, most therapeutic measures, such as salt and fluid restriction and the administration of antihypertensive and antibiotic drugs, are directed at controlling the complications.

Corticosteroids and immunosuppressive agents appear to have little value during the acute stage of glomerulonephritis. In fact, corticosteroids may be contraindicated because they tend to increase protein catabolism, sodium retention, and hypertension. Because inhibition of the immune response is presently difficult and often dangerous, some investigators have favored therapeutic methods directed at subsequent steps in the mediation of renal injury. One such approach is the use of anticoagulants.[13] In a small series of patients, the intravenous infusion of high doses of heparin resulted in a surprisingly rapid improvement in renal function. The rationale for this therapy is based on a presumed role for fibrinogen and related factors in the production of irreparable glomerular injury.

NONSTREPTOCOCCAL GLOMERULONEPHRITIS

The claim that other infective agents may induce a disease identical to acute poststreptococcal nephritis is not accepted by all investigators in the field However, there is little doubt that acute glomerulitis is seen in a variety of other diseases, and, under these circumstances, the lesions may be either focal or diffuse. Some of the diseases capable of producing non-streptococcal glomerulonephritis are listed in Table 6-3. In many, an immunologic mechanism has been implicated.

TABLE 6-3. Causes of Non-streptococcal Glomerulonephritis*

Other Infectious Agents
  Viruses
  Infectious mononucleosis
  Staphylococci (particularly associated with infected
    ventriculoatrial shunt)

Subacute bacterial endocarditis
Collagen-Vascular Diseases
  Systemic lupus erythematosus
  Polyarteritis nodosa
  Vasculitis (systemic non-suppurative)
  Cryoglobulinemia

Unknown Etiology
  Anaphylactoid purpura
  Goodpasture's syndrome
  Toxemia of pregnancy

Drugs
  Penicillin
  Drugs which produce lupus-like syndromes

Post-Transplantation Nephritis

---

* Diseases which have no known immunologic implications are excluded from the table.

Infectious Agents

It seems clear that other bacteria such as the staphylococcus may be associated with an immunologic nephritis. Several cases of nephritis with infected ventriculoatrial CSF shunt have been described in which there was a chronic coagulase-negative staphylococcal infection with bacteremia.[26] Fluorescent microscopy demonstrated low serum complement and IgM, IgG, and C3 distributed in a lobular fashion along the glomerular capillary wall. This provided good evidence for an immunologic pathogenesis.

In one case report, Coxsackie B virus was found by immunofluorescence at autopsy in the glomerulus of a patient with subclinical acute glomerulonephritis. In addition, a benign form of glomerulonephritis occurs in some patients with infectious mononucleosis. Otherwise, the evidence for a viral etiology of human glomerulonephritis remains inconclusive.

On the other hand, considerable experimental evidence has been collected for a viral etiology of nephritis in mice. In persistent, "tolerated," lymphocytic choriomeningitis virus (LCM) infection in mice, a nephritis occurs in which anti-LCM antibody, complement and the virus are localized along the glomerular basement membrane.[20] Under these circumstances, the renal disease appears to be due to immune complexes rather than to a direct effect of the virus or an autoimmune process. Recently, glomerulonephritis has been induced in mice with Echo 9 and Coxsackie B viruses. In both cases viral antigen was identified in the glomeruli, and in the Coxsackie B induced nephritis IgG was localized in the kidney.

Subacute Bacterial Endocarditis

The glomerulonephritis associated with subacute bacterial endocarditis may be focal or diffuse, and is now considered to be largely a manifestation of hypersensitivity rather than septic embolization of the kidney.

Collagen-Vascular Diseases

The renal lesions associated with collagen-vascular diseases are discussed in Chapter 8. Only in systemic lupus erythematosus is the pathogenetic mechanism well worked out. This disease appears to be due to an immune-complex process similar to that described for acute poststreptococcal glomerulonephritis.

Anaphylactoid Purpura (Henoch-Schönlein Syndrome)

Anaphylactoid purpura is a disease which presents clinically as acute or recurrent nonthrombocytopenic purpura. The basic lesion appears to be a vasculitis with a propensity to involve cutaneous and renal vessels.

Etiology.   A hypersensitivity mechanism has been suspected for a long time, but neither the etiologic agent nor the pathogenetic processes have been determined. Some investigators feel that bacterial infection with hypersensitivity to the organism concerned may play a significant role. This theory is based on the observations that: (1) infection is a common antecedent of the syndrome; and (2) in some cases exacerbations are apparently related to bacteremia, e.g., that which occurs after dental surgery. The β hemolytic streptococcus does not appear to be implicated as a causative agent.

Immunopathology.   The basic lesion is one of a severe necrotizing vasculitis with large numbers of polymorphonuclear leukocytes. Morphologically, the cutaneous vascular lesions look very much like those found in experimental Arthus vasculitis. The renal lesion is a diffuse proliferative glomerulonephritis. Polymorphonuclear leukocytes are generally prominent in the glomeruli and at times accumulate against the glomerular basement membrane in a fashion resembling acute nephrotoxic nephritis ("anti-GBM type" process) in animals.[11] Electron microscopy of the kidney reveals a number of changes, including a striking increase in the mesangial matrix, splitting of the GBM, endothelial cell swelling, and subendothelial electron dense deposits.[29] The absence of demonstrable subepithelial deposits is somewhat against an immune-complex mechanism in the pathogenesis of the renal lesions in anaphylactoid purpura.

Immunofluorescent studies in patients with renal involvement showed IgG and C3 deposited in a predominantly mesangial pattern, although some basement membrane orientated deposits were seen as well. No antigen has as yet been identified in the renal deposits.

Clinical Manifestations.   The cardinal clinical features of anaphylactoid purpura are nonthrombocytopenic purpura, arthralgias, colicky gastrointestinal pain, and nephritis. Constitutional symptoms such as fever and malaise may also be present.

The characteristic skin lesions may be ecchymotic, macular, or occasionally urticarial in nature. The renal lesions often lead to hematuria, proteinuria, and marked impairment of renal function. Renal involvement appears in approximately 40 per cent of patients with anaphylactoid purpura, and is not always a benign complication. Approximately 5 per cent of patients with kidney involvement die in acute renal failure, while up to 40 per cent may progress to chronic renal disease.

The serum complement levels are usually normal, and thus are of some value in distinguishing anaphylactoid purpura from acute poststreptococcal glomerulonephritis. A favorable response to azathioprine (1.5 to 2.5

mg/kg/day) and high dosage corticosteroid therapy has been reported in some patients who develop progressive renal disease after an episode of anaphylactoid purpura.[1a]

Goodpasture's Syndrome

Goodpasture's syndrome represents the human counterpart of the "anti-GBM type" of immunologic renal disease in animals.

Immunopathology.   On gross examination the lungs are typically large and hemorrhagic. The most characteristic microscopic lesions in the lung are nodular foci of septal fibrosis, intra-alveolar hemorrhage, and hemosiderin-laden macrophages.

The earliest renal lesion is a focal nephritis. However, there is usually rapid progression to a diffuse, severe disease not readily distinguishable from acute poststreptococcal glomerulonephritis. Certain features, such as intense proliferation of both the glomerular epithelial cells and the cells of the parietal layer of Bowman's capsule, are more common in Goodpasture's syndrome. The latter change leads to early "crescent formation." On the other hand, endothelial proliferation is substantially less. Other pathologic changes include the presence of amorphous, eosinophilic material in the glomerular capillary loops, and the fairly rapid destruction of glomeruli with progression to fibrosis.

Ultrastructural studies reveal extensive proliferative changes in capillary wall cells, masses of electron-dense fibrillar material in a subendothelial location, and thickening of the basement membrane with luminal deposits of membrane-like material. In some areas, masses are seen within the membrane itself. Subepithelial deposits similar to those found in acute post-streptococcal glomerulonephritis and systemic lupus erythematosus do not occur.

A considerable advance in our understanding of this disease and its underlying mechanism resulted from: (1) the demonstration of smooth, continuous, linear deposition of immune reactants along the glomerular basement membrane (Fig. 6-1); and (2) experiments which showed that the immunoglobulin distributed in this manner was antibody directed against the glomerular basement membrane. In addition, when this antibody was eluted from the kidney and injected into monkeys, it localized in a linear fashion along the monkey basement membrane and produced a severe glomerulonephritis.[15]

Linear deposition of IgG and C3 has also been demonstrated along the basement membrane of the pulmonary alveolar septae and capillaries in a manner very similar to that seen in the kidney.[3] Furthermore, antibodies eluted from lung tissue in Goodpasture's syndrome react with GBM, while those eluted from the kidney react with pulmonary alveolar septal membrane.[14] These observations suggest that similar and perhaps inter-related processes are operative in the lung and kidney. It is known that the lung and kidney basement membrane are antigenically related and that antisera to lung produced in experimental animals are capable of inducing both pulmonary and renal damage. The observation that the pulmonary lesion generally precedes clinical evidence of renal damage suggests that the initial tissue injury may take place in the lung.

The agent or agents which induce a patient to make antibodies reactive with his own GBM and pulmonary tissues are unknown. An increased number of cases of Goodpasture's syndrome seems to appear shortly after viral influenza pandemics, and virus-like particles have been demonstrated in the kidneys of two patients with the disease. However, there is no definite proof of a viral etiology.

Recently it has been found that all samples of normal rabbit and human urine contain soluble GBM antigens. Injection of autologous urinary GBM antigens into rabbits produces an "anti-GBM type" of renal disease similar to that found in Goodpasture's syndrome.[4] It is thus conceivable that altera-tion of a soluble glomerular basement membrane or pulmonary antigen, or a disturbance in their handling by the immune system could result in clinical disease.

Clinical Manifestations.   The characteristic clinical features of Goodpas-ture's syndrome consist of hemoptysis, anemia, and progressive renal failure, usually occurring in young males. Hemosiderin-laden macrophages can fre-quently be demonstrated in smears of sputum or gastric washings, but Goodpasture's syndrome can usually be distinguished from idiopathic hemo-siderosis by: (1) its occurrence in young males over the age of 16; (2) the presence of severe renal lesions; and (3) the absence of hepatomegaly.

The course is almost always a rapidly fatal one. Treatment with corti-costeroids (e.g., prednisone 40 to 60 mg, daily) may produce an occasional temporary remission, but does not appear to affect the ultimate outcome of the syndrome. Azathioprine in daily doses of 1.5 to 2.5 mg/kg has been administered with apparent benefit in some patients. A few patients have experienced dramatic improvement in their pulmonary lesions following total nephrectomy.

Cryoglobulinemia

The immunology and clinical features of cryoglobulinemia are discussed in Chapter 10. Renal disease is found primarily in patients with "mixed" cryoglobulinemia. The nephritis is of the immune complex type, and the glomeruli show deposition of IgG, IgM and C3 along the GBM in a granular pattern.

Drug-Induced Glomerulonephritis

Nephritis has been reported in patients receiving high doses of penicillin or methicillin. Fever and eosinophilia, as well as antibodies against penicillin, suggest a hypersensitivity mechanism. Most patients show an interstitial nephritis with round cell infiltration or an acute glomerulonephritis and arteritis. In one patient, in whom immunofluorescent studies were done, extensive linear staining of both tubular and glomerular basement membranes was seen with fluorescent antipenicilloyl antibody (see Chapter 20) and anti-Ig G antibodies. The significance of this finding is uncertain since there was no morphologic evidence of glomerulitis.[2]

Post-Transplantation Glomerulonephritis

Allografts. There is increasing evidence that a variety of glomerular changes which are distinct from the classic lesions of graft rejection (see Chapter 14) occur in renal allografts, particularly those which have been in place for several months. Abnormalities detected by electron or immunofluorescence miscroscopy are noted even in patients not undergoing an acute rejection episode, and these changes may be minimal on light microscopy.

The "transmission" of active glomerulonephritis has been described in a number of patients who received renal allografts. In the majority of cases, it is not yet clear whether the allograft nephritis represents a recrudescence of the recipient's own immunopathogenetic process, or whether it represents an immune response to new antigens in the graft. In one series of patients over 50 per cent of renal allograft recipients with an anti-GBM nephritis had a recurrence of the same type of renal disease, whereas approximately 25 per cent of patients with immune-complex nephritis had a recurrence of the original disease process.[5] The deposition of immunoglobulins in the glomeruli of the allografted kidneys is not clearly related to histocompatibility differences between donor and recipient, but there is a correlation between the deposition of immune reactants and azotemia or proteinuria.[16b] These observations would suggest that, in some instances, recurrent nephritis may present a greater threat to the survival of renal allografts than the rejection process. Allograft nephritis has also been reported in some patients who received kidney transplants because of congenital or infectious, rather than immunologic, renal disease. In this group of patients, the post transplantation nephritis is clearly unrelated to the original host disease.

Isografts. Although glomerulonephritis occurs in a minority of allografted recipients who are given immunosuppressive therapy, it is distressingly common in human renal isograft recipients where histocompatibility differences are theoretically nonexistent. In one series of 17 isografted patients whose original disease was glomerulonephritis, 11 developed recurrent glomerulonephritis.[9] Glomerular hypercellularity, glomerular deposition of IgG, C3, and fibrinogen, and both subendothelial and subepithelial deposits were found to underlie the hematuria, proteinuria, nephrotic syndrome, and progressive renal failure which occurred. Isograft nephritis always appears to be due to the same type of process which caused the original disease in the recipient.

Hyperacute Allograft Rejection. Several cases of hyperacute renal allograft rejection have been reported in which the hyperacute rejection phenomenon was attributed to a Shwartzman-like reaction (see Chapter 14). The rejected kidneys showed intravascular thrombi, marked infiltration with polymorphonuclear leukocytes, and deposition of fibrin in the glomeruli. There is also evidence that an Arthus-like mechanism might be operative in some acutely rejected kidney allografts. Heavy infiltrations of PMN's have been detected in the glomeruli, but immune reactants have not been demonstrated.[19]

SUBACUTE AND CHRONIC GLOMERULONEPHRITIS

Some of the disease entities that may produce subacute and chronic glomerulonephritis, such as Goodpasture's syndrome, have already been discussed earlier in this chapter. However, there remains a large group of relatively unclassifiable cases. Nowhere is the lack of understanding of the natural history of nephritis better exemplified than in this group of disorders, and their classification becomes an almost impossible problem.

Subacute nephritis may follow an overt attack of acute poststreptococcal glomerulonephritis and may be characterized by persistent edema, hematuria, hypertension, uremia, and a fatal termination in 6 to 18 months. Alternatively, there may be only persistent proteinuria after the acute attack with slow progression to renal failure in 10 to 40 years. These cases have been called Ellis type I nephritis in distinction to Ellis type II nephritis, where no acute episode is discernible. In the latter group of patients, there is insidious onset of proteinuria, edema, and the nephrotic syndrome, or else slow progression with hypertension and renal failure occurring in 10 to 20 years. The nephrotic syndrome will be discussed subsequently.

IMMUNOPATHOLOGY

The usual features of subacute nephritis are glomerular hypercellularity with crescent formation and a variable influx of inflammatory cells. The basic lesion is a proliferative one. With progression to chronic disease, there is contracture of the kidneys and scarring. The glomeruli show progressive fibrosis, hyalinization, and obliteration. In some cases, ultrastructural abnormalities have included the presence of electron-dense subepithelial deposits suggestive of immune-complex disease.

A variety of immunifluorescent changes may be seen. Some specimens show distinct deposition of immune reactants, including IgG, C3, and occasionally IgM in a membranous pattern, usually lumpy or focal. Fibrin or its products are seen in a membranous or patchy interstitial fashion in some glomeruli, while, in a few cases, diffuse localization in the epithelial crescents has been observed. Recently, several patients have been described in which the immune reactants were found in the kidney in a smooth, continuous, linear fashion along the glomerular basement membrane.

Thus, it appears that in some cases of subacute and chronic glomerulonephritis where immunologic factors are involved, at least two pathogenetic mechanisms may be operative: (*1*) the "immune-complex type" disease comparable to that found in systemic lupus erythematosus; or (*2*) the "anti-GBM type" disease comparable to that found in Goodpasture's syndrome. It is most important to note that the renal immunofluorescent pattern is not always clearly separable into either continuous linear or interrupted lumpy, granular patterns. In fact, both types of distribution may be seen in the one biopsy. It is not inconceivable that both immunopathogenetic mechanisms may be operative in the same patient—the one perhaps triggering the other (Fig. 6-2). In other patients, no immune reactants are demonstrable, and the etiology is even more obscure.

IMMUNOLOGY

The immunologic findings reflect the diversity of the disease processes encountered under the heading of subacute and chronic nephritis. Patients may have reduced complement levels, as measured by hemolytic complement activity, or normal levels of whole complement. The low serum complement levels are generally ascribed to excessive complement activation or consumption by antigen-antibody interaction. However, in at least one entity, progressive glomerulonephritis of childhood, there is a relatively selective deficiency of C3 which is due in part to a markedly decreased synthetic rate for this protein.

Circulating anti-GBM antibodies have been found in about 40 per cent of patients known to have glomerulonephritis mediated by anti-GBM antibodies, and are more readily detectable after total nephrectomy.[16a] It is assumed that these antibodies are absorbed in the kidney by exposed GBM antigens as long as the organs remain within the body. Evidence for immune complexes in the circulation has been indirect or circumstantial. Anticomplementary activity in the sera of certain patients with chronic glomerulonephritis has been taken as indirect evidence in favor of circulating immune complexes.[21]

CLINICAL MANIFESTATIONS

In the presence of a smoldering, subacute or chronic glomerulonephritis, the patient is frequently asymptomatic and the clinical evidence of disease consists almost entirely of an abnormal urinary sediment.

As the disease progresses, the signs and symptoms of chronic renal failure begin to appear. The cardinal signs of uremia consist of azotemia, anemia, and acidosis. The patient may have symptoms of extreme fatigue, nausea and vomiting, dyspnea, and pruritus. Severe hypertension may lead to headache, retinopathy, convulsions, and left heart failure. Terminal events may include muscle twitching, bleeding from mucous membranes, and semicoma.

The urine usually has a fixed low specific gravity, and contains small quantities of red blood cells, white blood cells, epithelial cells, and a few granular or waxy casts. Determination of serum electrolytes reveals findings typical of a metabolic acidosis, and there is often a normochromic anemia with hemoglobin levels as low as 6 to 9 gm/100 ml. The blood urea nitrogen and creatinine are markedly elevated.

TREATMENT

No entirely satisfactory treatment has been found for this group of patients. The usual treatment measures are directed towards the control of nephrotic syndrome, intercurrent infections, anemia, hypertension, and acidosis which may occur during the course of the disease.

Current thinking would suggest that chronic hemodialysis may be indicated: (1) for certain patients who are unsuitable for renal transplantation; and (2) for patients who are awaiting transplantation. The indications for renal transplantation are discussed in Chapter 14, and the role of corticosteroids and immunosuppresive agents will be discussed at the end of this chapter.

NEPHROTIC SYNDROME

The nephrotic syndrome is a clinical disorder characterized by marked proteinuria, hypoproteinemia, edema and usually hypercholesterolemia. A list of the more common causes of nephrotic syndrome is given in Tables 6-4 and 6-5. Some cases appear to have a distinct immunologic basis, while in others there is no clinical, serological, nor immunohistochemical evidence of an immune reaction. About 75 per cent of cases are due to primary renal disease, i.e., glomerulonephritis.

NEPHROTIC SYNDROME DUE TO PRIMARY RENAL DISEASE

Immunopathology

The renal lesions in patients with nephrotic syndrome due to primary renal disease generally fall into one of four pathologic categories depending on the nature of the glomerular abnormalities. These types are called the "foot-process type" (lipoid nephrosis, or minimal lesion nephrosis), membranous, proliferative, and mixed types of nephrosis. While the proliferative and mixed types may follow acute glomerulonephritis, the membranous and lipoid type are not usually preceded by an acute nephritic phase. There appears to be a clinical as well as pathologic basis for this separation into four categories, as patients beginning with one type tend to remain in that category, to pursue a course typical of it, and not to transform into other types.[23]

Lipoid Nephrosis.   The most clearly separable group are those with so-called lipoid nephrosis. Although this term is inaccurate, other more correct nomenclature tends to be rather awkward. The renal lesion is noteworthy for its lack of inflammatory changes or basement membrane alteration. The GBM is usually completely normal or minimally altered focally. Deposits are most unusual and the most striking change is fusion of the epithelial foot processes (podocytes). This latter change is not pathognomonic and is felt to reflect some sort of response to the massive protein leak across the basement membrane. Deposits of immunologic reactants are not demonstrable in the glomerular capillary loop area by the fluorescent antibody technique. The identification of myxovirus-like particles in glomerular epithelial cells in a few patients with lipoid nephrosis is of unknown significance at present, and the etiology of this disorder remains a mystery.

TABLE 6-4. Causes of Nephrotic Syndrome*

Primary Renal Diseases ("idiopathic")
  Membranous glomerulonephritis
  Proliferative glomerulonephritis (some cases)
  Idiopathic nephrotic syndrome of childhood
    ("lipoid" or minimal lesion nephrosis)
  Congenital familial nephrotic syndrome

Collagen-Vascular Diseases
  Systemic lupus erythematosus
  Sjögren's syndrome
  Polyarteritis nodosa
  Wegner's granulomatosis

Hypersensitivity Phenomena
  Insect stings
  Drugs†
  Pollen injections
  Anaphylactoid purpura
  Cyclical nephrotic syndrome of pregnancy
  Associated with tumors

Serum Sickness

Infectious and Postinfectious Causes
  Subacute (proliferative) glomerulonephritis,
    poststreptococcal
  Infected ventriculoatrial shunt
  Quartan malaria
  Subacute bacterial endocarditis
  Syphilis (active)

Multiple Myeloma

Amyloidosis

Waldenstrom's Macroglobulinemia

* Diseases which have no known immunologic implications are excluded from the table.
† See Table 6-5.

Membranous Type. In the membranous type of nephrosis, the glomerular lesion is also noninflammatory, but membrane changes are especially striking. The thickening and irregularity of the capillary walls may be seen under ordinary light microscopy. Ultrastructural examination usually reveals electron dense deposits, most prominently located on the epithelial side of the basement membrane, although they may also occur in subendothelial

Table 6-5. Drugs Which May Cause Nephrotic Syndrome

Inorganic mercurials	Phenindiones
Organic mercurials	Perchlorate
Trimethadione	Tolbutamide
Probenecid	Gold, bismuth and
Penicillamine	other heavy metals

and intramembranous locations. With time, these deposits appear to become covered by basement membrane whereupon they lose their distinct outline and become part of the grossly thickened membrane, so-called "membranous transformation." Immunofluorescent studies frequently reveal deposition of IgG and C3 in a discontinuous, granular fashion along the glomerular basement membrane. This finding coupled with the subepithelial deposits suggests an "immune-complex type" of mechanism, but the antigen has not been defined.

Proliferative Type. In the proliferative type of nephrosis, the pathologic lesions are quite different, and are characterized by a prominent proliferative, inflammatory component. In addition to cellular proliferation, there is a fairly normal GBM with occasional deposits, and a tendency for there to be lobulation of the glomerular tufts. This group of patients usually shows glomerular deposition of immune reactants along the GBM in a focal, linear, or mixed pattern.[7] Both the immune-complex and anti-GBM pathogenetic mechanisms are capable of producing a lesion of this type.

Mixed Type. Finally, a mixed lesion has been described which is likely a variant of proliferative glomerulonephritis with prominent membrane changes. Some patients with proliferative glomerulonephritis show various kinds of deposits in and around the glomerular basement membrane, but they are generally less dense and less discrete than those seen in classic membranous glomerulonephritis.

Immunology

Serum complement levels are low in the nephrotic syndrome associated with childhood progressive glomerulonephritis, proliferative glomerulonephritis, and, in some patients with membranous glomerulonephritis. Complement levels, however, are consistently normal in lipoid nephrosis. Immunoconglutinin levels are frequently elevated in children with steroid sensitive nephrotic syndrome. In all cases, the most marked serum protein abnormality is a moderate to extreme hypoalbuminemia. This change is generally accompanied by an elevation in serum lipoproteins and by a decrease in serum immunoglobulins.

The selective ability of the glomerulus to retain plasma proteins of different molecular weights has been used by some as a guide to diagnosis and prognosis as well as an indicator of the likelihood of response to corticosteroid therapy. The renal clearance ratio of various proteins, usually transferrin (M.W. 90,000), IgG (M.W. 150,000), and IgM (M.W. 950,000) is used to determine the selectivity of proteinuria. In some studies, low selectivity has been associated predominantly with membranous disease, a poor prognosis, and a failure to respond to corticosteroid therapy. Other investigators have been unable to correlate the selectivity of proteinuria with any pathologic lesion, and have found far advanced glomerular disease of any kind to be the main cause of low selectivity.

Clinical Manifestations

The basic pathophysiologic abnormality in the nephrotic syndrome is an increase in glomerular permeability due to basement membrane damage. The ensuing loss of plasma protein, mainly albumin, leads to hypoproteinemia, and a decreased plasma oncotic pressure. The latter, in turn, triggers salt and water retention which produces generalized edema and frequently ascites. Plasma lipids, especially cholesterol, are elevated with a few exceptions, most notably that of nephrotic syndrome in systemic lupus erythematosus. In children, increased susceptibility to intercurrent infection is common, and is possibly related to the urinary loss of γ-globulins. As the disease progresses, hypertension, renal failure, and azotemia appear. Nevertheless, massive proteinuria may continue.

The kidneys may excrete as much as 10 gm of protein per 24 hours. Electrophoresis of the urine usually reveals large amounts of albumin, and varying quantities of γ-globulin, depending on the degree of basement membrane damage. The urinary sediment contains casts, including the characteristic fatty and waxy varieties, renal tubule cells, some of which contain fatty droplets (oval fat bodies), and variable numbers of red blood cells.

Patients with lipoid nephrosis are usually children and do not as a rule show hematuria or hypertension. They constitute the largest single group of childhood nephrotics and generally have a good prognosis. In contrast, the membranous form of the nephrotic syndrome is generally seen in adults in whom the prognosis is somewhat poorer. Hematuria may occur, and hypertension is said to develop in about half the patients. The proliferative type of nephrotic syndrome occurs in both adults and children, may be clinically indistinguishable from other types, and is usually associated with a poor prognosis.

Treatment

The treatment of nephrotic syndrome is discussed at the end of the section which follows on nephrotic syndrome secondary to systemic diseases.

NEPHROTIC SYNDROME SECONDARY TO SYSTEMIC DISEASES

Collagen-Vascular Diseases

the nephrotic syndrome which occurs in association with collagen-vascular diseases is discussed in Chapter 8.

Hypersensitivity Syndromes

The nephrotic syndrome may occasionally occur following exposure to certain drugs (see Table 6-5). Particularly noteworthy is the high incidence in patients receiving trimethadione and paramethadione. Pathologically, the lesion resembles lipoid nephrosis. Whether or not these reactions represent true hypersensitivity states is uncertain. The argument for a hypersensitivity mechanism in the nephrotic syndrome which follows the injection of foreign proteins, pollens, insect stings, and plant products (e.g., poison ivy oleoresin) is perhaps stronger, in that other manifestations of hypersensitivity are often present. These include fever, arthralgias, and eosinophilic infiltration in the renal lesion itself. Nephrotic syndrome after D-penicillamine therapy is well documented, and the immunohistologic picture is characteristic of the "immune-complex type" of nephritis.

A cyclical nephrotic syndrome which occurs with repeated pregnancies has been postulated to be due to hypersensitivity or an immune response to unknown products of gestation.

An unusually high incidence of cancer, including lymphoma, has been noted in association with nephrotic syndrome. It has therefore been postulated that antitumor antibodies might cross-react with glomerular basement membrane, giving rise to renal injury.

An entity known as familial congenital or infantile nephrosis has been described based on the occurrence of nephrotic syndrome in multiple siblings in single families. In addition, there is a high incidence of allergy and urticaria in the same families. Immunofluorescent techniques have revealed a deposition of γ-globulin, C1 and C3 in some of the glomerular capillary loops. Other investigators have found evidence of maternal and fetal autoantibodies to kidney, and proposed that a basic immunologic incompatibility between mother and infant might be responsible for the disease.

Serum Sickness

The nephrotic syndrome occurs occasionally during the course of serum sickness. In experimental serum sickness the renal lesions are clearly related to the deposition of circulating immune complexes. A similar phenomenon may well occur in human serum sickness, although the reagin-mediated features of the disease frequently overshadow those due to immune complexes (see Chapter 2).

Infectious and Post-Infectious Causes

Some of these entities such as poststreptococcal glomerulonephritis, infected ventriculoatrial shunt (staphylococcal bacteremia), and subacute bacterial endocarditis have been discussed previously.

The nephrotic syndrome has been found to be epidemiologically related to *Plasmodium malariae* infection. The disease is particularly common in Nigeria around the fifth year of life when Plasmodium infection is also at a peak. Unlike the usual idiopathic childhood nephrotic syndrome, these patients are resistant to steroid therapy and have a relatively poor prognosis. The nephrotic syndrome in this disease appears to be due to the deposition of circulating soluble immune complexes of malarial antigen, its corresponding antibody and complement in the glomerular capillary loop.[30] In addition, the affected patients have remarkably high serum levels of IgM and antimalarial antibodies. Why other types of malarial parasites do not cause nephrotic syndrome with the same frequency is unclear at the present time. Nephrotic syndrome has also been described in association with active syphilis.

Multiple Myeloma

The pathogenesis of nephrotic syndrome secondary to multiple myeloma has not been well worked out. However, there does not appear to be an immunologic basis for the disorder in the usual sense of the word. Both glomerular and tubular lesions occur, and amyloidosis may be a complicating lesion (see Chapter 10).

Amyloidosis

Renal involvement is the most common and the most serious manifestation of amyloidosis. Pathologically, the major lesion is in the glomerulus where there is diffuse or nodular thickening of the basement membrane and eventually marked replacement of the entire glomerular structure with amyloid material (see Chapter 10).

Waldenstrom's Macroglobulinemia

Patients with Waldenstrom's macroglobulinemia may have proteinuria and even nephrotic syndrome. Pathologic changes include huge subendothelial deposits composed exclusively of IgM or the histologic picture of amyloidosis.

TREATMENT OF NEPHROTIC SYNDROME

In considering the response to treatment, the nature of the underlying lesion is of considerable importance. All nephrotics cannot be grouped together for therapeutic purposes.

In cases due to primary renal disease, those with the minimal lesion type (i.e., lipoid nephrosis), especially children, show the best response to corticosteroid therapy. In one series of 45 nephrotic children with the idiopathic type of disease, 40 per cent remained well for 5 years after only one short course of corticosteroid therapy (e.g., prednisone, 1 to 2 mg/kg/day, for 40 days), 53 per cent required one or more courses because incomplete response or relapse, and an additional 7 per cent showed no response at all.[1b]

Patients with membranous disease are usually not improved by corticosteroids.[23] In proliferative nephritis, the beneficial effect of corticosteroids is much less pronounced than in lipoid nephrosis. However, some patients, especially those with highly selective proteinuria, may improve on intensive corticosteroid therapy (e.g., prednisone, 40 to 60 mg, daily over a prolonged period of time).

Patients who do not respond to corticosteroids alone often benefit from the administration of immunosuppressive agents (cytotoxic drugs), either alone or in combination with corticosteroids. Satisfactory remissions have been obtained in over 80 per cent of nephrotic children with "minimal disease" by the use of cyclophosphamide alone.[18] However, since about half of all nephrotic children respond initially to corticosteroid drugs, immunosuppressive therapy should be reserved for those who are resistant or develop marked side-effects from corticosteroids.

Of considerable interest and of possible therapeutic significance is the observation that infection with measles may have a beneficial effect on the nephrotic syndrome in children. Recently, it has been shown that inoculations of measles-susceptible children with attenuated measles virus vaccine (see Chapter 21) will induce diuresis. However, the effect proved transient, lasting only 2 weeks on the average.[31]

MISCELLANEOUS RENAL DISORDERS OF IMMUNOLOGIC INTEREST

Hemolytic Anemia—Uremia Syndrome. This syndrome is characterized by hemolytic anemia, thrombocytopenia, and renal disease. In one patient, γ-globulin was demonstrated by the fluorescent antibody technique in a continuous linear pattern along the glomerular basement membrane in a manner similar to that seen in Goodpasture's syndrome. The renal lesion is usually that of bilateral cortical necrosis or glomerulitis.

Toxemia of Pregnancy. While there is no evidence for an immunologic abnormality in the renal disease accompanying toxemia of pregnancy, immunofluorescent studies have revealed a marked accumulation of fibrinogen-like products in the glomeruli. This material was found in focal deposits along the GBM and in swollen endothelial cells. Gammaglobulin was found only occasionally in small amounts and complement was not demonstrated. It is suggested that intravascular coagulation may play a role in the pathogenesis of this disease process.

Pyelonephritis. In experimental pyelonephritis in rabbits, a significant local immune response by the kidney has been demonstrated. It is possible that the local production of immunoglobulins (IgG) may be a factor in host resistance.

Nephritis Associated with Chronic Active Hepatitis. Recently, two patients with chronic active liver disease (see Chapter 16) were found to develop a lupus-like nephritis as a terminal event. In other patients, nephritis of an undetermined nature is often associated with chronic active hepatitis.

Renal Tubular Acidosis. The association between renal tubular acidosis and hypergammaglobulinemia is discussed in Chapter 10. Latent renal tubular acidosis has also been described in Sjögren's syndrome (see Chapter 8).

IMMUNOSUPPRESSIVE THERAPY OF RENAL DISEASE

Immunosuppressive agents have proven to be of therapeutic value in a variety of renal diseases. Unfortunately, at present, their mode of action is not entirely clear, and their use still remains somewhat empirical. The reasons for this are several. The agents themselves are generally cytotoxic drugs which have a variety of pharmacologic effects in addition to their immunosuppressive activity. Several of the common immunosuppressive agents also possess distinct anti-inflammatory properties. In addition, they are frequently used in combination with other multiaction drugs such as corticosteroids.

The mediation of immunologic (and nonimmunologic) tissue injury is a multistep, multicomponent process usually involving a variety of cellular and humoral factors.[24] It seems likely that these agents act at one or more stages in this process. It has been shown that no correlation can be found in most patients between the degree of immunosuppression and the clinical responses obtained. Therefore little explanation can presently be offered for the observed beneficial effect of drugs such as cyclophosphamide in the idiopathic childhood nephrotic syndrome, particularly as there is little or no evidence of immunologic abnormality. On the other hand, in some series the greatest improvement in chronic active renal disease attributable to immunosuppressive agents was found in those patients in whom immune reactants were demonstrable in the kidney.[17]

It would appear that immunosuppressive drugs such as azathioprine and cyclophosphamide, either alone or in combination with corticosteroids, *may* be of value in the following conditions:

1. Steroid resistant nephrotic syndrome, particularly in the lipoid or minimal lesion variety

2. Steroid resistant nephrotic syndrome associated with some cases of proliferative and membranous glomerulonephritis

3. Nephritis associated with anaphylactoid purpura

4. Some cases of chronic, active glomerulonephritis and persistent hypocomplementemic glomerulonephritis

5. Goodpasture's syndrome

6. Lupus nephritis (see Chapter 8)

7. Wegener's granulomatosis and certain other collagen-vascular diseases (see Chapter 8)

In all of these conditions, immunosuppressive agents are indicated only if corticosteroids fail to produce improvement, or are associated with disabling side-effects. Alternate day corticosteroid therapy probably reduces the severity of side-effects, but it is not known whether this regimen also reduces the therapeutic effect. Although optimal dosage levels of immunosuppressive drugs in renal disease are not firmly established, azathioprine is commonly employed in doses of 1.5 to 2.5 mgm/kg/day.

Improvement in a few patients with severe nephritis has recently been reported following treatment with antilymphocyte serum (ALS). These patients were apparently unresponsive to corticosteroids and azathioprine.

REFERENCES

1. Andres, G. A., Accini, L., Hsu, K., Zabriskie, J. B., and Seegal, B. C. Electron microscopic studies of human glomerulonephritis with ferritin-coated antibody. Localization of antigen-antibody complexes in glomerular structures of patients with acute glomerulonephritis. *J. Exp. Med. 123:*399, 1966.

1a. Ansell, B. M. Henoch-Schonlein purpura with particular reference to the prognosis of the renal lesion. *Brit. J. Derm. 82:*211, 1970.

1b. Arneil, G. C., and Lam, C. N. Long-term assessment of steroid therapy in childhood nephrosis. *Lancet 2:*819, 1966.

2. Baldwin, D. S., Levine, B., McCluskey, R. T., and Gallo, G. R. Renal failure and interstitial nephritis due to penicillin and methicillin. *New Eng. J. Med. 279:*1245, 1968.

3. Beirne, G. J., Octaviono, G. N., Kopp, W. L., and Burns, R. O. Immunohistology of the lung in Goodpasture's syndrome. *Ann. Intern. Med. 69:*1207, 1968.

4. Dixon, F. J. The pathogenesis of glomerulonephritis. *Amer. J. Med. 44:*493, 1968.

5. Dixon, F. J., McPhaul, J. J., Jr., and Lerner, R. Recurrence of glomerulonephritis in the transplanted kidney. *Arch. Intern. Med. 123:*554, 1969.

6. Dodge, W. F., Spargo, B. H., Bass, J. A., and Travis, L. B. The relationship between the clinical features of post-streptococcal glomerulonephritis. A study of the early natural history. *Medicine 47:*227, 1968.

7. Drummond, K. N., Michael, A. F., Good, R. A., and Vernier, R. L. The nephrotic syndrome of childhood: Immunologic, clinical and pathologic correlations. *J. Clin. Invest. 45:*620, 1966.

7a. Fish, A. J., Herdman, R. C., Michael, A. F., Pickering, R. J., and Good, R. A. Epidemic acute glomerulonephritis associated with type 49 streptococcal pyoderma. II. Correlative study of light, immunofluorescent, and electron microscopic findings. *Amer. J. Med. 48:*28, 1970.

8. Glassock, R. J., Edgington, T. S., Watson, J. I., and Dixon, F. J. Autologous immune complex nephritis induced with renal tubular antigen. II. The pathogenetic mechanism. *J. Exper. Med. 127:*573, 1968.

9. Glassock, R. J., Feldman, J. D., Reynolds, E. S., Dammin, G. J., and Merrill, J. P. Human renal isografts: A clinical and pathologic analysis. *Medicine 47:*411, 1967.

10. Goorno, W., Ashworth, C. T., and Carter, N. W. Acute glomerulonephritis with absence of abnormal urinary findings. *Ann. Intern. Med. 66:*345, 1967.

11. Hawkins, D., and Cochrane, C. G. Glomerular basement membrane damage in immunological glomerulonephritis. *Immunology 14:*665, 1968.

12. Herdman, R. C., Hong, R., Michael, A. F., and Good, R. A. Light chain distribution in immune deposits on glomeruli of kidneys in human renal disease. *J. Clin. Invest. 46:*141, 1967.

13. Kincard-Smith, P., Saker, B. M., and Fairley, K. F. Anticoagulants in "irreversible" acute renal failure. *Lancet 2:*1360, 1968.

14. Koffler, D., Sandson, J., Carr, R., and Kunkel, H. G. Immunologic studies concerning the pulmonary lesions in Goodpasture's syndrome. *Amer. J. Path.* 54:293, 1969.

15. Lerner, R. A., Glassock, R. J. and Dixon, F. J. The role of anti-glomerular basement antibody in the pathogenesis of human renal disease. *J. Exper. Med. 126:*989, 1967.

16. Lindberg, L., and Vosti, K. L. Elution of glomerular antibodies in experimental streptococcal nephritis. *Science 166:*1032, 1969.

16a. McPhaul, J. J., Jr., and Dixon, F. J. The presence of antiglomerular basement membrane antibodies in peripheral blood. *J. Immunol. 103:*468, 1969.

16b. McPhaul, J. J., Jr., Dixon, F. J., Brettschneider, L., and Starzl, T. E. Immunofluorescent examination of biopsies from long-term renal allografts. *New Eng. J. Med. 282:*442, 1970.

17. Michael, A. F., Vernier, R. L., Drummond, K. N., Levitt, J. I., Herdman, R. C., Fish, A. J., and Good, R. A. Immunosuppressive therapy of chronic renal disease. *New Eng. J. Med. 276:*817, 1967.

18. Moncrieff, M. W., White, R. H. R., Ogg, C. S., and Cameron, J. S. Cyclophosphamide therapy in nephrotic syndrome in childhood. *Brit. Med. J. 1:*666, 1969.

19. Myburgh, J. A., Cohen, I., Gecelter, L., Myere, A. M., Abrahams, C., Furman, K. I., Goldberg, B., and Van Blerk, P. J. F. Hyperacute rejection in human kidney allografts—Schwartzman or Arthus reaction? *New Eng. J. Med. 281:*131, 1969.

20. Oldstone, M. B. A., and Dixon, F. J. Pathogenesis of chronic disease associated with persistent lymphocytic choriomeningitis. viral infection. II. Relationship of the antilymphocytic choriomeningitis immune response to tissue injury in chronic lymphocytic choriomeningitis disease. *J. Exper. Med. 131:*1, 1970.

21. Pickering, R. J., Gewurz, H., and Good, R. A. Complement inactivation by serum from patients with acute and hypocomplementemic chronic glomerulonephritis. *J. Lab. Clin. Med. 71:*298, 1968.

22. Perlman, L. V., Herdman, R. C., Kleiman, H., and Vernier, R. L. Poststreptococcal glomerulonephritis: A ten year follow-up of an epidemic. *J.A.M.A. 194:*175, 1965.

23. Pollak, V. E., Rosen, S., Pirani, C. L., Muehrke, R. C., and Kark, R. M. Natural history of lipoid nephrosis and membranous glomerulonephritis. *Ann. Intern. Med. 69:*1171, 1968.

24. Schwartz, R. S. Therapeutic strategy in clinical immunology. *New Eng. J. Med. 280:*367, 1969.

25. Spitzer, R. E., Vallota, E. H., Forristal, J., Sudora, E., Stitzel, A., Davis, N. C., and West, C. D. Serum C' lytic system in patients with glomerulonephritis. *Science* *164:*436, 1969.

26. Stickler, G. B., Shin, M. H., Burke, E. C., Holley, K. E., Miller, R. H., and Segar, W. E. Diffuse glomerulonephritis associated with infected ventriculo-atrial shunt. *New Eng. J. Med. 279:*1077, 1968.

27. Treser, G., Semar, M., McVicar, M., Franklin, M., Ty, A., Sagel, I., and Lange, K. Antigenic streptococcal components in acute glomerulonephritis. *Science 163:*676, 1969.

28. Unanue, E. R., Dixon, F. J., and Feldman, J. D. Experimental allergic glomerulonephritis induced in the rabbit with homologous renal antigens. *J. Exper. Med. 125:*163, 1967.

29. Urizar, R. E., Michael, A., Sisson, S., and Vernier, R. L. Anaphylactoid purpura. II. Immunofluorescent and electron microscopic studies of the glomerular lesions. *Laboratory Invest. 19:*437, 1968.

30. Ward, P. A., and Kibukamusoke, J. W. Evidence for soluble immune complexes in the pathogenesis of the glomerulonephritis of quartan malaria. *Lancet 1:*283, 1969.

31. Yuceoglu, A. M., Berkowich, S., and Chiu, J. Effect of live measles virus vaccine on childhood nephrosis. *J. Pediat. 74:*291, 1969.

7

Clinical Immunology of the Heart

DAVID HAWKINS

In recent years, there has been increasing evidence that immune phenomena, perhaps of an autoimmune nature, are involved in a number of cardiac disorders.[10] For example, antibodies reactive with heart tissue are found in the sera of patients with diseases such as rheumatic fever, postcardiotomy syndrome, and postmyocardial infarction syndrome. In addition, immune reactants (e.g., immunoglobulins and complement) are occasionally deposited in the affected tissues.

ACUTE RHEUMATIC FEVER AND RHEUMATIC HEART DISEASE
ETIOLOGY AND PATHOGENESIS
Role of Streptococcal Infection

Acute rheumatic fever is invariably preceded by streptococcal infection due to group A organisms, usually of the β-hemolytic type. However, unlike glomerulonephritis, acute rheumatic fever does not appear to depend on particular bacterial strains such as the "nephritogenic" strains discussed in Chapter 6 or the "pyoderma" strains which contain specific M protein antigens.

The etiologic link between streptococcal infection and rheumatic fever has been firmly established on the basis of the following observations: (1) practically all patients with rheumatic fever have either bacteriologic or immunologic evidence of a recent streptococcal infection which usually takes the form of pharyngitis; (2) recurrences of rheumatic fever are largely prevented by prophylactic measures against streptococcal infections; (3) when rheumatic fever occurs despite prophylaxis or treatment of infections, it is usually possible to demonstrate that the organism has not been completely eradicated; and (4) acute rheumatic fever is more prevalent in the spring of the year after repeated winter epidemics of streptococcal infection.

A number of factors such as population density, economic status, and geography are known to influence the frequency of group A streptococcal infections. For example, infection appears to be more frequent in school children, military personnel, economically deprived persons, and those living in temperate climates. In general, streptococcal infections increase in frequency from infancy through childhood and then show a steady decline until adolescence, when a marked decrease in rate is noted.

The epidemiology of acute rheumatic fever more or less parallels that of group A streptococcal infections, but at a lower rate. However, acute rheumatic fever, unlike acute glomerulonephritis, is rare before the age of 2 years. The results of several surveys would suggest that the overall incidence of acute rheumatic fever in patients with evidence of recent streptococcal infection is less than 3 per cent.

Host Factors

Since only a relatively small percentage of group A hemolytic streptococcal infections are followed by rheumatic fever, host factors are obviously of considerable importance in its pathogenesis. The fact that multiple cases of rheumatic fever occur in single families cannot be attributed solely to heredity since these individuals frequently share the same environment. However, genetic factors have aroused considerable interest as host determinants. Of particular significance is the observation that the concordance rate for rheumatic fever in monozygotic twins approaches 20 per cent, whereas that for dizygotic twins is approximately 2.5 per cent. This finding suggests that genetic factors may be of some importance, although they are obviously not the sole determinant.

Immunopathogenetic Mechanisms

While it is generally accepted that the group A streptococcus is the etiologic agent responsible for rheumatic fever, the means whereby streptococcal infection produces tissue damage is presently not known with certainty. Three possible mechanisms have received considerable attention: (*1*) direct invasion of the affected tissue by the streptococcal organism; (*2*) production of extracellular cardiotoxins by the streptococcus in a manner comparable to that seen in diphtheria; and (*3*) induction of tissue injury by immunologic processes.

Although streptococcal organisms have occasionally been recovered from cardiac tissues in patients who have died of acute rheumatic fever, they have not been recovered consistently nor have they been found in joint fluids of patients with the arthritis of acute rheumatic fever. The latent period between infection and rheumatic manifestations is somewhat against direct invasion of affected tissues by the organism.

The streptococcus produces a wide variety of extracellular toxins some of which have cardiotoxic properties in vitro and in vivo.[12] However, there are a number of points which mitigate against toxins being important in the pathogenesis of rheumatic fever. The antibody levels to several streptococcal toxins and enzymes are at or near their peak when the manifestations of rheumatic fever occur. If the toxins were pathogenic under these circumstances it would have to be through the mechanism of antigen-antibody complex formation in a serum sickness-like fashion (see Chapter 1). There is little or no evidence for the participation of such complexes in rheumatic tissue injury. Furthermore, if toxins were important one would expect to find the greatest number of cases of rheumatic fever in patients with the most severe streptococcal infections. The latent period is also against a direct role for toxins in the causation of the lesions of rheumatic fever.

At present, immunologic mechanisms are considered most likely to be operative in the pathogenesis of acute rheumatic fever and rheumatic heart disease. However, the mechanism whereby heart-reactive antibodies produce cardiac damage is not as yet clear. It has been known for some time that the sera of patients with both acute rheumatic fever and rheumatic heart disease contain antibodies which are reactive with cardiac muscle. These antibodies may be detected by a variety of techniques including complement fixation, tanned red cell hemagglutination, immunofluorescence, immunoprecipitation, and antiglobulin consumption.

An important advance in this area occurred when it was shown by the immunofluorescence technique that antisera produced in rabbits against group A streptococci were capable of binding to cardiac muscle.[7] Initially, it was felt that the streptococcal antigen that showed cross-reactivity with human heart tissue was derived from the bacterial cell wall and was related to the M protein (see Chapter 6). However, later studies indicated that the antigen is widely distributed among group A streptococci including those which contain little or no M protein. Moreover, antibody to purified M protein does not react with human myocardium.

More recent work has provided evidence that antibodies to a streptococcal cross-reactive antigen also bind to human skeletal muscle, human smooth muscle cells from arteriolar media, and cardiac muscle from a variety of other species. It is also of significance that rheumatic and nonrheumatic heart tissue bind this antigen with equal intensity. Thus, the cross-reactive antigen is not species-specific but is moderately tissue-specific in that it is limited to cardiac, skeletal, and arteriolar smooth muscle. It is not found in other connective tissue elements such as joint synovium.

The cellular location and identity of the material in cardiac muscle which cross-reacts with streptococcal antigen(s) has not yet been determined with certainty. However, small amounts of sarcolemmal sheaths appear to be highly effective in absorbing out the heart-reactive antibody produced by immunizing animals with streptococcal cell membranes.[21] It has been suggested that the streptococcal antigen may be present in both the cell wall and in the cell membrane, that it acts as a hapten, and that different carrier proteins (e.g., M protein) are of importance depending on the source of the antigen.[10] On the other hand, there is evidence to suggest that it is the streptococcal cell membrane rather than the cell wall which is the sole source of antigen that displays cross-reactivity with mammalian muscle.[22]

It is also of interest that other streptococcal antigens react immunologically with human heart valve glycoprotein,[5] and with human connective tissue. These latter antigens are derived from the bacterial cell wall, and do not cross-react with muscle. In addition to those mentioned above, other streptococcal cross-reactive antigens include glomerular basement membrane, cartilage and transplantation antigens. Antibodies against structural glycoproteins of the heart valve have been demonstrated in a small number of children with rheumatic fever.

Several other observations are of possible significance in establishing the importance of heart-reactive antibodies in the pathogenesis of rheumatic fever. For example, when sera from patients with epidemic scarlet fever were examined 2 weeks after the onset of their illness, those patients who subsequently developed rheumatic fever had titers of heart-reactive antibodies twice as high as the group who did not develop rheumatic fever.[21] Furthermore, the decrease in titer of heart-reactive antibodies coincided with the clinical course of recovery in patients with acute rheumatic fever.[23]

Antibodies to group A streptococcal polysaccharides may persist at high levels for many years in patients with rheumatic heart disease, but not in patients with chorea or glomerulonephritis. It is also significant that the heart-reactive antibodies in patients with acute rheumatic fever can be readily absorbed out of the serum with streptococcal cell membranes and with cardiac tissue, whereas the heart-reactive antibodies in patients with non-rheumatic cardiac injury (Fig. 7-1) can be absorbed only with cardiac tissue.

Further evidence of a correlation between rheumatic fever and heart-reactive antibodies was provided by studies in a group of patients who were followed after their first attack of rheumatic fever. Usually heart-reactive antibody titers decrease fairly rapidly following the acute attack, and are barely detectable after 3 years. However, it was found that patients whose titer of heart-reactive antibodies did not decline in a normal manner appeared to be more susceptible to recurrent attacks of rheumatic fever. Furthermore when the titer of heart-reactive antibodies was increased by recurrent streptococcal infections, a critical level seemed to be reached at which time rheumatic fever made its appearance. On the other hand, it should be emphasized that levels of heart-reactive antibodies do not correlate well with the extent of valvular injury in rheumatic fever.

The production of autoimmune carditis in experimental animals has not contributed greatly to our understanding of related human conditions. The immunization of animals with either heterologous or homologous cardiac tissue in adjuvant results in the formation of autoreactive antiheart antibodies in a significant number of animals. However, the inflammatory lesions which develop in the heart tend to be rather sparse and unimpressive.[3] Furthermore, there is very little correlation between the titer of circulating antiheart antibodies and the severity of the experimental cardiac lesion.

Thus, the relationship between streptococcal infection and inflammatory cardiac disease appears to be well established, but little is understood concerning mechanisms of tissue damage. Two possible pathogenetic mechanisms for immunologic tissue injury in rheumatic fever are depicted schematically in Figure 7-1. The concepts expressed in the diagram are, of course, partly hypothetical.

Although the streptococcus is felt to be the major etiologic agent in rheumatic fever, evidence of viral infection has been found in an occasional patient with this disease. Recently it has been demonstrated that Coxsackie B$_4$ virus induces a carditis in monkeys that grossly resembles human rheumatic heart disease. Viral antigen is demonstrable by immunofluorescence at the sites of the acute lesions and chronic valvular lesions such as mitral stenosis may eventually occur in some animals.

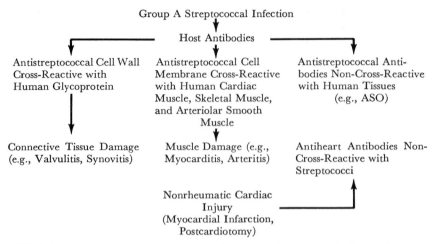

FIG. 7-1. Proposed mechanisms for the immunopathogenesis of rheumatic fever.

IMMUNOPATHOLOGY

Until recently most of the material available for histologic study came from patients dying of acute carditis. In these cases the heart is generally pale, flabby, and dilated, and occasionally shows vegetations on valve leaflets. The general cardiac dilatation results in enlargement of the valve orifices.

Microscopic examination of the heart reveals degeneration of muscle cells and "fibrinoid" changes in the collagenous tissues. Necrotic, non-myogenic Anitschkow cells are surrounded by mononuclear and giant cells and the resulting cluster constitutes the Aschoff body which is considered to be reasonably specific for rheumatic fever. By contrast, the Anitschkow cells have recently been found in the hearts of patients who do not have rheumatic heart disease and, thus, cannot be considered pathognomonic for this disease. In addition to these focal areas of inflammation there may be diffuse myocardial inflammatory change.

In those patients who go on to develop chronic rheumatic heart disease, the changes reflect the extent and type of valve involvement. The left side of the heart is characteristically more severely affected. Individual chamber enlargement and hypertrophy depends on the site and type of valve lesion. The valves themselves may be fibrotic, deformed, thickened, stenotic, or incompetent, and, in the late stages of the disease, may become calcified.

Since the advent of heart surgery, autopsy material is no longer the sole source of histologic material in rheumatic fever. The biopsy of atrial appendages has permitted the demonstration by the immunofluorescent technique of deposited immune reactants in approximately 20 per cent of patients undergoing surgery for rheumatic heart disease. For example, in one series, γ-globulin was found to be deposited in the myocardium and interstitial connective tissue of 18 per cent of patients.[9]

Of even greater interest is the finding of widespread deposition of immunoglobulins (IgG, IgA, and IgM) and complement in the myocardium of children who died with fulminating acute rheumatic fever. Immune reactants were deposited mainly in the sarcolemmal and subsarcolemmal areas, but were also found in vascular smooth muscle and interstitial connective tissue. While the distribution of bound immunoglobulin was of greater extent than the distribution of morphologic damage, the amount of deposited immunoglobulin correlated well with electrocardiographic and clinical evidence of widespread myocardial injury.[8] Immunoglobulins are also found in the connective tissue of the valves in patients with acute rheumatic fever. Unlike the myocardium, the valves bind only IgG; IgA, IgM, and complement are not involved.

Articular structures in patients with joint involvement show a diffuse inflammatory process with exudation, fibrin deposition, and leukocytic infiltration. The infiltrate is predominantly polymorphonuclear initially and later becomes monocytic in character. Destruction of joint structures and erosion of the joint surface similar to that found in rheumatoid arthritis do not occur. The subcutaneous nodules associated with acute rheumatic fever can generally be distinguished histologically from those which occur in rheumatoid arthritis. Characteristically the nodules show a considerable amount of fibrinoid material, edema, and a scant cellular infiltrate with little or no fibrosis.

In patients who die with chorea, changes in the brain include a focal arteritis in many areas, inflammatory cell infiltration, and occasional nerve cell degeneration. A less common finding is cerebral infarction due to embolization. Generally the neuropathologic abnormalities are not striking and there tends to be rather poor correlation between the pathologic changes and the observed clinical abnormalities of the nervous system. More than 50 per cent of patients with acute rheumatic fever show changes compatible with glomerulonephritis on renal biopsy. However, the ultrastructural abnormalities are not typical of the "immune-complex type" of post-streptococcal glomerulonephritis.

CLINICAL IMMUNOLOGY

Clinical immunologic procedures which may be useful in the diagnosis of rheumatic fever fall into three groups: (1) those which give nonspecific evidence of an immunologic reaction such as hypergammaglobulinemia and a change in serum complement levels; (2) those which provide specific evidence of a recent streptococcal infection; and (3) those which demonstrate the presence of heart-reactive antibodies in the sera.

Serum protein electrophoresis in acute rheumatic fever generally shows elevation of the α2-globulins (acute phase reactants), and an occasional increase in γ-globulin which is sometimes accompanied by a slight decrease in albumin. The serum complement is usually normal in acute rheumatic fever, but, for reasons which are poorly understood, it may occasionally be elevated or decreased. The occasional elevation of serum complement may be due to the fact that it behaves as an acute phase reactant. Another acute phase reactant, C-reactive protein (see Chapter 22), is frequently elevated as a non-specific manifestation of acute rheumatic fever.

Of more value are the specific streptococcal antibody tests, particularly those directed against "extracellular" antigens elaborated by the organism. The most useful of these is the anti-streptolysin O titer (see Chapter 22). While values for the test vary between laboratories, titers of at least 250 Todd units in adults and at least 333 Todd units in children over 5 years of age are considered to be significantly elevated. Since approximately 20 per cent of patients in the early stages of rheumatic fever have normal ASO titers, the use of other streptococcal antibody tests such as anti-hyaluronidase, anti-streptokinase, anti-DNAase and anti-NADase may be of value. Very few patients with acute rheumatic fever will fail to show an increase in streptococcal antibody titers when two or more tests are performed. The only possible exceptions to this general statement are those patients with pure chorea.[1]

The demonstration of elevated titers of heart-reactive antibodies may be of considerable assistance in the diagnosis of rheumatic fever. A number of other disorders such as SLE, rheumatoid arthritis, and sarcoidosis which may resemble rheumatic fever are not associated with the presence of these antibodies in high titer.

An indirect immunofluorescence test is usually employed for antibody detection. Cardiac muscle of animal origin is used as the substrate, and three immunofluorescent patterns are commonly recognized: sarcolemmal-subsarcolemmal, intermyofibrillar, and diffuse sarcoplasmic.[6a] The sarcolemmal-subsarcolemmal (SSL) pattern is the one generally observed in acute rheumatic fever and appears to be the most specific for this disease. The intermyofibrillar pattern is seldom seen, and the diffuse sarcoplasmic pattern is considered to be a non-specific response to inflammation. In a recent review,[6a] it was reported that antiheart antibodies of all three immunofluorescent patterns occur in 41 to 77 per cent of patients with acute rheumatic fever, in 12 to 21 per cent of patients with clinically inactive rheumatic heart disease, and in 0 to 4 per cent of normal individuals. The SSL pattern is also found in acute poststreptococcal glomerulonephritis and after uncomplicated streptococcal infections, but the antibody titers are much lower than in acute rheumatic fever.

Since the cardiac antibodies are probably multiple and the corresponding antigens are poorly defined, it is not surprising that antibody levels do not correlate well with disease activity. Nevertheless, the highest titers are often found: (1) in patients with carditis as opposed to those without, (2) in patients with active disease, and (3) in patients who have had multiple attacks of rheumatic fever.

CLINICAL MANIFESTATIONS

The symptoms and signs of rheumatic fever follow streptococcal infection after a latent period which may vary from 0 to 45 days, but usually averages approximately 18 days. The clinical manifestations have been divided into major and minor diagnostic criteria.[17] The major manifestations consist of carditis, polyarthritis, chorea, erythema marginatum, and subcutaneous nodules. The minor manifestations are divided into clinical and laboratory findings. The minor clinical manifestations include evidence of previous rheumatic fever or rheumatic heart disease, arthralgia, and fever. The laboratory manifestations consist of: (1) elevation of acute phase reactants such as C-reactive protein (see Chapter 22); (2) elevated erythrocyte sedimentation rate; (3) leukocytosis; and (4) prolongation of the P-R interval on the electrocardiogram.

The presence of two major criteria, or of one major and two minor criteria, is considered to be highly suggestive of the diagnosis of rheumatic fever *when supported by evidence of a preceding streptococcal infection.* This evidence may consist of a history of recent scarlet fever, a positive throat culture for group A streptococcus, or, more usually, immunologic evidence of a recent streptococcal infection.

Carditis is usually manifested clinically by the presence of a significant murmur in a patient without previous heart disease, or a change in a murmur in a patient with previous rheumatic disease. Cardiomegaly, pericarditis, and otherwise unexplained congestive heart failure may also be considered as manifestations of rheumatic carditis.

The polyarthritis of acute rheumatic fever is characterized by the usual signs of inflammation of joints, and it is typically migratory in nature. Although the large joints are most frequently affected, almost any joint in the body may be involved. Arthralgia without evidence of inflammation, tenderness, or limitation of joint movement is considered to be a minor manifestation.

Neurologic involvement in acute rheumatic fever takes the form of chorea and is characterized by involuntary movements, muscular weakness, and emotional lability. The abnormal movements may affect almost any muscle group, but most often involve the muscles of the hands and face. These involuntary movements tend to be purposeless and not rhythmic as in Parkinson's syndrome.

Two cutaneous manifestations are noted in rheumatic fever—erythema marginatum and subcutaneous nodules. The rash of erythema marginatum consists of serpiginous or circular areas of erythema with a pale center. The lesions occur mainly on the trunk and proximal portions of the limbs, but never on the face. They may be migratory, they are usually nonpruritic, and they tend to blanch on pressure. The subcutaneous nodules are firm, nontender, and occur mainly over the extensor surfaces of joints such as the elbows, knees, and wrists. Occasionally, subcutaneous nodules may be found in the occipital region and over the vertebral spinal processes.

Less common clinical manifestations may include fever, abdominal pain, malaise, anemia, and tachycardia. Erythema nodosum (see Chapter 5), pulmonary infiltrates (rheumatic pneumonia), and pleurisy have been described in a minority of patients. However, the existence of pulmonary involvement which is distinct from that associated with congestive heart failure has been questioned in recent years.

The duration of acute rheumatic fever is extremely variable, but most of the clinical findings tend to subside in 10 to 12 weeks, even in untreated patients.

PREVENTION AND TREATMENT

Prevention in Nonrheumatic Subjects

Rheumatic fever and rheumatic heart disease are theoretically preventable disorders, since the etiologic agent, the group A streptococcus, is well defined and can be eradicated. However, the fact that approximately one-third of the cases of acute rheumatic fever follow asymptomatic streptococcal infections makes effective prevention a difficult task. Essential to an adequate prevention program is the use of rapid techniques for throat culture in all patients with clinical pharyngitis and in all contacts of patients with known streptococcal infections. Present bacteriologic methods allow for identification of group A hemolytic streptococci within 1 to 2 days, and in most cases treatment can be withheld until the bacteriologic diagnosis is made. In patients with clinical signs of scarlet fever or obvious acute exudative pharyngitis, treatment may be instituted immediately after a throat culture is taken. Newer fluorescent antibody techniques may permit a much more rapid bacteriologic diagnosis to be made.

Once the diagnosis of group A streptococcal infection is established, effective prevention of rheumatic fever depends on maintaining adequate antibiotic blood levels for at least 10 consecutive days. This objective is most readily achieved by a single intramuscular injection of benzathine penicillin in a dose of 600,000 to 900,000 units for children and 900,000 to 1,200,000 units for adults. The disadvantage of oral penicillin in doses of 250,000 units, four times daily for 10 days, is that successful therapy depends entirely on complete patient cooperation. In those patients who are known to be allergic to penicillin, erythromycin in a dose of 125 to 250 mg, four times daily, is the recommended form of treatment.

Treatment

No therapeutic measure is known which is curative in acute rheumatic fever. However, a number of agents are available which will suppress the manifestations of the disease and certainly contribute to the patient's comfort. The treatment of rheumatic fever can be divided into general measures, antibiotic therapy, anti-inflammatory therapy, and therapy directed at specific organ dysfunction.

The most valuable general therapeutic measure is the judicious use of bed-rest. This form of therapy is certainly indicated in patients with severe polyarthritis and in those with congestive heart failure. In addition, it is probably indicated in all patients during the first 2 to 5 weeks of their illness. Patients who recover without residual cardiac disease should be allowed completely unrestricted physical activity.

Since many patients with acute rheumatic fever have either had an untreated recent streptococcal infection or still harbor the organism, many authorities feel that an eradicating dose of penicillin should be administered. However, well-controlled studies do not indicate any significant therapeutic effect from this form of therapy in terms of prevention of residual cardiac damage.[18]

Two groups of drugs, the salicylates and the adrenal corticosteroids, are capable of suppressing most of the acute manifestations of the disease. While there may be some continuing controversy about which of these agents is the more effective in controlling the acute manifestations, there now seems little doubt that there is no significant difference in residual cardiac damage between patients treated with corticosteroids, ACTH, or salicylates.[6] However, there is a general clinical impression that corticosteroids (e.g., prednisone, 40 to 80 mg, daily in divided doses) are more effective than salicylates in the treatment of patients with cardiac failure, despite their tendency to cause sodium and water retention. Otherwise, there seems to be little to be gained from the use of corticosteroids during acute rheumatic fever, and most patients can be adequately controlled on salicylates alone for 6 to 8 weeks. Acetylsalicylic acid in divided doses of 40 mg/lb of body weight per day for 2 weeks followed by 30 mg/lb day for 6 weeks is a commonly prescribed schedule for patients with moderate to severe arthritis or for patients who have carditis without congestive failure.

The clinical manifestations of chorea do not respond either to salicylates or to corticosteroids, but usually respond to mild sedative or tranquillizing drugs such as phenobarbital, the phenothiazines, or reserpine in doses commensurate with individual tolerance. Should congestive cardiac failure occur, the usual therapeutic measures such as bed rest, digitalis, sodium restriction, and diuretics are indicated.

At the end of a 6 to 8 week period, assuming the manifestations of the disease have come under control, medication should be discontinued gradually in order to avoid a severe recurrence of symptoms. If the recurrence which occurs is determined by laboratory evidence alone (e.g., elevated ESR or C-reactive protein) and is not accompanied by any clinical manifestations, then no additional therapy need be given. An acute exacerbation of the disease, particularly if accompanied by carditis, usually requires reinstitution of therapy.

Prevention of Recurrences in Rheumatic Patients

Since recurrences of rheumatic fever are clearly related to streptococcal infections of the group A type and tend to occur more frequently in individuals who have had a previous attack, continual prophylaxis against streptococcal infection is indicated in all patients who have had acute rheumatic fever. It has not yet been established when such prophylactic measures should be discontinued, if ever. Those at greatest risk are patients who had carditis during their first attack, those in the younger age groups, and those who have had an attack of acute rheumatic fever within the previous 5 years.

Prophylaxis is most effectively accomplished by a single monthly injection of 1.2 million units of benzathine penicillin. The oral administration of sulfadiazine, 1.0 gm daily, or oral penicillin, 400,000 units daily, is probably equally effective, but lack of patient cooperation may result in failure of prophylaxis.

The use of streptococcal vaccines may some day replace antibiotic prophylaxis, but, at present, their use is still experimental. Furthermore, vaccine administration, at least in a few patients, appears to have been followed by an attack of acute rheumatic fever.[11]

Patients with rheumatic heart disease have an increased susceptibility to subacute bacterial endocarditis following any disease process or any surgical procedure which is associated with bacteremia. Dental, upper respiratory tract, and genitourinary tract surgery are particularly hazardous, and require special preventive measures. The administration of 600,000 units of procaine penicillin intramuscularly on the day of surgery and for 2 days thereafter is considered mandatory. In those patients known to be allergic to penicillin, erythromycin may be substituted with satisfactory results.

POSTCARDIOTOMY AND POSTMYOCARDIAL INFARCTION SYNDROMES

The postcardiotomy syndrome was first described in patients who had recently undergone mitral commissurotomy, and, for a time, was believed to be due to reactivation of quiescent rheumatic fever. The subsequent occurrence of an identical syndrome after surgery for congenital heart disease, and after pericardiotomy for a variety of nonrheumatic disorders, rendered the reactivation theory highly unlikely. Very similar syndromes have been described after cardiac trauma and after acute myocardial infarction.

IMMUNOPATHOGENESIS

The pathogenesis of the postcardiotomy and postmyocardial infarction syndromes is unknown, but the latent period, clinical findings, response to corticosteroid therapy, and high incidence of antiheart antibodies strongly suggest an immune mechanism.

The incidence of heart antibodies after cardiac surgery appears to vary greatly depending on the method of detection. Incidences ranging from approximately 15 per cent of patients (antiglobulin consumption test) to 100 per cent of patients (immunofluorescence technique) have been reported.[19,21] The antibodies are usually present as a transient phenomenon in the postoperative period, and since they frequently occur in patients with no evidence of postcardiotomy syndrome, their pathogenetic significance is unclear. On the other hand, antiheart antibodies, often in high titer, are almost always present in the sera of patients with the clinical manifestations of the postcardiotomy syndrome.[10]

The heart antibodies show specificity for cardiac and skeletal muscle, and generally give a sarcolemmal-subsarcolemmal immunofluorescent staining pattern. In some patients, at least, the antibodies are absorbed by heart tissue, but, unlike the situation in rheumatic fever, they are not absorbed by streptococcal cell membranes.[21] It is conceivable that multiple heart antigens are involved, and perhaps certain antibodies are pathogenic while others are innocuous.

Antiheart antibodies are demonstrable in about one-half of the patients with the postmyocardial infarction syndrome,[19] and tend to disappear in quiescent periods between attacks. Antibodies are also found transiently in approximately one-quarter of all patients with myocardial infarction. The pathogenetic significance of these antibodies is thus unclear, and the same comments apply here as in the postcardiotomy syndrome. In both conditions, injury to the pericardium, myocardium, or skeletal muscle is presumed to be the stimulus to antibody production.

Other possible immunologic consequences of myocardial infarction include the development of a protein with "rheumatoid factor-like" activity and the appearance of small amounts of cryoprotein.[4] Both of these phenomena are generally transient.

CLINICAL MANIFESTATIONS

The postcardiotomy syndrome is characterized by fever, clinical manifestations of pericarditis (e.g., pain, friction rub), pleuritis, myalgia, arthralgia, and occasional pulmonary involvement. The clinical manifestations usually follow surgery after a 2 to 3 week latent period, but much longer latent periods have been described. The syndrome has a marked tendency to recur spontaneously.

The laboratory findings in the postcardiotomy syndrome are nonspecific and may include an elevated ESR, a positive test for C-reactive protein, and leukocytosis. The EKG may show evidence of pericarditis, and serous effusions may be detected on radiographic examination of the chest.

The postmyocardial infarction syndrome closely resembles the postcardiotomy syndrome. It occurs in approximately 3 per cent of patients with myocardial infarction and is characterized by fever, chest pain, pericarditis, pleuritis, and pneumonitis. The pericarditis is usually clinically apparent between the second and eleventh weeks of illness. The latent period, laboratory findings, and tendency to recurrence are all similar to those observed in the postcardiotomy syndrome.

TREATMENT

In mild cases of postcardiotomy or postmyocardial infarction syndrome, no specific treatment is necessary. However, restriction of activity is said to speed recovery. In more severely affected patients, corticosteroids (e.g., prednisone in divided doses of 10 to 40 mg daily) may provide dramatic symptomatic relief. It should be noted, however, that too rapid withdrawal may be followed by a severe relapse.

PERICARDITIS

ALLERGIC PERICARDITIS

Occasionally a form of benign pericarditis occurs in association with other allergic manifestations such as urticaria, bronchial asthma, allergic drug reactions, and after the administration of foreign proteins.[2] The mechanism of production of the pericardial inflammatory process is unknown.

RECURRENT ACUTE BENIGN PERICARDITIS

So-called "benign viral pericarditis" is often observed following an upper respiratory infection. The latent period, recurrent pattern, arthralgia, resemblance to the previously mentioned syndromes, and occasional eosinophilia have suggested a role for immune mechanisms in some of these patients. Antibodies reactive with cardiac tissue have been found in approximately one-half of patients with recurrent acute benign pericarditis,[10] and there is often a dramatic response to corticosteroid therapy.

IDIOPATHIC CARDIOMYOPATHIES

Antibodies to heart tissue and the deposition of γ-globulin in the ventricular myocardium have been described in patients with idiopathic primary myocardial diseases.[13,14] On the other hand, subsequent investigations have failed to disclose a significant difference in the incidence of antiheart antibodies between patients with various cardiomyopathies and control subjects.[10] Since a variety of basically different diseases are probably included in this category, the inconsistency of the immunologic findings is not too surprising.

ENDOMYOCARDIAL FIBROSIS

This disorder, which is quite common in Central Africa, has a number of interesting immunologic features. For example, antiheart antibodies are present in over 50 per cent of patients with endomyocardial fibrosis, and the incidence of antiheart antibodies shows a strong correlation with increased titers of antimalarial antibodies.[16,20] High serum levels of IgM are also noted in patients with antimalarial antibodies. Cryoglobulins of the mixed type are demonstrable in the majority of patients with endomyocardial fibrosis, and γ-globulin and fibrin have been found to be deposited in the myocardium of patients dying of this disease.

Of possible pathogenetic significance is the observation that there appears to be an unusual coexistence of rheumatic heart disease and endomyocardial fibrosis in African patients.[15] Furthermore, antibodies to heart, thyroid and gastric parietal cells have been demonstrated in patients with antimalarial antibodies. Thus, it is conceivable that an unusual immunologic response to a malarial, or even streptococcal, antigen gives rise to a variety of autoantibodies including an antimyocardial antibody (c.f., discussion in Chapter 6 on the relationship between quartan malaria and nephrotic syndrome). As yet, however, the pathogenetic potential of antiheart antibodies in endomyocardial fibrosis is not established.

REFERENCES

1. Ayoub, E. M., and Wannamaker, L. W. Streptococcal antibody titer in Syndenham's chorea. *Pediatrics 38:*946, 1966.

2. Clarkson, P. M., McCredie, K. B., and Fleishl, P. Allergic pericarditis. *Brit. Med. J. 1:*481, 1964.

3. Davies, A. M., Laufer, A., Gery, I., and Rosenmann, E. Organ specificity of the heart. III. Circulating antibodies and immunopathological lesions in experimental animals. *Arch. Path. 78:*369, 1964.

4. Finkelstein, A. E., Woerner, T. E., Smith, J. C., Bayles, T. B., and Levine, H. D. Abnormal globulins in myocardial infarction. With special reference to a material coating erythrocytes and a cold-insoluble protein. *Amer. J. Med. 35:*163, 1963.

5. Goldstein, I., Halpern, B., and Robert, L. Immunological relationship between streptococcus A polysaccharide and the structural glycoproteins of heart valve. *Nature 213:*44, 1967.

6. Joint Report Medical Research Council of Great Britain and American Heart Association: Natural history of rheumatic fever and rheumatic heart disease. Ten year report of a co-operative clinical trial of A.C.T.H., cortisone and aspirin. *Brit. Med. J. 2:*607, 1965.

6a. Kaplan, M. H. "Autoimmunity and Its Relation to Heart Disease. A Review," *In Progress in Allergy XIII,* ed. by Kallos, P., and Waksman, B. H., Basel, Karger, p. 408, 1969.

7. Kaplan, M. H. Immunologic relation of streptococcal and tissue antigens. I. Properties of an antigen in certain strains of group A streptococci exhibiting an immunologic cross-reaction with human heart tissue. *J. Immun. 90:*595, 1963.

8. Kaplan, M. H., Bolande, R., Rakita, L., and Blair, J. Presence of bound immunoglobulins and complement in the myocardium in acute rheumatic fever. *New Eng. J. Med. 271*:637, 1964.

9. Kaplan, M. H., and Dallenbach, F. D. Immunologic studies of heart tissue. III. Occurrence of bound γ-globulin in auricular appendages from rheumatic hearts. Relationship to certain histo-pathologic features of rheumatic heart disease. *J. Exp. Med. 113*:1, 1961.

10. Kaplan, M. H., and Frengley, J. D. Autoimmunity to the heart in cardiac disease. Current concepts of the relation of autoimmunity to rheumatic fever, post-cardiotomy and postinfarction syndromes and cardiomyopathies. *Amer. J. Cardiol. 24*:459, 1969.

11. Massel, B. F., Honikman, L. H., and Amezcua, J. Rheumatic fever following streptococcal vaccination. Report of three cases. *J.A.M.A. 207*:1115, 1969.

12. Reitz, B. A., Prager, D. J., Feigen, G. A. An analysis of the toxic actions of purified streptolysin O on the isolated heart and separate cardiac tissues of the guinea pig. *J. Exp. Med. 128*:1401, 1969.

13. Sanders, V. Viral myocarditis. *Amer. Heart. J. 66*:707, 1963.

14. Sanders, V., and Ritts, R. Ventricular localization of bound gamma globulin in idiopathic disease of the myocardium. *J.A.M.A. 194*:59, 1965.

15. Shaper, A. G. Endomyocardial fibrosis and rheumatic heart disease. *Lancet 1*:639, 1966.

16. Shaper, A. G., Kaplan, M. H., Foster, W. D., McIntosh, D. M., and Wilks, N. E. Immunological studies in endomyocardial fibrosis and other forms of heart disease in the tropics. *Lancet 1*:598, 1967.

17. Stollerman, G. H., Markowitz, M., Taranta, A., Wannamaker, L. W., and Whittemore, R. Jones criteria (revised) for guidance in the diagnosis of rheumatic fever. *Circulation 32*:664, 1965.

18. Vaisman, S. B., Guash, J. L., Vignau, A. I., Correa, E. T., Schuster, A. C., Mortimer, E. A., Jr., and Rammelkamp, C. H., Jr. Failure of penicillin to alter acute rheumatic valvulitis *J.A.M.A. 194*:1284, 1965.

19. Van der Geld, H. Anti-heart antibodies in the post-pericardiotomy and the post-myocardial infarction syndromes. *Lancet 2*:617, 1964.

20. Van der Geld, H., Peetom, F., Somers, K., and Kanyerezi, B. R. Immuno-histological and serological studies in endomyocardial fibrosis. *Lancet 2*:1210, 1966.

21. Zabriskie, J. B. Mimetic relationships between group A streptococci and mammalian tissues. *Advances Immun. 7*:147, 1967.

22. Zabriskie, J. B., and Freimer, E. H. An immunological relationship between the group A streptococcus and mammalian muscle. *J. Exp. Med 124*:661, 1966.

23. Zabriskie, J. B., Hsu, K. C., and Seegal, B. C. Heart-reactive antibody associated with rheumatic fever: characterization and diagnostic significance. *Clin. Exp. Immun. 7*:147, 1970.

8

Collagen-Vascular Diseases

DAVID HAWKINS

The collagen-vascular diseases are a group of disorders characterized by a multisystem nonsuppurative inflammatory process with a pronounced tendency to involve connective tissue and vascular structures. In most of the collagen-vascular diseases there is evidence of autoimmune phenomena or other features suggestive of an immunologic process. These immunologic abnormalities may include elevated serum immunoglobulin levels, deposition of immune reactants such as antigen, antibody and complement in affected organs, and altered serum complement levels. While the term "collagen disease" is not entirely accurate, it is widely used and serves to focus attention on the involvement of connective tissue and related structures.

A common feature of these diseases is their tendency to overlap in their clinical and laboratory manifestations. Nevertheless, a number of well-defined clinical entities are distinguishable.

SYSTEMIC LUPUS ERYTHEMATOSUS (SLE)

The most significant immunologic feature of systemic lupus erythematosus (SLE) is the tendency of the affected patient to form antibodies to a variety of tissue constituents, particularly nuclear components. As a result of recent studies of the immunopathogenesis of SLE, the abnormalities of this disorder are currently better understood than those in any of the other collagen-vascular diseases.

ETIOLOGY AND PATHOGENESIS

Although the etiology of SLE is unknown, there are several observations which provide insight into this area. The first is the ability of certain drugs to induce a syndrome resembling SLE, or to activate underlying SLE. One group of drugs appears to induce SLE as the direct result of their pharmacologic properties, whereas the others probably act through a hypersensitivity mechanism.[1]

The drugs which appear to act through pharmacologic mechanisms are listed in decreasing order of their potential for inducing SLE: (1) procainamide, (2) hydralazine, (3) isoniazid, and (4) several anticonvulsant agents such as dilantin, mesantoin, trimethadione, and primidone. As many as 65 per cent of patients receiving procainamide may develop antinuclear antibodies, and 8 to 13 per cent of patients receiving hydralazine may develop a lupus-like syndrome. A large percentage of patients who receive either procainamide or hydralizine show serologic abnormalities without the development of overt SLE.

The mechanism of activation of SLE in this group of patients may involve alteration of nuclear antigens in patients with an underlying lupus diathesis. The failure of regression of abnormalities in some patients on withdrawal of the initiating drug, as well as the greater prevalence of pre-existing immunologic abnormalities, tends to support this concept. The drug-induced SLE syndrome does not appear to differ from "spontaneous" SLE except for its greater occurrence in patients in the older age groups.

Those drugs that probably act by first giving rise to a hypersensitivity reaction, which initiates the manifestations of SLE, include: penicillin, the sulfonamides, α-methyl dopa, oral contraceptive agents, propylthiouracil, phenylbutazone, and reserpine.

Two further observations add weight to the contention that the SLE syndrome is genetically determined and depends on subsequent environmental factors (e.g., drugs, viruses, or sunlight) for its full manifestation. The first is the tendency for SLE and related collagen-vascular disorders to occur in single families and in identical twins. In addition, the immediate relatives of patients with SLE have a significant increase in the frequency of elevated immunoglobulin levels as compared with the immediate relatives of patients with rheumatoid arthritis.

The second observation is that of the occurrence of spontaneous systemic connective tissue disease in the inbred strain of New Zealand Black (NZB) mice. These mice develop autoimmune hemolytic anemia, thymic lesions, and occasionally malignant lymphoma. When these mice are bred to develop the NZB/NZW F_1 hybrid animals, they develop a syndrome which is remarkably similar to human SLE with glomerulonephritis. The immunopathology and pathogenesis of the renal lesions appear to be almost identical to that seen in human SLE.

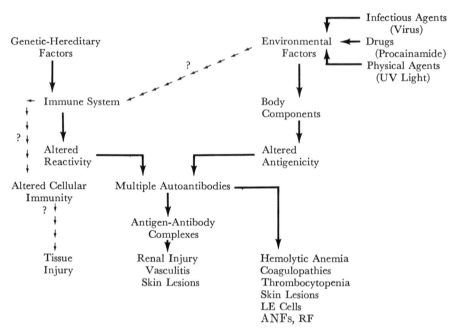

FIG. 8-1. Schematic representation of possible pathogenetic mechanisms in SLE.

Recently, there has been considerable interest in the role of naturally occurring virus-like agents in the production of SLE. Of particular interest is the report that a virus-like agent has been separated from lymphoma cells of NZB/Bl mice (see Chapter 12). Furthermore, evidence has been brought forward that a murine leukemia-like virus (muLV) is associated with the disorders of NZB mice. Such an agent has, through study of specific muLV group antigens, been found to be prevalent in extracts of spleen, kidney, and thymus throughout a substantial portion of the life span of these mice.[7] Murine leukemia-like virus group antigens and host immunoglobulins have been demonstrated by immunofluorescence in the glomerular lesions of NZB mice with renal disease.

Preliminary investigations suggest that viral agents may also be associated with human SLE. Significantly increased titers of antibodies to myxoviruses (e.g. parainfluenza I and measles) were found in some patients with SLE, particularly those with neurologic involvement.[8a] In addition, tubular structures morphologically similar to nucleoprotein strands liberated from myxoviruses were found in the endothelial cells of glomeruli in kidney biopsies from 45 patients with clinically proven SLE with renal involvement. These virus-like structures were not found in approximately 300 renal biopsies obtained from patients without SLE.[4,5a]

The possible roles of the genetic, environmental, and infectious factors in the etiology and pathogenesis of SLE are summarized in Figure 8-1. As yet, this scheme is largely hypothetical, and in any one patient not all factors may be operative. Furthermore, the effect of environmental agents may not be simply one of altering antigenicity, but may involve the production of cross-reactive antibodies or pathogenic antigen-antibody complexes (e.g., viral-antiviral antigen-antibody complexes). Thus, at least two basic immunopathogenetic mechanisms may be involved in the production of lesions in SLE: (1) the localization of antigen-antibody complexes in vascular structures in the kidney and other organs, and (2) the formation of specific antitissue or anticellular antibodies which damage their respective target organs (e.g., anti-erythrocyte antibodies).

IMMUNOPATHOLOGY

General Pathologic Changes in SLE

Despite the extensive clinical disease which can occur in terminal cases of SLE, the pathologic abnormalities may be remarkably less striking. Furthermore, of those seen, very few are actually pathognomonic of SLE.

Hematoxylin bodies which are round or oval masses found in a variety of tissues appear to be the tissue counterpart of the LE cell phenomenon. Hematoxylin bodies may be found in the skin, kidney, lung, lymph nodes, spleen, serous and synovial membranes, and heart. They are the only pathologic abnormality which can be considered in any way specific for SLE. These bodies appear to consist of deoxyribonucleic acid (DNA) complexed with γ-globulin; the latter, in all likelihood, represents antibody to nuclear constituents.

Other changes, while not specific for SLE, are highly suggestive of its presence. These include verrucous endocarditis, thickening of the glomerular capillaries of the kidney producing the so-called "wire-loop" appearance, concentric fibrosis of the central and penicillary arteries of the spleen giving the "onion skin" lesion, and deposition of fibrinoid material in a variety of organs. This latter substance, which has some of the tinctorial qualities of fibrin, has been found in different studies to contain protein material of nuclear origin, acid mucopolysaccharides, fibrin and related products, γ-globulin, and complement. Fibrinoid is most characteristically deposited along connective tissue fibers and in blood vessels. An inflammatory or necrotizing vasculitis may be seen in a variety of visceral lesions. The deposition of immune reactants and the frequent association of polymorphonuclear leukocyte infiltration in arteritic lesions suggests an Arthus-like phenomenon.

Skin

It is not possible to distinguish pathologically between chronic discoid lupus involving only the skin and the cutaneous lesions of SLE. Furthermore, there is no single specific cutaneous lesion in SLE. Nevertheless, the association of hyperkeratosis, keratotic plugging of hair follicles, epidermal atrophy, degeneration of the basal layer, hematoxylin bodies, fibrinoid necrosis, and a cellular infiltrate consisting mainly of lymphocytes is highly characteristic of the cutaneous lesions of SLE.

Immunofluorescent studies of skin biopsies from patients with the cutaneous lesions of SLE frequently reveal the following:

1. There is binding of γ-globulin and often complement to the nuclei of cells in the dermis and epidermis. The available evidence suggests that this binding actually occurs in vivo and may contribute significantly in the production of the lesion. Cells at the site of the skin lesions possibly are altered by permeability factors which permit penetration of antinuclear antibodies.

2. There are complexes of nuclear antigens and γ-globulin (presumably antinuclear antibody) which form aggregates at the dermal-epidermal junction. These deposits appear to be identical to the hematoxylin bodies seen in standard histologic preparations.

3. There is stippled deposition of γ-globulin and complement along the dermal-epidermal junction corresponding to the basement membrane area. The deposited γ-globulin may represent antibasement membrane antibody (see Chapter 5).

4. There is deposition of γ-globulin and complement in the walls of small cutaneous blood vessels; this is compatible with vasculitis of immunologic origin.

All of these observations support the contention that antibodies are of possible importance in the production of the pathologic lesions in the skin in SLE. It is noteworthy that none of these changes are found in skin biopsies obtained from patients with dermatomyositis, polymyositis, or drug-induced SLE. Areas of uninvolved skin in patients with SLE skin lesions are also devoid of immune reactants. It has recently been shown that exposure of human skin to ultraviolet irradiation results in rapid damage to DNA in epidermal nuclei.[11]

Kidney

In addition to the thickening of the glomerular capillary loops noted on light microscopy, a significant finding is the presence of subepithelial electron dense deposits on electron microscopic examination. As is the case in poststreptococcal glomerulonephritis, these changes are highly suggestive of an immune-complex type of process (see Chapter 6). Other renal ultrastructural changes include thickening of the glomerular basement membrane (GBM), endothelial cell swelling, subendothelial electron dense deposits, and virus-like structures in the glomerular endothelial cells.

The renal lesion in SLE appears to be due to deposition of circulating immune complexes along the GBM.[5] Kidney tissue from patients with lupus nephritis, when examined by fluorescent antibody techniques, shows γ-globulin and frequently complement in a nodular, discontinuous pattern along the GBM. Fibrin is found in focal deposits in the glomerular capillary lumina and in the area of the GBM. When the deposited γ-globulin is eluted from isolated glomeruli, it is found to contain a high concentration of antinuclear antibodies. Nuclear antigens have also been identified in glomerular deposits by immunofluorescence techniques.

In addition to nuclear constituents and their corresponding antibodies, mixed cryoglobulins consisting of IgG and IgM have been found deposited along the GBM in some patients with SLE and have been implicated in the production of both glomerulonephritis and vasculitis[10] (see Chapter 10).

Other Organs

Other organs have not been examined as extensively by immunopathologic techniques as have the skin and kidney. However, in many instances blood vessels in various tissues have been found to contain deposits of immune reactants, and thus there is further evidence in favor of an immunologic basis for the lesions. A discussion of the possible mechanisms of immunologic vascular injury is considered subsequently in this chapter under the vasculitic syndromes. (Also see Fig. 1-6.)

A point worthy of note is the appearance of lymph nodes in SLE which show disruption and necrosis of the sinuses with sparing of the follicles. This finding is in contrast to the changes in rheumatoid arthritis where follicular hyperplasia of the lymph nodes is common. In the synovial tissue, the presence of fibrin-like material adjacent to the synovium is the most characteristic finding. Damage to articular cartilage is much less striking than in rheumatoid arthritis.

CLINICAL IMMUNOLOGY

The LE Cell Phenomenon

The LE cell, which may be found in either the bone marrow or the peripheral blood, is a polymorphonuclear leukocyte which has phagocytized nuclear material, the latter having previously reacted with antinuclear antibody.[6] Antibodies to soluble nucleoprotein or DNA are capable of inducing this phenomenon in vitro. The LE test, as usually performed, requires the presence in the serum of the LE factor, damaged leukocytes, and normal leukocytes. In the indirect LE cell technique, leukocytes obtained from normal donors may be used to demonstrate the LE cell phenomenon.

The LE cell phenomenon is one of the most specific tests for SLE, and has greater diagnostic value than the demonstration of antinuclear antibodies by immunofluorescence or serologic techniques. However, the LE cell phenomenon is not pathognomonic for this disease, particularly in the adult where it may occur in patients with rheumatoid arthritis, chronic active liver disease, chronic ulcerative colitis, or leprosy.

Hypergammaglobulinemia

The commonest immunoglobulin abnormality in SLE is a broad-based or polyclonal hypergammaglobulinemia which may be associated with hypoalbuminemia if the nephrotic syndrome is also present (see Chapter 10). Occasionally, a monoclonal (M) peak may be superimposed on the polyclonal pattern. IgG is often disproportionately elevated as compared to IgA and IgM. On the other hand, patients with SLE and related collagen-vascular diseases sometimes catabolize IgG at an accelerated rate.

Antinuclear Antibodies

In patients with SLE, circulating antibodies have been detected against a number of tissue constituents, mostly nuclear. Not infrequently, more than one type of antibody is present in the same patient. For example, when double diffusion in agar is employed, antibodies may be found with specificity for DNA, soluble nucleoprotein, Sm antigen, ribosomal material, and cytoplasmic constituents.[1a] Antibodies with similar specificities may also be detected by complement fixation, passive agglutination, primary antigen-antibody binding, immunofluorescence, and antiglobulin consumption methods. Because techniques vary considerably among laboratories, it is not yet possible to establish with certainty the relative diagnostic value of the numerous tissue antibodies found in SLE. At present, it seems preferable for each institution to develop its own diagnostic criteria based on individual experience with a particular series of techniques.

In general, however, it may be said that anti-DNA antibody probably has a greater specificity for SLE than any other antibody. Furthermore, the diagnosis of SLE is highly unlikely if no antinuclear antibodies are detectable by any method. At least three types of antinuclear antibody systems have been defined in SLE: (1) anti-DNA antibodies, (2) anti-nucleoprotein antibodies, and (3) antibodies to Sm antigen.

Anti-DNA Antibodies.   The DNA–anti-DNA system shows considerable specificity for SLE. Anti-DNA antibodies, detected by double diffusion in agar gel or by complement-fixation techniques, may be found in the serum or joint fluid of patients with SLE. It is also of interest that both free DNA and antibodies to DNA may be detected in the serum of some patients with SLE. In some of these patients the appearance of free DNA in the circulation is associated with the disappearance of free antibodies to DNA, a marked exacerbation of the disease, fever, and deteriorating renal function. Thus, it is conceivable that the appearance of free DNA in the circulation represents a situation wherein soluble antigen-antibody complexes in antigen excess are being formed. The potential pathogenetic properties of circulating antigen-antibody complexes are discussed in Chapter 1.

It is felt that the source of the DNA in these patients is endogenous because free DNA is also seen in a number of diseases associated with tissue destruction such as hepatitis, metastatic carcinoma, and miliary tuberculosis. In SLE patients, both the skin and the joints have been considered possible sources of DNA for release into the circulation. However, the possibility must be considered that the DNA is exogenous in origin, e.g., microbial.

It has been suggested that free DNA, released during an exacerbation of the disease, must be altered in some way in order to be immunogenic or to combine with pre-existing antibodies. In some studies, anti-DNA antibodies were noted to react better with denatured (single-strand) DNA than with native (double-strand) DNA. An example of an agent capable of so altering DNA is ultraviolet irradiation. The skin lesions of lupus are not infrequently worsened by exposure to irradiation of this type and it is known that ultraviolet irradiated DNA acquires immunogenic properties which are not characteristic of native DNA.[11]

Antinucleoprotein Antibodies.   A second antigen-antibody system has been described in SLE. Antibodies to soluble nucleoprotein are detected by precipitation in agar gel in approximately 50 per cent of patients with SLE. The nature of the antigenic site on the soluble nucleoprotein moiety responsible for the reaction with the appropriate antibody has not been established but may depend on determinants on both DNA and nucleohistone.

Antibodies to Sm Antigen.   A third substance to which antibodies have been found in SLE is the Sm or phosphate extractable antigen of cell nuclei. Precipitins to the Sm antigen are demonstrable in 75 per cent of patients in the acute stage of the disease, but are not detected in the vast majority of patients with other connective tissue diseases such as scleroderma, dermatomyositis, rheumatoid arthritis, or in patients with various lymphoreticular malignancies. As yet the Sm antigen itself has not been found in the sera of patients with SLE, but it has been found in the urine.

Immunofluorescent Detection of Antinuclear Antibodies.   A valuable procedure for the detection of antinuclear antibodies (ANA or ANF) is the use of an indirect immunofluorescence technique utilizing a variety of substrates, usually murine liver. While this procedure does not have the specificity associated with the precipitin reaction in agar gel, it is a highly sensitive screening procedure. In a series of 100 cases of SLE, a positive test was found in *all* patients including those in remission for many years. By contrast, the LE cell test was positive in only 53 of the 100 patients and in only 12 per cent of those in complete remission.[3] In the same series it was found that IgG antinuclear factor was present in 96 per cent of patients, IgM in 81 per cent, and IgA in 51 per cent. There was no correlation between any particular type of immunoglobulin class of ANF and the clinical state of the patient.

A negative ANF by the immunofluorescence technique is considered by some to virtually exclude the diagnosis of SLE, but exceptions have been recorded. On the other hand, positive ANF tests have been reported in patients with a wide variety of disorders as listed in Table 8-1. Generally the titers in these diseases are lower than those observed in SLE. In patients with rheumatoid arthritis the ANF is frequently of the IgM type.

A variety of distinct nuclear staining patterns have been observed which include: (*1*) homogeneous (diffuse) staining produced by antibodies to particulate nucleoproteins; (*2*) shaggy (rim, peripheral) staining produced by antibodies to DNA; (*3*) speckled staining produced by antibodies to the Sm antigen; (*4*) nucleolar staining produced by a factor which reacts with nucleoli only. In general, the peripheral or shaggy pattern is found only in SLE, and correlates well with both disease activity and the LE

TABLE 8-1. Disorders Associated with Antinuclear
Antibodies

Collagen-Vascular Diseases
  Systemic lupus erythematosus
  Rheumatoid arthritis
  Juvenile rheumatoid arthritis
  Progressive systemic sclerosis
  Polymyositis
  Sjögren's syndrome

Hepatic Disease
  Chronic active liver disease

Lymphoproliferative and Myeloproliferative Disorders
  Hyperglobulinemic purpura of Waldenstrom
  Waldenstrom's macroglobulinemia
  Lymphoma
  Chronic leukemia

Pulmonary Disease
  Chronic bronchitis
  Tuberculosis
  Histoplasmosis
  Fibrosing alveolitis

Miscellaneous Disorders
  Chronic discoid lupus
  Hashimoto's thyroiditis
  Pernicious anemia
  Ulcerative colitis
  Chronic membraneous glomerulonephritis
  Lepromatous leprosy
  Neoplasms
  Drug reactions
  Myasthenia gravis
  Recurrent thrombophlebitis
  Infectious mononucleosis
  Idiopathic autoimmune hemolytic anemia
  Apparently healthy individuals

---

cell phenomenon. By contrast, diffuse or speckled patterns may be found in non-SLE disorders. For example, high titers of antinuclear antibody of the speckled variety are found in patients with scleroderma. In some patients progressive dilution of the serum may uncover antibody patterns which were masked by the presence of smaller amounts of other antibodies.

Other Antibodies

A variety of other antibodies and serologic abnormalities have been found in patients with SLE. Precipitating antibodies to ribosomal antigens have been described. Of interest is the fact that all patients with the antiribosomal anibody in one series manifested renal disease suggesting that ribosomal antigen-antibody complexes may be of pathogenetic significance in this disorder.

The sera of many patients with SLE demonstrate rheumatoid factor activity (anti-IgG), although the titers tend to be lower than those found in rheumatoid arthritis. Not infrequently there may be a positive Coombs' test associated with autoimmune hemolytic anemia, antibodies against neutrophils and platelets, cold agglutinins, and antithyroid antibodies. A biologic false-positive serologic test for syphilis is a frequent finding (see Chapter 21).

Intradermal tests to nuclear antigens have been correlated with anti-nuclear factors or clinical activity in SLE.[2] Out of 25 patients with SLE 21 gave positive reactions (generally delayed) to homologous leukocytes, 21 to calf-thymus nucleoprotein, 23 to calf-thymus histone, and 12 to calf-thymus DNA. Normal subjects gave negative intradermal reactions.

Circulating anticoagulants have been reported to occur in some patients with SLE (see Chapter 9). An increase in urinary γ-globulin has been described in patients with active SLE and nephritis of recent onset. The level of urinary γ-globulin tends to decrease with improvement in renal status. Mixed cryoglobulinemia is not uncommon in patients with SLE.

Serum Complement

That complement components may be important in both the production of pathogenic complexes and in the mediation of immunologic tissue injury is suggested by the recent finding that high complement-fixing activity of antinuclear antibodies was found in 15 patients with active nephritis. On the other hand, in 65 other patients with SLE, but without active nephritis, the relative complement fixing activity of their antibodies to nuclear antigens was much lower.[12] Very low serum complement levels and high titers of complement fixing antibody to DNA are frequently associated with active renal disease; the absence of these findings usually indicates inactive renal disease. In some patients, the fall in serum complement precedes the appearance of active renal disease.[9]

CLINICAL MANIFESTATIONS

Systemic lupus erythematosus usually appears in the second to fourth decade of life, but may occur at any age. It is several times more common in females than in males, although it should be noted that the sex difference is not as pronounced in drug-induced lupus-like syndromes and that in males there is no peak incidence in any particular decade. In females there is a greater risk of exacerbation of the disease process in the first few weeks after delivery. The puerperal period is particularly noteworthy for the severe renal involvement which may occur.

Constitutional symptoms are very common and include fever, malaise, weakness, weight loss, and anorexia. The major clinical features usually reflect involvement of one or more of the following systems: renal, cutaneous, musculoskeletal, hematologic, or nervous. The system initially affected often tends to remain the predominant one throughout the course of the disease, and multisystem involvement may only be clinically evident in the terminal stages.

Renal Disease

Renal disease is common, and, when present, is frequently the major contributor to morbidity and mortality. The kidney disorder may take the form of acute glomerulitis which may be focal or diffuse, subacute nephritis, nephrotic syndrome, or progressive renal failure (see Chapter 6). SLE causes 5 to 10 per cent of all cases of nephrotic syndrome and is the major cause of this disorder in females from 10 to 50 years old. A peculiarity of the nephrotic syndrome associated with SLE is the curious absence of the hypercholesterolemia so commonly seen in other forms of this disorder. Latent renal tubular dysfunction in the form of a subclinical defect of renal acidification may occur, or fully developed renal tubular acidosis may be found in association with hypergammaglobulinemia (see Chapter 10).

Cutaneous Lesions

The most characteristic skin lesion is an erythematous and violaceous eruption on the bridge of the nose and malar areas in the so-called "butterfly" pattern. Similar eruptions, sometimes with bluish discoloration, may be seen on exposed areas such as the face, neck, hands, and fingers. Exacerbations of the cutaneous eruptions are frequently produced by exposure to ultraviolet light.

Typical skin lesions may occur as an isolated finding without generalized systemic disease in the disorder known as chronic discoid lupus erythematosus. Its relationship to SLE is controversial, but there appears to be a higher frequency of systemic involvement in these patients than in normal individuals. However, the sex ratio is different than in SLE, males and females being almost equally affected, and serologic abnormalities are found less often. In one series, 42 of 120 patients with discoid lupus had positive tests for antinuclear factor, compared to 11 of 120 matched control subjects. In general, antinuclear antibody titers are lower in discoid lupus than in SLE. At present the two entities are considered to be distinct diseases.

A variety of other cutaneous abnormalities may be seen in SLE including nail destruction, retardation of hair growth along the anterior hairline, alopecia, urticaria, scleroderma, and a pemphigoid lesion known as Senear-Usher syndrome (see Chapter 5).

Polyserositis

Pericarditis occurs and may be associated with a pericardial effusion. Pleural involvement is not infrequent and may be bilateral. Peritoneal serositis, however, is relatively uncommon.

Articular Lesions

Articular symptoms are seen in the majority of patients, but the destructive bone changes so typical of rheumatoid arthritis are seldom observed. At times the articular involvement may appear identical to that seen in rheumatoid arthritis, and a distinction between the two diseases becomes impossible. This distinction is particularly difficult since many patients with severe rheumatoid arthritis show some of the serologic abnormalities which are considered to be characteristic of SLE. Subcutaneous rheumatoid-like nodules occur in a small percentage of patients with typical lesions of SLE.

Hematologic Abnormalities

In addition to involvement of any or all of the formed elements of the blood, a variety of coagulation defects have been described in SLE. The latter may be due to antibodies against coagulation factors such as factor VIII. Neutropenia is common, and a hemolytic anemia of the autoimmune variety may occur. Occasionally, SLE may present as an apparent idiopathic thrombocytopenic purpura and only subsequently may the fully developed systemic disease emerge. In a number of instances the diagnosis of SLE was established only after splenectomy and histologic examination. Splenomegaly and lymphadenopathy occur in a minority of adult patients, but lymphadenopathy and hepatosplenomegaly are much commoner in children with SLE.

Cardiovascular Lesions

Cardiovascular abnormalities include Raynaud's phenomenon, recurrent thrombophlebitis, thrombotic occlusion of arteries and arterioles, and cardiac arrhythmias, and conduction disturbances. A verrucous endocarditis, the Libman Sacks syndrome, is considered to be typical of SLE. However, because the heart valves are rarely destroyed, the syndrome is frequently not recognized during life and is diagnosed only at autopsy.

Pulmonary Lesions

Pulmonary involvement has been described in over 50 per cent of patients with SLE. Clinical symptoms such as dyspnea may be much more marked than might be suspected on the basis of radiographic changes. Impaired diffusing capacity is frequently found and is probably the most characteristic functional abnormality. Reduced vital capacity is also observed. The pulmonary disease may take the form of a pneumonitis, pulmonary fibrosis, or may be predominantly vasculitic in nature.

Nervous System Lesions

Systemic lupus erythematosus often involves the central nervous system, but rarely affects the peripheral nervous system. Convulsive disorders, aberrations of mental function, and cranial neuropathies are the commonest neurologic manifestations. In addition, there may be other CNS signs including hemiplegia, disorders of movement, and occasionally disorders of hypothalamic function. The peripheral neuropathy may take the form of sensory or motor disturbances, a polyneuritis (see Chapter 18) or a mononeuropathy. A myasthenia gravis-like syndrome has also been described.

Gastrointestinal Lesions

Gastrointestinal manifestations are seldom prominent, although disorders of esophageal motility, nonspecific colitis, and visceral vasculitides may be seen. While hepatomegaly may occasionally occur, extensive hepatocellular dysfunction as is found in chronic active liver disease is distinctly unusual.

The relationship between SLE and "lupoid hepatitis" is discussed in Chapter 16.

Eye Lesions

Retinopathy and corneal involvement are frequently encountered in SLE. Approximately 90 per cent of patients show abnormal staining of the cornea with fluorescein. The retinopathy is due to vascular involvement and is characterized by the presence of exudates, hemorrhages, and cytoid bodies.

Other Clinical Manifestations

In addition to these reasonably well delineated features of specific system dysfunction, there may be other disorders such as Sjögren's syndrome. There are also a group of patients with spontaneous painful ecchymoses of the arms and legs who demonstrate marked cutaneous hypersensitivity to either calf-thymus DNA or autologous leukocytic nuclear material. This syndrome has been called hemorrhagic cutaneous anaphylaxis, but there is little evidence at present to suggest an immunologic abnormality and the pathogenesis of the disorder remains unknown.

COURSE AND PROGNOSIS

The natural history of SLE seems to have changed somewhat over the past few decades. Whereas it once appeared to be a severe, unremitting, universally fatal disorder, much milder forms of the disease, with a better prognosis, are now recognized. Since better diagnostic techniques are presently available for the detection of SLE in mild and early stages, it is not clear whether there has been an actual change in the disease process or whether cases are now being diagnosed which were previously missed.

Several authors have suggested that SLE is not a uniformly fatal disease, even in children where the disease is recognized to be more severe than in adults. In general, increasingly poor prognosis is noted in groups of patients in the following order: (1) adults without renal disease; (2) adults with renal disease; (3) children without renal disease; and (4) children with renal disease.[8] Since the advent of corticosteroid therapy, the mean duration of the disease in all patients from the onset of disease until death has been estimated to range from 6 to 11 years. There appears to be little doubt that the outlook for patients with SLE has improved markedly since the introduction of corticosteroids.

TREATMENT

Patients with mild disease, such as those with arthralgia and minor constitutional symptoms, but without major systemic involvement or involvement of vital organs, may show satisfactory improvement on salicylates or antimalarial drugs such as quinacrine, chloroquine, or hydroxychloroquine. The latter agents carry a risk of drug-induced retinopathy which develops extremely insidiously and somewhat limits their usefulness. They may be particularly valuable, however, in the management of the cutaneous abnormalities in SLE and are of considerable therapeutic benefit in patients with chronic discoid lupus erythematosus. Common daily doses are: quinacrine, 100 to 300 mg, chloroquine, 250 to 500 mg; or hydroxychloroquine, 400 to 1600 mg, in divided doses.

Corticosteroids are generally indicated for patients with more severe systemic involvement such as pulmonary, renal or cerebral complications, autoimmune hemolytic anemia, or thrombocytopenic purpura. Prednisone administered in dosages of 40 to 60 mg per day will frequently produce improvement in these patients. Extremely high doses of prednisone (e.g., 100 to 500 mg daily) may be required for adequate control of severe central nervous system manifestations such as convulsions or psychosis.

There is some controversy as to the dose and duration of corticosteroid therapy required to treat the renal lesions of SLE. In the majority of patients, the glomerular lesion is focal rather than diffuse and responds well to doses of corticosteroids which are sufficient to suppress activity in other systems. Frequently, prednisone in doses of 10 to 15 mg per day are sufficient for this purpose. In most patients whose glomerular lesions are severe and diffuse, the administration of corticosteroids in larger doses (e.g., 60 to 100 mg per day) does not appear to significantly alter the course of the disease. In a few patients, favorable responses have been reported following the use of fairly high doses of corticosteroids, i.e., greater than 100 mg of prednisone per day for several months.

Recently, encouraging results in the treatment of SLE have been obtained with immunosuppressive agents such as azathioprine. For example, improvement in lupus nephritis has been reported in several series of patients who were no longer responsive to corticosteroids. (See Chapter 6 for a general discussion of the use of immunosuppressive drugs in renal disease). Beneficial responses have also been described in lupus nephritis with a combination of azathioprine and prednisone. In these patients the administration of azathioprine in doses of 1 to 3 mg/kg/day has permitted a reduction of corticosteroid dosage when the latter was causing serious untoward side-effects.

The autoimmune hemolytic anemia associated with SLE responds to both corticosteroid and immunosuppressive therapy (see Chapter 9).

In addition to these drugs, general supportive measures are of considerable value in the management of patients with SLE. The avoidance of factors which are frequently associated with exacerbations of the disease, such as infection, physical stress, sunlight, and emotional stress may prevent morbidity. Pregnancy should be avoided for at least three years after the diagnosis is made, and then should be permitted only if symptoms have been controlled during this period on less than 15 mg of prednisone daily.

Any of the drugs listed at the beginning of the chapter, which are capable of inducing the lupus-like syndrome, may also worsen the disease in patients with underlying SLE. The sulfonamides, in particular, may not only produce and precipitate an exacerbation of the disease, but may induce fatal illness. Their withdrawal in patients with drug-induced lupus-like syndrome is generally, but not invariably, associated with a gradual disappearance of all signs and symptoms.

RHEUMATOID ARTHRITIS

Rheumatoid arthritis is an inflammatory disease of connective tissue whose most striking clinical manifestation is its tendency to produce lesions in joints and periarticular structures. The discovery of rheumatoid factor (RF), an antibody which reacts with human γ-globulin, and the subsequent description of several other serologic aberrations in rheumatoid arthritis has led to the suggestion that immunologic abnormalities may be important in the pathogenesis of this disease.

ETIOLOGY AND PATHOGENESIS

The etiology of rheumatoid disease is essentially unknown and much of the ensuing discussion must necessarily be of a hypothetical nature. Currently, the focus of attention in rheumatoid disease has centered around three or four major possibilities: (1) that rheumatoid disease is an autoimmune phenomenon in which the body reacts against its own γ-globulin or other body constituents, (2) that immunologic mechanisms are important but the initial stimulus is an exogeneous agent such as a microorganism; (3) that an infectious agent is directly responsible for the disease; and (4) that there is some primary defect in connective tissue cells, whose altered metabolic properties initiate an inflammatory process. Finally, it is felt that there may be genetic determinants which predispose patients to develop the disease. These theories are not mutually exclusive and many investigators have proposed an interaction between an infectious agent, the immune system, and connective tissue cells in the production of the disease.

Although diffuse connective tissue disorders and immunoglobulin abnormalities frequently segregate in single families, there appears to be little firm data at present to support a genetic predisposition or genetic trait in the determination of rheumatoid arthritis.

Similarly there is no strong evidence to suggest a role for an infectious agent in the production of rheumatoid disease. The reported isolation of mycoplasma organisms from the joint fluids of patients with rheumatoid arthritis and patients with a variety of other diseases has not been confirmed by subsequent studies.[3] In addition to the studies on mycoplasma, attempts have been made to link virus-like agents and diphtheroid organisms to rheumatoid arthritis, but there has been no firm data to substantiate such a relationship.

Some interest has arisen in a possible antigenic cross relationship between certain components of bacterial cell walls and constituents of human connective tissue. While this may be of considerable importance in rheumatic fever, there is no evidence at present that antigenic cross relationships of this nature are significant in rheumatoid arthritis.

Because of the various immunologic abnormalities described in this disease, the possibility of an autoimmune process has received the greatest attention. In favor of such a theory is the clear, but not absolute, association of RF with rheumatoid arthritis. This factor reacts with 7S γ-globulin (IgG), can be detected in the sera and joint fluids of most adult patients with rheumatoid arthritis, and its titer tends roughly to correlate with the severity of the disease. Also of interest is the observation that the intraarticular injection of autologous IgG or heterologous IgG of a closely matching Gm type (see Chapter 1) will induce acute arthritis in patients with rheumatoid arthritis.

Despite these strong associations, there are a number of problems which cast uncertainty on the role of an autoimmune process in this disease. As far as RF is concerned, it is definitely found in the absence of arthritis in a number of connective tissue diseases where joint symptoms and signs fail to appear, and even in otherwise healthy individuals. From these observations there seems little doubt that RF alone is incapable of producing inflammatory arthritis. Not only may RF occur in the absence of arthritis, but fairly typical rheumatoid arthritis may occur in children in the absence of detectable RF. Moreover, a small proportion of adult patients with typical rheumatoid arthritis remain seronegative with respect to all known tests for anti-γ-globulins. Even more interesting is the occurrence of a rheumatoid arthritis-like syndrome in children with congenital agammaglobulinemia (see Chapter 11). While these children do have small amounts of circulating immunoglobulin, they do not appear to have RF. Furthermore, when they are treated with γ-globulin, there is frequently improvement in their inflammatory joint disease.

IMMUNOPATHOLOGY

The three major pathologic findings in rheumatoid arthritis are synovitis, the rheumatoid nodule, and vasculitis. None of the changes is pathognomonic for rheumatoid disease. However, the subcutaneous rheumatoid nodule is the most characteristic and occurs in few other disorders.

Synovitis

The basic joint lesion begins in the synovium with edema and exudation, fibrin deposition on the synovial surface, and the appearance of polymorphonuclear leukocytes into the edema fluid. The major synovial cellular infiltrate is lymphocytic in character. With progressive and long-standing disease the lymphocytes may be formed into nodular aggregates and eventually may form true lymphoid follicles. Later in the disease there may be infiltration of the synovium with plasma cells. Some of these cells have been demonstrated by the immunofluorescence technique to contain RF.[8] In addition to RF in plasma cells in joints, a variety of immune reactants have been found in articular tissues by immunofluorescence. These include RF complexed with IgG, and IgG complexed with complement.[9] At least two components of complement, C3 and C4, have been identified in these deposits.[11]

With the progression of the disease process there is villus hypertrophy of the synovial membrane to form a mass of granulation tissue known as pannus. The pannus is composed of proliferating vessels, synovial fibroblasts, and cellular infiltrates. Cartilage adjacent to the pannus is destroyed, and there is some evidence that enzymes which are capable of hydrolyzing articular cartilage are released from the pannus structure. In late disease the granulation tissue which forms the pannus may undergo change into fibrous tissue or even bone.

Subcutaneous Nodules

The subcutaneous nodule occurs in about 20 per cent of patients with rheumatoid arthritis and in its fully developed form is quite characteristic. There have been occasional reports of similar nodules occurring in patients without rheumatoid arthritis (e.g., rheumatic fever and SLE), and hence the lesion cannot be considered pathognomonic for rheumatoid disease. The typical nodule consists of a central area of necrosis surrounded by a palisade of connective tissue cells and this is in turn covered by a ring of granulation tissue containing lymphocytes and plasma cells. There is evidence that the primary lesion responsible for the production of the rheumatoid nodule is an acute vasculitis. It is of interest that patients with nodules are more likely to develop widespread systemic arteritis and to have a high titer of RF and low levels of serum complement.

Arteritis

The arteritic lesion in rheumatoid arthritis is not particularly characteristic histologically. Small arteries are generally affected and a spectrum of lesions from severe necrotizing vasculitis to a limited segmental arteritis may be seen. The demonstration of immune reactants by the fluorescent antibody technique in some of the arteritic lesions and subcutaneous nodules, as well as the morphologic resemblance to certain experimental vasculitities such as the Arthus phenomenon, suggest that a common mechanism may be involved in the production of tissue damage in these situations.

Mechanism of Tissue Damage

The pathogenesis of the articular lesions in rheumatoid arthritis is not understood at present. However, it seems likely that the final mediation of tissue injury is at least partly due to lysosomal enzymes and other inflammatory agents released from invading PMN's or synovial membrane lining cells. Immune-complexes present in the joint fluid and synovial structures may activate complement which, in turn, attracts PMN's. The mechanism by which the immune reaction localizes in the articular structures is not understood.

However, the phagocytosis of immune complexes by PMN's is known to lead to the release of enzymes such as collagenase and elastase as well as various permeability factors.[7a] Furthermore, synovial specimens obtained from patients with rheumatoid arthritis contain enzymes capable of degrading collagen in vitro. These enzymes are not elaborated by synovial tissues from patients with non-inflammatory joint diseases. The amount of synovial collagenolytic activity measured in culture appears to be closely related to both local and systemic disease activity.[10]

A similar immunopathogenetic mechanism involving complement and PMN's may be responsible for the arteritic-vasculitic lesions associated with rheumatoid arthritis.

Other Pathologic Lesions

In addition to these three more or less characteristic features of rheumatoid disease, a number of other pathologic lesions may be seen. Granulomatous lesions which occur in the heart are usually confined to the left side and may involve myocardium and the valves. A fibrinous pericarditis is found not infrequently on postmortem examination. In the lung there may be diffuse interstitial pulmonary fibrosis, granulomatous lesions resembling the subcutaneous nodule, or the larger silicotic type nodules found in Caplan's syndrome (see Chapter 4). In the lymph nodes, hyperplasia with formation of prominent germinal centers may be particularly striking. This is in contrast to SLE where the germinal centers are generally not affected. Local glomerulitis and interstitial changes are found in the kidneys of approximately 50 per cent of patients.

CLINICAL IMMUNOLOGY

Rheumatoid Factor

The single most striking immunologic feature of rheumatoid arthritis is the presence in the sera of a macromolecular factor capable of agglutinating a variety of particles which have been coated with human 7S γ-globulin. In eliciting RF activity the type of particle used is of no particular consequence. A variety of particles such as bacteria, sensitized sheep and human erythrocytes, latex, and bentonite have been employed. In all tests they are coated with either unaggregated or aggregated 7S γ-globulin (IgG), but the best reactions are usually obtained with denatured human γ-globulin.

The term rheumatoid factor has been applied to this agglutinating activity because it was first seen and occurs predominantly in patients with rheumatoid arthritis. However, it is not exclusive to rheumatoid arthritis, nor is it detected in every case of this disease. Other disorders in which RF activity may be demonstrated are listed in Table 8-2. The latex and bentonite flocculation tests for RF are widely utilized for screening purposes, but the high prevalence of false positive reactions severely limits their value as diagnostic procedures. On the other hand, the sensitized sheep cell agglutination test is considerably more specific for rheumatoid arthritis.

The RF itself is generally a 19S IgM immunoglobulin with antibody specificity for 7S IgG immunoglobulin. However, a few rheumatoid factors have been described which belong to the IgG or IgA class of immunoglobulins. While the majority of rheumatoid factors react with human γ-globulins, some also react with rabbit, horse, and bovine γ-globulin.

TABLE 8-2. Diseases Associated with Rheumatoid Factor
Activity

Frequent Association
  Rheumatoid arthritis (90%)
  Sjögren's syndrome (75%)
  Systemic lupus erythematosus (30%)
  Juvenile rheumatoid arthritis (25%)

Occasional Association
  Polyarteritis nodosa
  Systemic sclerosis
  Hypergammaglobulinemia due to any cause (see Chapter 10)
  Leprosy
  Fibrosing alveolitis (see Chapter 4)
  Chronic bronchitis
  Myocardial infarction
  Paroxysmal nocturnal hemoglobinuria
  Renal allografts
  Skin allografts
  Infectious mononucleosis
  Cryoglobulinemia (see Chapter 10)
  Syphilis
  Multiple transfusions
  Multiple vaccinations
  Endogenous depression
  Leukemia
  Normal individuals, particularly in the older age groups

For a time there was a question as to whether or not RF represented
a true autoantibody. However, recent evidence has shown RF to have autospecificity as well as isospecificity (e.g., Gm factor specificity). The demonstration of a 22S complex in some sera, which is dissociable into a 19S
and a 7S component, provides strong evidence that RF, the 19S component,
reacts in vivo with 7S γ-globulin.[6] Additional evidence in support of autospecificity came from the demonstration that when the 19S RF was removed
from the other serum components, particularly γ-globulin, it clearly showed
autospecificity. This finding also suggested that in certain sera the patient's
own γ-globulin may inhibit the autospecificity reaction.

In addition, a variety of other subspecificities have been described. Most
rheumatoid factors appear to react with an antigenic determinant present
on the Fc portion of the γ-globulin molecule (see Chapter 1). This observation is of particular interest since complement also appears to fix to the

Fc portion of the molecule. Because of its specificity for the Fc fragment of IgG, RF fails to react with other immunoglobulins such as IgM and IgA which have different Fc components, or with 7S IgG whose Fc fragment has been destroyed by proteolytic enzymes.

The production of RF is important in terms of understanding its specificity and biologic effects. Prolonged immunization of animals, or the occurrence of subacute bacterial endocarditis in humans leads to RF seropositivity. In patients with subacute bacterial endocarditis, the RF disappears when the infection is cured. These observations suggest that RF is directed against IgG which is complexed with an antigen derived from an infectious agent. The identity of this antigen, if one exists, in rheumatoid arthritis remains unknown. Presumably complexing of an antigen with IgG may subtly alter the antigenicity of IgG in a manner similar to that of complexed C3 (see discussion of immunoconglutinin in Chapter 1). A totally different hypothesis for the production of RF is that there may be an intrinsic structural defect in the IgG of patients with rheumatoid arthritis which is unrelated to complexing with antigen.

Synovial fluid leukocytes from patients with rheumatoid arthritis have been shown to contain intracytoplasmic inclusions of immunoglobulins. Because these cells are found with high frequency in rheumatoid arthritis they were designated RA cells. However they have subsequently been found in a variety of related disorders such as Reiter's syndrome and infectious arthritis, and therefore cannot be considered specific for rheumatoid arthritis. Similar inclusions have also been found in peripheral blood leukocytes in rheumatoid arthritis and a large group of completely unrelated disorders.[12]

Of perhaps more significance is the observation that homogenates of these synovial fluid cells give positive tests for RF in approximately 95 per cent of patients with rheumatoid arthritis, including patients who have no detectable RF in their sera or synovial fluids.[1] The synovial fluid frequently contains RF, occasionally in the absence of a positive serologic test for RF.

The biologic role of RF is uncertain despite many years of investigation. It is probably significant that patients with malignant systemic rheumatoid disease usually show extremely high titers of RF. These patients frequently have a widespread arteritis with localization of immune complexes in the arteritic lesions. The association of this syndrome with low serum complement levels suggests that circulating immune complexes containing RF, and capable of fixing complement, are important in its pathogenesis.

The recent observation that RF-IgG complexes can fix *human* complement supports the hypothesis stated above, and throws some doubt on the previously held theory that RF might exert a beneficial action by blocking the fixation of complement to potentially harmful antigen-antibody complexes.[4a] The largest amount of complement fixation appears to occur in joint fluids where the IgG-type of RF is most prevalent.[9] Thus the immunopathogenetic potential of RF may be more related to the IgG component than to the IgM antibody.

At present, it may be concluded only that RF represents a hallmark of rheumatoid disease and is of considerable diagnostic value. However, it is not known whether, in any individual patient, it is beneficial, deleterious, both, or neither.[7]

Immunoglobulins

Patients with rheumatoid disease frequently show elevated total serum immunoglobulin levels manifested by a polyclonal type of hypergammaglobulinemia on serum protein electrophoresis. Total immunoglobulins, IgA, and IgM levels are significantly, but not markedly, elevated in 50 to 60 per cent of patients with rheumatoid arthritis. However, there is no correlation between the elevated immunoglobulin levels and the sex or age of the patient, duration or stage of the disease, or RF titers.[2]

Complement Levels

The serum complement level in rheumatoid arthritis is usually normal or slightly elevated. The one exception to this general statement occurs in patients with widespread malignant rheumatoid arteritis who usually have low levels of serum complement. When total hemolytic complement activity is measured in joint fluid, it is frequently found to be significantly low as compared with serum levels. These findings suggest a local activation or consumption of complement components in the diseased joint.

Antinuclear Antibodies

Antinuclear antibodies (ANA) similar to those found in SLE have been described in 10 to 20 per cent of patients with rheumatoid arthritis. They are more likely to be of the IgM type as compared to SLE where most of the ANA is IgG. In addition, the ANA titers are generally lower than those found in SLE. There has been a suggestion that those patients with rheumatoid arthritis who have antinuclear antibodies tend to have more severe disease and are more prone to develop widespread systemic disease. DNA and antinuclear antibodies have also been found in the synovial fluids of patients with rheumatoid arthritis, and occasionally antinuclear antibodies are present in the joint fluid although absent from the serum. LE cells are found in less than 5 per cent of patients.

Other Serologic Abnormalities

Other serologic abnormalities in rheumatoid arthritis include the occasional occurrence of a biologic false-positive Wassermann reaction, but this finding is far less common than in SLE. Serum immunoconglutinin levels are usually elevated. This factor appears to represent an autoantibody against complement which has been fixed to either antigen-antibody complexes or γ-globulin aggregates. Approximately 5 per cent of patients have a positive direct Coombs' test.

CLINICAL MANIFESTATIONS

While rheumatoid arthritis is classically described as a disease of the joints, it is now apparent that widespread systemic involvement can occur in this disease. Furthermore, while the articular symptoms are usually the most prominent, they need not necessarily be the first to appear, nor may they be the most striking clinical manifestations. The variability in the clinical presentation and course of rheumatoid arthritis is similar to that found in SLE and has necessitated the formulation of a number of diagnostic criteria for classic, probable, and possible disease.

In general, the important diagnostic features may be summarized as follows: (1) a slowly progressive polyarthritis with a tendency to symmetrical joint involvement; (2) fusiform, soft tissue joint swelling early in the disease; (3) early morning stiffness; (4) subsequent development of typical deformities; (5) rheumatoid subcutaneous nodules; and (6) a positive test for RF. The differential diagnoses of nonsuppurative inflammatory diseases of the joints are presented in Table 8-3.

Despite these criteria, great difficulties are still encountered in epidemiologic studies which attempt to determine the prevalence of this disease. In most series, the prevalence of rheumatoid arthritis in the general population has been estimated to be in the range of 2 per cent. The disease may appear at any age and is 2 to 3 times more common in females than in males. The greatest incidence occurs between the ages of 30 and 50 years. Rheumatoid arthritis which occurs in juveniles has certain distinct differences from that which occurs in adults, both clinically and immunologically, and will be discussed as a separate entity.

In addition to the involvement of joints and muscles, there are frequently

TABLE 8-3. Differential Diagnoses of Nonsuppurative Inflammatory Diseases of the Joints*

Rheumatoid Arthritis and Its Variants
  Rheumatoid arthritis
  Juvenile rheumatoid arthritis
  Ankylosing spondylitis

Collagen-Vascular Diseases
  Systemic lupus erythematosus
  Rheumatic fever
  Polymyositis
  Sjögren's syndrome

Gastrointestinal Diseases
  Regional enteritis
  Ulcerative colitis
  Whipple's disease
  Bacillary dysentery

Mucocutaneous Diseases
  Psoriasis
  Reiter's syndrome
  Erythema nodosum
  Behçet's disease

Other Diseases
  Sarcoidosis
  Hypo- and agammaglobulinemia
  Gout
  Chondrocalcinosis (pseudo-gout)
  Familial Mediterranean fever
  Relapsing polychondritis
  Anaphylactoid purpura
  Hemochromatosis

* Predominantly degenerative diseases have been excluded.

systemic manifestations such as general malaise, fatigue, fever, and weight loss. Other systems not infrequently involved include the cardiovascular system, lungs, skin, blood, and nervous systems.

Joint Manifestations

The onset is usually insidious, but it may occur with dramatic suddeness. The distal joints are most commonly involved, particularly the proximal interphalangeal, metacarpal-phalangeal, toe, wrist, knee, and elbow joints. However, no joint is exempt and the larger joints such as the shoulder, hip, and spinal joints may eventually become involved. The usual symptoms are joint pain with swelling, stiffness after inactivity, and limitation of movement. The joint may appear red, hot, and swollen, and typically there is swelling of the periarticular structures which produces the classic spindle shaped appearance of the interphalangeal joints. Joint effusions of considerable magnitude may be seen, particularly in the larger joints such as the knee.

In far advanced disease, joint deformities occur with increasing limitation of movement and eventually there may be fibrinous and bony ankylosis of joints. A particularly characteristic deformity is seen in the hands where marked ulnar deviation occurs at the metacarpal-phalangeal joints due to the displacement of the extensor tendons.

Muscle wasting and weakness are frequently out of proportion to the activity of the disease or to the extent of involvement of the adjacent joints.

Radiologic examination of the joints in early cases reveals periarticular swelling associated with narrowing of the joint space and very occasionally periosteal elevation. As the disease becomes more advanced there is a loss of articular space, and erosions occur on the surface of the bone. Cystic areas may be seen underneath the joint cartilage, and eventually there may be complete destruction of the joint with bony ankylosis. Osteoporosis, which is initially only periarticular, becomes generalized.

Pulmonary Manifestations

Involvement of the lung and pleura have been described at postmortem examination in as many as 40 per cent of patients. Diffuse interstitial pulmonary fibrosis is the commonest manifestation, but is only rarely associated with the functional changes typical of restrictive pulmonary disease (see Chapter 4).

Cardiovascular Manifestations

Cardiovascular manifestations include pericarditis, interstitial myocarditis and coronary arteritis, aortic valvular disease due to rheumatoid granulomas in the aortic ring, and general vasomotor instability.

Cutaneous Manifestations

Skin changes such as atrophy, bronzing, liver palms, and the most characteristic cutaneous feature, subcutaneous nodules, are not uncommon. Nodules usually appear over points of pressure, are commonest on the ulnar aspect of the elbow, and are said to occur at some time in 20 to 25 per cent of patients. Purpura of the skin in rheumatoid patients is often associated with prolonged steroid therapy, or may occasionally form part of the purpura-arthralgia syndrome seen in association with the mixed type of cryoglobulinemia (see Chapter 4). The presence of tiny hemorrhage infarcts at the base of the nails or in the finger pulp is said to be specific for seropositive rheumatoid arthritis.

Neuromuscular Manifestations

In addition to muscle wasting and weakness, other neuromuscular manifestations include a distal symmetrical sensory loss, major peripheral nerve lesions at sites of nerve compression, and a polyneuropathy associated with vasculitis. A few patients with rheumatoid arthritis show a myopathic picture similar to polymyositis (see Chapter 19). Involvement of the cervical spine which occurs in a majority of patients with rheumatoid arthritis may lead to compression of the cervical cord. Central nervous system involvement is most uncommon.

Other Clinical Manifestations

Anemia is common in rheumatoid arthritis and tends to be of the normochromic and normocytic variety. A small group of patients have leukopenia associated with splenomegaly and occasionally hepatomegaly, pigmentation and ulceration of the legs. The selective neutropenia in these patients is felt to be a reflection of hypersplenism. This symptom complex was formerly known as Felty's syndrome, but there appears to be little justification for the use of this term at present. In most cases of rheumatoid arthritis, the leukocyte count is normal or slightly elevated.

Episcleritis and lacrimal hyposecretion associated with Sjögren's syndrome are the commonest ocular manifestations. Scleromalacia perforans, lenticular band keratitis, and retinal detachment due to choroid nodules are also found in patients with rheumatoid arthritis. In longstanding arthritics secondary amyloidosis may occur and may be associated with the nephrotic syndrome (see Chapter 10).

Impaired renal function, usually attributed to interstitial nephritis, is observed in many patients with rheumatoid arthritis. The pathogenesis of this complication remains uncertain.

Malignant Rheumatoid Disease

A small group of patients develop a more severe form of rheumatoid arthritis associated with widespread systemic disease. This syndrome is called malignant rheumatoid disease and the basic lesion appears to be an arteritic process. These patients frequently have rheumatoid nodules, very high titers of RF, low serum complement, and severe joint disease. The arteritis may give rise to purpuric or hemorrhagic skin lesions, episcleritis, pericarditis, peripheral neuropathy, and occasionally hemorrhagic infarcts in the nail fold and finger pulp areas. While this malignant form of rheumatoid disease was seen prior to the introduction of corticosteroids, its incidence seems to have increased considerably since then. However, no direct cause and effect relationship has been established between this class of drugs and the disease process.

Laboratory Findings

The significance of rheumatoid factor, hypergammaglobulinemia, antinuclear factors, complement levels, and other serologic abnormalities in the diagnosis of rheumatoid arthritis has been discussed previously in the section on clinical immunology.

Hematologic findings include a normochromic or hypochromic normocytic anemia which is sometimes associated with moderately decreased levels of serum iron. Leukocytosis may occur but is commoner in juvenile rheumatoid arthritics. An elevated erythrocyte sedimentation rate or increased levels of C-reactive protein may occur, and may be of some value in following the activity of the disease. Both of these tests, as well as the anemia, probably represent a nonspecific response to inflammation.

Analysis of the synovial fluid may be of considerable value in distinguishing rheumatoid arthritis from other diseases. The fluid is usually yellow to greenish in color, of low viscosity, and forms a poor mucin clot. The white cell count varies from 8 to 40,000, and approximately 70 per cent are polymorphonuclear leukocytes. The diagnostic significance of RA cells, RF, antinuclear antibodies, and complement in the synovial fluid has already been discussed in detail in the section on the clinical immunology of rheumatoid arthritis.

TREATMENT

Since the etiology of rheumatoid arthritis is unknown and its pathogenesis is still a matter of some controversy, it is not surprising that there is no specific therapy for the disease and no effective preventive measures are known. Nevertheless, a number of agents are available which provide substantial symptomatic relief. It is important to remember that rheumatoid arthritis is not simply a disease of joints but rather that it is a systemic disease and that an approach to the total patient is of great importance. The evaluation of antirheumatic therapy has proven to be difficult because of the tendency of the disease to pursue a variable course and to undergo spontaneous remissions and exacerbations.

Over the years a number of therapeutic agents have withstood the test of time and are now of established value in rheumatoid disease. The most widely used of these are the salicylates which in adequate dosage provide not only an analgesic but also an anti-inflammatory effect. Many patients with mild or moderate rheumatoid arthritis can be managed with acetylsalicylic acid alone, provided other adjuncts such as physiotherapy are provided. Most adults can tolerate 4 to 6 gm daily in divided doses without manifestations of toxicity such as gastric irritation and tinnitus.

Two other nonspecific anti-inflammatory agents, indomethacin and phenylbutazone, are occasionally of value in rheumatoid arthritis. The latter is of somewhat limited usefulness because of its occasional tendency to produce bone marrow depression. Indomethacin (150 to 200 mg daily in divided doses) does not appear to be much more effective than acetylsalicylic acid, and is not infrequently associated with a number of side-effects such as headache, nausea, heartburn, and vertigo.

Antimalarials such as quinacrine, chloroquine, and hydroxychloroquine are claimed to be of value in the treatment of rheumatoid disease. However, the occurrence of an insidiously developing and irreversible retinopathy in a significant number of patients represents a major obstacle to the widespread use of these agents in rheumatoid arthritis.

Gold salts have been shown to be beneficial in a controlled study.[5] Gold thiomalate or gold thioglucose may be given in weekly intramuscular doses of 10 mg the first week, 25 mg the second week, and 50 mg per week thereafter until toxic reactions appear, response is adequate, or a total dose of 1 gm has been given without improvement. Gold therapy may be complicated by nephrotoxicity in the form of nephrotic syndrome and a variety of adverse reactions such as dermatitis, agranulocytosis, purpura, hepatitis, and peripheral neuritis.

Corticosteroids, whether given systemically or intra-articularly, are unquestionably capable of producing considerable symptomatic relief and frequently objective improvement. The use of intra-articular steroids (e.g., hydrocortisone 25 to 50 mg) avoids some of the side-effects associated with systemic therapy. However, this method is not without risk either because of the danger of introducing infection or of producing changes in the joints secondary to the injection of the corticosteroids themselves. A Charcot-like arthropathy has been reported in association with this form of therapy.

The side-effects of systemic corticosteroids are well known. While intermittent or alternate day therapy may reduce some of the side-effects, this regimen is not always capable of suppressing the manifestations of the disease satisfactorily. Prednisone in divided doses of 10 to 15 mg daily will often produce considerable functional improvement in patients who do not respond favorably to conservative management or who are unable to tolerate other forms of medication. Despite the possible hazards, corticosteroids are probably the only therapeutic measure which appears to be of value in the management of the arteritis of rheumatoid arthritis.

Immunosuppressive drugs such as azathioprine and cyclophosphamide are beginning to be more widely employed in a variety of diffuse connective tissue diseases. However, their use has not been widely adopted in rheumatoid disease and sufficient clinical trials have not been conducted to permit a definite answer as to their usefulness.[4]

A variety of reconstructive surgical procedures have been used with increasing frequency and increasingly good results in the management of rheumatoid disease. In particular, synovectomy and reconstructive surgery of the hands have recently been employed with considerable benefit in many patients.

Physiotherapy and general supportive measures are often of primary importance in the conservative management of rheumatoid arthritis. Depending upon the individual circumstances and the stage of the disease these measures may include systemic rest, psychological support, appropriate orthopedic supports or splints, supervised exercises, local heat, and iron replacement.

ARTERITIS-VASCULITIS SYNDROMES

In a number of experimental conditions, such as the Arthus phenomenon and serum sickness arteritis, it has been clearly shown that immunologic mechanisms are essential to the production of vasculitic lesions. There are a number of syndromes occurring in humans which bear morphologic resemblance to these experimental models. However, in few of them have either the etiology or immunopathogenesis been clearly defined. As is the case with the collagen-vascular diseases in general, the disorders associated with arteritis, angiitis, and vasculitis tend to show considerable overlap in their clinical and pathologic features.

The basic unifying feature of the arteritis-vasculitis syndromes is the occurrence of a nonsuppurative angiitis which is frequently necrotizing. Many investigators feel that this group of disorders represents a continuous spectrum of pathologic changes from relatively pure angiitis at one end to almost pure granuloma formation at the other, with a number of diseases falling between the two. For this reason the classification of these syndromes in distinct groupings must necessarily be somewhat arbitrary (Table 8-4). Furthermore, except for the unifying feature of vascular inflammation, many of these diseases may be totally unrelated etiologically and pathogenetically. The nomenclature of the arteritis-vasculitis syndromes is also confusing because the terms arteritis, vasculitis, and angiitis have had slightly different meanings to different authors. In this section, the term which seems to be best established by common usage will be employed where applicable.

ETIOLOGY AND PATHOGENESIS

Since the vascular tree can react to noxious stimuli in a limited number of ways, the occurrence of a particular morphologic lesion cannot be inferred to be immunologic simply because a similar lesion can be produced experimentally by immunologic means. Nevertheless, immune mechanisms have long been felt to play an important role in the production of arteritis-vasculitis syndromes.

The evidence favoring an immunopathogenetic mechanism may be summarized as follows: (1) vasculitis is frequently seen in association with other collagen-vascular diseases (see Table 8-4); (2) many patients display evidence of immunologic abnormalities such as a polyclonal hypergammaglobulinemia or the occasional presence of rheumatoid factor; (3) in some patients the onset of vasculitis appears to have a definite relationship to the administration of a drug or protein antigen; (4) in some patients, immunologic reactants such as γ-globulin and complement have been identified by the immunofluorescent technique in the affected vessels; (5) some cases appear to follow exposure to microorganisms in a pattern suggestive of hypersensitivity (e.g., rheumatic arteritis following streptococcal infection); (6) immunization and hyperimmunization procedures have on occasion produced either a local vasculitis resembling the Arthus phenomenon or a diffuse necrotizing angiitis; and (7) in some patients, there are features such as bronchial asthma and eosinophilia which are frequently associated with hypersensitivity phenomena.

TABLE 8-4. The Arteritis-Vasculitis Syndromes

Vasculitis Associated with Collagen-Vascular Disease
    Polyarteritis nodosa
    Rheumatoid arthritis
    Systemic lupus erythematosus
    Systemic sclerosis
    Polymyositis
    Sjögren's syndrome

Vasculitis Associated with Hypersensitivity Phenomena
    Hypersensitivity angiitis
    Serum sickness arteritis
    Anaphylactoid purpura (Henoch-Schönlein syndrome)

Vasculitis Associated with Granulomatous Components
    Allergic granulomatous angiitis
    Wegener's granulomatosus
    Lethal midline granuloma
    Temporal arteritis
    Aortic arch syndrome (Takayasu's disease)

Vasculitis Associated with Cryoglobulinemia

Vasculitis Associated with Rheumatic Fever

Miscellaneous Diseases Occasionally Associated with Vasculitis
    Ulcerative colitis
    Postcoarctation resection
    Pulmonary hypertension
    Systemic hypertension
    Reticuloendothelial malignancies
    Goodpasture's syndrome
    Syphilis
    Erythema nodosum
    Nodular vasculitis
    Weber-Christian disease
    Cogan's syndrome
    Kolmier-Degos disease
    Drug abuse (Methamphetamine)

The occasional description of lesions similar to polyarteritis nodosa, limited to the pulmonary arteries, in patients with congenital heart disease and pulmonary hypertension would suggest that elevated intravascular pressure may sometimes play a role in the pathogenesis of the arteritis-vasculitis syndromes.

Because immunologic factors appear to be of considerable importance in the pathogenesis of the arteritis-vasculitis syndromes, comparable experimental models give some insight into the possible mechanism of immunologic injury in clinical cases. Two such models have been fairly well elucidated, the Arthus phenomenon and serum sickness arteritis.[3] A suggested mechanism for the production of various types of experimental vascular injury is outlined schematically in Figure 1-6. The essential features of this mechanism are antigen-antibody interaction followed by complement fixation, chemotaxis of PMN's, and finally the release of bioactive substances from the PMN.

IMMUNOPATHOLOGY

Polyarteritis Nodosa

In polyarteritis nodosa, the typical lesion involves medium and small arteries in a necrotizing inflammatory process which begins in the media and subsequently extends to involve all layers of the vessel. In the early lesions there is frequently an infiltration of polymorphonuclear leukocytes and disruption of the internal elastic lamina of the vessel. Eosinophils may also be seen, but are not present in every case. The lesions are frequently segmental and may involve only part of the circumference of the vessel.

Later there tends to be a more chronic inflammatory process with round cell infiltration, and eventually there may be healing with fibrosis or thrombosis with obliteration of the lumen. In addition, weakening of the vessel wall may occur leading to the formation of aneurysms and the occasional rupture of the artery. It is not unusual in any one case to see lesions in various stages of evolution. The nature of the fibrinoid material which is frequently seen in the vessel wall has not been determined, although there have been suggestions that it is in part composed of fibrin or fibrin-related products.

The usual lesion in the kidney is a glomerulitis with focal fibrinoid changes and marked proliferation of Bowman's capsule. Immunopathologic investigation of the involved vessels has shown deposition of immune reactants such as immunoglobulin and complement, as well as fibrin and occasionally albumin. The presence of the latter two proteins suggests that the deposition of these materials may be nonspecific, i.e., secondary to increased vascular permeability. The affected glomeruli may also contain γ-globulin and complement, but a consistent pattern of deposition has not been defined.

Hypersensitivity Angiitis

The major pathologic difference between hypersensitivity angiitis and polyarteritis nodosa is the size of the vessel affected. In the angiitidies associated with hypersensitivity, the venules, arterioles, and smallest arteries are involved in a necrotizing inflammatory process, whereas involvement of larger vessels is distinctly unusual. Frequently there is a very striking polymorphonuclear leukocyte infiltration. Involvement of cutaneous blood vessels is extremely common in this syndrome. Several years ago these patients were felt to represent variants of polyarteritis nodosa. However, there now seems to be sufficient pathologic justification for considering them as a separate entity. There have been few immunopathologic studies in hypersensitivity angiitis, but there is some evidence that immunoglobulin and complement are deposited in the affected vessels.

The vasculitis of cryoglobulinemia, particularly the mixed type, (see Chapter 10) resembles that of hypersensitivity angiitis and bears a rather striking resemblance to experimental Arthus vasculitis. Immunoglobulins and complement are found in the vascular lesions of cryoglobulinemia by immunofluorescence techniques.

Vasculitis with Granulomatous Components

Those arteritities with granulomatous components, namely allergic granulomatous angiitis, Wegener's granulomatosis, and those cases of polyarteritis nodosa with pulmonary involvement, share certain pathologic features. In addition to a multisystem necrotizing arteritis, there are extravascular granulomata, usually in the upper and lower respiratory tract and occasionally in the periglomerular region of the kidney.

In Wegener's granulomatosis, granulomatous invasion of the nervous system may occur. There may be involvement of medium and smaller sized arteries, and a more generalized focal vasculitis involving smaller arteries and veins, particularly in the lungs. In addition, there is a close morphologic similarity between the renal lesions found in anaphylactoid purpura (see Chapter 6) and those found in Wegener's granulomatosis and allergic granulomatous angiitis. Immunoglobulins and complement are frequently found in the lesions of allergic granulomatous angiitis, but are not found in Wegener's granulomatosis. In lethal midline granuloma, a necrotizing angiitis may be seen as well as focal granulomatous lesions of the upper respiratory tract.

In temporal or giant cell arteritis, the involved vessels usually show a panarteritis with proliferation and diffuse fibrotic thickening of the intima leading to narrowing, thrombosis, and occlusion of the lumen. The most marked inflammatory changes are in the media, and are often accompanied by necrosis, giant cell infiltration, and the formation of granulomata.

In the closely related aortic arch syndrome (Takayasu's disease), there is a mesarteritis of the aortic arch and its branches. In addition, the renal and pulmonary arteries may sometimes be involved. The initial inflammatory process is not infrequently complicated by necrosis of the media, and by thrombosis with obliteration of the vessel lumen.

CLINICAL IMMUNOLOGY

In polyarteritis nodosa, serum protein electrophoresis may show a polyclonal hypergammaglobulinemia and occasional elevated levels of α-globulin. Rheumatoid factor is present in a minority of patients and is most likely to be found in individuals whose vasculitis is associated with rheumatoid arthritis. Antinuclear antibodies and positive LE cell phenomena have occasionally been described. However, in view of the clinical overlap between the various collagen-vascular disorders, these findings are of limited diagnostic value.

Several investigators have noted the failure of sera from patients with polyarteritis nodosa to give a positive reaction with vascular basement membrane using an indirect fluorescent antibody technique. While this observation suggests that circulating antibasement membrane antibodies or antivascular antibodies are not present in large quantities, it does not necessarily exclude such a mechanism. As in the case of Goodpasture's syndrome (see Chapter 6), the large amount of vascular antigen accessible to the circulation may effect prompt removal of any antibody which is formed.

While an occasional patient with any of the arteritis-vasculitis syndromes may demonstrate polyclonal hypergammaglobulinemia, nothing more specific of an immunologic nature is generally found. At least one possible explanation for the lack of immunologic or immunopathologic findings in this group of disorders is the difficulty in obtaining suitable tissue material from active lesions.

CLINICAL MANIFESTATIONS

An extraordinarily wide variety of clinical manifestations may be associated with the arteritis-vasculitis syndromes. The clinical findings depend in large part on the site of vascular involvement, the rapidity and intensity with which the process develops, and the presence of associated conditions. As is the case with SLE, almost any organ in the body may be affected, but there are several clinical patterns which are characteristic of systemic vasculitis.

Polyarteritis Nodosa

Polyarteritis nodosa is a disease which occurs 3 to 4 times more often in males than in females, although it may appear in either sex. A significant percentage of patients appear to have preceding chronic respiratory infection or recent acute hemolytic streptococcal infection. Systemic manifestations are not uncommon, and fever and weight loss may be the presenting complaints.

Renal involvement occurs in 75 to 85 per cent of patients with polyarteritis nodosa, and lesions of the kidney are the greatest contributors towards mortality. The disease involves the larger renal arteries, or there may be glomerulitis with eventual renal failure. Proteinuria and hematuria are frequently found and hypertension eventually occurs in approximately 60 per cent of patients with the disease.

Neurologic signs and symptoms are common in polyarteritis nodosa. However, in contrast to SLE, peripheral neuropathy is far more common than central nervous system involvement. There is reasonable evidence that the peripheral neurologic lesions are primarily due to involvement of the vasa nervorum. The principal symptoms are burning pain, paresthesias, and muscle weakness in the extremities. Central nervous system involvement may lead to changes in behavior, seizures, upper motor neuron disease, cerebellar abnormalities, and occasional intracranial hemorrhage.

Musculoskeletal complaints are extremely common, particularly arthralgia and muscle soreness. Marked arthritis such as occurs in rheumatoid disease is unusual except in those cases where polyarteritis nodosa appears to complicate rheumatoid arthritis.

Gastrointestinal symptoms occur in the majority of patients, and abdominal pain is the most frequent presenting complaint when there is vasculitis of the digestive organs. Involvement of visceral arteries may lead to infarction of intra-abdominal organs or occasionally to bleeding or perforation of a viscus. A number of cases of acute pancreatitis, appendicitis, and cholecystitis have been found to be due to vasculitis of these organs. Polyarteritis nodosa is one of the commonest causes of massive hepatic infarction, and is the single most common cause of testicular infarction.

Involvement of the coronary arteries may lead to electrocardiographic findings similar to those seen in coronary arteriosclerosis, but more frequently involvement of small arteries leads to a clinical picture of insidious myocardial failure. Except for renal failure, congestive heart failure is the most common cause of death. Acute pericarditis has been reported to occur in approximately one-third of patients, whereas aneurysm formation or rupture of affected vessels is distinctly uncommon.

A variety of cutaneous lesions have been described, the most characteristic being tender subcutaneous nodules along the course of blood vessels. Purpuric eruptions may occur, but Raynaud's phenomenon and ischemic lesions of the extremities are more unusual.

Allergic Granulomatous Angiitis

Whether patients with striking pulmonary involvement should be classified as a variant of the polyarteritis nodosa syndrome or as a separate disease entity is still a matter of some controversy.[6] Many investigators feel that classic polyarteritis nodosa rarely involves the lungs, and that, when it does, there is usually a marked granulomatous component to the process.

In one series, 13 patients with disseminated angiitis had severe asthma, marked peripheral blood eosinophilia, extravascular granulomata, and prominent pulmonary manifestations.[2] All the patients had a history of severe asthma that preceded the fulminant terminal disease by a period of several years. Patients with polyarteritis nodosa and pulmonary involvement often have a specific respiratory illness preceding the systemic disease. Renal, cutaneous and neurologic involvement are fairly common. The term allergic granulomatosis and angiitis has been used to distinguish this entity from polyarteritis nodosa even though the pathologic lesions in the vessels are quite similar. Other authors have referred to the same syndrome as allergic granulomatous arteritis or angiitic granulomatosis.

Wegener's Granulomatosis

Wegener's granulomatosis is characterized by necrotizing granulomatosis of the upper and lower respiratory tract, necrotizing angiitis of the pulmonary vessels, and focal glomerulitis. Thus it bears a certain resemblance to allergic granulomatous angiitis. Wegener's granulomatosis occurs in young or middle-aged adults and the usual clinical features consist of rhinitis, sinusitis, fever, cutaneous vasculitis, arthralgia, peripheral neuropathy, and nephritis. It usually pursues a fairly relentless course, over a period of several weeks to several years, until death. Eosinophilia, asthma, and cardiac involvement are extremely uncommon and, if they occur, their presence suggests that the patient has allergic granulomatous angiitis. A series of patients have been described with most of the features of Wegener's granulomatosis, but none of them had glomerulitis. Thus, limited forms of Wegener's granulomatosis may exist in which the prognosis is better than in those with the classic disease.[1]

Lethal Midline Granuloma

In midline granuloma the granulomatous component predominates, although occasionally vasculitis may be associated with the lesion. The relationships between lethal midline granuloma, Wegener's granulomatosis, allergic granulomatous angiitis, polyarteritis with pulmonary manifestations and pulmonary infiltration with eosinophilia (see Chapter 4) remain somewhat arbitrary at present. In fact, some authors have suggested that the P.I.E. syndrome may well represent a benign variant of one of the other diseases in this category.

Hypersensitivity Angiitis

A group of patients has been described in which involvement of the vessels follows a pattern rather distinct from that of classic polyarteritis nodosa. In many of these patients, there appears to be an extrinsic precipitating agent which suggests that a hypersensitivity phenomenon may be involved. Most frequently this agent is a drug; occasionally it is microbial. Of particular significance is the tendency of the process to involve much smaller blood vessels including the smallest arterioles and venules. A variety of

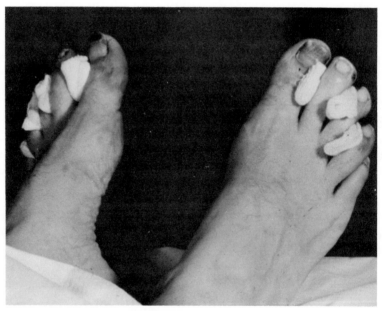

FIG. 8-2. Ischemic lesions in the toes of a patient with hypersensitivity angiitis.

names have been attached to this vasculitis of small vessels such as hypersensitivity angiitis, allergic vasculitis, and anaphylactoid purpura.

Typical clinical manifestations may include ischemic lesions in the tips of the fingers to toes (Fig. 8-2), arthralgia, edema, purpura, fever, weight loss, subcutaneous nodules, pulmonary involvement, muscle tenderness, urticaria, polyneuritis, gastrointestinal bleeding, and renal failure. The renal manifestations of anaphylactoid purpura are discussed in Chapter 6.

It is well known that, in experimental animals, the injection of a foreign protein can lead to serum sickness with involvement of a variety of large blood vessels. The aorta and coronary arteries are most commonly affected. In man, the reagin-mediated manifestations of serum sickness usually outweigh those due to arteritis, although the latter have occasionally been reported (see Chapter 2).

Temporal Arteritis

A more clearly separable group of patients are those with temporal arteritis (cranial arteritis, giant cell arteritis). This form of arteritis usually involves one or more of the branches of the carotid artery and occurs predominantly in older people. The disease is not infrequently associated with systemic manifestations such as fever, arthralgia, weakness, and weight loss, but the most prominent symptom is headache in the temporal area. When the temporal artery itself is affected it may be tortuous and tender, and the overlying skin may be red in appearance.

Of particular importance is the tendency of the disease process to involve the arteries of the eye in approximately 50 per cent of patients. The ocular fundi may show signs of occlusive arteriolar disease. Unfortunately, and not infrequently in the untreated patient, blindness is the ultimate outcome.

The relationship of temporal arteritis to the syndrome of polymyalgia rheumatica is not entirely resolved. Polymyalgia rheumatica, in its typical form, occurs in elderly patients and is characterized by the presence of fatigue, weight loss, fever and marked elevation of the erythrocyte sedimentation rate. Diffuse pain, stiffness, and tenderness, in the absence of muscle wasting, are usually most pronounced in the proximal limb muscles. The syndrome occurs commonly in association with temporal arteritis, but many patients with temporal arteritis do not have polymyalgia rheumatica. Another characteristic feature of polymyalgia rheumatica is the often dramatic response to corticosteroid therapy.

Aortic Arch Syndrome (Takayasu's Disease)

At the opposite end of the spectrum from patients with hypersensitivity angiitis are a group of patients in whom involvement of the aortic arch and its branches is predominant. The aortic arch syndrome (Takayasu's disease, pulseless disease, brachial arteritis) was first described in young Japanese females, but it is now recognized to occur more widely.

The clinical symptoms result from occlusion of the aortic arch branches and include absence of pulses in the head, neck, and upper extremities. There may also be signs of circulatory insufficiency to the upper limbs, a low or unobtainable blood pressure in the arms, and a variety of trophic changes in the upper half of the body such as loss of hair and facial ulceration. Other symptoms include headache, visual disturbances, fever, and weight loss.

Arteritis Associated with other Diseases

An acute necrotizing vasculitis with rather prominent polymorphonuclear leukocyte infiltration has been described in the skin lesions of patients with mixed cryoglobulinemia (see Chapter 10).

A variety of other disorders occasionally associated with vasculitis are shown in Table 8-4. However, in most of them there is little or no evidence to suggest that an immunologic aberration plays any part in the process.

Thrombotic thrombocytopenic purpura, a disorder characterized by fever, hemolytic anemia, purpura, neurologic signs, and renal disease, is worthy of mention because of the extensive vascular involvement which occurs. However, the major defect in this disease appears to be related to intra-vascular deposition of fibrin with little or no evidence of an inflammatory process in the vessels or kidney. Thus, the disorder cannot be considered as a primary vasculitic process. Immunofluorescent studies of splenic and renal tissue in thrombotic thrombocytopenic purpura reveal the subendo-thelial deposition of fibrin and IgG in arteries, arterioles, veins, and glomeruli. The deposition of fibrin is felt to be of primary importance, whereas the deposition of IgG most likely represents a nonspecific phenomenon.

Recently, a necrotizing angiitis indistinguishable from polyarteritis nodosa was described in young persons who were habitual users of methamphetamine.

DIAGNOSIS

The histologic diagnosis of the arteritis-vasculitis syndromes is usually made by obtaining biopsies of muscle, skin, testicle, or kidney. Unfortunately, positive biopsies are obtained in only a small percentage of patients, pre-sumably due to the tendency of the disease process to affect blood vessels in a segmental fashion. Recently, there have been reports that multiple suction biopsies of the rectal mucosa results in a higher frequency of positive biopsies than are obtained by conventional methods.[5]

TREATMENT

There is no specific therapy for the human vasculitides. In those cases where the development of vasculitis is related to exposure to an obvious offending antigen, such as a drug or a foreign protein, the withdrawal of this agent frequently, but not invariably, results in the reversal of the disease process. The only therapeutic agents which have been extensively used and found to be of value in the treatment of vasculitis are the corticosteroid drugs. When administered in sufficient dosage (e.g., prednisone, 20 to 80 mg per day in divided doses), they appear to have a beneficial effect on the course of most of the arteritis-vasculitis syndromes. Indeed, in some patients may be life saving. On the other hand, it has been suggested that corticosteroids may occasionally be responsible for or may aggravate the vasculitis associated with malignant rheumatoid disease.

In temporal arteritis, once severe ocular manifestations have developed, they may not be reversed by corticosteroid therapy. However, early diagnosis and prompt treatment with corticosteroids appears to be highly effective in preventing visual loss. In the closely related disorder of polymyalgia rheumatica, corticosteroids are often dramatically effective in relieving symptoms.

The treatment of polyarteritis nodosa with corticosteroids is somewhat less satisfactory. While there may be a striking improvement initially in symptoms and signs, the results of long-term studies suggest that the overall prognosis may not be significantly altered.

Wegener's granulomatosis usually pursues an inexorable course towards death. However, in some cases of limited forms of this disease favorable responses have been obtained with corticosteroid therapy. Recently, there have been several reports of apparently favorable responses to combined immunosuppressive and corticosteroid therapy.

In the aortic arch syndrome (Takayasu's disease) the prognosis is generally poor, although there have been sporadic reports of good results with corticosteroid therapy.

Two patients with severe rheumatoid vasculitis have been reported who appeared to respond well to penicillamine.[4] The exact mechanism of action of penicillamine on this disease process is unknown. However, it was noted that the clinical improvement was associated with a significant fall in the RF titer in both cases.

PROGRESSIVE SYSTEMIC SCLEROSIS

Progressive systemic sclerosis (scleroderma) is a disease of connective tissue, the most characteristic feature of which is sclerosis or thickening of the skin. For many years it was considered to be primarily a dermatologic condition, but the systemic nature of the disease is now clearly recognized. In fact, patients have been described in whom only the visceral lesions of progressive systemic sclerosis are present.

The sclerotic lesions may be a minor feature in many cases, whereas atrophic, vascular, and inflammatory changes may be much more pronounced. The disorder has a slight, but definite, tendency to overlap with diseases such as SLE, polymyositis, Sjögren's syndrome, thyroiditis, and rheumatoid arthritis. However, the immunologic abnormalities in progressive systemic sclerosis are usually much less striking than those seen in the other collagen-vascular disorders.

ETIOLOGY AND PATHOGENESIS

The etiology of progressive systemic sclerosis is unknown and very little is understood about the pathogenesis. Interest in possible etiologic factors has centered on four major areas: genetic, immunologic, primary connective tissue disorder, and an autonomic nervous system abnormality with primary effects on the vasculature.

Some studies have shown that immunologic abnormalities such as antinuclear antibodies occur in unusually high incidence in the relatives of patients with progressive systemic sclerosis. This suggests that there may be a hereditary predisposition to develop abnormal immunologic reactivity.

The role of the immune system in progressive systemic sclerosis is unclear, and none of the immunologic changes are specific for this disease. Nevertheless, antinuclear antibodies occur consistently in a high proportion of patients, and produce a characteristic "speckled" immunofluorescent pattern. The fact that vascular and inflammatory changes occur in progressive systemic sclerosis cannot be taken as conclusive evidence of an immunologic process, even though there may be a superficial morphologic resemblance to the experimental vasculitides. The limited variety of responses of vascular tissue to a number of noxious stimuli prohibits such a conclusion. Furthermore, the absence of demonstrable immune reactants in the vascular lesions of progressive systemic sclerosis is against the hypothesis that immunologic mechanisms play a causative role in tissue damage.

The scleroderma-like changes which occur in rats with runt disease (see Chapter 14) is also of uncertain relevance to the human disorder. The immunologic changes in progressive systemic sclerosis may be merely epi-phenomena as no definite autoimmune processes involving either vascular tissue or collagen are yet evident.

Attempts to demonstrate a primary metabolic disorder of connective tissue have been generally disappointing. The total amount of collagen in the skin is generally not increased, although variations in the amount of soluble collagen have been reported. The collagen fibrils themselves appear to be structurally normal. Hexoses and hexosamines are bound in increased amounts in the affected skin and the hydroxyproline content is diminished. However, other reports of an abnormal amino acid composition of collagen and altered mucopolysaccharide metabolism have not been consistent.

Scleroderma-like changes have been reported in patients with carcinoid syndrome and increased levels of circulating serotonin. Furthermore, drugs such as methysergide, which are known to affect vasoactive amine metabo-lism, can produce mediastinal and retroperitoneal fibrosis. It is also of inter-est that dermal fibrosis has been produced in animals by the subcutaneous injection of serotonin.

An increase in serotonin production might result from altered tryptophan metabolism. That this might occur is suggested by the finding of increased urinary excretion of certain tryptophan metabolites in patients with progres-sive systemic sclerosis. In addition, patients with progressive systemic scle-rosis demonstrate an increased response to the intra-arterial injection of serotonin as manifested by a decrease in digital temperature. The signifi-cance of these observations in relation to progressive systemic sclerosis is unclear, but they may have a bearing on the unusual vascular changes which occur in this disease.

It is conceivable, but unproven, that a disturbance in autonomic nervous system control, which is not related to abnormal serotonin metabolism, may account for the changes in the pulmonary, systemic, renal, and digital blood vessels. Other smooth muscle changes such as occur in the esophagus and bowel are not associated with any consistent morphologic change in the autonomic nervous system, although they too suggest a disturbance in nerve supply.

The calcinosis which is often associated with progressive systemic sclerosis does not seem to be due to any basic or primary disturbance in calcium metabolism, and the reports of hyperparathyroidism in association with this disease are probably coincidental. The calcific deposition is possibly secondary to disordered connective tissue metabolism.

Despite the extensive description of these immunologic, metabolic, vascu-lar, and genetic abnormalities, they have yet to be molded into a workable hypothesis which can explain the etiology and pathogenesis of progressive systemic sclerosis.

PATHOLOGY

The pathologic lesions in progressive systemic sclerosis include sclerosis or fibrosis, vascular alterations, atrophy, and inflammation. These are found predominantly in the skin, lungs, kidney, gastrointestinal tract, skeletal muscle, and heart. In many organs the blood vessels may show intimal fibrosis, endothelial proliferation, hyperplasia of the media, and adventitial sclerosis. It is impossible at present to determine whether the collagen changes or the vascular changes are primary, or whether both result from a common basic abnormality.

Skin changes in advanced disease include an increase in dermal collagen, epidermal atrophy, and loss of dermal appendages. Eventually, homogenization of collagen occurs, and vessels in the skin become hyalinized. In the gums, the periodontal membrane is 2 to 4 times its normal thickness, and shows uniform widening with loss of the normal arrangement of the collagen bundles.

Interstitial fibrosis is the common pulmonary lesion at autopsy, while pulmonary arteriolar thickening due to medial hypertrophy or intimal proliferation is also frequently noted.[2] Ultrastructural studies show thickening of both alveolar and vascular basement membrane. These findings provide a morphologic basis for the restrictive abnormalities and impaired gas exchange which are frequently found in progressive systemic sclerosis (see Chapter 4).

The renal lesions are varied and may include (1) hyperplasia of interlobular arteries; (2) fibrinoid necrosis of intralobular arteries and glomerular tufts; (3) diffuse glomerular basement membrane thickening which is generally not of the "wire-loop" type; (4) cortical infarcts; and (5) tubular degeneration. The clinicopathologic correlation in the kidney, especially with regard to hypertension, is not absolute, as any of these lesions may occur without hypertension.

In the gut, muscular atrophy and fibrosis are found in the esophagus and the large and small bowel. The smooth muscle atrophy, especially in the esophageal circular muscle ring, is most striking, and the fibrosis seems to appear as a secondary effect. Thus the fibrotic process replaces existing tissue and does not reflect a primary proliferative disorder. Intimal sclerosis of esophageal vessels is a common finding.

There is frequently skeletal muscle atrophy and occasional evidence of chronic myositis. Electron microscopic changes include capillary endothelial proliferation, luminal narrowing, muscle fiber degeneration, and evidence of damage to most elements of the muscle fiber.

The primary articular lesion is a synovitis manifested by infiltration of chronic inflammatory cells, lymphocytes, and plasma cells. The most striking feature is an intense fibrosis leading to synovial sclerosis which resembles the dermal lesions. Tendonitis, sclerosis of vessels, and lining cell atrophy may occur but, in contrast to rheumatoid arthritis, pannus formation, ankylosis, and bone destruction are usually absent.

True "scleroderma heart disease" is an unusual clinicopathologic entity, but a small number of patients have been described in whom there is evidence of a patchy myocardial fibrosis. More commonly, the predominant myocardial changes are those of left and right ventricular hypertrophy secondary to systemic and pulmonary hypertension. Pulmonary hypertension in progressive systemic sclerosis may be due to primary pulmonary vascular changes, vascular occlusion due to pulmonary fibrosis, and reflex pulmonary arterial spasm secondary to hypoxia.

In contrast to the rarity of primary myocardial lesions, pericarditis of the chronic adhesive variety is quite common. It occurs in over one-third of patients and may be associated with a pericardial or pleural effusion. There is also a high incidence of chronic fibrous pleuritis.

CLINICAL IMMUNOLOGY

Immunologic abnormalities are unquestionably present in the majority of cases of progressive systemic sclerosis, but their etiologic and pathogenetic significance is unclear. Furthermore, none is entirely specific for progressive systemic sclerosis.

Hypergammaglobulinemia of the polyclonal type is found in about 50 per cent of patients with progressive systemic sclerosis. RF is present in low titer in approximately 35 per cent of patients, and biologic false-positive tests for syphilis or positive LE cell phenomena are found in a small minority of patients.

The most common immunologic aberration is the presence of antinuclear antibodies in at least 60 per cent of patients,[4] and the most characteristic immunofluorescent pattern is a fine or coarse speckled nuclear stain. Antinuclear titers in this disease do not correlate with clinical severity or duration of symptoms, but tend to be higher in patients with other serologic abnormalities such as hypergammaglobulinemia and a positive test for RF. The presence of antinucleolar antibodies has been reported occasionally.

CLINICAL MANIFESTATIONS

The disease may occur at any age including in childhood, although it is commonest in the fourth and fifth decades. It is twice as common in females as it is in males. The occurrence of more than one case in a single family is rare.

Constitutional symptoms, apart from weight loss, are uncommon. The disease is generally insidious in onset and slowly progressive. Raynaud's phenomenon is a frequent presenting complaint and may precede the appearance of other symptoms by several years.[1]

Skin involvement, another frequent early sign, usually starts in the terminal digits and eventually involves the upper extremities, head, neck, face, and anterior chest. In some patients, the skin over the entire body may be involved. Early changes include swelling of the digits and a reddish discoloration which is usually followed by gradual sclerosis accompanied by a taut, "bound-down" feeling to the skin. Cutaneous appendages such as the hair follicles and sweat glands are lost and finally atrophic changes become apparent. The skin appears tight and shiny, and limitation of movement may be extreme. The face becomes immobile, pinched, and expressionless (Fig. 8-3).

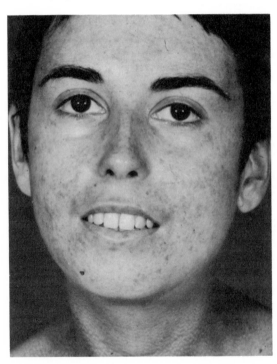

FIG. 8-3. Typical facial appearance of a 20-year-old girl with advanced progressive systemic sclerosis.

Pigmentary changes include hyperpigmentation and depigmentation which commonly resemble vitiligo. Cutaneous telangiectasia is also a common feature of progressive systemic sclerosis. Calcium deposits may be seen scattered throughout the subcutaneous tissues, but are particularly common in the finger tips where ulceration may occur. Gangrene of the digits and resorption of phalanges may eventually result in striking deformities of the hands.

Dysphagia due to esophageal aperistalsis is a frequent symptom and is often associated with Raynaud's phenomenon. Ulceration of the esophagus, esophagitis, and stricture of the esophagus may also occur. The esophageal abnormalities can be detected readily and early by performance of motility studies and appropriate radiologic examinations. In addition to esophageal involvement, the entire gastrointestinal tract may show motor abnormalities. Intestinal malabsorption is not unusual late in the disease and may contribute to the general debility of the patient. Dilation of any portion of the gut and large pseudodiverticula of the colon are common findings.

Pulmonary involvement leads initially to dyspnea and cough, and later to pulmonary hypertension and right-sided cardiac failure. Lung disease is common and usually takes the form of diffuse interstitial pulmonary fibrosis with pulmonary vascular alterations (see Chapter 4). In addition, thoracic wall movement may be reduced by dermal sclerosis and intercostal muscle atrophy. In many patients with progressive systemic sclerosis, radiologic changes and clinical findings in the lungs frequently lag behind abnormalities found in respiratory function tests. Typical changes in pulmonary function may include an impaired diffusing capacity as well as evidence of restrictive and obstructive lung disease. There have been occasional reports of an association between progressive systemic sclerosis with pulmonary lesions and alveolar cell carcinomas of the lung.

Renal disease is a frequent contributor to mortality in progressive systemic sclerosis. Although the clinical picture closely resembles that of malignant hypertension, renal failure occasionally occurs in the absence of hypertension,[2] and the degree of renal functional impairment is greater than might be expected, even when hypertension is present. Fulminant malignant hypertension may appear at any time during the course of the disease.

Muscle atrophy is frequent and is often severe in the late stages of progressive systemic sclerosis. Some patients have elevated muscle enzymes and probably represent cases which overlap clinically with polymyositis (see Chapter 19). Many patients present initially with articular symptoms, and a symmetrical arthritis of the hands, feet, and knees is eventually found in approximately 50 per cent of patients.

In addition to Raynaud's phenomenon, a number of other cardiovascular abnormalities may occur, such as pericarditis with or without effusion, congestive cardiac failure, and cardiac arrhythmias. Electrocardiographic changes, if present, usually reflect ventricular hypertrophy or conduction defects.

Radiologic studies may reveal: (1) pulmonary infiltration, fibrosis, and cystic changes; (2) widespread subcutaneous calcium deposition; (3) absorption of the terminal phalanges and osteoporosis; (4) rheumatoid changes without bone destruction; and (5) widening of the periodontal membrane.

Progressive systemic sclerosis usually pursues a progressive course until death occurs in a few years. In one series, 50 per cent of the patients were dead 5 to 13 years after the onset of the disease.[3] Cardiac and renal involvement and an elevated erythrocyte sedimentation rate were the findings most frequently associated with a poor prognosis. In addition, hypertension, aspiration pneumonia, inanition, intestinal malabsorption, and pulmonary insufficiency may contribute significantly to mortality. Limited, nonprogressive forms of the disease, such as isolated dermal sclerosis, or true scleroderma, probably exist, and their relationship to progressive systemic sclerosis may be compared to that previously discussed for discoid lupus and SLE. Another relative benign variant is the syndrome of calcinosis, Raynaud's phenomenon, sclerodactyly and telangiectasia (CRST syndrome).

TREATMENT

No effective form of treatment exists. A formidable variety of agents including corticosteroids, relaxin, chelating agents, potassium para-aminobenzoate, and penicillamine have all achieved limited success in a few selected cases. However, none of these drugs has proven consistently beneficial or has been shown to affect overall prognosis. Sympathectomy has proven disappointing.

Supportive measures may be of considerable value. These include antibiotics for the treatment of intercurrent infections, antihypertensive agents when indicated, physiotherapy, protection from cold, and esophageal dilatation.

SJÖGREN'S SYNDROME

Sjögren's syndrome is a clinical symptom complex consisting of keratoconjunctivitis sicca, xerostomia, and a collagen-vascular disease, most commonly rheumatoid arthritis. Any two of these three features are considered necessary to make the diagnosis. In addition to rheumatoid arthritis, any of the other collagen-vascular diseases such as SLE, progressive systemic sclerosis, polyarteritis nodosa or polymyositis may occur in association with Sjögren's syndrome. Furthermore, the sicca complex of Sjögren's syndrome has been reported to occur alone without coexisting collagen-vascular disease, and has also been reported in association with chronic discoid lupus.

ETIOLOGY AND PATHOGENESIS

Little is known concerning either the etiology or pathogenesis of Sjögren's syndrome. The obvious clinical overlap with other diseases of a suspected immunologic nature suggests that immune processes may be important in this disorder. However, the evidence at present is entirely circumstantial and there is no direct proof of immunologic tissue injury.

The lymphocytic infiltration in the salivary glands has an obvious similarity to Hashimoto's disease, but it is not known whether the infiltrating lymphocytes are pathogenic. Although a variety of autoantibodies, including antisalivary duct antibodies, have been detected in Sjögren's syndrome, there has been no convincing demonstration that they are other than epiphenomena.

There is an infrequent but definite association between neoplasia and Sjögren's syndrome. Some patients with lymphoma, leukemia, and Waldenström's macroglobulinemia develop salivary disease apparently due to infiltration of the glands by neoplastic cells. On the other hand, a few patients with Sjögren's syndrome have developed reticulum cell sarcoma after the disease process was present for a number of years. It is of possible significance that some of these latter patients also received radiation therapy.

There is some evidence that hereditary factors may play a role in the production of Sjögren's syndrome. Close relatives have been found who had Sjögren's syndrome, lymphosarcoma, rheumatoid arthritis, thyroid disease, or hypergammaglobulinemia. Moreover, the association of salivary duct pathology, renal collecting duct dysfunction (hyposthenuria), and pancreatic dysfunction in patients with Sjögren's syndrome suggests that there may be a widespread intrinsic defect in duct function in this disorder. Possibly the interplay of genetic, immunologic, and lymphoproliferative processes is necessary for full expression of Sjögren's syndrome.

PATHOLOGY

The pathology of Sjögren's syndrome as reflected in the salivary glands is diverse. Proliferative changes in the duct lining cells are fairly common and involve both epithelial and myoepithelial cells. The formation of epimyoepithelial islands, considered by some to be characteristic of Sjögren's syndrome, is seen in less than 50 per cent of patients.[1] This finding cannot, therefore, be invariably relied upon to distinguish Sjögren's syndrome from malignant lymphoma involving the salivary glands. The acini show some degree of atrophy and infiltration with mature lymphocytes. At times the infiltration may be massive and germinal lymphoid centers may be found.

In other patients the infiltrate may be sparse and the atrophied acini replaced by adipose tissue. In addition to these changes, dilatation of the salivary ducts (sialectasis) is a very frequent finding in Sjögren's syndrome.

Similar histologic changes may be found in the lacrimal glands, and, less frequently, in the mucous glands of the pharynx, larynx, trachea, bronchi, esophagus, and vagina.

CLINICAL IMMUNOLOGY

Immunoglobulin Abnormalities

A polyclonal hypergammaglobulinemia is the most common immunoglobulin abnormality in Sjögren's syndrome. It is most pronounced in patients who have the sicca complex alone and may be associated with hyperglobulinemic purpura (see Chapter 10). On the other hand, hypogammaglobulinemia has been noted in an occasional patient with Sjögren's syndrome complicated by reticulum cell sarcoma.

Serologic Abnormalities

Rheumatoid factor is found by the tanned sheep cell agglutination method in approximately 75 per cent of patients with Sjögren's syndrome. The highest titers of RF are detected in the patients with the sicca syndrome alone and the levels are matched only by patients with severe rheumatoid arthritis and subcutaneous nodules. In addition, mixed cryoglobulins have been found in a few patients with Sjögren's syndrome (see Chapter 10). The specificity of rheumatoid factors in patients with the sicca complex alone appears to differ significantly from that found in patients whose Sjögren's syndrome is associated with rheumatoid arthritis. A higher incidence of anti-Gm factor specificity is found in the latter group of patients.

Antinuclear antibodies, as detected by immunofluorescence, have been found in over 50 per cent of patients with Sjögren's syndrome. In one series, antinuclear antibodies were found in 88 per cent of patients with the sicca complex alone.[1] More recently anti-DNA antibodies have been found in approximately 25 per cent of patients with Sjögren's syndrome using the ammonium sulfate co-precipitation technique of antibody determination.[2] The LE cell phenomenon is found only in a small percentage of patients, and is more common in those with associated rheumatoid arthritis.

Antibodies to salivary gland excretory duct antigens, but not to acinar antigens, have been demonstrated by indirect immunofluorescence in the majority of patients with Sjögrens syndrome. The antibody appears to be specific for the salivary system, but its pathogenetic significance is unclear.[3] In addition, antithyroid antibodies and a positive Coombs' test are found in a small percentage of patients.

CLINICAL MANIFESTATIONS

Sjögren's syndrome occurs predominantly in middle-aged women and pursues a benign chronic course. While the onset is usually around the fifth decade of life, cases have been reported which began at any age from childhood to the eighth decade. In most patients with associated rheumatoid arthritis, the joint symptoms precede the development of the sicca complex.

The symptoms and signs of the sicca complex are basically due to hyposecretion of the salivary and lacrimal glands. Patients with keratoconjunctivitis sicca generally complain of a foreign body sensation or burning in the eyes. Inability to tear appropriately is also frequently mentioned. Physical signs of corneal abnormalities are often minimal, but slit lamp examination of the cornea is extremely helpful in detecting minute breaks which stain with fluorescein. Furthermore, the bulbar conjunctiva usually stains visibly on instillation of Rose Bengal dye. Lacrimal hyposecretion is confirmed by the Schirmer test which shows decreased wetting of a strip of filter paper inserted into the outer third of the unanesthetized conjunctival sac. Occasionally anterior uveitis, corneal thinning, ulceration, and perforation may occur.

Xerostomia results in oral dryness, decreased salivary flow, difficulty with mastication, and a variety of dental problems such as increased caries and breakdown of dental restoration. An increased fluid intake is not uncommon. Parotid gland enlargement occurs in approximately 50 per cent of patients with Sjögren's syndrome. Examination of the oral cavity may reveal few abnormalities, or the mucous membrane may appear dry, the lips cracked, and the angles of the mouth fissured. Chronic parotitis is a common complication and is probably due to poor salivary drainage.

Quantitative estimation of salivary flow reveals marked diminution, particularly in those patients with the sicca complex alone. Sialectasis, as demonstrated by secretory sialography, is almost invariably noted in patients who otherwise fulfill the diagnostic criteria for Sjögren's syndrome.

Upper respiratory findings include nasal crusting and dryness, bilateral otitis media due to Eustachian canal obstruction, decreased hearing, sinusitis, hoarseness and cough. There is a higher incidence of pleurisy, pneumonia, and atelectasis in patients with Sjögren's syndrome, presumably due to poor bronchial drainage and secondary infection.

Several patients have been described with latent renal acidosis or with hyposthenuria which is resistant to the action of vasopressin. These manifestations are probably a further reflection of the widespread defect in tubular and duct function which occurs in this disease.

A striking feature of Sjögren's syndrome is the unusually high incidence of drug allergy. In one series, 63 per cent of patients had some evidence of drug hypersensitivity. Penicillin was the drug most frequently implicated, while other drugs responsible for adverse reactions included gold salts, antibiotics, acetylsalicylic acid and barbiturates.[1]

Sjögren's syndrome is a benign disease and the ultimate fate of the patient is usually determined by the associated collagen-vascular disease, or by complications such as drug reactions or superimposed malignancy. The benign course of Sjögren's syndrome should not be confused with the syndrome of salivary involvement which occurs occasionally in leukemia and lymphoma.

TREATMENT

No therapeutic measure is available which will correct or reverse the sicca syndrome. Therefore, conservative methods, such as the instillation of methylcellulose drops into the eyes, are the most satisfactory form of treatment for Sjögren's syndrome. The unusually high incidence of adverse drug reactions which occurs in this disorder necessitates considerable care in the choice and use of any therapeutic agent. Because the incidence of lymphoma appears to be higher in patients who have received therapeutic radiation to the salivary glands, this form of treatment is not recommended.

POLYMYOSITIS AND DERMATOMYOSITIS

Polymyositis and dermatomyositis are considered in detail in Chapter 19 on the Clinical Immunology of Skeletal Muscle.

MISCELLANEOUS DISORDERS RELATED TO COLLAGEN-VASCULAR DISEASES

A number of diseases have clinical, pathologic, or laboratory findings which resemble one or more of the major collagen-vascular syndromes. In large part they are disorders of unknown etiology and pathogenesis which have minimal or no immunologic features. These conditions are included in this section primarily because they may be of importance in the differential diagnosis of collagen-vascular diseases.

ANKYLOSING SPONDYLITIS (MARIE-STRUMPELL'S SPONDYLITIS, RHEUMATOID SPONDYLITIS)

Ankylosing spondylitis is an inflammatory disorder which involves predominantly spinal and sacroiliac joints. For many years it was considered to be a variant of rheumatoid arthritis. However, it differs sufficiently to warrant classification as a distinct clinical entity.

This disease shows a striking predilection for males, usually appears in the third decade of life, and displays a remarkably high familial incidence. It is characterized by back pain, limitation of spinal movement, and eventually by ankylosis of the affected joints. The sacro-iliac joints, posterior apophyseal joints of the spine, and costovertebral articulations are usually affected, although peripheral joint involvement, which is essentially indistinguishable from that of rheumatoid arthritis, occurs in about one-fifth of patients.

An important feature of the disease is an aortitis, due to destruction of the elastica in the aortic root, which is often associated with aortic valvular insufficiency. This type of lesion is not seen in rheumatoid arthritis where granulomatous lesions tend to involve the valves themselves. There also appears to be a strong association between involvement of the sacro-iliac joints in this disorder and nonspecific intestinal inflammatory disease.

In contrast to rheumatoid arthritis, tests for rheumatoid factor are negative in the great majority of patients, and no other immunologic abnormalities are demonstrable.

JUVENILE RHEUMATOID ARTHRITIS

While juvenile rheumatoid arthritis is probably a true variant of rheumatoid arthritis occurring in a younger age group, there are a number of features which are quite distinctive to the juvenile disorder. The major contrasting features are summarized in Table 8-5. In addition, splenomegaly and lymphadenopathy are more common in the juvenile form of rheumatoid arthritis, whereas subcutaneous nodules and vasculitis are less common.

Juvenile rheumatoid arthritis usually occurs between the ages of 6 months and 15 years, and most patients either "burn out" or go into remission before early adulthood. An occasional patient will experience a severe flare-up with joint destruction many years after remission of the juvenile disease.

There are no diagnostic laboratory tests which are specific for juvenile rheumatoid arthritis. A polymorphonuclear leukocytosis is frequently present and may be of considerable magnitude. Tests for rheumatoid factor are positive in less than one-third of patients. Seropositivity associated with late onset and disease of the small joints is said to herald a poorer prognosis. Other relatively nonspecific laboratory findings include elevation of the erythrocyte sedimentation rate and a positive test for C-reactive protein.

TABLE 8-5. Contrasting   Features   in   Juvenile   and   Adult   Rheumatoid
          Arthritis*

	Juvenile rheumatoid arthritis (%)	Adult rheumatoid arthritis (%)
Systemic		
High fever (temperature of 102–106°F.)	25	1
Evanescent rash	25–40	1–6
Chronic iridocyclitis	8–15	1
Articular		
Absence of joint pain	25	(Unusual)
Monarticular onset	25–30	8
Nonarticular		
Subcutaneous nodules	6	20
Abnormalities of growth	50	(Not applicable)
Laboratory		
Leukocytosis	50	25
Rheumatoid factor	10–30	65–85

* Adapted from Calabro, J. J., and Marchesano, J. M. *New Eng. J. Med.* 277: 696, 1967.

Antinuclear antibodies are detected by the indirect immunofluorescence technique in approximately 50 per cent of female patients with juvenile rheumatoid arthritis, but are found in less than 10 per cent of male patients.[5] The only clinical correlation is the occasional reversion of a positive to a negative test during remission. Serum protein electrophoresis may show elevated levels of α2-globulin and γ-globulin. Synovial biopsy and synovial fluid analysis reveal changes very similar to those found in adult rheumatoid arthritis except that the levels of complement in the joint fluid tend to be closer to normal limits.[1]

Little more can be added that is not included in the discussion of adult rheumatoid arthritis except for the curious observation that a clinical picture virtually indistinguishable from rheumatoid arthritis occurs frequently in children with agammaglobulinemia or marked hypogammaglobulinemia.

Although the synovial fluid in some of these children contains considerably higher levels of immunoglobulins than the serum, the frequent association of the two disorders and the occasional favorable response to treatment with γ-globulin suggest a direct connection between the immunologic deficiency state and the inflammatory joint disease (See Chapter 11).

PSORIATIC ARTHRITIS

An unusually high degree of association between psoriasis and inflammatory joint disease has been noted for many years. While some of these patients present a clinical picture almost identical to rheumatoid arthritis, there appears to be reasonable justification for separating off a group of patients who have an arthropathy which is characteristic of psoriasis.

The features which distinguish psoriatic arthritis from classic rheumatoid arthritis are: (1) the frequent involvement of the distal interphalangeal joints of both hands and feet; (2) the asymmetrical joint involvement; (3) the absence of a positive test for rheumatoid factor; (4) the absence of subcutaneous nodules; and (5) the tendency of the arthritis and the cutaneous lesions to parallel each other in terms of activity.

REITER'S SYNDROME

This disorder consists of a clinical triad of urethritis, conjunctivitis, and arthritis often accompanied by mucocutaneous abnormalities. The syndrome usually occurs in young males, and occasionally follows sexual exposure, venereal disease, or diarrhea.

Although the etiology and pathogenesis of Reiter's syndrome are unknown, the not infrequent association with preceding urethritis or enteritis has prompted a search for an infectious agent. In recent years particular interest has been focussed on the mycoplasma and Bedsonia group agents (see Chapter 21) as the result of the following observations: (1) both types of agents have been isolated from urethral secretions and synovial biopsies in patients with Reiter's syndrome; (2) inclusion particles compatible with Bedsonia group agents have been seen in synovial fluid cells and in synovial biopsies; and (3) arthritis has been induced in a monkey by the injection of a Bedsonia agent recovered from a patient with Reiter's syndrome. However, it should be emphasized that none of these findings occurs consistently or exclusively in this disease, and the case for an infectious agent is not yet proven.[6] Elevated titers of myxovirus antibodies have recently been demonstrated in some patients with Reiter's syndrome.

Antibodies to a prostatic antigen were found in the sera of over 50 per cent of patients with Reiter's syndrome in one series,[3] but were also found in a number of patients with ankylosing spondylitis, uncomplicated prostatitis, and rheumatoid arthritis. The significance of these antibodies is unclear, as is the clinical overlap of Reiter's syndrome with ankylosing spondylitis and psoriatic arthritis.

BEHÇET'S SYNDROME

This relatively rare disorder is characterized by uveitis, oral and genital mucosal ulceration, thrombophlebitis, erythema nodosum, and a variety of neurologic abnormalities. Esophageal ulceration, joint involvement, and obliterative vasculitis of the ocular veins may also occur.

Hypogammaglobulinemia has been reported in some patients with Behçet's syndrome, and positive intradermal or hemagglutination tests with aggregated human γ-globulin have also been described.[7] In addition, cytoplasmic staining with fluorescein labelled antihuman γ-globulin antibodies has been demonstrated in cells obtained from oral ulcers and in peripheral blood polymorphonuclear leukocytes. Despite these findings, the etiology of the disorder is unknown, and the significance of the immunologic findings is uncertain.

SARCOIDOSIS

Joint manifestations, usually arthralgic rather than arthritic in nature, occur in about one-fifth of patients with sarcoidosis (see Chapter 12 for a detailed discussion of sarcoidosis).

RELAPSING POLYCHONDRITIS

Relapsing polychondritis is an unusual disease characterized by inflammation, destruction, and atrophy of cartilage at multiple sites in the body. Any area of cartilage may be affected, but the cartilage of the ears, nose, tracheobronchial tree, and costochondral articulations are most usually involved. The disease occurs in both sexes, generally in the mid-decades, and tends to pursue a remitting, relapsing course. In addition to cartilage involvement, other common features include fever, ocular lesions (e.g., episcleritis, anterior uveitis, conjunctivitis), aortic aneurysms, hearing impairment, nonspecific skin lesions, lymphadenopathy, and leg edema.[2]

In one series 30 per cent of the patients had a positive test for RF, while an occasional patient showed a positive LE cell phenomenon or a positive serologic test for syphilis.[2] Leukocytosis occurs in nearly one-half of the patients, eosinophilia in one-fifth, and albuminuria in one-third. There may be mild abnormalities of liver function, hyperglycemia and elevated levels of serum α2-globulin and γ-globulin. However, no specific renal or hepatic lesions have been described in this syndrome.

ENTERITIC COLITIC ARTHROPATHY

Joint involvement is not uncommon in association with nonspecific inflammatory disease of the gastrointestinal tract, particularly in patients with ulcerative colitis or regional ileitis (see Chapter 16). Arthritis may also occur in Whipple's disease (intestinal lipodystrophy) and bacillary dysentery. Unlike typical rheumatoid arthritis, subcutaneous nodules are absent, tests for rheumatoid factor are negative, and erosive joint changes are lacking. Arthritis occurs more often in those patients with other systemic manifestations such as erythema nodosum, uveitis, and pyoderma gangrenosum.

NODULAR PANNICULITIS

Weber-Christian disease was originally described as a relapsing, febrile, nonsuppurative panniculitis of the skin. However, in recent years it has become apparent that there is often involvement of fatty tissues in the mesenteric and retroperitoneal areas in addition to the skin. Furthermore, visceral lesions may occur even in the absence of skin lesions. For this reason, the more general term of nodular panniculitis would appear to be preferable to Weber-Christian disease.

Although the etiology and pathogenesis of this disorder is not understood, it is of interest that vasculitis may often be detected in biopsy specimens obtained from affected areas. In addition, a similar lesion may be produced in the adipose tissue of animals by immunologic methods. Nodular panniculitis is occasionally associated with SLE or tuberculosis.[4]

DISSEMINATED EOSINOPHILIC COLLAGEN DISEASE (DECD)

This syndrome, perhaps related to polyarteritis nodosa, is characterized by muscle pain, tenderness, stiffness and weakness; arthralgia; hepatomegaly; dermal edema, erythema and pruritis; and myocarditis with cardiac failure. Many organs, including the heart, show dense infiltrates of neutrophils and eosinophils. The peripheral blood picture is that of an eosinophilic leukemoid reaction.

REFERENCES

Systemic Lupus Erythematosus

1. Alarcon-Segovia, D. Drug induced lupus syndromes. *Mayo Clin. Proc.* *44*:666, 1969.

1a. Alarcon-Segovia, D., Fishbein, E., Alcala, H., Olguin-Palacios, E., and Estrada-Parra, S. The range and specificity of antinuclear antibodies in systemic lupus erythematosus. *Clin. Exp. Immun.* *6*:557, 1970.

2. Azoury, F. J., Jones, H. E., Derbes, V. J., and Gum, O. B. Intradermal tests and antinuclear factors in systemic lupus erythematosus. A comparative study. *Ann. Intern. Med.* *65*:1221, 1966.

3. Gonzalez, E. N., and Rothfield, N. F. Immunoglobulin class and pattern of nuclear fluorescence in systemic lupus erythematosus. *New Eng. J. Med.* *274*:1333, 1966.

4. Györkey, F., Min, K. W., Sincovics, J. G., and Györkey, P. Systemic lupus erythematosus and myxovirus. *New Eng. J. Med.* *280*:333, 1969.

5. Koffler, D., and Kunkel, H. G. Mechanisms of renal injury in systemic lupus erythematosus. *Amer. J. Med.* *45*:165, 1968.

5a. Kowano, K., Miller, L., and Kimmelsteil, P. Virus-like structure in lupus erythematosus. *New Eng. J. Med.* *281*:1228, 1969.

6. McDuffie, F. C. Twenty years of the lupus erythematosus cell. *Ann. Intern. Med.* *70*:413, 1969.

7. Mellors, R. C., Aoki, T., and Hubner, R. J. Further implications of murine leukemia-like virus in the disorders of NZB mice. *J. Exp. Med.* *129*:1045, 1969.

8. Meislin, A. G., and Rothfield, N. Systemic lupus erythematosus in childhood. Analysis of 42 cases, with comparative data on 200 adult cases followed concurrently. *Pediatrics* *42*:37, 1968.

8a. Phillips, P. E., and Christian, C. L. Myxovirus antibody increases in human connective tissue disease. *Science* *168*:982, 1970.

9. Schur, P. H., and Sanson, J. Immunologic factors and clinical activity in systemic lupus erythematosus. *New Eng. J. Med.* *278*:533, 1968.

10. Statsny, P., and Ziff, M. Cold-insoluble complexes and complement levels in systemic lupus erythematosus. *New Eng. J. Med.* *280*:1376, 1969.

11. Tan, E. M., and Stoughton, R. B. Ultraviolet light induced damage to desoxyribonucleic acid in human skin. *J. Invest Derm.* *52*:537, 1969.

12. Tojo, T., and Friou, G. J. Lupus nephritis: Varying complement-fixing properties of immunoglobulin G antibodies to antigens of cell nuclei. *Science* *161*:904, 1968.

Rheumatoid Arthritis

1. Astorga, G., and Bollet, A. J. Diagnostic specificity and possible pathogenetic significance of inclusions in synovial leukocytes. *Arthritis Rheum. 8:*511, 1965.

2. Barden, J., Mullinax, F., and Waller, M. Immunoglobulin levels in rheumatoid arthritis: Comparison with rheumatoid factor titers, clinical stage, and disease duration. *Arthritis Rheum. 10:*228, 1967.

3. Barnett, E. V., Balduzzi, P., Vaughan, J. H., and Morgan, H. R. Search for infectious agents in rheumatoid arthritis. *Arithritis Rheum. 9:*720, 1966.

4. Baum, J., and Vaughan, J. H. Immunosuppressive drugs in rheumatoid arthritis. *Ann. Intern. Med. 71:*202, 1969.

4a. Editorial. Biological significance of rheumatoid factor. *Lancet 1:*1034, 1970.

5. Empire Rheumatism Council. Gold therapy in rheumatoid arthritis. Final report of a multi-centre controlled trial. *Ann. Rheum. Dis. 20:*315, 1961.

6. Franklin, E. C., Holman, H. R., Müller-Eberhard, H. J., and Kunkel, H. G. An unusual protein component of high molecular weight in the serum of certain patients with rheumatoid arthritis. *J. Exp. Med. 105:*425, 1967.

7. Hamerman, D. Views on the pathogenesis of rheumatoid arthritis. *Med. Clin. N. Amer. 52:*593, 1968.

7a. Harris, E. D., Jr., Evanson, J. M., DiBonna, D. R., and Krane, S. M. Collagenase and rheumatoid arthritis. *Arthritis Rheum. 13:*83, 1970.

8. Hollander, J. L., Fudenberg, H. H., Rawson, A. J., Abelson, N. M., and Torralba, T. P. Further studies on the pathogenesis of rheumatoid joint inflammation. *Arthritis Rheum. 9:*675, 1966.

9. Kinsella, T. D., Baum, J., and Ziff, M. Immunofluorescent demonstration of an IgG–β_{1c} complex in synovial lining cells of rheumatoid synovial membrane. *Clin. Exp. Immun. 4:*265, 1969.

10. Lazarus, G. S., Decker, J. L., Oliver, C. H., Daniels, J. R., Multz, C. V., and Fullmer, H. M. Collagenolytic activity of synovium in rheumatoid arthritis. *New Eng. J. Med. 279:*914, 1968.

11. Rodman, W. S., Williams, R. C., Jr., Bilka, P. J., Jr., and Müller-Eberhard, H. J. Immunofluorescent localization of the third and fourth component of complement in synovial tissues from patients with rheumatoid arthritis. *J. Lab. Clin. Med. 69:*141, 1967.

12. Vaughan, J. H., Barnett, E. V., Sobel, M. V., and Jacox, R. F., Intracytoplasmic inclusions of immunoglobulins in rheumatoid arthritis and other diseases. *Arthritis Rheum. 11:*125, 1968.

Arteritis-Vasculitis Syndromes

1. Carrington, C. B., and Leibow, A. A. Limited forms of angiitis and granulomatosis of Wegener's type. *Amer. J. Med. 41:*497, 1966.

2. Churg, J., and Strauss, L. Allergic granulomatosis, allergic angiitis and periarteritis nodosa. *Amer. J Path. 27:*277, 1951.

3. Cochrane, C. G. "Immunologic Tissue Injury Mediated by Neutrophilic Leukocytes," in *Advances in Immunology 9*, New York, Academic Press, 1968, p. 97.

4. Jaffe, I. A., and Smith, R. W. Rheumatoid vasculitis—Report of second case treated with penicillamine. *Arthritis Rheum. 11:*585, 1968.

5. Schneider, R. E., and Dobbins, W. O. Suction biopsy of the rectal mucosa for diagnosis of arteritis in rheumatoid arthritis and related diseases. *Ann. Intern. Med. 68:*651, 1968.

6. Rose, G. A., and Spencer, H. Polyarteritis nodosa. *Quart. J. Med. 26:*43, 1957.

Systemic Sclerosis

1. Bianchi, F. A., Bistue, A. R., Wendt, V. E., Puro, H. E., and Keech, M. K. Analysis of twenty-seven cases of progressive systemic sclerosis (including two with systemic lupus) and a review of the literature. *J. Chron. Dis. 19:*953, 1966.

2. D'Angelo, W. A., Fries, J. F., Masi, A. T., and Shulman, L. E. Pathologic observations in systemic sclerosis (scleroderma). A study of fifty-eight autopsy cases and fifty-eight matched controls. *Amer. J. Med. 46:*428, 1969.

3. Farmer, R. G., Gifford, R. W., Jr., and Hines, E. A. Prognostic significance of Raynaud's phenomenon and other clinical characteristics of systemic scleroderma. *Circulation 21:*1088, 1960.

4. Rothfield, N. F., and Rodnan, G. P. Serum antinuclear factors in progressive systemic sclerosis (scleroderma). *Arthritis Rheum. 11:*607, 1968.

Sjögren's Syndrome

1. Block, K. J., Buchanan, W. W., Wohl, M. J., and Bunim, J. J. Sjögren's syndrome. A clinical, pathological and serological study of sixty-two cases. *Medicine 44:*187, 1965.

2. Pincus, T., Schur, P. H., Rose, J. A., Decker, J. L., and Talal, N. Serum DNA-binding activity in systemic lupus erythematosus. *New Eng. J. Med. 281:*701, 1969.

3. Whaley, K., Chisholm, D. M., Goudie, R. B., Downie, W. W., Dick, W. C., Boyle, J. A., Williamson, J. Salivary duct autoantibody in Sjögren's syndrome: Correlation with focal sialadenitis in the labial mucosa. *Clin. Exp. Immun. 4:*273, 1969.

Miscellaneous Disorders Related to Collagen-Vascular Diseases

1. Calabro, J. J., and Marchesano, J. M. Juvenile rheumatoid arthritis. *New Eng. J. Med. 277:*696, 1967.

2. Dolan, D. L., Lemmon, G. B., Jr., and Teitelbaum, S. L. Relapsing polychondritis. Analytical literature review and studies on pathogenesis. *Amer. J. Med.* *41:*285, 1966.

3. Grimble, A., and Lessof, M. H. Anti-prostate antibodies in arthritis. *Brit. Med. J. 2:*263, 1965.

4. Macdonald, A., and Feiwal, M. A review of the concept of Weber-Christian panniculitis with a report of five cases. *Brit. J. Derm. 80:*355, 1968.

5. Miller, J. J., 3rd, Heinrich, V. L., and Brandstrup, N. E. Sex difference in incidence of antinuclear factors in juvenile rheumatoid arthritis. *Pediatrics 38:*916, 1966.

6. Schachter, J., Barnes, M. G., Jones, J. P., Jr., Engleman, E. P., and Meyer, K. F. Isolation of Bedsoniae from the joints of patients with Reiter's syndrome. *Proc. Soc. Exp. Biol. Med. 122:*283, 1966.

7. Shimizu, T., Katsuta, Y., and Oshima, Y. Immunological studies on Behçet's syndrome. *Ann. Rheum. Dis. 24:*494, 1965.

9

Immunohematology

JOSEPH SHUSTER

Some of the earliest and most reliable observations in clinical immunology have been derived from studies of immune disorders of blood and blood forming organs. Many of the concepts which originated in this area are basic to our understanding of pathogenetic mechanisms in immune disorders, and it is for this reason that the immunologic aspects of hematology will be discussed in some detail. The nature of the isoantigens of human erythrocytes, leukocytes, and platelets is discussed in Chapter 1.

BASIC CONCEPTS IN IMMUNOHEMATOLOGY

FATE OF ANTIBODY COATED BLOOD CELLS

Before dealing with specific clinical syndromes, the fate of antibody coated cells will be considered. Most of the information in this area has been derived from studies on erythrocytes, but it seems reasonable to assume that similar mechanisms are probably operative for the other formed elements of the blood.

The sensitization of the formed elements of the blood is mediated by circulating antibodies directed against the surface antigens of one or more peripheral blood cell types. Although the mechanisms of antigen-antibody interaction has been well defined for isosensitization reactions, the nature of the antigenic stimulus is poorly understood in relation to other conditions such as the autoimmune blood disorders.

264

It is customary to divide the in vivo mechanisms of cell destruction into two general categories: intravascular hemolysis and extravascular cell destruction. However, it should be remembered that these two mechanisms are not mutually exclusive, and both may occur during the course of the same immunologic reaction (Fig. 9-1).

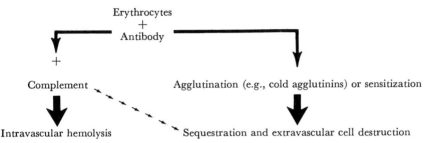

FIG. 9-1. Schematic representation of mechanisms of destruction of antibody coated blood cells.

Intravascular Hemolysis

During the sensitization process, complement components become fixed and activated at the cell surface. Activation of complement components fixed to antibody coated cell membranes usually results in the appearance of small holes in the membrane. If the holes are sufficiently small to retain macromolecules such as hemoglobin, water will enter in response to the colloid osmotic pressure of the intracellular proteins. The cells then swell and rupture, or the holes stretch sufficiently to permit the loss of colloids. In either case, the final result is that of cell death due to *colloid osmotic lysis*. Larger holes in the cell membrane may result in direct loss of intracellular protein or *nonosmotic lysis*. Clinically, this form of erythrocyte destruction results in hemoglobinemia.

It is more than likely that there are other mechanisms of complement induced intravascular hemolysis, but these are not completely understood at present. Furthermore, it is well established that erythrocytes sensitized by complement-fixing antibody may participate in the process of extravascular cell destruction (Fig. 9-1).

Extravascular Cell Destruction

The extravascular type of cell destruction occurs primarily in the liver and spleen. During this process, cells which have been sensitized by antibodies are first sequestered in the cells of the reticuloendothelial system, and the process of disruption of the cell membrane occurs as a final event. Red cells and platelets are primarily trapped within the spleen and liver, whereas leukocytes may be sequestered in the spleen, liver, or lung.

It appears to be the amount of antibody attached to the cell membrane which determines whether the principal site of sequestration will be the reticuloendothelial cells of the spleen or of the liver. For example, erythrocytes sensitized by a high ratio of antibody to red cell mass are rapidly trapped within the liver, whereas those sensitized by small amounts of antibody are primarily sequestered in the spleen. A possible mechanism for the recognition of sensitized erythrocytes has been described recently. Human monocytes, and probably human tissue macrophages, contain receptors which recognize cells sensitized by IgG antibody molecules and C3.[19] Presumably, the recognition of sensitized cells by receptors in the reticuloendothelial system leads to in vivo sequestration.

It has been suggested that the unique architecture of the spleen may contribute to the entrapment of minimally sensitized cells that escape destruction elsewhere in the reticuloendothelial system.[37] Cells entering the macrophage-lined Billroth cords return to the venous system via a slow, tortuous path. Thus, the movement of antibody and complement coated cells through this delayed transit phase of the splenic circulation permits maximum exposure to macrophages.

Although there is no delayed transit component to the hepatic circulation, the efficiency of sequestration is attributed to the large fraction of the cardiac output entering this organ, the low pressure of the hepatic circulation, and the large surface area of the macrophage-lined hepatic sinusoids. It has been estimated that the liver is capable of removing sensitized erythrocytes at the rate of 20 to 30 per cent per minute, whereas the spleen, with its lesser blood flow, is capable of removing 3 to 4 per cent per minute.

The precise mechanism by which sensitized leukocytes are trapped within the pulmonary microcirculation is not understood at present.

Once sequestration has taken place, immunologically mediated cell death may occur through one or more unrelated and poorly understood mechanisms:

Phagocytosis.   Phagocytosis by tissue macrophages and other reticuloendothelial cells is one of the numerous factors which contribute to the death of sensitized cells.

Mechanical Stress.   Sensitized cells, upon exposure to macrophages, frequently undergo fragmentation due to the loss of a portion of the cell membrane. The fragmented cells become more spherical and more rigid, but there is no loss of hemoglobin. If these cells re-enter the circulation, they are more susceptible to osmotic or mechanical stress, and, thus, intravascular hemolysis may be the end result. Furthermore, the altered cells are predisposed to re-entrapment and subsequent destruction by the spleen.

Metabolic Factors.   Erythrocytes are very sensitive to the metabolic consequences of stasis. In this connection, it should be noted that glucose is a major red cell substrate essential for cellular viability. Depletion of the available substrate glucose has been demonstrated within the spleen when erythrostasis has occurred, even though the circulating blood glucose levels are normal. It is now believed that the metabolic death of erythrocytes secondary to the depletion of glucose is a significant cause of lysis and death of antibody sensitized red cells.

Cell Lysis.   Although difficult to prove, it is conceivable that complement dependent cell lysis similar to that which takes place during extravascular hemolysis may occur in sequestered cells.

COMPLETE AND INCOMPLETE ANTIBODIES

The term complete antibodies is commonly used to describe isoantibodies which agglutinate erythrocytes suspended in saline or which hemolyze erythrocytes in the presence of fresh complement. On the other hand, incomplete antibodies are those which require modification of the physicochemical conditions of the agglutination reaction or the use of the Coombs' (antiglobulin) test for their demonstration (see Table 9-2). Although there is probably no basic difference in the molecular structure of complete or incomplete antibodies, the distinction between the two types of antibodies in the laboratory has certain practical implications which will become apparent in the subsequent sections of this chapter.

THE COOMBS' (ANTIGLOBULIN) TEST

Direct Coombs' Test

The direct Coombs' test is a procedure for detecting antibodies fixed to the surface of the patient's own erythrocytes. The antibodies demonstrated by this technique are incomplete because they do not, in themselves, cause agglutination of erythrocytes in vitro. The test is performed by exposing the patient's washed erythrocytes to a specific antiserum directed against one of the major immunoglobulin classes or against the third (C3) or fourth (C4) components of complement. If any of these substances are present on the red cell surface, agglutination will occur on exposure to the appropriate antiserum. Thus, the direct antiglobulin test merely indicates that antibodies or complement are present on the red cell surface, and therefore a positive test is not necessarily an indication of hemolysis. For example, mild immunologic injury may not be associated with hemolysis, or false-positive tests may be brought about by drugs (e.g., cephaloridine) which cause nonspecific absorption of antibodies to the red cell surface.

Indirect Coombs' Test

The indirect Coomb's test is used to detect the presence of erythrocyte autoantibodies which are "free" in the serum. Human erythrocytes of known phenotype obtained from another donor are exposed to the incomplete antibodies of the patient's serum. If the cells become coated with antibody, they will agglutinate on exposure to a specific antiglobulin serum.

BLOOD TRANSFUSION REACTIONS

Adverse reactions to blood transfusion may occur as the result of both immunologic and nonimmunologic factors. A classification of the common causes of transfusion reactions is presented in Table 9-1.

TABLE 9-1. Classification of Blood Transfusion Reactions

Nonimmunologic Reactions
  1. Air or fat embolism
  2. Thrombophlebitis at the site of transfusion
  3. Febrile reactions resulting from pyrogenic material contaminating improperly cleaned tubing or improperly prepared diluting fluids
  4. Circulatory overload
  5. Transmission of infectious disease (e.g., viral hepatitis, malaria, syphilis, brucellosis, trypanosomiasis, and bacteremia with shock)
  6. Metabolic abnormalities resulting from administration of large amounts of acid-citrate-dextrose (A.C.D.) (e.g., hyperkalemia, hypocalcemia, acidosis, and alkalosis)
  7. Transfusion hemosiderosis
  8. Hypotension and hypothermia due to cold blood

Immunologic Reactions
  1. Reactions due to plasma proteins
  2. Reactions due to erythrocytes
  3. Reactions due to leukocytes
  4. Reactions due to platelets

Immunologically mediated blood transfusion reactions will be discussed under four headings: (*1*) reactions due to plasma proteins; (*2*) reactions due to erythrocytes; (*3*) reactions due to leukocytes; and (*4*) reactions due to platelets.

REACTIONS DUE TO PLASMA PROTEINS

Immunology

The clinical features of urticaria, angioedema, bronchospasm, and serum sickness would suggest that some of the manifestations of allergic-type transfusion reactions may be mediated by reagins which react with soluble antigens in the donor blood. In favor of this hypothesis is the increased incidence of this type of transfusion reaction in atopic individuals as compared to the normal population.

Plasma proteins would appear to be the most likely source of antigen in allergic-type transfusion syndromes. It is well recognized that immune responses can be elicited in humans due to genetic differences between the plasma proteins of the donor and the recipient. This form of immune response has been ascribed to incompatibilities of the Gm factors of human IgG immunoglobulins.[33] For these reasons, genetic differences between plasma proteins will undoubtedly prove to be of increasing clinical significance in the future. For example, specific replacement therapy using whole plasma or partially purified plasma protein concentrates (e.g., normal human immunoglobulin, antihemophilic globulin, and factor IX enriched fractions) is now much more commonly employed in the treatment of a variety of clinical disorders than previously. The repeated use of such preparations can unquestionably lead to sensitization. It is also conceivable that allergic manifestations in the recipient may result from reagins in the donor blood directed against allergens to which the recipient is exposed, but ordinarily not sensitive.

However, it should be emphasized that reagins have not been demonstrated in most patients with the clinical picture of allergic-type transfusion reactions. Furthermore, many of the same symptoms can be produced by immunologic reactions mediated by other types of antibodies. For instance, antibodies to IgA have been implicated in transfusion reactions.[34] Two groups of patients have been described: (*1*) those patients who had normal serum IgA levels; and (*2*) those who were congenitally deficient in this immunoglobulin fraction. In the group with normal immunoglobulin levels, wheezing and urticaria developed following transfusion. These allergic-type symptoms were associated with the appearance of anti-IgA antibodies and decreased levels of serum complement. On the other hand, the patients with IgA deficiency tended to develop symptoms of generalized anaphylaxis. It is conceivable that both types of reaction, which differ only in their severity, may be mediated by the complement-induced release of substances such as anaphylatoxin (see Chapter 1).

The pathogenesis of serum sickness which occasionally occurs in association with transfusion reactions is poorly understood. Plasma proteins are ideal antigens for the experimental production of serum sickness in heterologous species. In animals, however, the disease process is difficult to induce by the injection of homologous plasma proteins. It is possible that, in rare instances, transfusion of blood containing aggregated γ-globulin or drugs bound to serum proteins may serve as a sufficient stimulus for the production of syndromes resembling serum sickness (see Chapter 2).

Clinical Manifestations

Typical symptoms consist of urticaria, angioedema, and bronchospasm which usually occur within 30 minutes of the onset of the transfusion. Generalized anaphylaxis and serum-sickness-like syndromes are less frequent manifestations of allergic-type transfusion reactions.

The diagnosis is usually based on the characteristic clinical picture and the absence of demonstrable immune reactions against erythrocytes, leukocytes, or platelets.

Treatment

Allergic-type reactions to blood transfusions may often be prevented entirely, or reduced in severity, by the administration of oral antihistamines (e.g., chlorpheniramine maleate, 8 mg) prior to transfusion in patients with severe atopy or a previous history of urticaria after transfusion. The addition of antihistamines to the transfused blood is not a recommended procedure because it offers no particular therapeutic advantage. It has also been observed that slowing the rate of infusion of whole blood or plasma will often diminish symptoms of urticaria and angioedema.

When symptoms appear, urticaria or angioedema may be treated with chlorpheniramine maleate, 10 mg, intravenously, and bronchospasm may be relieved by the subcutaneous injection of 0.5 ml of aqueous epinephrine, 1:1000. The use of washed erythrocytes, if further blood transfusions are required, may help prevent subsequent allergic-type reactions.

REACTIONS DUE TO ERYTHROCYTES (HEMOLYTIC TRANSFUSION REACTIONS)

Immunopathology

The probability of hemolysis following incompatible blood transfusions depends on: (1) the incidence of a particular blood group antigen in the population considered; and (2) the potency of the antigen. For instance, when the incidence of an antigen approaches 50 per cent, the possibility of an antigenic challenge in random transfusions is markedly increased. Considering these factors, the blood group antigens which are of major importance in transfusion practice are the ABO and Rh systems (see Table 1-6).

Naturally occurring isoantibodies directed against blood group antigens are generally IgM, whereas most immune antibodies belong to the IgG class of immunoglobulins. However, examples of IgA isoantibodies have been described in the ABO system. Both IgM and IgG classes of antibody fix complement, an absolute requirement for intravascular hemolysis.

The acute local symptoms observed in hemolytic transfusion reactions are possibly due to complement mediated release of vasoactive amines. Anti-A or anti-B isoantibodies usually produce intravascular hemolysis, whereas anti-Rh isoantibodies are normally associated with splenic sequestration of erythrocytes. However, in many patients, the distinction between intravascular and extravascular hemolysis is not clear and considerable clinical overlap occurs. For example, hemoglobinemia, which is the hallmark of intravascular hemolysis, may occur in some patients with Rh incompatibility.

Passive transfer of isoantibodies can occasionally be a cause of hemolysis. Transfusion of group O, Rh-negative blood, so-called universal donor blood, into recipients of any other ABO group is usually innocuous, since the anti-A and anti-B antibodies in the donor blood are diluted by the recipient's plasma and are distributed over a large mass of recipient cells. However, in some instances, transfusion of plasma or blood from type O individuals with high titers of immune anti-A and anti-B antibodies will result in overt hemolysis. In general, the use of "universal donor" blood in emergency situations is a practice to be discouraged.

Bleeding due to increased intravascular coagulation is an infrequent complication of incompatible blood transfusions. This syndrome is characterized by thrombocytopenia, prolongation of the prothrombin time, hypofibrinogenemia, and low levels of factor V and VIII. There is some evidence that antigen-antibody interaction may activate the fibrinolytic system, and thus contribute to the bleeding tendency.

The oliguric state which develops as a consequence of intravascular hemolysis is due to a combination of factors which are poorly understood. A decreased glomerular filtration rate secondary to anoxia, hypotension, and impaired renal blood flow would appear to be the most important cause of oliguria. However, it is possible that the toxic effects of free hemoglobin on the kidney and anoxia may also be of significance. It is unknown if intrarenal thrombosis, which may occur as a consequence of intravascular coagulation, contributes to the pathogenesis of the oliguria of transfusion reactions.

Prevention

A summary of the various techniques used to study isoantibodies are shown in Table 9-2. As will be noted from the table, IgM isoantibodies are generally complete, whereas, IgG isoantibodies tend to be incomplete.[24] In practice, both donor and recipient blood are cross-matched for antigens of the ABO and Rh (D) systems since the other blood group antigen systems possess limited immunogenicity and are seldom involved in sensitizing the recipients of blood transfusions. In addition to determining the ABO and Rh groups of the donor and recipient, it is essential that the donor's red cells be tested against the patient's serum to rule out unusual blood group incompatibilities.

TABLE 9-2. Techniques Used to Detect Erythrocyte Isoantibodies

Technique	Antibody class	System
Agglutination in saline	IgM	ABO
Agglutination in 22% albumin	IgG	Rh
Agglutination of enzyme treated cells	IgG	Rh
Indirect antiglobulin test	IgG	Rh
Hemolysis of red cells	IgG	ABO

In some instances, antibodies capable of bringing about destruction of red cells in vivo exist at antibody concentrations which are too low to be detected by in vitro tests. In addition, failure to detect isoantibodies may be due to anticomplementary properties of the patient's serum, or to the use of antiglobulin serum which reacts poorly with the antibody coated cells in the Coombs' test.

Clinical Manifestations

The symptoms of acute intravascular hemolysis occur shortly after the onset of transfusion. They are characterized locally by a sensation of heat or pain along the vein through which the blood is being transfused, and systemically by a feeling of restlessness and apprehension. Subsequently, flushing of the face, fever, chills, nausea and vomiting, and pain in the extremities or lumbar region may occur. In more severe cases, constricting chest pain, air hunger, hypotension, and shock may take place. A transient decrease in urine output is a common manifestation of hemolytic transfusion reactions. However, in patients with severe hypotension, marked oliguria and even complete anuria may occur. In patients under general anesthesia, the only signs of a hemolytic transfusion reaction may be hypotension and bleeding.

In some patients, acute erythrocyte destruction due to primary immunization to blood group antigens may occur only after a delay of 7 to 10 days. On the other hand, erythrocyte destruction due to an anamnestic response to blood group antigens may occur after 3 to 5 days. The bleeding tendency associated with intravascular coagulation is another serious complication.

The symptoms of extravascular destruction of red cells are more subtle. The patients may be completely asymptomatic, or mild jaundice and failure to increase the red cell count after transfusions may be the only manifestations.

Diagnosis

The most characteristic laboratory finding in acute intravascular hemolysis is the occurrence of hemoglobinemia. Hemoglobinuria usually appears after the serum haptoglobins are saturated with hemoglobin. If intravascular hemolysis is suspected, an anticoagulated blood sample should immediately be obtained from a site other than that used for infusion, and the plasma examined for the presence of hemoglobin. Great care should be exercised to prevent mechanical hemolysis during the handling of the blood sample. Intravascular hemolysis will also result in a decrease of serum haptoglobin levels below the normal range of 140 to 200 mg/100 ml.

Hemoglobinuria occurs when the plasma level of hemoglobin exceeds 150 mg/100 ml. Free hemoglobin may be reabsorbed by the renal tubules and the released iron stored as hemosiderin in the tissues. Consequently, iron laden cells and free hemosiderin may sometimes appear in the urine.

Unconjugated hyperbilirubinemia is often the sole laboratory manifestation of extravascular sequestration and destruction of erythrocytes. Neutropenia followed by leukocytosis has been reported in some patients with extravascular hemolysis. It is possible that these latter two manifestations may be the result of a phenomenon analogous to the in vitro demonstration of immune adherence (see Chapter 1).

In the rare cases of hemolytic transfusion reactions due to the passive transfer of donor isoantibodies, symptoms of anemia, jaundice, and hemoglobinuria frequently develop within a few hours. Spontaneous agglutination of whole blood samples withdrawn from the recipient may be noted. The direct Coombs' test becomes positive, and its specificity is directed against antibodies absorbed by the recipient's red blood cells.

If a hemolytic transfusion reaction is suspected, the clinical impression of donor-recipient incompatibility should always be confirmed serologically by cross-matching blood obtained from the recipient and from the donor bottle. Rechecking of the cross-match with some of the minor blood group antigens may be necessary to uncover the source of incompatibility.

Treatment

If still running, the transfusion should, of course, be discontinued. The intravenous infusion of mannitol (100 to 200 ml of a 20% solution) may help promote diuresis. Plasma or plasma expanders such as dextran are preferable to whole blood for the treatment of shock. Acute renal failure can usually be managed conservatively without the use of peritoneal dialysis or hemodialysis.

REACTIONS DUE TO LEUKOCYTES

Febrile transfusion reactions may occur when the recipient has circulating isoantibodies directed against leukocytes in the donor blood.

Immunology

Naturally occurring leukocyte isoantibodies are extremely rare (Table 1-9). Antigenic challenge in the form of either (1) fetomaternal isoimmunization during pregnancy or (2) multiple transfusions is a necessary prerequisite for the formation of leukocyte isoantibodies.[23] Usually at least seven transfusions are required before leukocyte isoantibodies can be detected in the recipient serum. Like erythrocyte isoantibodies, leukocyte isoantibodies are of two types: complete (leukoagglutinating) and incomplete. The incidence of antileukocyte antibodies in pregnant women varies from 17 to 65 per cent depending upon whether a search is made for incomplete antibodies as well as leukoagglutinins. Ordinarily, one searches for the latter because of the simplicity of their detection.

As expected, febrile transfusion reactions due to antileukocyte antibodies are observed primarily in multiparous females and in individuals who have received multiple blood transfusions.[28] It is of undoubted pathogenetic significance that the occurrence of adverse reactions parallels the development of leukoagglutinins. Further proof of the significance of leukocyte antibodies is provided by the observation that buffy coat preparations infused into recipients with detectable leukoagglutinins produce febrile reactions, whereas washed red cells from the same donor have no adverse effects. A high titer of leukocyte antibodies and a minimum number of leukocytes $(1$ to $4 \times 10^9)$ appear to be necessary before a febrile reaction will take place. It is postulated that the destroyed transfused leukocytes liberate an endogenous pyrogen which is at least partly responsible for the characteristic febrile symptoms.

Indirect leukocyte transfusion reactions may occasionally result from leukoagglutinins in the donor plasma reacting against recipient leukocytes. This type of reaction is more common when multiparous females serve as blood donors.

Clinical Manifestations

Immunologic transfusion reactions due to leukocyte incompatibility usually begin 30 to 90 minutes after the transfusion has commenced, and may last up to 8 hours. The severity of the reaction appears to be dependent on the dose of antigen, the titer of antibody, and the rate of infusion. The initial symptoms are often characterized by flushing, palpitations, tachycardia, and a feeling of tightness in the chest. Subsequently, chills and fever may occur which are often followed by apathy and weakness persisting for several hours.

Neutropenia may be evident during the early stages of the reaction, whereas leukocytosis with a shift to the left may occur several hours after the transfusion. Fibrinolysis, similar to that previously described for reactions due to erythrocyte incompatibility, may occur in a small number of patients with high titers of antileukocyte antibodies.

Treatment

There is no specific treatment. The transfusion should be discontinued and acetylsalicylic acid prescribed for symptomatic relief of febrile symptoms. If subsequent transfusions are required, the use of washed red cells is often effective in preventing further febrile reactions.

REACTIONS DUE TO PLATELETS (POST-TRANSFUSION PURPURA)

Immunology

Isosensitization to platelets during pregnancy is probably the initiating factor in this syndrome, and it is postulated that transfusion may produce an anamnestic response to platelet antigens. Antibody specificity, as determined by complement-fixation and agglutination techniques, is directed against *donor* platelets. However, due to factors which are only partially understood, both donor and recipient platelets are destroyed.[8]

Clinical Manifestations

The characteristic clinical features consist of petechiae, hemorrhage, and ecchymoses which occur 5 to 7 days after transfusion. The patients are almost invariably multiparous women over the age of 40. It is of interest that some of the reported cases had never received previous blood transfusions.

Treatment

In most patients, spontaneous recovery takes place in 3 to 4 weeks. However, in some instances, hemorrhagic manifestations may be sufficiently severe to require prednisone, 40 to 60 mg, daily in divided doses. In one case report, exchange transfusion resulted in the return of the platelet count to normal within 3 days.

ISOIMMUNIZATION OF PREGNANCY

Isoimmunization during pregnancy occurs because of differences in antigenic composition between fetal and maternal blood cells or plasma proteins. In other words, paternal antigens inherited by the fetus, but absent in the mother, are a potential source of antigenic stimulation in the mother. The isoimmunization which occurs during pregnancy may be due to antigens associated with: (*1*) plasma proteins; (*2*) erythrocytes; (*3*) leukocytes; and (*4*) platelets.

ISOIMMUNIZATION DUE TO PLASMA PROTEINS

Although genetic differences among serum γ-globulins can lead to the production of anti-allotype antibodies (see Chapter 1), no clinical syndromes have been attributed directly to them thus far. However, the transient physiologic hypogammaglobulinemia of infancy (see Chapter 11) may be due to maternal isoantibodies with specificity for the Gm and Inv antigens of fetal immunoglobulins (see Table 1-1).

ISOIMMUNIZATION DUE TO ERYTHROCYTES (HEMOLYTIC DISEASE OF THE NEWBORN)

Maternal isoimmunization with fetal red cells, which is the most common form of isoimmunization during pregnancy, occurs in 1 per cent of live births and is responsible for a significant number of stillbirths. IgG maternal antibodies produced as a result of antigenic stimulation with fetal erythrocyte antigens of paternal type cross the placenta, coat fetal red cells, and subsequently lead to their accelerated destruction. Since the prognosis and clinical manifestations of isoimmunization with antigens of the Rh and ABO blood groups differ significantly, they will be considered separately.

Hemolytic Disease of the Newborn Due to Rh Incompatibility

Immunology.   The time at which maximum maternal sensitization takes place has been the subject of considerable investigation and controversy. It has been demonstrated that the incidence of mothers with fetal cells in their circulation increases from approximately 7 per cent in the first trimester to 14 per cent in the second, and to 30 per cent in the third trimester of pregnancy. In the immediate postpartum period, the figure rises to 60 per cent. Furthermore, it has been shown that the incidence of immunization increases in direct relationship to the volume of fetal blood in the maternal circulation during the postpartum period.[39] These observations have led to the hypothesis that transplacental hemorrhage at or near the time of labor is the cause of maximum sensitization.

On the other hand, other investigators maintain that Rh-negative women are at risk throughout pregnancy due to repeated antepartum transplacental hemorrhage, and that the trauma of delivery is relatively unimportant in the pathogenesis of Rh isoimmunization. These latter conclusions are based on the observation that only 1 out of 8 mothers who developed Rh isoantibodies has a history of large transplacental hemorrhage during the immediate postpartum period.[42] In evaluating the significance of these conflicting points of view, it is worth remembering that a volume of blood in the range of 0.5 to 1.0 ml constitutes a large transplacental hemorrhage.

It is rare for Rh antibodies to be found during the first pregnancy unless isoimmunization has occurred due to a previous incompatible blood transfusion. Despite the fact that maternal exposure to fetal antigens may occur as early as the first trimester, antibody production is not demonstrable until several months postpartum. There is no completely satisfactory explanation for the apparent failure of the mother to respond immunologically to Rh fetal cells during the first pregnancy, but this fact is of relevance in the prophylaxis of Rh hemolytic disease of the newborn.

Diagnosis.   Rh typing of both parents should be routinely performed during the prenatal period, and, in Rh incompatible pregnancies, the development of maternal anti-Rh antibodies should be assessed throughout the pregnancy. However, it should be noted that the Rh titer, as measured by the indirect Coombs' test, does not necessarily rise as an Rh incompatible pregnancy progresses, and is thus not a reliable guide to the course of the disease.[13] Nevertheless, there appears to be a critical level for the Coombs' titer below which stillbirths or neonatal deaths are rare. A titer of 1:16 has been suggested as the critical level, but, because of variations in techniques among laboratories, each laboratory must determine its own standard values. The titer of Rh antibodies is a reliable guide to prognosis only during the first pregnancy in which sensitization occurs. In subsequent pregnancies, the anamnestic response to fetal Rh antigens makes the results of this test extremely difficult to interpret.

Prevention.   One of the most exciting advances in clinical immunology has been the prevention of Rh isoimmunization through the use of high titer human anti-Rh_o (D) immunoglobulin. An intramuscular injection of 1.0 ml of anti-Rh immunoglobulin containing 300 μg of antibody is usually given in late pregnancy or within 72 hours of delivery to non-immunized Rh-negative mothers bearing Rh-positive infants. The studies reported showed almost complete suppression of antibody formation in the initial and subsequent exposures of Rh-negative mothers to Rh-positive fetuses. An average failure rate of less than 0.2 per cent was recorded in a series of clinical trials carried out by several groups of investigators. It is, of course, necessary to repeat the immunization procedure with each pregnancy.

The possibility that passive immunization with anti-Rh antisera might be an effective method of preventing Rh isosensitization was first suggested by studies on ABO incompatibility between mother and fetus. Although there is no satisfactory explanation, it is well established that women who bear ABO incompatible fetuses are much less susceptible to Rh isoimmunization than women with ABO compatible infants. The protection offered by ABO incompatibility was originally explained by the hypothesis that fetal cells crossing the placenta into the maternal circulation at the time of delivery became sensitized with maternal ABO antibodies. The sensitized cells were then thought to be rapidly sequestered in the liver where there is little or no antibody production.

It is conceivable that a similar mechanism might account for the efficacy of passive immunization with anti-Rh immunoglobulin. According to this theory, fetal Rh-positive cells in the maternal circulation at the time of birth become sensitized by passively administered Rh antibodies, and are rapidly sequestered by the cells of the reticuloendothelial system. However, there is no conclusive evidence in favor of this supposition and other possible mechanisms should be considered. For example, there is considerable experimental data to suggest that the passive administration of antibody results in a negative feed-back mechanism which specifically inhibits further antibody production.[32] It is also conceivable that passively administered antibody inhibits the processing of antigen by the macrophage and thus prevents the ultimate transfer of information to antibody producing cells (see Chapter 1). At present, one can only speculate regarding the mode of action of passive immunization with anti-Rh immunoglobulin.

As might be expected, the use of anti-Rh immunoglobulin is not effective in suppressing the secondary antibody response in mothers who are already sensitized. Repeated plasmaphoresis of the mother has been employed in this situation in an attempt to reduce the titer of maternal anti-Rh antibodies, but the efficacy of the procedure as a therapeutic measure remains to be established.[7]

A number of studies have shown an increase in the number of fetal cells in the maternal circulation after abortion has taken place. Sufficient fetomaternal hemorrhage occurs, particularly in abortions associated with curettage or hysterotomy, that maternal Rh sensitization may be induced. Therefore, if Rh incompatibility exists, anti-Rh immunoglobulin should be administered to nonimmunized mothers at the time of abortion in order to prevent possible sensitization. Because the possibility of spontaneous or therapeutic abortion is always present, Rh typing should be performed very early in pregnancy in order to recognize this potential hazard.

Clinical Manifestations. Hemolytic disease of the newborn due to Rh incompatibility formerly occurred in approximately 0.5 per cent of pregnancies, and the incidence of stillbirths was approximately 12 per cent. When passive immunization with anti-Rh antisera becomes widely available, the prevalence of this disease, after a period of years, should be almost negligible.

Infants with severe anemia at birth are often grossly edematous (hydrops fetalis) due to a combination of congestive heart failure, increased central venous pressure, and hypoalbuminemia. Other common clinical findings are marked pallor, cardiomegaly, and hepatosplenomegaly. In severe cases, hemoglobin levels are extremely low, and considerable numbers of nucleated red cells and reticulocytes are seen in the peripheral blood smear.

Jaundice may not be apparent at birth since the fetus can excrete bilirubin via the placenta in utero. A yellowish appearance of both the vernix and the amniotic fluid provides strong evidence in favor of red cell destruction in utero and, under these circumstances, jaundice usually becomes evident within a few hours after birth. Thus, the onset of jaundice within 24 hours after birth should always suggest a hemolytic process. In infants with hemolytic disease of the newborn, elevated concentrations of unconjugated bilirubin can produce kernicterus—a syndrome associated with permanent and often fatal brain damage.

Treatment.   In most institutions, an indirect Coombs' titer of 1:16 or greater is an indication for amniocentesis, regardless of the past history of disease. Once amniocentesis is considered necessary, future management is based almost entirely upon the results of spectrophotometric analyses of the amniotic fluid for bile pigments. The values obtained are interpreted as reflecting the current status of the fetus in terms of probable survival or death.

Mildly affected infants are usually induced at 38 weeks, and moderately affected infants are often induced between 35 and 38 weeks of gestation. Severely affected infants of more than 34 weeks of gestation are delivered immediately, but their chances of survival are poor. Severely affected infants of less than 34 weeks are treated as early as 24 to 26 weeks by a series of intrauterine fetal transfusions with group O, Rh-negative, washed red blood cells. Intrauterine transfusion corrects the anemia and permits the infants to reach a sufficient stage of gestation so that the hazards of prematurity can be reduced.

Following delivery, treatment is primarily directed towards decreasing the levels of bilirubin in an attempt to prevent kernicterus. The most important form of therapy at this stage is the use of exchange transfusions which: (1) removes large numbers of antibody sensitized red cells destined to have a short life-span; (2) reduces bilirubin levels and maternal antibody titers; and (3) corrects the anemia. The use of ultraviolet light to oxidize bilirubin (phototherapy), or albumin infusions to bind circulating bilirubin constitute useful ancillary measures.

Hemolytic Disease of the Newborn Due to ABO Incompatibility

The incidence of ABO incompatibility between mothers and their fetuses is approximately 20 per cent. A detectable hemolytic process attributable to ABO incompatibility occurs in 0.5 to 3 per cent of pregnancies. However, only 1 out of 3000 newborn infants requires treatment for hemolysis due to ABO incompatibility.

Immunology. ABO disease arises whenever the mother has anti-A or anti-B isoantibodies of the IgG immunoglobulin class, and the fetus inherits an A^1 or B phenotype (see Table 1-7) from the father. Weaker antigenic expressions of the A or B antigens do not produce clinical disease. Invariably, the mothers are of group O blood type, reflecting the fact that IgG anti-A and anti-B isoantibodies are found more frequently in group O than in group A or group B mothers. In contrast to Rh disease, clinical manifestations may occur during the first pregnancy.

Diagnosis. The diagnosis of fetomaternal ABO incompatibility is often difficult to establish by standard serologic methods. The direct Coombs' test performed on washed cord red blood cells is usually negative or weakly positive. A possible explanation for the negative test is that the ABO antigens have a wide distribution in the tissues and circulation, and, thus the fetal erythrocytes constitute only a small fraction of the total antigen present. Therefore, tissue and circulating ABO antigens compete with erythrocytes for maternal antibodies.

However, the diagnosis should be suspected whenever ABO incompatibility exists between infant and mother, especially if the mother is type O. After birth, free antibodies are sometimes demonstrable in the infant's serum. In addition, it has been observed that ^{51}Cr-labelled erythrocytes of the same ABO type as the infant undergo destruction if transfused into an infant with hemolytic disease due to ABO incompatibility.

Clinical Manifestations. Although jaundice usually develops within the first 24 hours of neonatal life, it may be absent in some infants. Typical laboratory findings include mild anemia, microspherocytosis on blood smear, and an increased osmotic fragility of the erythrocytes.

Treatment. ABO incompatibility probably never causes intrauterine death, and thus premature termination of pregnancy is not indicated. The anemia is seldom severe and recovery is usually spontaneous. One of the major indications for treatment is hyperbilirubinemia in excess of 20 mg/100 ml. Treatment in this situation consists of exchange transfusion using fresh type O blood of the same Rh type as the infant with added AB substance, and phototherapy.

ISOIMMUNIZATION DUE TO LEUKOCYTES (NEONATAL NEUTROPENIA)

Immunology

As noted previously in the section on blood transfusion reactions due to leukocytes, antileukocyte antibodies increase in incidence and titer in multiparous mothers. Despite the relative frequency of maternal leukocyte antibodies, isoimmune neonatal neutropenia is a relatively uncommon disorder. This is in part due to the compensatory leukocyte production in the fetus in sufficient numbers to overcome low titer maternal isoantibodies.

In addition, the pathogenetic effect of maternal antileukocyte antibodies on the fetus must also be related to the class and serologic specificities of the antibody, and to the tissue distribution of leukocyte antigens. For instance, antibodies which have specificity only for neutrophil antigens are the most likely to be pathogenic. Maturation arrest in the myeloid series may occasionally result from specific leukocyte antibodies binding to precursor cells in the bone marrow. If the leukocyte antigens are indeed transplantation antigens with a wide tissue distribution, the antibodies are likely to be fixed on different tissues and their deleterious effects minimized.[23]

Clinical Manifestations

Neonatal neutropenia due to leukocyte isoimmunization may result in a transient form of neutropenia which may persist as long as 4 months. The neutropenia may or may not be complicated by secondary infection. The prognosis depends largely on the nature, site, and severity of intercurrent infections. Typical laboratory findings include neutropenia and maturation arrest in the myeloid series on examination of the bone marrow.

Treatment

Symptomatic therapy with antibiotics is usually the only form of treatment required.

ISOIMMUNIZATION DUE TO PLATELETS (ISOIMMUNE NEONATAL THROMBOCYTOPENIC PURPURA)

Immunology

Fetomaternal incompatibility of platelet antigens results in an immune response analogous to that observed with the other formed elements of the blood. Considering the frequency with which the three major transplantation and platelet antigens Zw^a, H-LA2, and C1 (H-LA type not yet established) occur on platelets, the statistical probability of genetic incompability is approximately 1:3 (see Tables 1-9 and 1-10). However, the incidence of this syndrome is low, occurring in not more than 1:5,000 to 1:10,000 births. The low incidence of this disease, despite the high risk of platelet antigen incompatibility, has not been unexplained. Unlike hemolytic disease of the newborn, 20 percent of cases occur in primiparas without a history of prior sensitization by blood transfusion or hematologic disease.

Clinical Manifestations

Generalized petechiae and ecchymoses over the bony prominences and the presenting fetal parts are often absent at birth but may appear within 1 hour after delivery. Intracranial hemorrhage is a potentially serious complication. Melena and hematuria are rare, and hepatosplenomegaly does not occur. However, jaundice may appear 24 to 48 hours after birth as a manifestation of occult hemorrhage due to thrombocytopenia. A negative past history of maternal idiopathic thrombocytopenic purpura (ITP) distinguishes this entity from cases of thrombocytopenia seen in infants born of mothers with ITP. The immediate mortality rate of iso-immune neonatal thrombocytopenic purpura is approximately 12 per cent.

Laboratory investigations generally reveal platelet counts less than 30,000/mm^3, with parallel abnormalities in the bleeding and coagulation studies. Thrombocytopenia is also evident in the cord blood. The white cell count is usually normal despite the fact that platelets and granulocytes may share common antigens (see Chapter 1). The normal white counts are presumably due to a compensatory increase in the production of white cells. The infants are usually not anemic. However, the presence of circulating nucleated red blood cells and reticulocytes provides evidence for increased red cell production that is probably secondary to occult hemorrhage. The bone marrow demonstrates normal or reduced numbers of megakaryocytes, depending on the severity of the disease process.

Treatment

The lack of availability of diagnostic reagents for the determination of platelet antigens and the comparative rarity of the disease makes routine antenatal studies unfeasible. If a mother has previously delivered a thrombocytopenic infant, treatment of the mother with corticosteroids (e.g., prednisone, 40 to 60 mg, daily) 2 weeks before the expected due date may be of value. Birth trauma should be minimized as much as possible.

In infants with moderate thrombocytopenia, the continuation of prednisone therapy in doses of 10 mg/day orally in divided doses may be the only treatment that is required. In more severe cases, exchange transfusion with washed platelets of maternal origin should be performed in an attempt to prevent intracranial hemorrhage.[1] Thus, the lack of availability of antisera for platelet typing does not preclude exchange transfusion in this situation.

AUTOIMMUNE HEMOLYTIC ANEMIAS

The term autoimmune hemolytic anemia (AIHA) is used to describe a group of disorders associated with the formation of antibodies against the patient's own erythrocytes. Although autoimmune hemolytic anemia may appear as a secondary manifestation of some underlying disease process (see Table 9-3), there is no associated primary disease in 50 to 70 per cent of patients.[12] This latter group of patients is usually classified as suffering from idiopathic autoimmune hemolytic anemia. (AIHA caused by drugs will be discussed in Chapter 20.)

TABLE 9-3. Autoimmune Hemolytic Anemias

	Warm antibodies	Cold antibodies
Idiopathic	+	+
Collagen-vascular disease	+	
Infectious diseases (mostly viral)	+	+
Liver disease	+	+
Lymphoreticular malignancies	+	+
Solid neoplasms	+	
Idiopathic thrombocytopenic purpura	+	
Drugs (α-methyl dopa)	+	
Primary agammaglobulinemia	+	
Infectious mononucleosis		+
Ulcerative colitis	+	
Thyroid disease	+	
Cardiac prosthetic valves	+	

The idiopathic and secondary autoimmune hemolytic anemias may be divided into two broad groups, "warm" and "cold" antibody types, on the basis of the optimum temperature at which the autoantibody sensitizes the erythrocytes (see discussion later in this section). Such thermal differences are usually associated with distinct clinical syndromes.

ETIOLOGY

The mechanism of autoantibody production in this heterogeneous group of disorders is largely unknown. However, there are several possible explanations for autologous red cells becoming antigenic. Particularly enlightening in this respect is the chain of events which leads to hemolysis following the administration of α-methyl dopa (see Chapter 20). Symptoms of hemolysis do not appear until the drug has been administered for at least 4 months, a period approximately equal to the life-span of the erythrocyte. It is possible that the drug sufficiently modifies the red cell membrane at some point during the maturation of the erythrocyte so that it is recognized by the immune system as a new antigen.[40]

Similarly, viruses may modify the erythrocyte surface and generate neoantigens. For example, it has long been known that the influenza virus can attack and presumably modify the erythrocyte surface through the activity of the enzyme neurominadase contained in the viral organisms. In the autoimmune hemolytic anemias associated with viral disease, the erythrocyte autoantibodies do not cross-react with the presumed viral etiologic agent. This observation would suggest that the viruses act indirectly by modifying the antigenic properties of the erythrocyte. Another example of an analogous phenomenon is provided by the transient modification of the erythrocyte membrane which occurs in leukemia. For example, erythrocyte ABO antigens may disappear when the leukemic process is in relapse, but return with remission following treatment.

Thus, it is conceivable that a common feature of many autoimmune hemolytic anemias is an alteration of the erythrocyte membrane associated with the creation of neo-antigens. The AIHA which is occasionally superimposed on the mechanical hemolysis found in patients with artificial heart valves may reflect a similar surface alteration secondary to mechanical trauma.

An additional hypothesis has been proposed on the basis of the frequent association between AIHA, other autoimmune diseases, thymoma, and lymphoreticular malignancies in both humans and NZB mice. For example, in one series of patients it was reported that approximately 50 per cent of patients with AIHA had an associated lymphoreticular malignancy.[29] It has been proposed that some individuals have a basic defect in their immune apparatus which permits the prolonged survival of abnormal or foreign cells. The cells of the lymphoreticular system are more likely to develop mutations because of their high turnover rate, or, alternatively, abnormal cells may result from viral infection. Thus, it has been suggested that a clone of abnormal lymphoreticular cells arising in susceptible individuals may produce antibodies against normal cellular constituents, or may undergo malignant transformation.

AUTOIMMUNE HEMOLYTIC ANEMIA—WARM ANTIBODY TYPE

Immunology

Warm antibodies are usually defined as hemolytic antibodies which optimally sensitize erythrocytes at 37° C. Occasionally, the warm antibodies are complete as demonstrated by: (*1*) spontaneous agglutination in peripheral blood smears; or (*2*) autohemolysis which occurs when the patient's cells are incubated in vitro for 48 hours. However, in the vast majority of cases the warm autoantibodies are of the incomplete type and can be demonstrated only by the direct Coombs' reaction.

Three patterns of direct Coombs' reactions are encountered in autoimmune hemolytic anemias: (*1*) those due to sensitization of cells with autologous IgG alone; (*2*) those due to sensitization with both IgG and complement; and (*3*) those due to sensitization with complement alone. Positive direct Coombs' tests for IgA and IgM antibodies have been described infrequently in autoimmune hemolytic anemias of the warm antibody type.

In those cases where the Coombs' test is positive for complement alone, prior sensitization of the erythrocytes with antibodies of the IgM class is required.[20] Failure to detect IgM antibodies may be due to small numbers of IgM antibody molecules fixed to the cell surface. However, each IgM molecule is capable of mediating the binding of several hundred C3 molecules at other sites on the cell surface.[26] The result is that a positive Coombs' test for complement may be obtained despite the fact that the IgM molecules themselves cannot be detected on the red cell surface. This type of reaction is sometimes referred to as the non-γ-antiglobulin test or the complement Coombs' test. Using techniques more sensitive than the conventional direct Coombs' test, it has recently been possible to demonstrate IgG, as well as IgM, on the erythrocytes of AIHA patients with a positive non-γ-antiglobulin reaction.[15a]

In about one-third of patients with autoimmune hemolytic anemia of the warm antibody type, the serologic specificity of the IgG antibodies is directed toward the antigens of the Rh blood group system.[24] However, in most cases, the autoantibodies lack well defined blood group antigen specificity. In this context, they are called panantibodies and are assumed to be directed against universal antigens invariably present on human red cells.

Clinical Manifestations

As noted previously, the majority of cases fall into the idiopathic category and may occur in any age group. However, the prevalence of the secondary forms of AIHA tends to increase with age because the causes of this syndrome are more common in the older age groups.

The clinical picture is extremely variable. Typical presenting signs and symptoms include pallor, jaundice, fever, and unexplained abdominal pain. Splenomegaly of moderate size occurs in 60 to 70 per cent of patients, but hepatomegaly is less pronounced and less common. There may also be evidence of a hyperkinetic circulation, reflecting the degree of anemia present. Not infrequently, there is a history of a recent upper respiratory infection prior to the onset of symptoms.

Laboratory investigation discloses a positive Coombs' test of the warm antibody type. Other common hematologic findings include a macrocytic or normocytic anemia of variable degree, reticulocytosis, spherocytosis, and the presence of nucleated red blood cells in the peripheral blood smear. Examination of the peripheral blood may also reveal evidence of autoagglutination or erythrophagocytosis. Either leukopenia or leukocytosis may occur. A much less frequent manifestation of autoimmune hemolytic anemia is thrombocytopenia with purpura (Evans' syndrome).

Examination of bone marrow aspirations usually reveals a normoblastic hyperplasia. However, megaloblastic changes in the bone marrow are found in about 10 per cent of patients and may be the result of folic acid or B_{12} deficiency.

An elevated serum bilirubin, which is primarily indirect in type, is found in about 75 to 85 per cent of patients. Other manifestations of erythrocyte destruction may include hemoglobinemia and increased levels of urine urobilinogen, but hemoglobinuria is rare. Decreased or absent levels of serum haptoglobins reflect the increased binding of this component of the serum proteins by free hemoglobin.

A variety of serum immunoglobulin abnormalities are detected in AIHA of the warm antibody type. Approximately 50 per cent of patients have low levels of one or more immunoglobulin classes, particularly IgA. Elevated levels of IgM are most common in the idiopathic cases. Low serum complement levels are occasionally detected in the acute phases of all types of AIHA. Recently, a form of chronic AIHA has been described in children which is characteristically associated with immunoglobulin deficiencies, recurrent opportunistic infections, lymphadenopathy, thrombocytopenia, neutropenia, and a poor prognosis.

Treatment

Corticosteroids (e.g., prednisone, 60 to 100 mg, daily in divided doses) are remarkably effective in the vast majority of cases.

Splenectomy is usually reserved for those patients who do not respond to corticosteroids or who are unable to maintain a remission once the steroid levels are reduced to maintenance doses. Survival studies of ^{51}Cr, which demonstrate increased splenic sequestration, are often useful in predicting a favorable response to splenectomy. However, the absence of significant splenic sequestration does not necessarily preclude a satisfactory response to splenectomy.

In general, splenectomy is not as effective in the secondary forms of autoimmune hemolytic anemia as it is in the idiopathic type. Therapy in such patients is usually most profitably directed towards the primary disease process. Although the autoantibodies are generally panagglutinins, which makes successful crossmatching extremely difficult, blood transfusions should not be withheld when required.

Despite the dramatic effects of corticosteroids and splenectomy, about 30 to 50 per cent of patients with the idiopathic form eventually succumb to the disease. When other forms of therapy are unsuccessful, azathioprine in doses of 100 to 150 mg daily may be added to the treatment plan.

In evaluating any form of treatment in this rather diffuse and ill-defined group of diseases, it is worth remembering that spontaneous remissions may occur.

AUTOIMMUNE HEMOLYTIC ANEMIA–COLD ANTIBODY TYPE (COLD AGGLUTININ DISEASE)

Immunology

The characteristic laboratory finding in autoimmune hemolytic anemia of the cold antibody type is autoagglutination of the patient's own cells in the cold (less than 20° C), a phenomenon which is completely reversed by warming.[31] The cold agglutinins belong to the IgM class of antibodies, and may have cryoglobulin properties (see Chapter 10). In addition, they may be reversibly dissociated from the red cells leaving complement attached to the cell membrane. The complement Coombs' test is usually positive at 37° C, and complement dependent hemolysis can be demonstrated after slight acidification (pH 6 to 7) at temperatures of 20 to 30° C. These are the optimum conditions for antibody and complement fixation, and for the lytic activity of complement.

In the idiopathic variety of autoimmune hemolytic anemia, the cold agglutinins are invariably IgM molecules of kappa light chain type, usually directed against the I blood group antigen (see Table 1-6).[16] In the secondary forms, the cold agglutinins are usually IgM molecules of either the kappa or lambda chain type and may have serologic specificity other than anti-I. For example, in infectious mononucleosis, mixed IgM-IgG and IgM-IgA cold agglutinins with anti-i specificity have been described (See

Chapter 12). Because cord blood erythrocytes contain i antigen, and practically no I antigen, differential titers between adult and cord blood erythrocytes are often performed in patients with the secondary forms of cold agglutinin disease.

The degree of hemolysis, as detected by standard hematologic techniques, is usually proportional to the titer of cold agglutinins.

Clinical Manifestations

Autoagglutination of the patient's erythrocytes occurs in the superficial blood vessels upon exposure to cold. The clinical result is pallor and acrocyanosis of the ears, nose, fingers, and toes, all of which are readily reversed on warming of the affected parts. A mild to moderate chronic hemolytic anemia may result from repeated exposure to the cold and may even occur at skin temperatures which fail to produce clinically evident red cell agglutination and vascular occlusion. The acute hemolytic episodes occasionally result in hemoglobinuria which may be followed by acute renal failure.

Unlike Raynaud's phenomenon, which affects the distal parts of the extremities only, occlusion of larger and more central blood vessels may sometimes appear in this disorder. Hepatomegaly and splenomegaly are not prominent features. The disease may remain clinically latent in warm climates.

In patients with high titers of cold agglutinins but with minimal laboratory evidence of hemolysis, the clinical picture is that of typical cold-induced acrocyanosis and a mild hemolytic anemia.[11] However, these patients do not have acute hemolytic episodes induced by cold. In those rare patients in which the degree of hemolysis is out of proportion to the titer of cold agglutinins, a chronic hemolytic anemia is the major clinical manifestation.

The findings on peripheral blood smear, as well as the erythrocyte, leukocyte, and platelet counts, are similar to those found in the warm antibody type of autoimmune hemolytic anemias. Bone marrow aspiration may show hyperplasia of the erythropoietic cells, which may be normoblastic or macronormoblastic in type, and there may be considerable lymphocytic infiltration.

On electrophoresis, a monoclonal peak may be observed in some patients in the fast γ or β regions. The monoclonal peak is usually found to be a 19S component in the ultracentrifuge, and the level of the abnormal component can usually be correlated with the titer of cold agglutinins.[38]

Treatment

The major principle of treatment is the avoidance of excessive contact with cold. Acute episodes are commonly managed with bed rest alone.

Corticosteroids, immunosuppressive agents, and chelating agents have not met with well documented success as a form of treatment. However, a significant reduction in symptoms, titers of cold agglutinins, and IgM levels were recently reported after therapy with chlorambucil given continuously or intermittently in doses of 10 mg/day.[18a]

In lymphoproliferative malignancies associated with the production of cold agglutinins, therapy is directed primarily towards the underlying disorder. The cold agglutinins which follow viral infections are a transient occurrence and usually disappear spontaneously within a few weeks.

The outlook for long-term survival is good in the idiopathic form of autoimmune hemolytic anemia. However, a number of patients with apparently idiopathic disease eventually develop a malignant lymphoma after the hemolytic process has been present for a number of years.

PAROXYSMAL COLD HEMOGLOBINURIA

This rare form of autoimmune hemolytic anemia is characterized by the presence of antibodies with unique thermal characteristics. The disease is unusual today, but may occur: (1) in congenital syphilis; (2) in latent syphilis; (3) transiently following viral infections; and (4) as an idiopathic phenomenon.

Immunology

In contrast to the cold antibody type of autoimmune hemolytic anemia where a single temperature change is sufficient to demonstrate agglutination by IgM antibodies, two steps are required to demonstrate the presence of antibodies (Donath-Landsteiner antibodies) in paroxysmal cold hemoglobinuria. Furthermore, the primary in vitro manifestation of antigen-antibody interaction in paroxysmal cold hemoglobinuria is that of hemolysis rather than agglutination. The antibodies in paroxysmal cold hemoglobinuria have anti-P(Tj[a]) specificity (see Table 1-6).

In the initial step, which must be carried out at temperatures below 20° C, IgG antibodies are fixed to the erythrocyte surface in the presence of complement. The second step consists of warming the sensitized cells to 37° C in order to produce hemolysis.[36] The direct Coombs' test is usually positive for IgG and complement when erythrocytes are tested during an acute hemolytic episode.

Clinical Manifestations

The symptoms of paroxysmal cold hemoglobinuria are characteristically precipitated by exposure to cold temperatures. There is considerable individual variation in the temperature and length of exposure required to produce hemolysis. Thus, the disease may become manifest as a form of chronic hemolytic anemia or there may be acute hemolytic episodes which occur with varying frequency in different patients. The laboratory findings are similar to those previously described for other forms of hemolytic anemia.

Treatment

Management consists essentially of transfusion during acute hemolytic crises, and the treatment of active syphilis, when it exists, with penicillin. Because of the relative rarity of the disease in the modern era, the efficacy of corticosteroids in the management of acute paroxysmal cold hemoglobinuria has not been established.

PAROXYSMAL NOCTURNAL HEMOGLOBINURIA

Paroxysmal nocturnal hemoglobinuria (PNH) is a rare form of hemolytic anemia resulting from an acquired intrinsic defect in the erythrocyte membrane, and is characterized by chronic intravascular hemolysis which is accentuated during sleep. PNH is not an immunologic disease in the classic sense, but is included in this chapter because the erythrocytes are unusually susceptible to the action of complement.[41] A similar defect has recently been found in the platelets and granulocytes of patients with PNH, suggesting that the fundamental lesion may reside at the level of a multipotential stem cell.

Immunopathology

Red cells from PNH patients are rapidly destroyed when transfused into normal individuals. On the other hand, normal red cells transfused into patients with PNH have a normal survival time. Thus, PNH cells appear intrinsically defective and the defect appears to reside in the membrane rather than in the hemoglobin molecule or in other intracellular proteins.[18] The antigenic composition and morphology of PNH cells are normal, and no enzyme abnormality of pathogenetic significance has been detected in PNH cells. However, a deficiency of the enzyme acetylcholinesterase in PNH erythrocytes is sufficiently characteristic to be considered diagnostic of the condition. Recently, an experimental model of PNH was produced by treating normal erythrocytes with sulfhydryl compounds.[22] This observation suggests that the basic defect in PNH may be an abnormality of the erythrocyte membrane, and that the deficiency of acetylcholinesterase may represent a secondary manifestation of the changes in the cell membrane.

In the normal individual, there is continuous activation of trace amounts of C1 in the plasma which, in turn, activate small numbers of C3 molecules. The biologically active C3 components are rapidly inactivated unless they are bound to a cell surface (see Chapter 1). In PNH, the erythrocytes, platelets, and granulocytes are capable of binding trace amounts of activated C3 (and the subsequent components of the complement sequence) to the cell surface in the absence of antibody.

The observations described in the preceding paragraphs explain three characteristics of PNH hemolysis: (1) the serum complement levels are normal and the Coombs' tests are negative; (2) the levels of erythrocyte acetylcholinesterase are decreased; and (3) the acid hemolysis (Ham) test is positive, but is very sensitive to dilution of serum since only trace amounts of activated C3 are generated in normal serum. (The acid hemolysis test is carried out by incubating erythrocytes in homologous serum which is acidified to pH 6.5 in order that optimum complement-fixation may occur. The degree of hemolysis is then measured. A positive acid hemolysis test may occasionally be found in conditions other than PNH.)

Any system (e.g., antigen-antibody reactions or aggregated γ-globulin) which is capable of activating C1 esterase, and through it the cascade system of complement reactions, will potentiate the chronic hemolytic state and will acutely accentuate cellular destruction. This is the reason why hemolytic crises may be precipitated when PNH patients develop infections, receive drugs, or are given blood transfusions. The mechanism by which hemolysis is accentuated during sleep remains obscure, but may be related to the slight acidification of the blood which occurs during sleep.

Clinical Features

The term paroxysmal nocturnal hemoglobinuria is actually a misnomer because accentuated hemolysis will occur during the day if the patient's sleep patterns are reversed. The disease affects patients of both sexes of all ethnic groups, is not genetically determined, and usually begins in the third or fourth decade of life.

In patients with severe disease, the acute hemolytic crises are characterized by fever which is often associated with abdominal, lumbar, or substernal pain. In addition, the first urine passed in the morning is dark with hemoglobin, but successive urine samples become progressively lighter. In the majority of patients, however, the disease does not present so dramatically, although the diurnal variation in hemoglobin excretion can still be demonstrated in the urine. In fact, most patients manifest symptoms of a chronic anemia, rather than an acute hemolytic state.

The clinical and laboratory findings in PNH are similar to those previously described for other forms of hemolytic anemia. The syndrome may occasionally occur is association with aplastic anemia or acute leukemia. This latter observation has led some observers to suggest that PNH be included among the myeloproliferative disorders. An increased susceptibility to infection secondary to granulocytopenia and a thrombotic tendency secondary to intravascular hemolysis are additional clinical features of the PNH syndrome.

The membrane defect in PNH can be demonstrated by the acid hemolysis test previously described, or, more simply, by screening tests which are based on the ability of aggregates of autologous IgG to fix complement in low ionic strength sucrose solutions (e.g., the sugar-hemolysis or sugar-water tests).

Treatment

The management of PNH is essentially symptomatic. Acute or chronic anemia may be corrected by transfusions of washed erythrocytes. Anticoagulants may be utilized to prevent thrombosis during acute hemolytic episodes.

PERNICIOUS ANEMIA

Pernicious anemia and several diseases characterized by hypofunction of endocrine glands (e.g., Hashimoto's thyroiditis, primary adrenal atrophy, primary hypoparathyroidism, and diabetes mellitus) have remarkably similar histopathologic and immunologic features as well as a high degree of coexistence within the same patient[10] (see Table 9-4). Furthermore, there is considerable evidence to suggest that antibodies to intrinsic factor may contribute to the pathogenesis of pernicious anemia.

PATHOPHYSIOLOGY

Deficient absorption of dietary vitamin B_{12} may be due to any pathologic process which results in either (1) deficient production of intrinsic factor (a glycoprotein of 50,000 molecular weight) by the gastric parietal cells, or (2) a selective failure of vitamin B_{12} absorption in the ileum. Addisonian pernicious anemia is the consequence of an irreversible atrophic process of the stomach which results in the loss of parietal cells and an inadequate secretion of intrinsic factor. The active absorption of dietary vitamin B_{12}

TABLE 9-4. Percentage of Different Types of Autoantibodies in Pernicious Anemia and Various Endocrine Disorders

Diagnosis	Parietal cell antibodies*		Intrinsic factor antibodies		Thyroid microsomal antibodies		Adrenal antibodies (immuno-fluorescence)	Parathyroid antibodies (immuno-fluorescence)	Associated diseases
	Complement-fixation	Immuno-fluorescence	Binding	Blocking	Complement-fixation	Immuno-fluorescence			
Pernicious anemia	62–75	80–90	20–47	33–70	16–37	55	0	0	Grave's disease, primary hypo-thyroidism, Hashimoto's thyroiditis, non-toxic goiter
Chronic thyroiditis (Primary hypothy-roidism and Hashi-moto's thyroiditis)	15–30	30	0	3–10	78	87	0	12	Pernicious ane-mia, hypopara-thyroidism, pri-mary adrenal atrophy
Grave's disease	17	24	0	3–6	34	83	0	†	Pernicious anemia
Primary adrenal atrophy	35	10–40	0	20	37	46	60	26	Thyroid disease, pernicious ane-mia, diabetes mellitus, hypo-parathyroidism
Primary hypopara-thyroidism	†	13–22	0	†	†	13	12	41	Thyroid disease, primary adrenal atrophy, perni-cious anemia
Chronic hypochro-mic anemia	0	100	0	2	†	12	†	†	
Normal controls	3	5–13	0	0	4–13	13	†	†	

* Directed against microsomal antigens.
† Figures not available.

in the ileum requires the complexing of vitamin B_{12} to intrinsic factor, and it has been established that one molecule of intrinsic factor binds one molecule of vitamin B_{12}. Only about 1 per cent of the normal daily output of intrinsic factor is required to achieve absorption of the 1 μgm daily dietary requirement of vitamin B_{12}. Thus, at least 99 per cent of the intrinsic factor secreting capacity of the parietal cells must be lost before impaired B_{12} absorption results in Addisonian pernicious anemia.

Although the precise mechanism underlying the development of atrophic gastritis is uncertain, genetically determined factors may contribute to the failure in adult life of the stomach to secrete adequate amounts of intrinsic factor. The importance of hereditary factors is suggested by the significantly increased incidence of pernicious anemia in the immediate families of patients with this disease.

Microscopic examination of the gastric mucosa in pernicious anemia characteristically reveals marked atrophy of the mucosa, reduction in the number of parietal cells, and infiltration with numerous lymphocytes and other inflammatory cells. The histologic picture of atrophy and lymphocytic infiltration is not dissimilar to that seen in Hashimoto's thyroiditis and other autoimmune disorders.

The pathophysiologic consequences of vitamin B_{12} deficiency are chiefly reflected by changes in the gastrointestinal, hematopoietic, and central nervous systems. The pathogenesis of the neurologic manifestations of pernicious anemia is not well understood, but has been attributed by some investigators to methyl malonic acid, a metabolite which accumulates in vitamin B_{12} deficiency.

IMMUNOLOGY

Parietal Cell Antibodies

Gastric parietal cell antibodies which can be demonstrated by complement-fixation or immunofluorescent techniques are present in the sera of a high proportion of patients with pernicious anemia (see Table 9-4). The antibodies are predominantly IgG, are usually directed against microsomal antigens, fix complement, and do not cross-react with other microsomal tissue antigens such as those found in the thyroid, adrenal, and parathyroid glands. On the other hand, parietal cell antibodies may be detected in the sera of patients with Hashimoto's thyroiditis, Graves' disease, and primary adrenal atrophy (see Table 9-4, and Chapter 15).

The stimulus for the production of gastric parietal cell antibodies in other diseases or for the appearance of other organ specific antibodies in pernicious anemia is not well understood. Although the figures presented in Table 9-4 are obtained from a highly selected series of patients, the presence of a spectrum of antibodies directed against similar organs suggests the possibility of a common, but unknown, pathogenesis. In all instances, the highest incidence of autoantibodies is found to be directed against the primary disease organ.

The presence of parietal cell antibodies in pernicious anemia, thyroiditis, and other disorders is invariably associated with some degree of gastric atrophy, diminished numbers of parietal cells, variable degrees of lymphocytic infiltration, and reduced secretion of hydrochloric acid. In no way can the presence or titer of parietal cell antibodies be used to predict the level of impaired secretion of intrinsic factor, or the severity of the histopathologic changes. In pernicious anemia, the titer of parietal cell antibodies has no relation to the duration of the disease, and, curiously, the antibody titers remain constant even after virtually all the gastric antigens have disappeared due to mucosal atrophy.[15]

Intrinsic Factor Antibodies

Two types of anti-intrinsic factor antibodies have been found, using radioimmunoassay techniques, in the serum of patients with pernicious anemia.[30]

The so-called *blocking* antibody (Type I antibody) prevents vitamin B_{12} from attaching to intrinsic factor. The assay is performed by incubating the serum to be tested with gastric juice prior to the addition of vitamin B_{12}. Immunochemical studies have demonstrated that blocking antibody is bound to an antigenic determinant of intrinsic factor at or very near the site of vitamin B_{12} attachment. On the other hand, *binding* antibody (Type II antibody) has the capacity to bind preformed intrinsic factor-B_{12} complexes; that is, it will attach to intrinsic factor regardless of the sequence in which serum and vitamin B_{12} are reacted with gastric juice. Presumably, the binding antibody is directed towards an antigenic determinant remote from the site of attachment of B_{12} to intrinsic factor.

The incidence of intrinsic factor antibodies varies depending on the methods used for their detection. A single pernicious anemia serum may contain either blocking antibodies alone, both blocking and binding antibodies, or no intrinsic factor antibodies at all. However, it is unusual to find binding antibodies alone.

While parietal cell antibodies do not appear to play a role in the pathogenesis of pernicious anemia, intrinsic factor antibodies probably contribute to the pathogenesis of the disease. In vivo experiments have shown that oral B_{12} absorption can be prevented when serum containing both forms of intrinsic factor antibodies are added to normal gastric juice.

Intrinsic factor antibodies, usually IgG in type, have been found in the gastric juice of the majority of pernicious anemia patients, and, in this location, it is conceivable that they influence the absorption of vitamin B_{12}.[13a] However, it is unlikely that circulating intrinsic factor antibodies prevent vitamin B_{12} absorption in the gastrointestinal tract. Recently, a secretory IgA antibody which binds intrinsic factor was demonstrated in the gastric juice of a patient with pernicious anemia.[15] The IgA antibody is probably produced locally in the gastric mucosa,[4] because IgA antibodies against intrinsic factor cannot be detected in the sera of pernicious anemia patients.

It is possible that intrinsic factor antibodies may also contribute to vitamin B_{12} malabsorption once the secretion of intrinsic factor is reduced by the primary disease process. An interesting example of this phenomenon is provided by infants born to mothers with pernicious anemia. In these infants, maternal intrinsic factor antibody crosses the placenta and is present in both the serum and gastric juice. Normally, intrinsic factor is present in the gastric juice in birth, but in infants born to mothers with pernicious anemia it often cannot be demonstrated during the first 1 to 3 months of life. Thus, suppression of intrinsic factor production may be another mode of action of intrinsic factor antibodies.

Antibodies to Vitamin B_{12}

Patients with pernicious anemia treated parenterally with long-acting vitamin B_{12} preparations may develop an IgG antibody of low affinity directed towards transcobalamin II, a B_{12} binding protein found in serum. This antibody is of no practical clinical significance.

Parietal Cell Antibodies and Iron Deficiency Anemia

A glycoprotein secreted by the stomach, but distinct from intrinsic factor, appears to be required for intestinal absorption of organic iron. Therefore, iron deficiency anemia associated with achlorhydria and parietal cell antibodies may result from a gastric atrophic process similar to that of pernicious anemia.[35]

Role of Antibodies in the Pathogenesis of Pernicious Anemia

Although tissue specific antibodies are a prominent feature of pernicious anemia and related diseases, it has not been established whether immune mechanisms are of primary importance in the pathogenesis of atrophic gastritis. The occasional development of pernicious anemia in patients with primary agammaglobulinemia mitigates against a primary role for circulating antibodies in the pathogenesis of atrophic gastritis.[6] However, cell-mediated immune responses which may lead to target organ destruction have not been extensively investigated in this disease.

As noted previously, there is a strong hereditary factor in pernicious anemia. Prospective family studies which relate the development of antibodies to the onset of atrophic gastritis may eventually clarify the role of immune mechanisms in the pathogenesis of the disease.

CLINICAL MANIFESTATIONS

Pernicious anemia generally begins in adults over 40 years of age and increases in incidence in each decade thereafter. It occurs with approximately equal frequency in both sexes. The usual clinical presentation is that of an elderly individual who has not felt well for several months or years, and eventually seeks medical attention because of symptoms of weakness, easy fatiguability, digestive disturbances, or neurologic manifestations.

Typical gastrointestinal symptoms include episodic abdominal pain, constipation or diarrhea, flatulence, heartburn, vomiting, malabsorption syndrome, painful red tongue, and weight loss. The tongue may be beefy red in appearance, ulcerated or smooth, glazed, and devoid of papillae. The general physical appearance may be that of an individual with yellowish skin and prematurely grey hair. Other signs and symptoms may be secondary to severe anemia and include dyspnea, palpitations, tachycardia, and angina pectoris. Fever and hepatomegaly may occur, but the spleen is not usually palpable.

The neurologic manifestations of vitamin B_{12} deficiency (subacute combined degeneration of the cord) are due to demyelinating lesions in the posterior and lateral columns of the upper thoracic and cervical regions of the spinal cord. The patient first notices weakness and paresthesias which usually begin in the distal portions of the lower extremities and then ascend gradually. The neurologic changes are invariably symmetrical and constant, and may eventually result in marked unsteadiness of gait. On neurologic examination in advanced disease, the loss of vibration sense is extensive and position sense is impaired. Motor signs include weakness, spasticity, absent or hyperactive reflexes, and extensor plantar responses. The contribution of a peripheral neuropathy to these signs and symptoms is controversial. Mental changes are not infrequent in patients with pernicious anemia and may include irritability, lability of mood, intellectual deterioration, and, occasionally, overt psychosis.

A normochromic, macrocytic anemia characterized by anisocytosis and poikilocytosis is almost always present. In addition, examination of the peripheral blood may reveal megaloblasts, hypersegmented polymorphonuclear leukocytes, neutropenia, and a moderate thrombocytopenia. Examination of the bone marrow characteristically demonstrates megaloblastic erythroid hyperplasia and a reduction or reversal of the normal M/E ratio.

Histamine fast achlorhydria is nearly always present in pernicious anemia. However, it should be remembered that achlorhydria may occur in normal individuals, particularly in the older age groups where the incidence of pernicious anemia is maximal. Thus, 14 per cent of individuals in the fourth decade and 28 per cent in the seventh decade of life demonstrate histamine fast achlorhydria. In both normal individuals and patients with pernicious anemia, atrophic gastritis or gastric atrophy are morphologic correlations of the failure to produce hydrochloric acid.

The serum level of indirect bilirubin is often elevated in pernicious anemia. Serum immunoglobulin levels are usually normal, but serum complement levels are reduced in approximately 40 per cent of patients as a consequence of the ability of gastric parietal cell antibodies to fix complement. The serum lactic acid dehydrogenase (LDH) is often markedly elevated due to the release of this enzyme from destroyed red blood cells.

DIAGNOSIS

Since the signs and symptoms of pernicious anemia are nonspecific, the diagnosis is usually not made on a clinical basis unless characteristic neurologic changes are present. The demonstration of typical findings on examination of the peripheral blood and bone marrow in conjunction with histamine fast achlorhydria provides suggestive, but inconclusive, evidence in favor of the diagnosis of pernicious anemia.

Schilling Test

More direct evidence of vitamin B_{12} absorption is obtained with the Schilling test. This test is based on the observation that less than 5 per cent of a fixed dose of orally administered, radiolabelled vitamin B_{12} is absorbed from the intestine in patients with pernicious anemia. However, if exogenous intrinsic factor of either hog or human origin is administered simultaneously with the radiolabelled vitamin B_{12}, the vitamin B_{12} absorptive defect reverts to normal levels.

Serum B_{12} Levels

In pernicious anemia, serum B_{12} levels as measured by microbiologic assay are usually less than 100 $\mu\mu$gm/ml. Normal levels are greater than 200 $\mu\mu$gm/ml.

Immunologic Assay

There are, however, some equivocal cases in which the Schilling test gives borderline values between 5 and 10 per cent and the serum B_{12} values are low, but not below 100 $\mu\mu gm/ml$. In such instances, immunologic assay for circulating intrinsic factor antibodies and direct immunoassay of the gastric juice for intrinsic factor may help clarify the diagnosis.[21] Intrinsic factor antibodies are rarely found in other disorders and hence, if present, are highly suggestive of pernicious anemia.

Urine Methyl Malonic Acid

The B_{12} deficiency state causes an increase in the urinary excretion of methyl malonic acid. Thus, the accumulation of this metabolite is specific for B_{12} deficiency, but the routine assay is time consuming and is of little value as a diagnostic procedure.

TREATMENT

After the diagnosis of pernicious anemia has been established, treatment consists of the chronic parenteral administration of vitamin B_{12} (cyanocobalamin). Patients in relapse should be given 100 μgm of vitamin B_{12} intramuscularly 1 to 3 times a week until the anemia is corrected. Thereafter, a monthly maintenance dose of 100 μgm is administered for the rest of the patient's life. It has been suggested that larger amounts of vitamin B_{12} may be needed if there is neurologic involvement, but the evidence for increased benefit is not well established. In general, the neurologic changes are reversible if they have been present for less than 6 months, but may be permanent if they have existed for a longer period of time.

JUVENILE (CONGENITAL) PERNICIOUS ANEMIA

Several forms of isolated B_{12} deficiency occur in childhood and can be attributed to two different pathophysiologic mechanisms.[14]

The first type, due to intrinsic factor deficiency, can be subdivided into two distinct types. (1) In some children there is a congenital lack of intrinsic factor secretion which occurs in association with normal HCl production, normal pepsinogen production, and a normal gastric biopsy. The disease has its onset in infancy and is not characterized by the presence of autoantibodies. (2) In other children there is an acquired defect of intrinsic factor production with histologic and immunologic features similar to adult onset pernicious anemia. Some children with this form of defect (usually females) have associated endocrine abnormalities such as hypoparathyroidism and adrenal insufficiency. There is evidence that replacement of the deficient endocrine hormone results in the reversal of gastric lesions and the return of intrinsic factor production.

A second major juvenile form of pernicious anemia is due to a selective failure of the gastrointestinal tract to absorb vitamin B_{12}. This recessively inherited disorder is associated with normal gastric histology, normal gastric function, and an absence of gastric antibodies. Albuminuria is common, and frequently there is a nonspecific amino-aciduria which persists even after vitamin B_{12} therapy. These findings suggest the presence of defective reabsorption mechanisms in both the gastrointestinal tract and the kidneys.

IMMUNOLOGIC NEUTROPENIA

Immunologic neutropenia may occur (*1*) in diseases characterized by the presence of antileukocyte antibodies, or (*2*) in a variety of developmental abnormalities of the immune system in which there is an associated neutropenia, but no detectable leukocyte antibodies (see Table 9-5).

TABLE 9-5. Classification of Immunologic Neutropenias

I. **Neutropenias associated with the presence of antileukocyte antibodies**
   Neonatal neutropenia
   Drug-induced neutropenia
   Collagen vascular diseases, e.g., SLE, rheumatoid arthritis
   Lymphomas, lymphoproliferative diseases

II. **Neutropenia found in immunologic deficiency diseases—antileukocyte antibodies usually absent (see Chapter 11)**

   Thymic aplasia and lymphopenia
   Immunologic deficiency, short-limbed dwarfism, and ectodermal dysplasia
   Dysgammaglobulinemia—low IgG, low IgA, elevated IgM

IMMUNOPATHOLOGY

In neonatal neutropenia and drug-induced neutropenia (see Chapter 20), the nature of the antigenic stimulus is quite clear. In other forms of immunologic neutropenia associated with leukocyte antibodies, the immunopathogenic mechanisms are less well understood.[23]

Antileukocyte antibodies have been found, using the antiglobulin consumption test, in almost 100 per cent of patients with systemic lupus erythematosus. The antiglobulin consumption test is a somewhat complex variation of the Coombs' test, and is used to demonstrate γ-globulin absorption on leukocytes and platelets. Therefore, the results of the antiglobulin consumption test should be interpreted with considerable caution as the test is highly sensitive, and merely detects the presence of γ-globulin fixed to the surface of the leukocyte. Thrombocytopenia and leukopenia are frequently found together in systemic lupus erythematosus, and it is quite possible that antibodies with specificity for antigens common to both types of cells may be involved (see Chapter 1). It is also possible that hyperplenism may be a factor in some cases of leukopenia which occur in the collagen-vascular diseases (e.g., Felty's syndrome).

Sporadic examples of positive antiglobulin consumption tests have been described in the leukopenias found in some patients with Hodgkin's disease, lymphosarcoma, and acute leukemia.

A second category of immunologic neutropenias is found in association with a variety of developmental disorders of the immune system (see Chapter 11). The neutropenia which occurs in these immunologic deficiency states is a reflection of a common underlying lesion at the level of the stem cell.

CLINICAL MANIFESTATIONS

Neutropenia need not always be symptomatic. However, agranulocytosis or granulocytopenia is frequently associated with an increased susceptibility to infections, generally of the bacterial type, which may occur at any site within the body.

In some patients with agranulocytosis, the initial clinical manifestations may consist of the sudden and dramatic onset of high fever, chills, rigors, prostration, and sore throat. Numerous ulcers of the oropharynx, often covered with a membrane, frequently accompany the sore throat. Less commonly, similar ulcerative lesions are found in the skin and mucous membranes in other regions of the body. Jaundice and regional adenopathy may occur in some patients with agranulocytosis. This rapidly disseminating form of sepsis which is secondary to severe granulocytopenia or agranulocytosis carries a high mortality rate.

Characteristic laboratory findings in severe cases include white blood cell counts which are usually less than 2000/mm³, with neutropenia predominating. In those entities associated with immune mediated destruction of neutrophils, compensatory bone marrow hyperplasia occurs. On the other hand, neutropenia found in association with immune deficiency diseases is usually the result of decreased production of neutrophils, and the bone marrow is hypoplastic on examination.

TREATMENT

In patients with drug-induced immunologic neutropenia, the suspected drugs should, of course, be discontinued. Otherwise, the management is symptomatic. Acute infections should be treated with appropriate antibiotics, but prophylactic antibiotics are not necessary in all patients with neutropenia since many patients may remain asymptomatic for months or years. Maintenance of good oral hygiene is important in order to prevent or reduce the incidence and severity of infected ulcerations of the oropharynx.

IMMUNOLOGIC THROMBOCYTOPENIC PURPURA

A number of diverse disorders characterized by: (1) thrombocytopenia; (2) accelerated platelet destruction mediated by immunologic mechanisms; and (3) increased numbers of megakaryocytes in the bone marrow are grouped together under the heading immunologic thrombocytopenic purpura. The mechanism of platelet destruction appears to be extrinsic in nature inasmuch as donor platelets infused into patients with the disease are destroyed as rapidly as the patient's own platelets. Furthermore, plasma from affected individuals transfused into normal recipients can produce profound thrombocytopenia.

ETIOLOGY

Several entities which meet the criteria outlined above have been discussed previously in this chapter, and include post-transfusion purpura, isoimmune neonatal thrombocytopenic purpura, and Evans' syndrome. Other forms of thrombocytopenia are drug-induced (see Chapter 20) or are associated with a variety of disease entities such as systemic lupus erythematosus or other collagen-vascular diseases, the lymphoproliferative disorders, viral diseases,[27] and septicemias. A great many cases of thrombocytopenia have no known cause and are therefore termed idiopathic thrombocytopenic purpura (ITP)[3] (see Table 9-6).

IMMUNOLOGY

The probable immunologic nature of ITP was first demonstrated by exchange transfusion experiments.[17] In 60 per cent of patients, plasma or

TABLE 9-6. Causes of Immunologic Thrombocytopenic Purpura

Idiopathic (ITP)
Post-transfusion purpura
Neonatal thrombocytopenic purpura
Autoimmune hemolytic anemia (Evans' syndrome)
Systemic lupus erythematosus
Other collagen vascular diseases
Lymphoproliferative disorders
Drug-induced
Viral diseases
Septicemia

---

blood obtained from patients with ITP caused sustained thrombocytopenia when infused into normal recipients. The antiplatelet factor demonstrated in this manner was found to be associated with the IgG immunoglobulin fraction, and could be transmitted through the placenta. Furthermore, the thrombocytopenic factor was found to be species specific, but capable of destroying both autologous and homologous platelets. It should be emphasized that this factor was found mostly in chronic cases of ITP. More recent studies using a highly sensitive assay technique demonstrated the presence of an antiplatelet factor in the plasma of 73 per cent of patients with ITP and in 85 per cent of patients with systemic lupus erythematosus.[22a]

Delineation of the properties of the antiplatelet factor is hampered by difficulties in applying current in vitro immunologic procedures to the study of the problem. Most in vitro techniques for measuring platelet antibodies give either negative or occasionally positive tests with ITP sera. The reason that platelet antibodies are not consistently found in immunologic thrombocytopenic purpura is not entirely clear. However, it is possible that the antibodies exist in low titer and have a great affinity for platelets or other tissues. Another, more indirect, approach to the demonstration of antiplatelet factors is to measure the survival of autologous platelets labelled with ^{51}Cr. In most instances, the half-life of ^{51}Cr-labelled platelets is significantly reduced from the normal 8 to 10 days.

The thrombocytopenic factor observed in chronic ITP appears to possess the characteristics of an antibody, but there is no obvious extrinsic antigen. The association of chronic ITP with systemic lupus erythematosus, a condition associated with a multiplicity of autoantibodies, suggests an "autoimmune" etiology. In chronic lymphatic leukemia, one may speculate that there is proliferation of a clone of lymphocytes which has lost the capacity for self-recognition, and that antiplatelet antibodies are formed as a result of cross-reactivity between platelet and leukocyte antigens.[29]

The peripheral platelet counts in ITP appear to depend exclusively on the survival time of the platelets, indicating that there is little compensatory increase in platelet production. This observation contrasts with the findings in autoimmune hemolytic disorders and suggests that the immune mechanism may also affect megakaryocyte function.

CLINICAL MANIFESTATIONS

Acute idiopathic thrombocytopenic purpura (ITP) is predominantly a disease of childhood which most commonly occurs under the age of 8 years. The onset is sudden, is often preceded by an acute infectious process, and is characterized by petechial and purpuric lesions of the skin and mucous membranes. Intracranial hemorrhage may be a serious complication. Usually the spleen is not palpable. Platelet counts below 10,000 are not uncommon in the acute forms of ITP. Most acute cases undergo spontaneous remission over a period of 1 week to 3 months, but in 10 per cent of patients the disease may progress to the chronic form. Recurrent, acute, -self-limited episodes constitute an uncommon clinical variant.

The chronic form of ITP is more common in young adult females and is more insidious in onset. Typical clinical findings include prolonged menses, a long history of easy bruising, and hematuria. Splenomegaly is an infrequent finding. The platelet counts are usually in the range of 40,000 to 80,000 and even during remission rarely return to normal levels. In managing patients with chronic ITP, it is difficult to relate the hemorrhagic tendency to the level of the platelet counts. The clinical course is extremely variable. The natural history of the disease is characterized by repeated relapses, often precipitated by acute infections, and by spontaneous remissions. Although associated with a high morbidity, the chronic disease is not generally life-threatening.

Common laboratory findings include thrombocytopenia which is often associated with a prolonged bleeding time, poor clot retraction, and a positive Rumpel-Leede phenomenon. Anemia, if present, is proportional to the extent of the blood loss, and leukocytosis is observed only during hemorrhagic episodes. Examination of bone marrow aspirates frequently reveals hyperplasia and decreased budding of the megakaryocytes. Serum immunoglobulins and serum complement levels are usually normal.

The determination of platelet survival times may sometimes be of assistance in distinguishing between the acute and chronic forms of ITP. The platelet survival tends to be shorter in the acute form of the disease.

TREATMENT

The initial aim of therapy is to control the bleeding tendency and to maintain the patient's health until a remission occurs either spontaneously or with splenectomy. Corticosteroids are frequently highly effective in achieving this objective. The presumed mode of action of these drugs in thrombocytopenic purpura is to inhibit sequestration in the reticuloendothelial system and to lower the titer of antiplatelet antibodies. Prednisone therapy may be started at doses ranging from 20 to 60 mg per day in divided doses. When bleeding manifestations have been controlled and a satisfactory platelet response is obtained (60,000 to 100,000 platelets/mm^3), the dose of prednisone may be tapered slowly to maintenance levels which are sufficient to control bleeding.

In the acute form of ITP, splenectomy has almost no place in the treatment program. Usually, corticosteroid therapy alone is continued until a remission occurs. In the chronic form of the disease, corticosteroids do not produce a complete cure in most instances and cessation of therapy almost inevitably results in a prompt return of symptoms. Thus, splenectomy is usually required in an attempt to prevent serious hemorrhagic complications, but, unfortunately, the results cannot be predicted with any degree of certainty. Preliminary reports of the treatment of refractory ITP with azathioprine in daily doses of 1.5 to 2 mg/kg/day have been encouraging.

Platelet transfusions are effective in controlling acute hemorrhagic episodes, although the very nature of the defect in ITP reduces the life-span of the transfused cells. Therefore, platelet transfusions should be reserved for life-threatening episodes, or for preparation of patients for surgery.

CIRCULATING ANTICOAGULANTS

Within the last decade, a series of hemorrhagic disorders have been defined which are characterized by the presence of circulating anticoagulants in the blood. The circulating anticoagulants have many of the properties of antibodies, and are found most commonly in two broad groups of patients: (1) patients with a congenital deficiency of blood clotting factors (e.g., hemophilia) who have received replacement therapy in the form of fresh plasma or plasma concentrates on numerous occasions; and (2) patients with a variety of disease processes with immunologic features.[5]

IMMUNOLOGY

Congenital Deficiency of Essential Blood Clotting Factors

Hemorrhagic manifestations can be due to congenital deficiency of any one of the many components essential for the blood clotting mechanism. Most of the work on circulating anticoagulants has been done on patients with hemophilia (absence or deficiency of factor VIII), and the subsequent discussion will be devoted to the abnormalities found in hemophilic patients.

The circulating anticoagulant appears to develop after replacement therapy is initiated with fresh plasma or antihemophilic globulin (AHG). Multiple infusions are required before the anticoagulants appear, and they are specific for the blood clotting factor the patient lacks. Thus, the stimulus for production, the time of appearance, and the specificity of the inhibitor substance all provide strong evidence in favor of an immune response. Furthermore, the circulating anticoagulants have the physical properties of an IgG immunoglobulin, and the anticoagulant activity can be removed by absorbing the patient's sera with antisera specific for immunoglobulins. However, it should be emphasized that only about 20 per cent of hemophiliacs who receive replacement therapy develop antibodies to the coagulation factor that they lack. Circulating anticoagulants have also been reported in a small proportion of patients with factor IX deficiency (Christmas disease).

Other Causes of Circulating Anticoagulants (Acquired Hemophilia)

Hemorrhagic manifestations associated with circulating anticoagulants develop for no obvious reason in otherwise normal individuals in the older age groups or in association with a variety of other diseases which may include systemic lupus erythematosus, ulcerative colitis, paraproteinemias, severe penicillin allergy, and bullous skin diseases. These circulating anticoagulants may be directed against factors present in almost any stage of the clotting mechanism.

On rare occasions, women may develop a severe bleeding tendency within a year after parturition which is accompanied by the appearance of a circulating anticoagulant. The nature or source of this anticoagulant is not understood, but it may persist for periods of from 6 months to 11 years after the initial appearance.

CLINICAL MANIFESTATIONS

The presence of a circulating anticoagulant should be suspected (1) in any individual with a history of congenital deficiency in the coagulation system who suddenly becomes refractory to therapy, and (2) in all other patients in whom acquired hemophilia develops. The presence of circulating anticoagulants is associated with the usual clinical manifestations of hemophilia. Prolonged bleeding occurs spontaneously or with minimal trauma and virtually any site within the body may be involved.

Before an attempt is made to confirm the diagnosis by elaborate coagulation studies, the presence of thrombocytopenia, afibrinogenemia, or the use of anticoagulant drugs should be excluded. Determination of the prothrombin time and the partial thromboplastin time are useful screening procedures where circulating anticoagulants are suspected. The specificity of the circulating anticoagulant may be determined by incubating the patient's plasma with normal plasma and determining which clotting factor becomes deficient as measured by the thromboplastin generation test.

TREATMENT

The management of congenital hemophilia is made considerably more difficult by the development of circulating anticoagulants. The usual form of treatment consists of local measures to control bleeding, and correction of anemia by transfusions of washed red cells. Encouraging results have recently been reported with azathioprine in doses of 1 to 3 mg/kg daily.

PERIPHERAL BLOOD EOSINOPHILIA

Despite extensive investigation and considerable speculation, the origin and function of the eosinophilic leukocyte remain largely unknown. Nevertheless, the presence of increased numbers of eosinophils in the tissues and peripheral blood is considered to be a characteristic feature of numerous hypersensitivity syndromes.

PATHOPHYSIOLOGY

In guinea pigs, it was shown that the injection of minute amounts of antigen into the footpad results in the accumulation of eosinophils in the draining lymph nodes within 24 hours.[25] This finding would suggest that the presence of antigen is a stimulus to the accumulation of eosinophils in the tissues. It was also demonstrated that, under special circumstances, eosinophils are able to phagocytose antigen-antibody complexes in vivo, but it is difficult to generalize from this isolated experimental observation. Another group of investigators showed that horse eosinophils block the action of histamine and, thus, it has been postulated that eosinophils may function as a source of naturally occurring antihistamine substances.[2] Neither of these experimental models has been thoroughly investigated in humans.

CLINICAL CORRELATIONS

A list of the common causes of peripheral blood eosinophilia is presented in Table 9-7. Some of the hypersensitivity states associated with eosinophilia will be described in more detail in the section which follows.

TABLE 9-7. Common Causes of Eosinophilia

Bronchial asthma and allergic rhinitis
Drug hypersensitivity
Parasitic infestations
Polyarteritis nodosa
Pulmonary infiltration with eosinophilia
Pemphigus, dermatitis herpetiformis, and other dermatoses
Eosinophilic leukemia
Hodgkin's disease
Sarcoidosis
Malignant tumors
Irradiation
Acute viral, mycotic, and bacterial infections
Plasma cell dyscrasias

Bronchial Asthma and Allergic Rhinitis

In patients with allergic rhinitis, increased numbers of eosinophils are frequently found in nasal polyps, in smears of the nasal secretions, and in the peripheral blood. It is of interest that the eosinophilia associated with allergic rhinitis is often found in the absence of any obvious extrinsic allergen.

In bronchial asthma, eosinophils are found in the bronchial mucosa on biopsy, in the sputum, and in the peripheral blood. The Charcot-Leyden crystals which characteristically appear in the sputum in bronchial asthma represent crystallized proteins extruded from eosinophils in the lower respiratory tract. In general, there is a higher percentage of eosinophils in the peripheral blood of patients with intrinsic asthma than there is in those with extrinsic asthma. However, eosinophilia over 25 per cent is not usually found in bronchial asthma due to any cause and, when present, would suggest that the clinical signs of airway obstruction are more likely to be caused by a collagen-vascular disease or the P.I.E. syndrome (see Chapter 4).

It is also a common clinical observation that bronchial asthma, nasal polyps, aspirin disease (see Chapter 20) and peripheral blood eosinophilia frequently occur together in patients over the age of 40 years. The mechanisms underlying this association are entirely unknown.

It has recently been reported that vacuolization of peripheral blood eosinophils occurs in approximately two-thirds of symptomatic asthmatic patients.[9] The abnormal human eosinophils have a marked morphologic resemblance to the guinea pig eosinophils which participate in the phagocytosis of antigen-antibody complexes.

Drug Hypersensitivity

Peripheral blood eosinophilia, with or without fever, is a frequent accompaniment of adverse reactions to drugs. This syndrome may occur as the sole manifestation of putative drug hypersensitivity, but is more commonly associated with other systemic or cutaneous manifestations of drug allergy (see Chapter 20). Contrary to expectation, eosinophilia is found only rarely in serum sickness and urticaria.

Parasitic Infestations

Peripheral blood eosinophilia of a marked degree is a frequent accompaniment of parasitic infestations of all types. The periorbital edema and eosinophilia which sometimes occurs in trichinosis occasionally leads to a mistaken diagnosis of angioedema due to extrinsic allergens or drugs.

Collagen-Vascular Diseases

Peripheral blood eosinophilia occurs most commonly in polyarteritis nodosa, but may be found occasionally in other diseases in this category (see Chapter 8).

P.I.E. Syndrome

The syndrome of pulmonary infiltration with eosinophilia is fully discussed in Chapter 4.

REFERENCES

1. Adner, M. M., Fisch, G. R., Starobin, S. G., and Aster, R. H. Use of "compatible" platelet transfusions in treatment of congenital immune thrombocytopenic purpura. *New Eng. J. Med. 280:*244, 1969.

2. Archer, R. K. The eosinophil leukocytes. *Series Haematologica I 4:3*, 1968.

3. Baldini, M. Idiopathic thrombocytopenic purpura. *New Eng. J. Med. 274:1245*, 1966.

4. Bauer, S., Fisher, J. M., Strickland, R. G., and Taylor, K. B. Autoantibody-containing cells in gastric mucosa in pernicious anemia. *Lancet 2:887*, 1968.

5. Bidwell, E. Acquired inhibitors of coagulants. *Ann. Rev. Med. 20:63*, 1969.

6. Clark, R., Tornyos, K., Herbert, V., and Twomey, J. J. Studies on two patients with concomitant pernicious anemia and immunoglobulin deficiency. *Ann. Intern. Med 67:403*, 1967.

7. Clarke, C. A., Elson, C. J., Bradley, J., Donohoe, W. T. A., and Jones, N. C. Intensive plasmaphoresis as a therapeutic measure in rhesus-immunized women. *Lancet 1:793*, 1970.

8. Colombani, J. Auto- and iso-immune thrombocytopenia. *Seminars Hemat. 3:74*, 1966.

9. Connell, J. T. Morphologic changes in eosinophils in allergic disease. *J. Allergy 41:1*, 1968.

10. Doniach, D., Roitt, I. M., and Taylor, K. B. Autoimmune phenomena in pernicious anemia. Serological overlap with thyroiditis, thyrotoxicosis, and systemic lupus erythematosus. *Brit. Med. J. 1:1374*, 1963.

11. Evans, R., S., Turner, E., Bingham, M., and Woods, R. Chronic hemolytic anemia due to cold agglutinins. II. The role of C' in red cell destruction. *J. Clin. Invest. 47:691*, 1968.

12. Eyster, M. E., and Jenkins, D. E., Jr. Erythrocyte coating substances in patients with positive direct anti-globulin reactions. Correlation of γG globulin and complement coating with underlying diseases, overt hemolysis and response to therapy. *Amer. J. Med. 46:360*, 1969.

13. Freda, V. J. Antepartum management of the Rh problem. *Progr. Hemat. 5:266*, 1966.

13a. Goldberg, L. S., and Bluestone, R. Hidden gastric antibodies to intrinsic factor in pernicious anemia. *J. Lab. Clin. Med. 75:449*, 1970.

14. Goldberg, L. S., and Fudenberg, H. H. Familial selective malabsorption of vitamin B_{12}. *New Eng. J. Med. 279:405*, 1968.

15. Goldberg, L. S., and Fudenberg, H. H. The autoimmune aspects of pernicious anemia. *Amer. J. Med. 46:489*, 1969.

15a. Guilliland, B. C., Leddy, J. P., and Vaughan, J. H. The detection of cell-bound antibody on complement coated human red cells. *J. Clin. Invest. 49:898*, 1970.

16. Harböe, M., and Lind, K. Light chains in transiently occurring cold hemagglutinins. *Scand. J. Haemat. 3:269*, 1966.

17. Harrington, W. J., Sprague, C. C., Minnich, V., Moore, C. V., Aulvin, R. C., and Dubach, R. Immunologic mechanisms in idiopathic and neonatal thrombocytopenic purpura. *Ann. Intern. Med. 38:433*, 1953.

18. Hinz, C. F., Jr. The hemolytic reaction in paroxysmal nocturnal hemoglobinuria. *Progr. Hemat. 5:*60, 1966.

18a. Hippe, E., Jensen, K. B., Oleson, H., Lind, K., and Thomson, P. E. B. Chlorambucil treatment of patients with cold agglutinin syndrome. *Blood 35:*68, 1970.

19. Huber, H., Polley, M. J., Linscott, W. D., Fudenberg, H. H., and Müller-Eberhard, H. J. Human monocytes: Distinct receptor sites for the third component of complement and for immunoglobulin G. *Science 162:*1281, 1967.

20. Hudgins, W. R., Wordlaw, L. L., and McDuffie, F. C. Relationship of the anticomplement Coombs' test to the classes of immunoglobulins. *Vox Sang. 12:*401, 1967.

21. Irvine, W. J., Cullen, D. R., Scarth, L., and Simpson, J. D. Intrinsic-factor secretion assessed by direct radioimmunoassay and by total-body counting in patients with achlorhydria and in acid secretors. *Lancet 2:*184, 1968.

22. Kann, H. E., Jr., Mengel, C. E., Merriwether, W. D., and Ebert, L. Production of in-vitro characteristics of paroxysmal nocturnal hemoglobinuria in normal erythrocytes. *Blood 32:*49, 1968.

22a. Karpatkin, S., and Siskind, G. W. In-vitro detection of platelet antibody in patients with idiopathic thrombocytopenic purpura and systemic lupus erythematosus. *Blood 33:*795, 1969.

23. Lalezari, P. Clinical significance of leukocyte iso- and auto-antibodies. *Seminars Hemat. 3:*87, 1966.

24. Leddy, J. P. Immunological aspects of red cell injury in man. *Seminars Hemat. 3:*48, 1966.

25. Litt, M. "Studies in Experimental Eosinophilia. VIII. Induction of Eosinophilia by Homologous 7Sγ1 Antibody and by Extremely Minute Doses of Antigen," in *Proceedings of the Sixth International Congress of Allergology,* Amsterdam, Excerpta Medica Foundation, 1968, p. 38.

26. Müller-Eberhard, H. J., Dalmasso, H. J., and Caleate, M. A. The reaction mechanism of β_{1c}-globulin (C'3) in immune hemolysis. *J. Exp. Med. 123:*33, 1966.

27. Myllylä, C., Valieri, A., Vesikari, T., and Penttinen, K. Interaction between human blood platelets, viruses and antibodies. IV. Post-rubella thrombocytopenic purpura and platelet aggregation by rubella antigen-antibody interaction. *Clin. Exp. Immun. 4:*323, 1969.

28. Perkins, H. A., Payne, R., Ferguson, J., and Wood, M. Non-hemolytic febrile transfusion reactions. *Vox Sang. 11:*578, 1966.

29. Pirofsky, B. Autoimmune hemolytic anemia and neoplasia of the reticuloendothelium with a hypothesis concerning etiologic relationships. *Ann. Intern. Med. 68:*109, 1968.

30. Samloff, M., Kleinman, M. S., Turner, M. D., Sobel, M. V., and Jeffries, G. H. Blocking and binding antibodies to intrinsic factor and parietal cell antibody in pernicious anemia. *Gastroenterology 55:*575, 1968.

31. Schubothe, H. The cold hemagglutinin disease. *Seminars Hemat. 3:*27, 1966.

32. Siskind, G. W. Immunologic suppression of primary Rh antibody formation. *Transfusion 8:*127, 1968.

33. Vierucci, A., Blumberg, B. S., Dettori, M., and Levene, C. Isoantibodies to inherited types of β-lipoproteins (Ag) and immunoglobulins (Gm and Inv). *J. Pediat. 72:*776, 1968.

34. Vyas, G. N., and Fudenberg, H. H. Isoimmune anti-IgA causing anaphylactoid transfusion reactions. *New Eng. J. Med. 280:*1073, 1969.

35. Waxman, S., Pratt, P., and Herbert, V. Malabsorption of hemoglobin iron in pernicious anemia: Correlation with intrinsic factor-containing substances. *J. Clin. Invest. 47:*1819, 1968.

36. Weiner, W., Gordon, E. G., and Rowe, D. A Donath-Landsteiner antibody (non-syphilitic type). *Vox Sang. 9:*684, 1964.

37. Wennberg, E., and Weiss, L. The structure of the spleen and hemolysis. *Ann. Rev. Med. 20:*29, 1969.

38. Wollheim, F. A., Williams, R. C., Jr., and Polesky, H. F. Studies on the macroglobulins of human serum. III. Quantitative aspects related to cold agglutinins. *Blood 29:*203, 1967.

39. Woodrow, J. C., and Finn, R. C. Transplacental hemorrhage. *Brit. J. Haemat. 12:*297, 1966.

40. Worlledge, S. M., Carstairs, K. C., and Dacie, J. V. Autoimmune hemolytic anemia associated with α-methyl dopa therapy. *Lancet 2:*135, 1966.

41. Yachnin, S., and Ruthenberg, J. M. The initiation and·enhancement of human red cell lysis by activators of the first component of complement and by first component esterase; studies using normal red cells and red cells from patients with paroxysmal nocturnal hemoglobinuria. *J. Clin. Invest. 44:*518, 1965.

42. Zipursky, A., and Israels, L. G. The pathogenesis and prevention of Rh immunization. *Canad. Med. Ass. J. 97:*1245, 1967.

10

Disorders Associated with Hypergammaglobulinemia and Paraproteinemia

JOSEPH SHUSTER

In contrast to hypogammaglobulinemia, hypergammaglobulinemia is a frequent laboratory finding in a wide variety of clinical disorders.[1] The term *monoclonal* gammopathy is used to describe immunoglobulin abnormalities characterized by tall, narrow, homogeneous peaks on electrophoresis, since it is believed that the abnormal proteins are the product of a single clone of antibody producing cells (see Chapter 1). Because *m*onoclonal peaks are frequently associated with *m*yeloma, *m*acroglobulinemia, or *m*alignant lymphoma, the term M proteins is sometimes used to describe the abnormal proteins (paraproteins) found in these conditions. On the other hand, the term *polyclonal* gammopathy is used to describe diffusely increased γ-globulin fractions which are broad-based and heterogeneous, and which are believed to be the products of several clones of antibody producing cells (see Figs. 10-1, 10-2, 10-3, and 10-4).

POLYCLONAL GAMMOPATHIES

In most instances, the polyclonal type of immunoglobulin pattern is believed to reflect an antibody response to antigenic stimulation. Liver disease appears to be an exception to this general concept because significant immunoglobulin abnormalities may occur in both primary liver disease and in systemic diseases with liver involvement in the absence of obvious antigenic stimulation.

The disorders which may produce a polyclonal gammopathy are listed in Table10-1. Most of the disease entities in this category are described in detail in the chapters devoted to the clinical immunology of organ systems. However, some of the more common causes of polyclonal gammopathy, as well as causes which are not described elsewhere in the book, will be discussed below.

INFECTIOUS DISEASES

Significant hypergammaglobulinemia occurs mainly in association with chronic bacterial infections such as lung abscess, osteomyelitis, and other protracted pyogenic infections. Under these circumstances, the duration and extent of the disease process usually results in a marked immunologic response. The hypergammaglobulinemia is restricted predominantly to the IgG class of immunoglobulins because most antibacterial antibodies are IgG in nature. However, in trypanosomiasis, there is a pronounced elevation of IgM which is sufficiently characteristic to be considered as diagnostic of the disease. Elevated IgM levels in the neonatal period are considered to be an indication of intrauterine infection.[2b]

COLLAGEN–VASCULAR DISEASES

Immunologic mechanisms are believed to play a prominent role in the pathogenesis of most of the collagen-vascular diseases (see Chapter 8), and therefore a polyclonal gammopathy is relatively common in this group of disorders. For example, marked hypergammaglobulinemia occurs in the majority of patients with systemic lupus erythematosus, and usually involves the IgG class of immunoglobulins to the greatest extent. It is of interest that the levels of IgG show a rough correlation with the anemia which is frequently associated with this disease.

About 50 per cent of patients with rheumatoid arthritis show elevated immunoglobulins, usually of the IgM type. The increase in IgM immunoglobulins is probably related to the fact that rheumatoid factor is an IgM

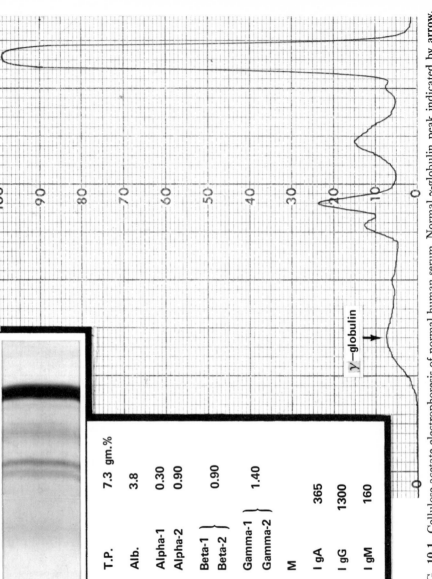

T.P.	7.3 gm.%
Alb.	3.8
Alpha-1	0.30
Alpha-2	0.90
Beta-1 }	
Beta-2 }	0.90
Gamma-1 }	
Gamma-2 }	1.40
M	
I gA	365
I gG	1300
I gM	160

FIG. 10-1. Cellulose acetate electrophoresis of normal human serum. Normal γ-globulin peak indicated by **arrow.**

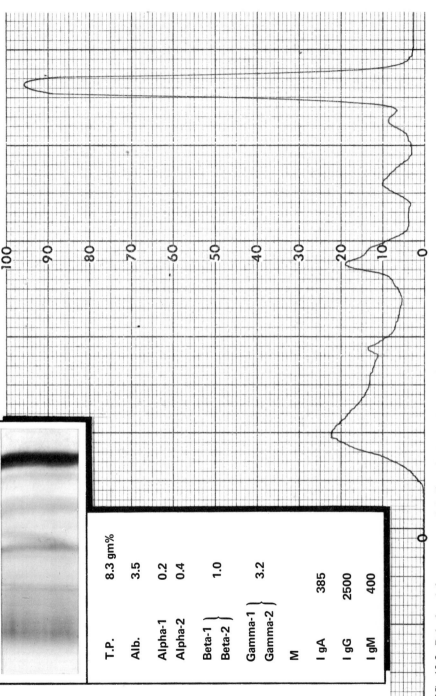

T.P.	8.3 gm%
Alb.	3.5
Alpha-1	0.2
Alpha-2	0.4
Beta-1 ⎱ Beta-2 ⎰	1.0
Gamma-1 ⎱ Gamma-2 ⎰	3.2
M	
IgA	385
IgG	2500
IgM	400

FIG. 10-2. Polyclonal hypergammaglobulinemia in patient with systemic lupus erythematosus.

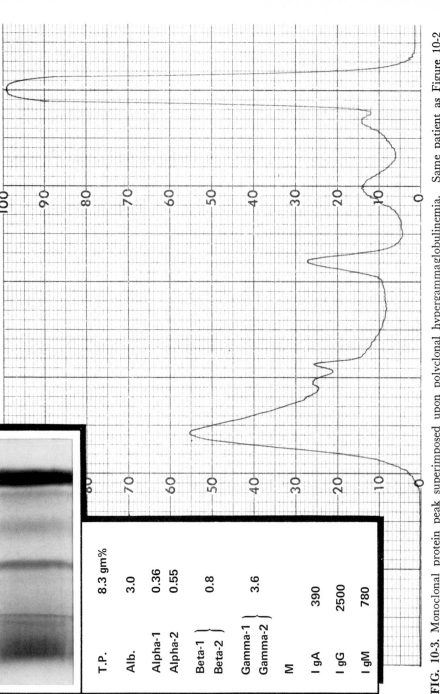

T.P.	8.3 gm%
Alb.	3.0
Alpha-1	0.36
Alpha-2	0.55
Beta-1 } Beta-2 }	0.8
Gamma-1 } Gamma-2 }	3.6
M	
I gA	390
I gG	2500
I gM	780

FIG. 10-3. Monoclonal protein peak superimposed upon polyclonal hypergammaglobulinemia. Same patient as Figure 10-2 but at a later stage in her disease.

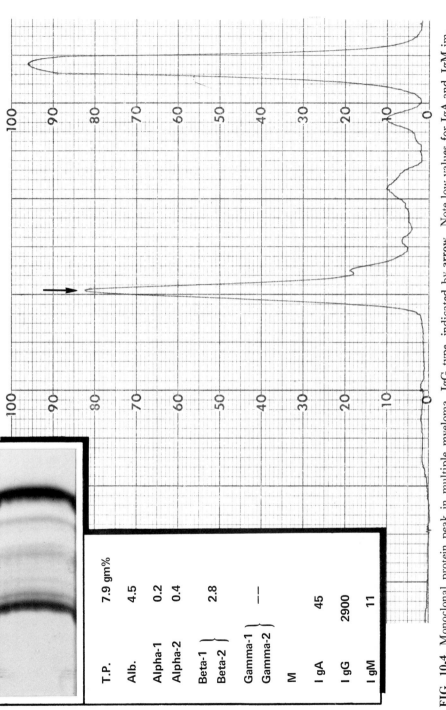

T.P.	7.9 gm%
Alb.	4.5
Alpha-1	0.2
Alpha-2	0.4
Beta-1 ⎫ Beta-2 ⎭	2.8
Gamma-1 ⎫ Gamma-2 ⎭	— —
M	
I gA	45
I gG	2900
I gM	11

FIG. 10-4. Monoclonal protein peak in multiple myeloma, IgG type, indicated by **arrow.** Note low values for IgA and IgM immunoglobulins.

TABLE 10-1. Classification of Polyclonal Gammopathies

Collagen-Vascular Diseases
  Systemic lupus erythematosus
  Rheumatoid arthritis
  Polyarteritis nodosa
  Sjögren's Syndrome

"Autoimmune" Organ System Diseases
  Thyroiditis
  Primary adrenal atrophy
  Aspermatogenesis
  Polymyositis
  Myasthenia gravis
  Sympathetic ophthalmia

Infectious Diseases
  Chronic bacterial infections
  Trypanosomiasis

Liver Diseases
  Alcoholic cirrhosis
  Cryptogenic cirrhosis
  Biliary cirrhosis
  Chronic active liver disease
  Other forms of parenchymal liver damage

Gastrointestinal Disease
  Ulcerative colitis
  Regional enteritis

Renal Disease
  Acute glomerulonephritis

Miscellaneous
  Neoplasms
  Histiocytoses and lipid storage diseases
  Hypergammaglobulinemic purpura of Waldenstrom
  Sarcoidosis
  Mongolism

---

macromolecule. The other collagen-vascular diseases are less frequently associated with hypergammaglobulinemia, and the levels are usually lower. In most of the collagen-vascular disorders, the immunoglobulin levels tend to increase or decrease in proportion to the severity of the disease.

HEPATIC DISEASE

Parenchymal liver disease is often accompanied by a striking diffuse hypergammaglobulinemia which affects all classes of immunoglobulins. Although there are many exceptions, alcoholic cirrhosis is frequently associated with increased levels of IgG and IgA, whereas biliary cirrhosis is associated with increased IgM values. The hypergammaglobulinemia which is a characteristic feature of chronic active liver disease reaches values not often attained in any other form of hypergammaglobulinemia, and monoclonal peaks have also been reported in this condition.[31] (see Chapter 16). In all forms of liver disease, the degree of immunoglobulin elevation provides an approximate indication of the severity of the damage to the liver parenchyma.

It is not understood why hypergammaglobulinemia occurs in hepatic diseases, but a number of theories have been advanced as possible explanations. For example, it has been postulated that hypergammaglobulinemia may occur as the result of autoantibodies formed against damaged liver cells. Other investigators suggest that it may be a compensatory mechanism to maintain the plasma osmotic pressure following the reduction in serum albumin levels which occurs during the course of liver disease.

HYPERGAMMAGLOBULINEMIC PURPURA OF WALDENSTROM

This unusual syndrome is characterized by diffuse hypergammaglobulinemia and recurrent purpura of the lower extremities. Despite the similar eponyms, the hypergammaglobulinemic purpura of Waldenstrom should not be confused with Waldenstrom's macroglobulinemia. The hypergammaglobulinemic purpura of Waldenstrom occurs predominantly in middle-aged women, and may appear as an isolated disease process or in association with systemic lupus erythematosus, Sjögren's syndrome, sarcoidosis, cirrhosis, or chronic pulmonary disease. Anaphylactoid purpura (see Chapter 6) and hypergammaglobulinemic purpura may occasionally coexist in the same patient.

Serum protein electrophoretic patterns disclose a diffuse hypergammaglobulinemia which may show fluctuating changes in both the concentration and shape of the γ-globulin region. In the ultracentrifuge, the serum frequently shows intermediate sedimenting components of 9S to 15S, but the nature of the individual constituents contributing to these complexes is unknown.[3] Serologic tests for rheumatoid factor are invariably positive. Histologically, there is evidence of arterial necrosis, but the pathogenetic mechanisms responsible for the purpuric lesions remain unclear.

Acute attacks are often precipitated by mechanical factors which promote stasis in the lower extremities. Examples of precipitating factors are: (1) prolonged walking, dancing, or standing; (2) protracted sitting in a cramped position, such as occurs on long airplane trips; or (3) the wearing of tight garments over the lower extremities. The purpuric eruptions are often painful and are frequently accompanied by systemic manifestations of fever and arthralgia. Coagulation studies are invariably normal.

There is no specific treatment except the avoidance of factors which promote vascular stasis in the lower extremities. It has been reported that the wearing of a fitted waist-high leotard may reduce the number of acute episodes.

HYPERGAMMAGLOBULINEMIA AND RENAL TUBULAR ACIDOSIS

Renal tubular acidosis occurs occasionally in association with monoclonal gammopathies, but is more common in patients with polyclonal gammopathies. In one series of patients with hypergammaglobulinemia due to a variety of causes, impaired renal acidification and impaired concentrating capacity were found in over 50 per cent of patients tested.[22] Nephrocalcinosis was often detected radiologically. These findings coupled with the absence of aminoaciduria, the absence of glycosuria, th eabsence of proteinuria, and the normal handling of HCO_3^- strongly suggest an abnormality of the distal tubule.

There is no correlation between the incidence of this disorder and elevation of a specific immunoglobulin class. Although the data suggest that the hypergammaglobulinemia is responsible for the defect in renal acidification, the exact pathogenetic relationships are not established.

MONOCLONAL GAMMOPATHIES

By definition the M proteins found in the monoclonal gammopathies belong to a single immunoglobulin class and contain only one light chain type of either the kappa or lambda variety (see Chapter 1). The monoclonal γ-globulins are usually first detected by demonstrating the M protein on paper or cellulose acetate electrophoresis. The serologic characteristics of the paraprotein may then be determined by immunoelectrophoresis against antisera specific for the heavy chains of IgG, IgA, IgM, IgD, and IgE, and the kappa and lambda determinants of light chains.

Serologically, structurally, and chemically, the M proteins are similar to normal serum immunoglobulins, but differ from the total serum γ-globulins in their extreme homogeneity.[5] Thus, it would appear that the M proteins are the product of a single clone of antibody producing cells.[24] However, an obvious source of antigenic stimulation is invariably absent. These abnormal proteins are most frequently associated with disorders such as multiple myeloma or macroglobulinemia which are characterized by the neoplastic proliferation of plasma cells or by lymphocytoid plasma cells. To date, all of the homogeneous proteins produced by the proliferating plasma cells have been structurally unique to the patients in which they occur. In this section, the plasma cell dyscrasias will be classified according to the type of M protein produced, because characteristic clinical syndromes are frequently correlated with specific forms of paraproteinemia (see Table 10-2.)

TABLE 10-2. Diseases Associated with Monoclonal Gammopathies

Plasma cell dyscrasias
 (Multiple myeloma, macroglobulinemia, light chain disease,
 heavy chain disease, plasmacytomas)
Benign monoclonal gammopathies
Carcinoma
Lymphoreticular malignancy
Amyloidosis
Histiocytoses and lipid storage diseases
Papular mucinosis (see Chapter 5)
Monoclonal gammopathy superimposed on a polyclonal gammopathy
 (e.g., liver disease, collagen-vascular diseases)

MULTIPLE MYELOMA

Multiple myeloma is the most common of the plasma cell proliferative disorders. Although the great majority of the paraproteins detected in this disease belong to the IgG or IgA class of immunoglobulins, there have been rare case reports of patients who have IgD or IgE myeloma proteins in their sera.[11] The prevalence of the various types of myeloma proteins coincides with the relative quantities of normal immunoglobulins detected in normal serum. This observation would suggest that the neoplastic process results from the random proliferation of a single clone of plasma cells.

However, on rare occasions two different classes of myeloma proteins are found in the same patient.

Etiology

The etiology of multiple myeloma is unknown. Nevertheless, the occasional association between antecedent carcinoma or chronic biliary tract infection and the subsequent development of a plasma cell dyscrasia presents intriguing possibilities.[24] Both of these clinical observations suggest a possible relationship between chronic stimulation of the immune system and neoplastic proliferation of plasma cells. The experimental production of multiple myeloma in BALB/c mice by the intraperitoneal injection of Freund's adjuvant or mineral oil lends further support to this hypothesis.

Pathology

The bone marrow invariably demonstrates an increase in plasma cells. However, several bone marrow aspirations may sometimes be necessary to demonstrate morphologic changes because the myeloma lesions are frequently patchy in their distribution. A plasma cell count of 25 per cent or greater is usually considered essential to distinguish multiple myeloma from other causes of plasmacytosis such as rheumatoid arthritis, tuberculosis, chronic infection, cirrhosis, carcinomatosis, and nonmyelomatous disorders associated with M proteins.[21] Apart from the unusually high proportion of plasma cells, there are no specific morphologic features in the bone marrow which are pathognomonic of multiple myeloma. The abnormal or immature plasma cells which are often seen in multiple myeloma may occasionally be found in other diseases associated with plasmacytosis.

Immunology

The elaboration of M type γ-globulins is frequently associated with a concomitant decrease in production and increase in catabolism of normal immunoglobulins and antibodies. However, there appears to be little correlation between the severity of the decreased antibody response and the reduction in the concentration of normal serum immunoglobulins. The primary antibody response to new antigens is poor, but the secondary response to antigens to which the patient has had previous contact is usually intact. There is an increased susceptibility to bacterial infections in most patients with multiple myeloma, and deficient delayed type hypersensitivity responses have been noted in occasional patients with the disease. Peripheral blood lymphocytes obtained from patients with multiple myeloma and macroglobulinemia often show a diminished response to stimulation with PHA.

The abnormal proteins which appear in multiple myeloma and in macroglobulinemia were regarded by some investigators as not being true antibodies since they had no antibody specificity. However, within the last few years, several examples of paraproteins in both humans and experimental animals have been shown to have antibody specificity for the Fc fragment of IgG, 2, 4-dinitrophenol, pneumococcal polysaccharides, serum lipoproteins, and other antigenic determinants.

Clinical Manifestations

There is a great diversity of clinical patterns in multiple myeloma. In some patients, the appearance of an M protein, often associated with plasmacytosis and an elevated sedimentation rate, may precede the characteristic clinical signs and symptoms by many years. In more typical cases, the presenting features of multiple myeloma consist of bone pain, anemia, hypercalcemia, and renal insufficiency.

The usual skeletal symptoms are transient bone pain caused by the presence of plasma cell tumors in the ribs, sternum, spine, skull, shoulder, or pelvic girdle. Less commonly, a pathologic fracture, usually of the vertebrae or ribs, is the first clinical sign of bony involvement. Radiologically, the bone lesions are usually osteolytic (punched-out lesions), and tend to increase in size as the disease progresses. About 20 per cent of patients demonstrate diffuse osteoporosis as the first radiologic sign of skeletal involvement, but osteolytic lesions eventually become apparent in these individuals as well. Very infrequently, an osteoblastic reaction, in the absence of an obvious fracture, is seen. Hypercalcemia and hypercalciuria secondary to the bony changes are frequent findings in multiple myeloma. Anemia due to decreased erythropoiesis, accelerated erythrocyte destruction, and a bleeding tendency is present initially in most patients, and eventually occurs in all individuals with the disease.

Multiple myeloma is the disorder which is most frequently associated with amyloidosis. Other clinical manifestations which are more directly related to the presence of a paraprotein include: (1) symptomatic cryoglobulinemia; (2) hyperviscosity syndrome; and (3) coagulation defects due to the chelation of coagulation factors (V, VII, VIII, Ca^{++}, and fibrinogen) to the M proteins. (Amyloidosis, cryoglobulinemia, and the hyperviscosity syndrome are discussed in detail in subsequent sections of this chapter.)

In multiple myeloma, renal insufficiency may result from hypercalcemia, hyperviscosity, hyperuricemia, or amyloidosis. In addition, there is a unique form of renal disease, known as myeloma kidney, which is usually associated with the presence of free light chains in the urine. Current theories regarding the pathogenesis of myeloma kidney are discussed in the section on light chain disease in this chapter. Rarely, a secondary Fanconi syndrome may appear during the course of multiple myeloma.

Polyneuropathy may occur due to the infiltration of nervous tissue by plasma cells or by amyloid deposits. In addition, a polyneuropathy and myopathy similar to that observed in other neoplastic diseases (e.g., bronchogenic carcinoma) may develop during the course of multiple myeloma or may even precede the other clinical manifestations. Paraplegia due to compression of the spinal cord is another common neurologic finding. There have been several case reports of rheumatoid arthritis preceding or occurring in association with multiple myeloma.[30]

Bacterial infections such as pyodermas, pyelonephritis, septicemias, and pneumococcal pneumonia are common manifestations of multiple myeloma. In fact, renal failure and overwhelming infection are the most common causes of death in this disease. Plasma cell leukemia is a rare clinical variant of multiple myeloma, and has been the mode of presentation of two reported cases of IgE myeloma.[26]

Abnormal laboratory findings may include a normochronic, normocytic anemia, erythrocyte sedimentation rates in the range of 130 to 160 mm/hr (Westegren), rouleaux formation in smears of the peripheral blood and bone marrow, bone marrow plasmacytosis greater than 25 per cent, and occasional thrombocytopenia or leukopenia. Plasma cells may be demonstrated on careful examination of the buffy coat, and peripheral blood eosinophilia is noted in a small percentage of patients. Examination of the serum proteins shows the presence of M proteins, low values for normal (i.e., nonmyeloma) immunoglobulins, and frequent hypoalbuminemia.

In less than 1 per cent of the plasma-cell proliferative disorders a monoclonal peak is not detectable in either the blood or the urine, and the serum of these so-called "dry" or "nonsecretory" myeloma patients often contains normal amounts of immunoglobulins. Nevertheless, the typical skeletal and other manifestations of multiple myeloma are present. The probable pathophysiologic explanation for this rare variant of multiple myeloma is the failure of the neoplastic plasma cells to secrete the paraprotein into the extracellular space. In support of this hypothesis is the observation that myeloma proteins can be demonstrated in the plasma cells of the bone marrow by immunofluorescence techniques.[13]

In patients over the age of 70 years, a benign monoclonal gammopathy which never progresses to multiple myeloma is not an uncommon occurrence.[2] In this age group, mild anemia and osteoporosis are not unusual findings, and, thus, the detection of an M protein in the serum may lead to a mistaken diagnosis of multiple myeloma. In our experience, elderly patients with benign monoclonal hypergammaglobulinemia may be distinguished by the following laboratory and clinical findings: (1) the paraprotein peak is usually low (less than 1 gm/100 ml) ; (2) the serum levels of normal immunoglobulins are not decreased; (3) the electrophoretic pattern remains constant over a period of years; (4) the plasmacytosis in the bone marrow is less than 25 per cent; and (5) there is no progression of anemia and osteoporosis (see Table 10-3).

TABLE 10-3. Differential Diagnosis of Monoclonal Gammopathies*

	Plasma cell dyscrasias	Other causes of monoclonal gammopathy
Symptoms	Characteristic of myeloma or lymphoma	No symptoms or symptoms of underlying disease
Anemia	Almost always present	Absent in benign disorders; may be present in other associated diseases
Bone lesions	Osteolytic lesions very common	Uncommon except in metastatic bone disease
Bone marrow	Plasmacytosis 25 per cent or more; morphology normal or abnormal	Plasmacytosis less than 25 per cent; morphology usually normal
Concentration of M components	Often more than 2 gm/100 ml; increases with progression of disease	Usually less than 1 per cent; remains stable
Concentration of normal immunoglobulins	Decreased	Increased or normal
Free light chains	Often present in serum and urine	Rare

*Adapted from Michaux, J. L., and Heremans, J. F. *Amer. J. Med. 46*:562, 1969.

Treatment

Local irradiation is often effective in relieving pain due to nerve compression or due to localized bone lesions.

Currently, the systemic treatment of choice is phenylalanine mustard given orally in doses of 50 µgm/kg of body weight per day. Because of the danger of severe leukopenia and thrombocytopenia, the white blood count and platelet counts should be determined 2 to 3 times per week. If there is a good response to therapy, as judged by a reduction in the paraprotein content of the serum, 1 to 2 mg of phenylalanine mustard may be given on alternate days as maintenance therapy. Relief of bone pain may occur within a week of beginning therapy, and calcium levels may return to normal within 10 days. A trial of cyclophosphamide may be attempted in patients who are refractory to phenylalanine mustard. In addition, corticosteroids may be used with good effect to treat acute hypercalcemic episodes. An alternate method of controlling hypercalcemia is the use of neutral phosphate buffer in doses of 1 to 4 gm daily by mouth.

Despite the temporary improvement which is achieved with chemotherapy in some patients, the prognosis in multiple myeloma is still very poor.[12] Most patients succumb to their disease within 2 years.

MACROGLOBULINEMIA

The paraprotein or M protein in macroglobulinemia (Waldenstrom's macroglobulinemia) is a 19S immunoglobulin of the IgM class. The clinical and pathologic features of macroglobulinemia are more similar to those of a lymphoma than they are to multiple myeloma. Approximately 80 per cent of reported cases occur over the age of 50, and two-thirds of these are males.[18]

Pathology

Examination of the bone marrow readily distinguishes macroglobulinemia from multiple myeloma. The characteristic cell population is heterogeneous and is composed of plasmacytoid lymphocytes, small lymphocytes, or plasma cells. Electron microscope studies show that the abnormal cells contain significant endoplasmic reticulum. This observation would suggest that the cells which appear to be lymphocytes by light microscopy are actively synthesizing protein in a manner similar to plasma cells. It is for this reason that the term lymphocytoid plasma cells is often used to describe them. Predominantly lymphocytic infiltrations in the bone marrow are occasionally difficult to differentiate from lymphocytic leukemia.

Characteristic changes in the lymph nodes include destruction of the normal architecture of the node, infiltration with mature or lymphoblastic lymphocytes, and the presence of foci of plasma cells or lymphocytoid plasma cells. PAS-positive cytoplasmic droplets, which may represent accumulations of paraproteins, are sometimes observed in atypical cells in the lymph nodes and bone marrow.

Immunology

The M protein in macroglobulinemia usually migrates in the intermediate or β-globulin region on paper or cellulose acetate electrophoresis. The levels of normal immunoglobulins, humoral immune responses, and cell-mediated immunity are not impaired to the same extent as in multiple myeloma. Ultracentrifugal, chromatographic, and immunologic studies have provided conclusive evidence that the paraprotein in macroglobulinemia belongs to the IgM class of immunoglobulins. The recent finding that a significant proportion of the paraprotein consists of 7S monomer IgM would indicate that there is a defective assembly of 7S monomer IgM units into 19S polymer IgM.

Hyperviscosity of the plasma is usually more pronounced in macroglobulinemia than in the other plasma cell dyscrasias.[15] Although the increased protein concentration undoubtedly contributes to viscosity, the physicochemical properties of the paraproteins such as size, shape, degree of hydration, and cryoprecipitability are also important factors.[17a] Hyperviscosity is also a feature of multiple myeloma due to the concentration and aggregation of IgG and IgA paraproteins. Nevertheless, hyperviscosity is a much more prominent feature of macroglobulinemia because the intrinsic viscosity of IgM molecules is approximately 3 times greater than that of IgG molecules.

Clinical Manifestations

Fatigue, weakness, and weight loss are the most common presenting symptoms. Lymphadenopathy, epistaxis, gingival bleeding, and blurring of vision are less common initial manifestations. Frequently the disorder is diagnosed in an asymptomatic state on the basis of serum electrophoretic findings. The most prominent physical findings are slight hepatosplenomegaly and lymphadenopathy.

The hyperviscosity syndrome is characterized clinically by mucous membrane bleeding, blurred vision, congestive heart failure, and central nervous system manifestations such as delirium, depression, and confusion. The relative viscosity of normal plasma is usually less than 1.65 times that of water. Symptoms of hyperviscosity do not occur in patients with relative viscosity values less than 6, although the threshold varies from patient to patient.

The ocular and central nervous system findings are related to changes in small blood vessels secondary to hyperproteinemia and hyperviscosity. On funduscopic examination, there may be retinal hemorrhage, microaneurysms, venous stasis, and distended, tortuous retinal veins. Relative viscosity values in the range of 8 to 10 are frequently associated with hemorrhagic manifestations. The bleeding tendency is due to a variety of factors including the chelation of clotting factors to paraproteins, interference with platelet function, and a direct effect of sludging and stasis on the capillaries.

Raynaud's phenomenon is an occasional feature of macroglobulinemia associated with significant cryoglobulinemia. Skeletal manifestations are not common in macroglobulinemia, although generalized osteoporosis and osteolytic lesions have been described in occasional patients.

Typical laboratory findings include a normochromic, normocytic anemia, an elevated erythrocyte sedimentation rate, rouleaux formation, and mild thrombocytopenia. The white blood count may be increased or decreased; the plasma volume is usually increased; and an autoimmune hemolytic anemia is sometimes present.

Cellulose acetate electrophoresis, immunoelectrophoresis, and quantitative immunoglobulin determinations are usually sufficient to demonstrate the macroglobulin characteristics of the paraprotein. Analytic ultracentrifugation shows a preponderance of 19S sedimenting material and polymers in the 27 to 31S range. The Sia water test is an unreliable method of determining macroglobulins because there is a high percentage of both false-negative and false-positive results.

The clinical course of the disease is extremely variable. Macroglobulinemia may be present for many years before clinical symptoms occur. On the other hand, some patients run a more rapidly progressive downhill course manifested by the appearance of clinical abnormalities early in the disease. A reticulum cell sarcoma is not an infrequent terminal event.

Treatment

Many of the clinical manifestations of macroglobulinemia are temporarily reversed by reducing the plasma viscosity through plasmaphoresis. This relatively simple procedure is often effective because 80 per cent of IgM is intravascular, whereas significant quantities of IgG are distributed throughout the extravascular space. Chlorambucil in an initial dose of 6 to 12 mg/day for 2 to 3 weeks, followed by a maintenance dose of 2 to 8 mg/day is often beneficial. If therapy with chlorambucil is instituted, blood counts should be performed at frequent intervals to prevent the occurrence of severe thrombocytopenia or leukopenia. Cyclophosphamide in doses of 2 mg/kg per day may sometimes produce a remission in patients refractory to chlorambucil.

LIGHT CHAIN DISEASE

Light chain disease is a variant of multiple myeloma in which there is an asynchronous synthesis of light chains in comparison to the rate of production of heavy chains.[29]

In the older literature Bence-Jones proteinuria was described as one of the characteristic features of multiple myeloma. In patients with Bence-

Jones proteinuria, a white cloudy precipitate appears when the urine is heated to temperatures of 50 to 60° C, but disappears when the temperature is raised to near the boiling point. Recent studies have shown that Bence-Jones proteins are, in fact, free light chains which may be secreted: (*1*) in association with other M proteins; or (*2*) as an isolated phenomenon (light chain disease). Free light chains are secreted in the urine in about 25 per cent of cases of multiple myeloma associated with the presence of a serum IgG or IgA paraprotein. However, the presence of free light chains in the urine is rare in macroglobulinemia.

In light chain disease, the characteristic immunochemical findings include the presence of free light chains in the concentrated urine, the frequent presence of free light chains in the serum, and hypogammaglobulinemia. Because free light chains have a relatively low molecular weight, they are rapidly excreted in the urine by the normal kidney. It is only after the onset of renal failure that they can be detected in the serum because: (*1*) excretion is impaired; and (*2*) the kidney is the primary site of catabolism of light chains.[17] The presence of free light chains in the urine or serum is associated with monoclonal peaks demonstrable by paper or cellulose acetate electrophoresis.

Clinically and pathologically, light chain disease is identical to multiple myeloma. From a diagnostic standpoint, light chain disease must be distinguished from those very rare cases of multiple myeloma which are characterized by hypogammaglobulinemia and the absence of detectable M proteins in the serum or in the concentrated urine ("dry" myeloma). Another rare source of diagnostic confusion is the IgD myelomas where the M peaks may be obscured on electrophoresis by the normal β-globulin peaks. In the latter instance, the true diagnosis can be established by immuno-electrophoresis using anti-IgD antisera.[8]

The majority of cases of myeloma kidney are associated with the presence of detectable free light chains in the urine. Myeloma kidney is characterized pathologically by atrophy and degeneration of the renal tubules, the deposition of tubular casts within the kidney, and secondary tubular degeneration. The tubular cells appear swollen and their cytoplasm contains hyaline deposits. Recent immunofluorescent studies of myeloma kidney disease have demonstrated the presence of light chains in the tubular cytoplasm and in the casts.[16] In addition, the casts may contain albumin, γ-globulin, and fibrinogen. However, as yet, there is no clear correlation between the quantities of light chains excreted in the urine, the histologic findings by light microscopy or by immunofluorescent techniques, and the severity of the renal disease. Thus, the pathogenesis of this type of renal failure remains obscure.

Occasionally, renal failure in multiple myeloma or light chain disease is precipitated by the performance of an intravenous pyelogram. It has been suggested that this form of renal impairment occurs as the result of the dehydration prescribed to prepare the patient for the pyelogram, or as the result of an unknown effect of the dye.[6] It is also of interest that IgD myelomas are almost invariably associated with the presence of free light chains in the urine and that there is a high incidence of renal failure in this form of myeloma.

HEAVY CHAIN (FC FRAGMENT) DISEASE

Structurally and immunologically, the M proteins in this rare disease are very similar to Fc fragments (see Chapter 1). They react with antisera directed against the Fc fragment, but not with anti-Fab or anti-light chain antisera.[9] Furthermore, the molecular weight of the paraproteins is approximately 55,000 which is similar to that of Fc fragments produced by the proteolytic digestion of IgG. Hence, the term heavy chain disease is actually a misnomer, but is widely accepted in the literature.

Of the 12 cases described to date, 8 were characterized by paraproteins with antigenic characteristics similar to the heavy chains of IgG (γ-chains), and 4 were antigenically similar to the heavy chains of IgA (α-chains). A single case of μ-chain disease has been reported,[2a] and it might be anticipated that plasma cell dyscrasias associated with the abnormal production of M proteins antigenically similar to δ-chains and ϵ-chains will eventually be described.

Pathology

The bone marrow and lymph nodes are infiltrated by atypical plasma cells, and cells which are intermediate between lymphocytes, reticulum cells, and plasma cells. In some instances, the histologic picture is very similar to that found in Hodgkin's Disease (see Chapter 12).

Immunology

The disorder is characterized by a disturbance in the control of γ-globulin synthesis inasmuch as the abnormal proliferating cells do not secrete light chains. Amino acid sequence data suggest that several different mechanisms are involved in the elaboration of heavy chain disease paraproteins.

Clinical Features

The clinical features of γ-heavy chain disease resemble a lymphoma more closely than they do multiple myeloma. Typical findings consist of fever, painful lymphadenopathy, hepatosplenomegaly, and recurrent infections. Edema and erythema of the uvula is an unusual and pathognomonic clinical sign. A spontaneous waxing and waning in the size of lymph nodes is present in some patients with heavy chain disease. Abnormal laboratory findings may include a moderate degree of anemia, leukopenia, thrombocytopenia, and eosinophilia as well as hyperuricemia and azotemia. Rheumatoid arthritis frequently occurs in association with γ-heavy chain disease.

All of the 4 reported cases of α-heavy chain disease presented with the clinical features of both an abdominal lymphoma and infiltration of the small intestine with lymphocytoid plasma cells.[27]

The specific diagnosis is made by the presence of an M peak in the serum and concentrated urine, and by the detection of Fc fragments in the serum and urine through the use of specific antisera. The disease may be distinguished from multiple myeloma by the characteristic immunologic findings and by the absence of skeletal lesions.

PLASMACYTOMAS

Solitary Plasmacytoma

About 80 per cent of solitary plasmacytomas involve the bone and soft tissues of the head and neck.[25] The serum proteins are usually not abnormal at this stage. However, disseminated lesions of the skeleton ultimately develop and a paraprotein is demonstrable in the serum.

Multiple Plasmacytomas

Another clinical variant consists of the simultaneous appearance of multifocal solitary nodules. These lesions usually progress slowly and respond well to surgery or radiation therapy.

Extramedullary Plasmacytoma

A plasmacytoma which is predominantly extraosseous represents another uncommon manifestation of the plasma cell dyscrasias.[7] Pathologically, the tissues show infiltration with plasma cells of varying degrees of maturity, or the abnormal cells may resemble reticulum cells by light microscopy. However, electron microscopic studies frequently demonstrate an abundant endoplasmic reticulum and thus reveal the plasmacytoid nature of the cells. Extraosseous tumors which extend directly from the bone or occur as solitary nodules in the soft tissues are a frequent manifestation of IgD myelomas. The common clinical manifestations of extraosseous plasmacytomas include anemia, renal impairment, unusual susceptibility to infections, amyloidosis, cryoglobulinemia, and the presence of M components in the serum and urine.

MISCELLANEOUS CAUSES OF MONOCLONAL GAMMOPATHIES

Monoclonal γ-globulin peaks are found in a variety of disorders (see Table 10-2) in which there is no overt evidence of multiple myeloma. The majority of patients in this category have underlying lymphoreticular malignancies or carcinomas. The benign monoclonal gammopathy which is occasionally found in elderly individuals has been discussed in the section on multiple myeloma in this chapter.

In addition, there is a heterogeneous group of obscure disorders characterized by a bone marrow plasmacytosis of over 25 per cent and nonprogressive paraproteinemia. Affected individuals have varied manifestations of their disease including a mild stable anemia, hypogammaglobulinemia, increased susceptibility to infections, and, less commonly, an associated polyneuropathy and myopathy.

This diverse group of patients has been described in the literature under a number of names such as premyeloma, cryptogenic myeloma, dysimmunoglobulinemia, lanthic disease, and benign (or essential) monoclonal gammopathy. It has been suggested that some of these cases may represent a form of dysgammaglobulinemia (see Chapter 11) rather than a latent type of multiple myeloma.

CRYOGLOBULINEMIA

Cryoglobulins are plasma proteins which have the property of reversible precipitation in the cold. Several plasma proteins are cryoprecipitable, but from the practical standpoint the cryoglobulins of greatest clinical significance are those which contain immunoglobulins. Cryofibrinogenemia will be considered separately.

IMMUNOLOGY

Several distinct types of cryoglobulins have been described on the basis of immunochemical analyses of the cryoprecipitate.[19]

Simple Type.   The simple type of cryoglobulin consists of a single immunoglobulin species which is usually IgG or IgM. The simple cryoglobulins occur, for the most part, in the plasma cell dyscrasias and in the lymphoproliferative disorders.

IgG Polymers. This type of cryoglobulin is usually found in multiple myeloma where the IgG paraprotein appears to have antibody activity directed against the Fc fragment of normal IgG. Polymers of IgG with the property of cryoprecipitability are believed to result from this interaction.[10]

Mixed Type. The mixed type of cryoglobulin is probably of the greatest clinical significance. The mixed IgM—IgG type of cryoglobulin is the most common variety and may be found in association with the collagen-vascular diseases, lymphoproliferative disorders, chronic infections such as subacute bacterial endocarditis and kala-azar, infectious mononucleosis, liver disease, and a unique syndrome characterized by nonthrombocytopenic purpura and arthralgia. The IgM components of the mixed IgM—IgG cryoglobulins almost always have rheumatoid factor activity, and the mixed cryoglobulins may contain complement components. It has been demonstrated that the IgM molecule recognizes antigenic determinants on the Fc fragment of IgG and, thus, it has been postulated that an antigen-antibody reaction is the basis for the formation of this type of cryoglobulin. The mixed IgM—IgG cryoglobulins which sometimes occur in systemic lupus erythematosus may demonstrate antinuclear activity in both the IgM and IgG components, and it is sometimes possible to demonstrate the presence of DNA in the cryoprecipitates.[28]

Mixed cryoglobulins due to IgG—IgA interaction have been reported as a rare occurrence in association with syphilis.

The mechanism responsible for the cold-induced precipitation of cryoglobulins has not been elucidated. The clinical importance of cryoglobulinemia appears to depend primarily on two factors: the thermal characteristics of the cryoprecipitate, and the ability to fix complement (C1q, C3, and C4). For example, cryoprecipitation at room temperature (20 to 30° C) may lead to symptoms in the absence of exposure to cold. Mixed cryoglobulins usually fix complement and constitute a form of immune-complex disease. Complement-fixing mixed cryoglobulins may lead to vasculitis or renal lesions on precipitation in the small blood vessels or in the kidney (see Chapters 6 and 8). In addition, cryoglobulins of all types may contribute to a hyperviscosity syndrome, to erythrocyte aggregation, and to sludging in small blood vessels.

CLINICAL MANIFESTATIONS

The simple type of cryoglobulinemia may lead to Raynaud's phenomenon, or it may be completely asymptomatic. The mixed type of cryoglobulins are the most likely to produce clinical manifestations, although their precise contribution to the pathogenesis of the vasculitis already present in collagen-vascular diseases is difficult to establish.

The purpura-arthralgia syndrome appears to be etiologically related to the presence of mixed type cryoglobulins.[20] Typical clinical features consist of nonthrombocytopenic purpura, arthralgia, lymphadenopathy, hepatosplenomegaly, a positive test for rheumatoid factor, and low serum complement levels. Glomerulonephritis and vasculitis have been reported in some patients with this syndrome (see Chapters 6 and 8). Cold urticaria due to the presence of a cryoglobulin which activates C1 esterase and triggers the complement cascade has been reported in some patients with cryoglobulinemia (see Chapter 5).

Whenever cryoglobulinemia is suspected, a fresh sample of nonheparinized blood should be allowed to clot at 37°C. Thereafter, an aliquot of serum should be stored at 4°C for at least 48 hours and examined for precipitation or gel formation. Subsequently, the type of cryoprecipitate should be determined, if possible, by immunochemical analysis. Other abnormal laboratory findings in cryoglobulinemia may include hyperviscosity, rouleaux formation, and decreased serum complement levels.

TREATMENT

There is no specific therapy for cryoglobulinemia. Treatment should be directed against the primary disorder.

CRYOFIBRINOGENEMIA

Cryofibrinogenemia is a rare disorder which is characterized by the occurrence of cryoprecipitation in the plasma, but not in the serum. Although the cryoprecipitates consist primarily of fibrinogen, significant quantities of γ-globulin, albumin, and other serum proteins can also be detected. These latter constituents may be present as the result of nonspecific coprecipitation. Cryofibrinogenemia may occur alone or in association with metastatic carcinoma, lymphomas, collagen-vascular diseases, diabetes, disseminated intravascular coagulation, thromboembolic disorders, and pregnancy.[23] It is of interest that small quantities of cryofibrinogen may be found in the sera of approximately 40 per cent of nonpregnant females who take oral contraceptive agents.[32]

The clinical manifestations may include Raynaud's phenomenon, ischemic skin lesions, purpura, a tendency to thromboembolic phenomena, and a bleeding tendency. The comparative rarity of this disorder makes the evaluation of treatment difficult. Heparin in relatively large doses is sometimes effective in inhibiting the formation of cryofibrinogen and in controlling intravascular coagulation. In this situation, it is believed that heparin acts as an antithrombin and inhibits the formation of cryofibrinogen due to the partial action of thrombin on fibrinogen.[24]

PYROGLOBULINEMIA

Certain paraproteins found in multiple myeloma precipitate in vitro upon heating. This property does not appear to be of clinical significance.

AMYLOIDOSIS

Amyloidosis is a disease of unknown etiology characterized by the deposition of protein-polysaccharide complexes of varying composition in the tissues of the body. Although almost any organ may be infiltrated with amyloid material, the small arterioles, the renal glomeruli, the liver, the spleen, and the adrenals are most commonly affected. The disease may occur as a primary disorder or may be associated with multiple myeloma, rheumatoid arthritis, familial Mediterranean fever, or chronic infectious and inflammatory diseases.

PATHOLOGY

On gross examination, amyloid is an amorphous, translucent material which transmits the color of the underlying tissues. On light microscopy, it is a hyaline-like material which accumulates in connective tissue or between parenchymatous cells. Amyloid can be distinguished from other forms of hyaline by: (1) its ability to stain with Congo red; (2) its extracellular deposition; (3) a characteristic birefringence on examination of unstained sections by light microscopy; and (4) the presence of a fibrillar ultrastructure on examination by polarization microscopy or by electron microscopy.

ETIOLOGY AND PATHOGENESIS

Although a cause and effect relationship has been postulated between the presence of paraproteins and the deposition of amyloid material, there is little evidence to support this hypothesis. However, its relationship to chronic inflammatory and infectious diseases, and the fact that it can be produced experimentally in animals by repeated injections of bacterial toxins or substances such as casein suggest that immune mechanisms may be important in the production of amyloidosis. It is possible that prolonged antigenic stimulation may be a factor of major importance in the pathogenesis of the disease.

In some patients, immunoglobulins and complement have been demonstrated by the immunofluorescence technique in the area of amyloid deposition. However, the bulk of the available evidence suggests that this deposition is nonspecific since a number of other serum proteins are also found in a similar distribution.

Furthermore, amyloid itself appears to be a fibrous protein with a characteristic ultrastructure quite distinct from that of γ-globulin or collagen. Thus, current experimental data does not suggest a direct role for an immune mechanism in the production of tissue injury in amyloidosis. However, it is conceivable that a variety of stimuli to the reticuloendothelial stem cell may result in the production of the abnormal fibrous protein.[4] One of these stimuli could well be immunologic.

CLINICAL MANIFESTATIONS

The clinical manifestations of systemic amyloidosis are extremely variable. Amyloidosis which occurs in patients without known pre-existing disease usually affects individuals of middle-age or beyond, and is characterized by involvement of the muscles of the heart, tongue, and gastrointestinal tract and the media of small blood vessels. Typical signs and symptoms include macroglossia, congestive heart failure, malabsorption syndrome, purpura, and peripheral neuropathy.

In patients with involvement of parenchymatous organs secondary to another disease process, the cardinal clinical manifestations are hepatosplenomegaly, nephrotic syndrome (see Chapter 6), and adrenal insufficiency. Rarely, amyloidosis may occur as an isolated process involving the larynx in the absence of underlying disease and without evidence of amyloidosis in other tissues.

The diagnosis of amyloidosis is best established by a biopsy of the rectal mucosa since the arterioles in this region are involved in almost all clinical types. Examination of unstained sections for birefringence by polarization microscopy sometimes discloses amyloid deposits not seen after staining with Congo red or other special dyes. All patients with suspected amyloidosis should be investigated for evidence of multiple myeloma or one of the other plasma cell dyscrasias. The rapid disappearance of Congo red after intravenous injection is no longer considered a reliable diagnostic procedure.

TREATMENT

There is no effective treatment of systemic amyloidosis, and death usually occurs within 1 to 3 years. The prompt treatment of chronic pyogenic infections may reduce the prevalence of amyloidosis in the future, but there is little evidence to suggest that the treatment of multiple myeloma with chemotherapeutic agents is effective in controlling amyloidosis once the process has been initiated. Localized amyloid deposits in the larynx are treated by surgical excision.

REFERENCES

1. Alper, C. A., Rosen, F. S., and Janeway, C. A. Hypergammaglobulinemia. *New Eng. J. Med. 275:*591, 1966.

2. Axelsson, V., Bachmann, R., and Hallen, J. Frequency of pathological proteins (M-components) in 6995 sera from an adult population. *Acta Med. Scand. 179:*235, 1966.

2a. Ballard, H. S., Hamilton, L. M., Marcus, A. J., and Illes, C. H. A new variant of heavy-chains disease (μ-chain disease). *New Eng. J. Med. 282:*1060, 1970.

2b. Blankenship, W. J., Cassady, G., Schafer, J., Straumfjord, J. V., and Alford, C. A., Jr. Serum gamma-M globulin responses in acute neonatal infections and their diagnostic significance. *J. Pediat. 75:*1282, 1969.

3. Carr, R. D., and Heisel, E. B. Purpura hyperglobulinemia. *Arch. Derm. 94:*536, 1966.

4. Cohen, A. S. Pathogenesis of amyloidosis. *Ann. Intern. Med. 70:*418, 1969.

5. Cohen, S. The nature of myeloma proteins. *Brit. J. Haemat. 15:*211, 1968.

6. Cwynarski, M. T., and Saxton, H. M. Urography in myelomatosis. *Brit. Med. J. 1:*486, 1969.

7. Edwards, G. A., and Zawadski, Z. A. Extraosseous lesions in plasma cell myeloma. A report of 6 cases. *Amer. J. Med. 43:*194, 1967.

8. Fahey, J. L., Carbone, P. P., Rowe, D. S., and Bachmann, R. Plasma cell myeloma with D myeloma protein (IgD myeloma). *Amer. J. Med. 45:*373, 1968.

9. Franklin, E. C., Lowenstein, J., Bigelow, B., and Meltzer, M. Heavy chain disease—A new disorder of serum γ-globulins. *Amer. J. Med. 37:*332, 1964.

10. Grey, H. M., Kohler, P. F., Terry, W. D. and Franklin, E. C. Human monoclonal γG-cryoglobulins with anti-γ-globulin activity. *J. Clin. Invest. 47:*1875, 1968.

11. Hobbs, J. R. Immunochemical classes of myelomatosis. *Brit. J. Haemat. 16:*599, 1969.

12. Hobbs, J. R. Growth rates and responses to treatment in human myelomatosis. *Brit. J. Haemat. 16:*607, 1969.

340   Clinical Immunology

13. Hurez, D., Preud'homme, J. L., and Seligmann, M. Intracellular "monoclonal" immunoglobulin in non-secretory human myeloma. *J. Immunol. 104:*263, 1970.

14. Komp, D. M., and Donaldson, M. H. *In-vitro* and *in-vivo* effects of heparin on cryofibrinogen. *New Eng. J. Med. 279:*1439, 1968.

15. Kopp, W. L., Beirne, G. J., and Burns, R. O. Hyperviscosity syndrome in multiple myeloma. *Amer. J. Med. 43:*141, 1967.

16. Levi, D. F., Williams, R. C., Jr., and Lindstrom, F. D. Immunofluorescent studies of the myeloma kidney with special reference to light chain disease. *Amer. J. Med. 44:*922, 1968.

17. Lindstrom, F. D., Williams, R. C., Jr., Swaim, W. R., and Freir, E. F. Urinary light-chain excretion in myeloma and other disorders—An evaluation of the Bence-Jones Test. *J. Lab. Clin. Med. 71:*812, 1968.

17a. Mackenzie, M. R., Fudenberg, H. H., and O'Reilly, R. A. The hyperviscosity syndrome. The role of protein concentration and molecular shape. *J. Clin. Invest. 49:*15, 1970.

18. McCallister, B. D., Bayrd, E. D., Harrison, E. G., Jr., and McGuckin, W. F. Primary macroglobulinemia. *Amer. J. Med. 43:*394, 1967.

19. Meltzer, M., and Franklin, E. C. Cryoglobulinemia—A study of twenty-nine patients. *Amer. J. Med. 40:*828, 1966.

20. Meltzer, M., Franklin, E. C., Elias, K., McCluskey, R. T., and Cooper, N. Cryoglobulinemia—A clinical and laboratory study. Cryoglobulins with rheumatoid factor activity. *Amer. J. Med. 40:*837, 1966.

21. Michaux, J. L., and Heremans, J. F. Thirty cases of monoclonal immunoglobulin disorders other than myeloma or macroglobulinemia. *Amer. J. Med. 46:*562, 1969.

22. Morris, R. C., and Fudenberg, H. H. Impaired renal acidification in patients with hypergammaglobulinemia. *Medicine 46:* 57, 1967.

23. Mosessan, M. W., Colman, R. W., and Sherry, S. Chronic intravascular coagulation syndrome. Report of a case with special studies of an associated plasma cryoprecipitate. *New Eng. J. Med. 278:*815, 1968.

24. Osserman, E. F., and Fahey, J. L. Plasma cell dyscrasias. Current clinical and biochemical concepts. *Amer. J. Med. 44:*256, 1968.

25. Pascoe, H. R., and Dorfman, R. F. Extramedullary plasmacytoma of the submaxillary gland. *Amer. J. Clin. Path. 57:*501, 1969.

26. Pruzanski, W., Platts, M. E., and Ogryzlo, M. A. Leukemic form of immunocytic dyscrasia (plasma cell leukemia). *Amer. J. Med. 47:*60, 1969.

27. Seligmann, M., Mihaesco, E., Hurez, D., Mihaesco, C., Preud'homme, J. L., and Rimbaud, J. C. Immunochemical studies in four cases of alpha chain disease. *J. Clin. Invest. 48:*2374, 1969.

28. Stastiny, P., and Ziff, M. Cold-insoluble complexes and complement levels in systemic lupus erythematosus. *New Eng. J. Med. 280:*1376, 1969.

29. Williams, R. C., Jr., Brunning, R. D., and Wollheim, F. A. Light-chain disease. An abortive variant of multiple myeloma. *Ann. Intern Med.* 65:471, 1966.

30. Zawadski, Z. A., Benedek, T. G., Ein, D., and Easton, J. M. Rheumatoid arthritis terminating in heavy chain disease. *Ann. Intern. Med.* 70:335, 1969.

31. Zawadski, Z. A., and Edwards, G. A. Dysimmunoglobulinemia associated with hepatic biliary disorders. *Amer. J. Med.* 48:196, 1970.

32. Zlotnick, A., Shahin, W., and Rachmilewitz, E. A. Studies in cryofibrinogenemia. *Acta Haematol.* 42:8, 1969.

11

Immunologic
Deficiency Disorders

JOSEPH SHUSTER

Within the past two decades, experimental studies have shed considerable light on the ontogeny and phylogeny of the immune response (see Chapter 1). The studies of the development of the immune system in animals have been supported or extended by human models of immunologic deficiency diseases. These human models are, in effect, "experiments of nature." However, it should be emphasized that data obtained in animals cannot always be applied to humans, and hence our knowledge of the development of the immune system in humans is still far from complete. It is for this reason that a functional classification of immunologic deficiency diseases is not possible at the present time. Despite the fascinating theoretic implications of the primary immunologic deficiency diseases, it should be emphasized that the secondary immunologic deficiency syndromes are encountered much more frequently in clinical practice.

PRIMARY IMMUNOLOGIC DEFICIENCY DISEASES

The development of immunologically competent lymphocytes depends on the interaction between central (e.g., thymus) and peripheral (e.g., spleen

342

and lymph nodes) lymphoid tissues. The central lymphoid tissue influences lymphoid cells or their precursors so that the immunologic potential of a lymphoid cell is directed along cellular or humoral mediated lines (see Chapter 1).

This concept is best illustrated in chickens where the central lymphoid tissue includes the bursa of Fabricius and the thymus gland. The bursa of Fabricius is required for full maturation of the antibody synthesizing system, whereas the thymus gland is required for full expression of cell-mediated immunity. Removal of the bursa of Fabricius profoundly impairs the capacity of the animal to produce circulating antibodies. In addition, there is poor development of the germinal centers in the spleen, and a reduction in the numbers of lymphocytes and plasma cells in the paracortical regions and medullary cords of the lymph nodes. Cell-mediated immunity remains intact.

Thymectomy, on the other hand, results in marked diminution of cell-mediated immune mechanisms, and is associated morphologically with reduction in the lymphoid elements in the deep cortical areas of the lymph nodes and in the splenic white pulp. Thus, both structurally and functionally, the peripheral lymphoid system is organized into bursa and thymus dependent areas.

Although a bursa analogue has not been defined in man, the structural and functional arrangement of the peripheral lymphoid system into "thymus dependent" and "bursa dependent" areas is a useful concept when considering the immune deficiency diseases. For example, it has been postulated that the lymphoid stem cell in humans originates in the bone marrow and then enters the thymus gland. A population of immunologically competent cells develops under the influence of the thymus gland or as the result of the secretion of a thymic hormone. It is these "thymus dependent" cells which express the immunologic functions of delayed-type hypersensitivity, graft rejection, and graft-versus-host reactivity (see Chapter 1).

In man, developmental abnormalities at the level of any one of the cells associated with the maturation of the immune response may be responsible for one of the immunologic deficiency syndromes. A normal child is born with its mother's IgG, and is thus passively protected during the first few months of life against organisms to which the mother has circulating IgG antibodies. As the maternal IgG is catabolized, the normal child begins to secrete his own immunoglobulins. Antibodies belonging to the IgG class of immunoglobulins first appear at about 3 months of age, whereas IgM antibodies are produced at a much earlier date. In contrast to the limitations of humoral immunity in infancy, the capacity to develop cell-mediated immunity is present soon after birth. A classification of cellular and humoral immunologic deficiency diseases is presented in Table 11-1.

TABLE 11-1. Cellular and Humoral Deficiency Diseases

1. Third and fourth pharyngeal pouch syndrome (Di George's syndrome)
2. Thymic hypoplasia and hypothyroidism
3. Thymic aplasia and lymphopenia
    a. X-linked form with agammaglobulinemia
    b. Autosomal recessive form with agammaglobulinemia (Swiss type)
    c. Autosomal recessive form with normal immunoglobulins (Nezelof's syndrome)
    d. Autosomal recessive form with agammaglobulinemia and agranulocytosis
    e. Progressive failure of lymphoid and hematopoietic systems.
4. Cell-mediated immune deficiency, short-limbed dwarfism, and ectodermal dysplasia
5. Antibody deficiency syndromes
    a. Primary agammaglobulinemia
    b. Dysgammaglobulinemias
    c. Hypercatabolism of IgG and albumin
    d. Circulating anti-IgG
    e. Down's syndrome in infants
    f. Transient hypogammaglobulinemia of infancy
6. Wiskott-Aldrich syndrome
7. Ataxia telangiectasia
8. Circulating lymphocytotoxic factor
9. Chronic mucocutaneous candidiasis

THIRD AND FOURTH PHARYNGEAL POUCH SYNDROME
(DIGEORGE'S SYNDROME)

DiGeorge's syndrome is the result of a defect in the maturation of the third and fourth pharyngeal cleft pouches which are the embryonic anlage of the thymus and parathyroid glands.[18]

Pathology

The thymus and parathyroid glands may be completely absent or vestigial, or, in some patients, miniature ectopic glands of normal morphology may be detected. The deep cortical areas of the lymph nodes, and the periarteriolar sheaths of the spleen ("thymus dependent" areas) demonstrate lymphocyte depletion. By contrast, the "bursa dependent" areas of peripheral lymphoid tissue are normal.

Immunology

The manifestations of delayed hypersensitivity are markedly reduced (Table 22-7), and in vitro lymphocyte transformation with phytohemagglutinin is diminished. In contrast to the lymphopenic forms of primary immunologic deficiency, the peripheral blood lymphocyte count is usually within normal limits. Although immunoglobulin levels are normal, some patients show deficient responses to antigenic stimulation.

Transplantation of thymus tissue from human female fetuses promptly corrected the immunologic deficits in at least two male infants with DiGeorge's syndrome.[1a] Prior to transplantation the infants were unable to respond immunologically to sensitization with DNFB, whereas sensitization was achieved with relative ease shortly after transplantation. This observation, plus the fact that the responding cells were male (i.e., of recipient origin), would suggest that the basic defect in DiGeorge's syndrome lies not in the recognition and processing of antigen, but in the efferent limb of the cell-mediated immune response (see Chapter 1).

Clinical Manifestations

Hypocalcemia and neonatal tetany secondary to hypoparathyroidism are common presenting features. In addition, these infants frequently suffer from repeated episodes of bacterial sepsis, monilial infections, and *Pneumocystis carinii* infections (see Chapter 4). Affected infants often have a characteristic facies consisting of increased distance between the orbits (ocular hypertelorism), low set and notched ear pinnae, shortened vertical groove in the median portion of the upper lip (philtrum), micrognathia, and clefts in the nose. Other congenital anomalies of the heart and great vessels may be found in the same patient.

Treatment

Most patients with DiGeorge's syndrome die in early infancy. While alive, appropriate antibiotics are used to treat bacterial infections, and replacement therapy with calcium gluconate is used to control seizures due to hypocalcemia. The long-term results of further thymic transplants are awaited with interest.

THYMIC HYPOPLASIA AND HYPOTHYROIDISM

The syndrome of thymic hypoplasia and hypothyroidism is characterized by the presence of defective cellular immunity, hypothyroidism and antithyroglobulin antibodies in newborn infants.[14] Parathyroid function and humoral immunity are normal. Two pathogenetic mechanisms have been proposed for this syndrome (1) there may be a defect in the development of the embryonic anlage of the second and third pharyngeal pouches from which the thyroid and thymus glands arise, or (2) the basic defect is hypoplasia of the thymus gland, and secondary destruction of the thyroid is due to autoimmune or infectious processes.

THYMIC APLASIA AND LYMPHOPENIA

Several clinical syndromes characterized by a vestigial thymus, lymphopenia, and markedly deficient cellular immune responses are included in this category: X-linked thymic alymphoplasia with agammaglobulinemia, autosomal recessive alymphocytic agammaglobulinemia (Swiss-type agammaglobulinemia), autosomal recessive lymphopenia with normal immunoglobulins (Nezelof's syndrome), autosomal recessive lymphopenia with variable immunoglobulins, and lymphopenia-agammaglobulinemia with agranulocytosis.[15] The clinical variants of this syndrome differ primarily in their mode of inheritance, the morphology of the peripheral lymphoid system, and the degree to which humoral antibody responses are affected. A syndrome of rapidly progressive failure of the lymphoid and hematopoeitic system during the second year of life may represent an additional variant of this group of disorders.[24a] The basic defect in all of these syndromes appears to reside at the level of the bone marrow stem cell.

Pathology

In all of the syndromes listed above, the thymus gland is small, and is composed of poorly developed lobules of epithelial stroma cells. Lymphocytes and Hassall's corpuscles are absent. Both the X-linked and autosomal recessive forms of lymphopenia associated with agammaglobulinemia show a marked deficiency of lymphoid follicles and germinal centers in the spleen, lymph nodes, tonsils, and gastrointestinal tract. These changes are less pronounced in the X-linked variety where occasional aggregates of lymphoid cells may be found in the peripheral lymphoid tissue. Plasma cells are usually absent, but may occasionally be found in small numbers.[22]

Immunology

Both cellular and humoral immune responses are profoundly diminished (Table 22-7). In the X-linked and autosomal recessive varieties, there is a virtual absence of immunoglobulins. The other clinical entities associated with lymphopenia and thymic dysplasia have either normal immunoglobulin levels (Nezelof's syndrome), dysgammaglobulinemia, or even hypergammaglobulinemia. In Nezelof's syndrome, antibody synthesis is deficient despite normal immunoglobulin levels.

Clinical Manifestations

In contrast to infants with congenital agammaglobulinemia as the sole immunologic defect, the infants in this group are usually ill or fail to thrive from birth, and die within 2 years. They are particularly affected by infections with organisms which are only mildly pathogenic for normal individuals (e.g., Pseudomonas, varicella, Candida, and *Pneumocystis carinii*). Generalized BCG infections and progressive vaccinia are frequent and serious complications of routine immunization procedures in this group of children, and appear to be particularly related to the deficient cell-mediated immune responses. Chronic diarrhea, with or without malabsorption syndrome, and exanthems of undetermined origin are frequent clinical findings. A hemolytic-uremic syndrome occurs occasionally in this group of patients.

In keeping with the pathologic findings, the degree of lymphopenia and the severity of the illness are often less prounounced in the X-linked variety than in the autosomal recessive forms.

Treatment

Early reports of therapy with thymus and bone marrow transplants have, in general, been disappointing. However, a single case report described the apparent success of buffy coat and bone marrow transplantation in the X-linked form of thymic aplasia, lymphopenia, and agammaglobulinemia. The beneficial result obtained was attributed to careful histocompatibility matching of donor and recipient antigens.[10]

It is questionable whether γ-globulin replacement therapy contributes significantly to management in this group of patients. Antibiotics are used for the treatment of bacterial infections, and pentamidine isethionate is the most useful agent available for the treatment of *Pneumocystis carinii* infections (see Chapter 4). Patients with thymic aplasia and lymphopenia should not be immunized with vaccines containing live organisms (see Chapter 21).

Graft-versus-host reactions (see Chapter 14) may occur following attempted bone marrow or thymus transplants, or following blood transfusions with viable immunologically competent cells. In order to prevent the latter complication, it has been recommended that blood transfusions should be carried out only with irradiated blood or with blood from which the buffy coat has been carefully removed. On the other hand, it has been shown that significant lymphocyte function may remain in blood even after irradiation or after storage for periods up to 12 days.

IMMUNOLOGIC DEFICIENCY, SHORT-LIMBED DWARFISM, AND ECTODERMAL DYSPLASIA

A number of patients have been described who share a constellation of developmental defects: (1) immunologic deficiency; (2) short-limbed dwarfism distinct from achondroplasia; and (3) ectodermal dysplasia (e.g., fine hair, early loss of hair, erythroderma, and ichthyosiform skin lesions.)[18a] The pattern of immunologic deficiency is extremely variable. It may resemble the recessive form of thymic aplasia with lymphopenia and agammaglobulinemia, Nezelof's syndrome, or may consist of predominantly cell-mediated immune defects. Malabsorption syndrome and neutropenia were frequent findings amongst the original group of patients described in the Old Order Amish.

PRIMARY AGAMMAGLOBULINEMIA

This category of immune deficiency syndromes includes several entities in which there is a deficiency of all the major immunoglobulin classes (IgG, IgA, IgM, IgD, and IgE), but no deficiency in cell-mediated immunity. The clinical manifestations are quite similar, but the patterns of inheritance, age of onset, immunoglobulin levels and coexistence of "autoimmune" diseases varies considerably within the group.[25]

The immunoglobulin deficiency may manifest itself clinically during the first 2 years of life, or may not become apparent until the patient is an adult. Formerly, the primary agammaglobulinemias were separated on this basis into the "congenital" and "acquired" types. However, it is now believed that genetic abnormalities are probably responsible for both variants, and that the difference in the age of onset does not necessarily imply a different pathogenesis.

Genetics

Two patterns of inheritance are observed in patients whose disease begins in infancy. In most cases, the disease affects male children and is transmitted as an X-linked recessive disorder (Bruton type agammaglobulinemia). However there are sporadic cases which affect both male and female infants.

The adult onset type of primary agammaglobulinemia affects both males and females. The fact that the kindred of patients with the disease often demonstrate immunoglobulin abnormalities or an increased incidence of "autoimmune" diseases would suggest that genetic influences are operative. Furthermore, there is evidence from studies of the mode of expression of Gm factors and heavy chain sub-classes that structural and regulatory gene abnormalities exist in this group of patients and their families.[21a]

The delay in the onset of clinical symptoms may reflect, in part, an abnormal, genetically determined decline of antibody production with age (abiotrophy). It is also conceivable that the autoimmune manifestations detected in the patients or in their close relatives may result from an increased susceptibility to infectious agents similar to those which have been implicated in the etiology of experimental "autoimmune" diseases.

Pathology

Characteristic findings in the peripheral lymphoid tissues include absent germinal centers and plasma cells, and diffuse hyperplasia of reticulum cells. In children, the absence of plasma cells in the bone marrow is not a reliable diagnostic feature because the bone marrow contains very few plasma cells at birth and does not reach adult levels until the age of 5 years. On the other hand, the failure to detect plasma cells in lymph nodes following antigenic challenge is typical of agammaglobulinemic syndromes.

Immunology

In patients whose disease begins in infancy, the immunoglobulin levels are usually less than 200 mg/100 ml. In the adult onset group of patients, however, the immunoglobulins may occasionally reach levels as high as 500 mg/100 ml. In both groups of patients, there is usually a significant decrease in all of the immunoglobulin classes. However, many patients with the adult onset type of primary hypogammaglobulinemia have normal IgD levels, but reduced levels of all the other immunoglobulin classes.

Patients with primary agammaglobulinemia fail to make antibodies following the administration of microbial antigens such as poliovirus, typhoid, and tetanus vaccines. In addition, they have extremely low titers of "naturally occurring" anti-A and anti-B isoantibodies.

Cell-mediated immunity, including allograft rejection, is usually intact. However, it is of interest that a few individuals with primary agammaglobulinemia demonstrate a delayed first set rejection, although second set rejection usually occurs in the normal way. These findings serve to illustrate the complexity of the immune response in graft rejection, and might be interpreted as evidence in favor of the hypothesis that humoral factors play a role in the rejection of allografts (see Chapter 14).

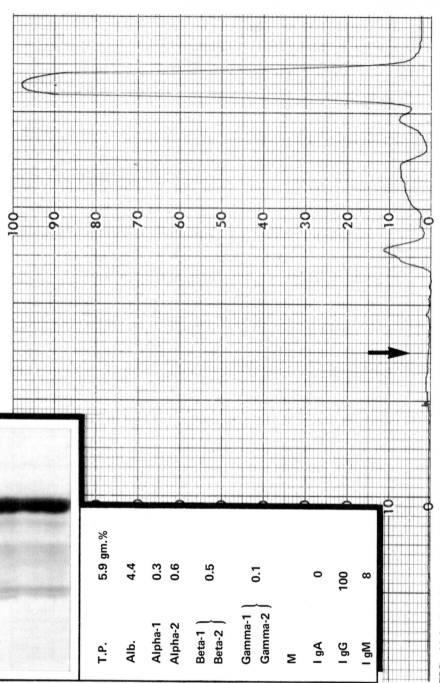

T.P.	5.9 gm.%
Alb.	4.4
Alpha-1	0.3
Alpha-2	0.6
Beta-1 ⎫ Beta-2 ⎭	0.5
Gamma-1 ⎫ Gamma-2 ⎭	0.1
M	
I gA	0
I gG	100
I gM	8

FIG. 11-1. Cellulose acetate electrophoresis and quantitative immunoglobulin determinations in a patient with primary agam-

Studies of the response of peripheral blood lymphocytes to stimulation with phytohemagglutinin have yielded conflicting results. In some patients with primary agammaglobulinemia, a normal response was obtained, whereas in others the response was diminished. There is evidence to suggest that decreased lymphocyte transformation occurs predominantly in the X-linked form of the disease, and that the carrier state can be detected in the mothers by a diminished response to phytohemagglutinin.

Clinical Manifestations

In contrast to the immunologic deficiency syndromes associated with thymic aplasia and lymphopenia, infants with primary agammaglobulinemia are usually asymptomatic during the first few months of life. It is assumed that the transplacental passage of maternal γ-globulin provides passive protection against infectious agents during this period.

A cyclic leukopenia is frequently detected in primary agammaglobulinemia, and failure to find adenoidal tissue in the nasopharynx constitutes a useful radiologic sign.

When symptoms begin, these children are extremely susceptible to infection with pyogenic organisms such as staphylococci, pneumococci, streptococci, meningococci, and *H. influenzae*. The clinical syndromes most commonly seen as the result of pyogenic infection include recurrent episodes of otitis media, pyoderma, pneumonia, meningitis, septicemia, and bronchiectasis. Infection with *P. carinii* should be suspected when refractory, bilateral pneumonia occurs in a patient with primary agammaglobulinemia. These children usually demonstrate relatively normal resistance to viral, fungal, and protozoal infections. However, there have been occasional reports of children with repeated attacks of measles, mumps, herpes zoster, and herpes simplex, and there is an unexpectedly high incidence of viral hepatitis and tuberculosis.[20]

Although "autoimmune" disorders occur occasionally in association with the childhood type of primary agammaglobulinemia, they are more characteristic of the adult onset type. Rheumatoid arthritis and dermatomyositis have been described occasionally in children with primary agammaglobulinemia. Of particular interest is the well documented observation that the symptoms of rheumatoid arthritis respond to treatment with normal human immunoglobulin. Other clinical associations in this group of children include an increased incidence of chronic active liver disease, malabsorption syndrome, and disaccharidase deficiency (see Chapter 16).

The "autoimmune" manifestations most frequently encountered in the adult group of patients include systemic lupus erythematosus, pernicious anemia, autoimmune hemolytic anemias, and thrombocytopenia. Another frequent complication in the adult onset group is a sprue-like syndrome which occurs despite a normal small intestinal biopsy. The prevalence of lymphoreticular malignancy is higher than in the normal population.

Sporadic cases of primary agammaglobulinemia have been reported in infants in whom there is no apparent family history of immunologic disorders. These children frequently have higher levels of IgG and a higher incidence of hepatosplenomegaly and lymphadenopathy than the usual patient with primary agammaglobulinemia.

Treatment

The intramuscular administration of normal human immunoglobulin (IgG) (see Chapter 21) is often effective in preventing the recurrent pyogenic infections which occur in patients with primary agammaglobulinemia. An initial dose of normal human immunoglobulin of 1.8 ml/kg of body weight of a solution containing approximately 15 to 16 gm/100 ml raises the serum immunoglobulin levels by approximately 300 mg/100 ml. The objective is to raise the serum immunoglobulins by 200 to 300 mg/100 ml. Thereafter, a monthly maintenance injection of 0.6 ml/kg of body weight is usually sufficient to maintain adequate serum immunoglobulin levels.

Adverse reactions to injected normal human immunoglobulin preparations eventually occur in about 20 per cent of patients, and typically consist of dyspnea, tightness of the chest without wheezing, hypotension, diffuse erythema, and facial swelling. These reactions have been attributed to aggregates of γ-globulin in immunoglobulin preparations (see Chapter 2). Special preparations of normal human immunoglobulins, which contain fewer aggregates, are available for patients who experience severe reactions.

In some centers, fresh frozen plasma is preferred because it supplies IgA, IgM, and nonspecific serum opsonins in addition to IgG. The major disadvantage of fresh frozen plasma is the inconvenience of transfusion in small children, and the increased risk of serum hepatitis.

TRANSIENT HYPOGAMMAGLOBULINEMIA OF INFANCY

About 90 per cent of the maternal antibodies transmitted through the placenta are catabolized by the third month of life. At about this time, the normal infant begins to secrete his own immunoglobulins. However, in some infants, the synthesis of IgG may be delayed for periods which may extend up to the fifteenth month. During the interval of depressed immunoglobulin synthesis, symptoms may occur which closely resemble those of primary agammaglobulinemia. The etiology of this disorder is unknown, but it has been suggested that maternal antibodies directed against Gm allotypic antigens (see Chapter 1) on the infant's immunoglobulins may be responsible for the delayed onset of antibody synthesis. In this respect, it is of interest that anti-allotype antisera has been shown to depress antibody synthesis in experimental animals.

Therapy with human normal immunoglobulin is usually effective in controlling symptoms.

THE DYSGAMMAGLOBULINEMIAS

The term dysgammaglobulinemia refers to hypogammaglobulinemia which is restricted to one or more immunoglobulin classes, the remainder being normal or elevated. The numerous possible combinations of alterations in the serum levels of IgG, IgA, and IgM which have already appeared in the literature have been designated by a numerical system which is unnecessarily cumbersome. Undoubtedly, new combinations of immunoglobulin abnormalities will be discovered in the future, and there is considerable overlap between most of the clinical syndromes in this group.

As in the case with primary agammaglobulinemia, genetic factors appear to be of major importance in the pathogenesis of the dysgammaglobulinemias. These entities demonstrate several modes of inheritance, but may not become apparent until adult life. Clinically, the patients in this group have an increased susceptibility to pyogenic infections, and an increased incidence of associated "autoimmune" disorders. For the present, it seems simplest to refer to all of these varied immunoglobulin abnormalities as dysgammaglobulinemias without attempting further subclassification.

Isolated IgA Deficiency

Isolated IgA deficiency will, however, be described in more detail because it occurs in association with a wide variety of disorders which include ataxia telangiectasia, recurrent respiratory tract infection, gluten-induced enteropathy, malabsorption syndrome, collagen-vascular disease, autoimmune hemolytic anemias, thrombocytopenia, fatal hemorrhagic varicella, hypersplenism, and cirrhosis of the liver. In addition, it occurs in completely asymptomatic individuals.[13] There is also a statistically significant, but poorly understood correlation between isolated IgA deficiency and the development of milk precipitins (see Chapter 16).

Pathologically, this group of patients usually has less numerous lymphoid follicles and germinal centers in the peripheral lymphoid tissues. Secretory IgA, the major immunoglobulin in the external secretions, is produced locally by plasma cells in the submucosae of tissues exposed to the external environment (see Chapter 1). In isolated IgA deficiency, there is often a marked reduction of IgA producing plasma cells. However, the epithelial cells continue to produce secretory piece which can be found free in external secretions such as the saliva.

A form of malabsorption syndrome associated with low IgA and the presence of lymphoid nodules in the lamina propria of the small bowel has been shown to improve after the infusion of whole plasma. It is not clear whether the response to plasma is due to replacement of IgA or due to replacement of nonspecific opsonins.[12]

Isolated IgG Deficiency

Isolated IgG deficiency is associated with at least three apparently unrelated conditions: (1) a familial disorder characterized by hypercatabolism of IgG and albumin; (2) a relative immunologic deficiency state characterized by the presence of an IgM autoantibody with anti-IgG specificity (Rheumatoid factor); and (3) there has been a recent report of low IgG levels in infants with Down's syndrome.[20a] The latter observation is somewhat surprising since thyroid autoantibodies and elevated serum IgG levels have been described in adults with Down's syndrome (see Chapter 15). It is possible that there may be a relationship between the IgG deficiency and the increased susceptibility of mongoloid infants to infection.

WISKOTT-ALDRICH SYNDROME

The Wiskott-Aldrich syndrome is characterized by the clinical triad of thrombocytopenia, eczema, and multiple infections. In most instances, the disease is transmitted as an X-linked recessive disorder, but sporadic cases have been reported in males with an apparently normal family history.[19]

Pathology

In the thymus, the numbers of small lymphocytes are decreased and corticomedullary distinction is lacking. The lymph nodes show depletion of small lymphocytes. The lymphoid follicles are present, but the germinal centers may be absent in some patients during the late stages of the disease. The plasma cells are normal.

Immunology

The pattern of immunologic deficiency in the Wiskott-Aldrich syndrome varies considerably between patients.

Cell-mediated immunity is frequently impaired. Failure to achieve skin sensitization with dinitrochlorobenzene (DNCB) occurs in about 90 per cent of cases. In addition, allograft rejection is frequently abnormal.

The most consistently demonstrable immunoglobulin abnormality is a decrease in IgM. The serum levels of IgG and IgA may be normal, or the level of IgA may sometimes be slightly increased. The low values for IgM have been shown to be due to decreased synthesis rather than increased catabolism of this class of immunoglobulins. The reduced titers of anti-A and anti-B isoagglutinins found in many patients with the Wiskott-Aldrich syndrome is thought to be a reflection of decreased IgM synthesis. In addition, many affected individuals display markedly reduced antibody responses when challenged with carbohydrate antigens, but show normal responses to protein antigens. It has been postulated that the genetically determined defect in this disease lies in the afferent limb of the immune responses (see Chapter 1), and is characterized by either a failure to recognize or process carbohydrate antigens.

Recently, the thrombocytopenia found in this disorder was shown to be the result of rapid platelet destruction caused by an intrinsic defect in the platelets.[4] The bone marrow, the levels of serum complement, and phagocytosis are normal. Mixed cryoglobulins (see Chapter 10) have been found in a small number of patients.

Clinical Manifestations

The clinical manifestations have their onset at the time of birth, and most children with the disease die in infancy. However, a few sporadic cases, which follow a milder course, have been reported in older children.

The characteristic clinical findings consist of thrombocytopenia, splenomegaly, eczema, and severe recurrent infections with all classes of microorganisms. Lymphopenia occurs not infrequently, but it should be noted that considerable fluctuation in the levels of circulating lymphocytes may occur in individual patients. The most common causes of death are hemorrhage or fulminating sepsis. Children who survive past infancy are particularly prone to lymphoreticular malignancy.

Treatment

Infections should be treated with appropriate antibiotic agents. Splenectomy is contraindicated as a form of treatment for the thrombocytopenia because of the high postoperative mortality rate.[7] There is a single case report of bone marrow transplantation from a female donor to a male infant with the Wiskott-Aldrich syndrome.[2] The recipient developed chimerism of the peripheral blood cells, and there was some increase in the number of platelets. Dramatic clinical improvement and immunologic reconstitution was recently reported in a single patient treated with "transfer factor" (See Chapter 1). This relatively simple therapeutic procedure requires no histocompatibility matching and virtually eliminates the problem of graft versus host reactions.

ATAXIA TELANGIECTASIA

Ataxia telangiectasia is inherited as an autosomal recessive disease, and is characterized by immunologic deficiency, cutaneous, and neurologic manifestations.[5]

Pathology

In most patients, the thymus is small, markedly deficient in lymphocytes and Hassall's corpuscles, and shows poor corticomedullary demarcation. The findings in the peripheral lymphoid tissue consist of poorly developed or absent lymphoid follicles, a decrease in plasma cells, and an increase in stromal elements. In the brain, the major pathologic abnormalities are found in the cerebellum where there is degeneration of the Purkinje cells, and increased tortuosity of the cerebellar blood vessels. In the skin, the characteristic cutaneous telangiectasia is formed by dilated veins in the papillary venous plexus.

Immunology

The pattern of immunologic deficiency in ataxia telangiectasia varies considerably from patient to patient. However, about 80 per cent of affected individuals have: (1) low or absent serum and secretory IgA levels; (2) low or absent IgE levels; (3) normal or low serum IgG levels; and (4) normal serum IgM levels. Reduced antibody responses to a number of common antigens have been reported and anti-IgA antibodies have been found in two patients. Children with ataxia telangiectasia generally show diminished responses to cutaneous sensitization with DNCB; skin homografts persist for prolonged periods; and the in vitro response of peripheral blood lymphocytes to phytohemagglutinin is reduced.

The fundamental defect which underlies the various immunologic and clinical manifestations of this disorder has not been determined. Furthermore, it has not been established whether the immunologic abnormalities are present at birth, or develop progressively after birth. It has been speculated that the basic defect lies in the mesenchymal tissue which is required for the normal development of many organ systems. It is conceivable that a failure of development of mesenchymal tissue at a specific point during the ontogeny of the immune system, brain, and other tissues might result in the constellation of defects found in ataxia telangiectasia.

Clinical Manifestations

The affected children are usually normal for the first year of life. Telangiectasia of the bulbar conjunctivae, ears, butterfly area of the face, neck, antecubital fossae, and other areas of the skin is often the first sign of the disease. It is frequently an important clinical feature in distinguishing between ataxia telangiectasia and other heredofamilial ataxias. Cerebellar ataxia, which is relentlessly progressive, may become apparent when the child first begins to walk. Despite the poor cell-mediated responses, these children suffer mainly from repeated bacterial infections of the respiratory tract rather than from unusual viral or fungal diseases. The increased susceptibility to respiratory tract infections appears to be found only in those children with combined IgA and IgE deficiency. Gonadal dysgenesis and an increased incidence of lymphoreticular malignancies are common associated findings. Peripheral blood lymphopenia is present in approximately one-third of patients.

Treatment

Children with ataxia telangiectasia invariably become incapacitated by their neurologic disorder, but may survive to early adult life if bacterial infections are mild or brought under control with antibiotic therapy. On the other hand, the results of treatment of acute or chronic bacterial infections with antibiotics or with replacement of normal human immunoglobulins is often disappointing in this syndrome.

CIRCULATING LYMPHOCYTOTOXIC FACTOR

An autosomal recessive disorder of newborn infants, which was recently described, consists of deficient cell-mediated immunity, absent immunologic memory, episodic lymphopenia, eczema, and normal immunoglobulins.[17] A complement dependent lymphocytotoxic factor, somewhat similar to ALS, was found in the sera of these patients.

SECONDARY IMMUNOLOGIC DEFICIENCY DISEASES

There are a number of disorders in which immunologic deficiency occurs as a secondary manifestation of the underlying disease process. The immunologic implications of the nephrotic syndrome, multiple myeloma, Waldenstrom's macroglobulinemia, Hodgkin's disease, lymphosarcoma, chronic lymphocytic leukemia, and leprosy are discussed in Chapters 6, 10, and 12. The remaining disorders in this category will be discussed in this chapter. The abnormalities of cell-mediated and humoral immunity that may be found in some of these conditions are summarized in Table 11-2.

TABLE 11-2. Secondary Immunologic Deficiency Diseases

	Deficient responses	
Diseases	Humoral	Cellular
Multiple myeloma	++	+
Waldenstrom's macroglobulinemia	+	
Chronic lymphatic leukemia	++	+
Lymphosarcoma	+	
Reticulum cell sarcoma	+	+
Hodgkin's disease		+
Giant follicular lymphoma	+	
Thymoma	+	
Leprosy		+
Protein-losing gastroenteropathy	+	+
Drug-induced	+	+
Viral infections	+	++
Nephrotic syndrome	+	
Sarcoidosis		++

PROTEIN-LOSING GASTROENTEROPATHY

Protein-losing gastroenteropathy is a syndrome characterized by the loss of albumin, γ-globulin, and other proteins in the gut in association with a heterogeneous group of primary disorders.

Immunopathology

Patients with the clinical manifestations of protein-losing gastroenteropathy can be divided into two broad categories: (1) those in whom there is peripheral blood lymphopenia; and (2) those in whom the circulating lymphocytes are present in normal numbers.

The lymphopenic type is found in association with intestinal lymphagiec-tasia, Whipple's disease, regional enteritis, and congestive heart failure (particularly constrictive pericarditis). Congenital intestinal lymphangiectasia is probably the most common disease entity within this group.[28] Pathologically, all of the patients demonstrate dilated lymphatic channels in the small intestine, and, therefore, it is assumed that both the lymphocytopenia and the hypoproteinemia are due to structural abnormalities of the lymphatics. Affected individuals often have a severe hypogammaglobulinemia secondary to the loss of all classes of immunoglobulins in the gut, but they respond normally to antigenic challenge. Immunoglobulin synthesis is normal, although there is no apparent increased synthesis to compensate for the gastrointestinal loss of antibody molecules. A profound defect of cell-mediated immunity is present in many patients with the lymphopenic form of protein-losing gastroenteropathy (see Table 22-7). Allografts, for example, may survive indefinitely. Despite the marked deficiency in humoral and cell-mediated immunity, this group of patients is not unusually susceptible to infection.

The nonlymphopenic type of protein-losing gastroenteropathy is found most commonly in gluten-induced enteropathy (see Chapter 16), primary hypogammaglobulinemia, nephrotic syndrome (see Chapter 6), nonspecific granulomatous disease of the small bowel, carcinomas of the gastrointestinal tract, giant hypertrophy of the gastric mucosa, thymoma, ulcerative colitis (see Chapter 16), and allergic gastroenteropathy (see Chapter 16).

Clinical Manifestations

Protein-losing gastroenteropathy should be suspected in any patient with hypoproteinemia which occurs in the absence of proteinuria, exudative dermatitis, multiple myeloma, or liver disease. The major clinical manifestations of gastrointestinal protein loss are edema, growth retardation in children, mild diarrhea, and hypochromic anemia. Chylous effusions may occur in those entities which are associated with lymphatic obstruction. The diagnosis of gastrointestinal protein loss may be confirmed by clearance studies employing ^{131}I polyvinylpyrrolidone (PVP) in conjunction with ^{51}Cr albumin.

Treatment

Protein-losing gastroenteropathy is often reversed by the successful treatment of the primary disease process.

THYMOMA

Tumors of the thymus may be associated with one or more of the following clinical syndromes: (1) hypogammaglobulinemia; (2) aregenerative

anemia or pancytopenia; and (3) a varied group of disorders with immunologic features such as the collagen-vascular diseases (see Chapter 8),
myasthenia gravis (see Chapter 19), or autoimmune hemolytic anemia (see
Chapter 9).

The significance of these associations is unclear. In one series, 7 of 169
patients with thymomas had hematologic disorders, and one of this group
had agammaglobulinemia.[23] Clearly then, thymomas are only infrequently
associated with immunologic deficiency. However, because of the rarity
of agammaglobulinemia itself, it is likely that the coexistence of thymoma
and hypogammaglobulinemia is significant.

Thymic tumors usually occur over the age of 40. It is often difficult
to determine on histologic grounds whether the thymoma is benign or malignant, and, in this respect, the clinical course of the tumor appears to be
the only useful guide. Most of the thymic tumors associated with immunologic deficiency syndromes or hematologic disorders pursue a benign clinical
course.

The hypogammaglobulinemia-thymoma syndrome is similar to primary
agammaglobulinemia from both a clinical and pathologic standpoint. Diarrhea occurs in about one-third of patients and protein-losing gastroenteropathy may be a feature. Skin allografts are rejected, but at a slower
rate than in normal individuals.

Thymectomy constitutes the only form of specific treatment. After thymectomy, there is often a marked improvement in the anemia, but the immunologic deficiency usually continues without change.

MYOTONIC DYSTROPHY

Low serum IgG levels and increased catabolism of IgG are common findings
in myotonic dystrophy.[30] The clinical syndrome is a dominantly inherited
disorder which is characterized by wasting of the muscles of the face and
neck, myotonia, alopecia, cataracts, and gonadal atrophy. The precise relationship between the hypercatabolism of IgG and the other manifestations
of this inherited syndrome have not been established.

VIRAL INFECTIONS

Transient depression of cell-mediated immune responses may occur during
the course of viral infections, particularly those which follow the administration of live attenuated poliovirus vaccine or measles virus vaccine[9] (see
Chapter 21). Humoral antibody responses are normal, but cell-mediated
immune responses such as delayed-type cutaneous hypersensitivity, the passive transfer of tuberculin hypersensitivity, and the in vitro lymphocyte

response to microbial antigens are often decreased or absent. In addition, a peripheral blood lymphopenia is not infrequently associated with this state of immunologic hyporeactivity. Because the pattern of immunologic deficiency is almost identical to that seen in Hodgkin's disease, these observations have been interpreted by some as indirect evidence in favor of a viral etiology for Hodgkin's disease (see Chapter 12).

Congenital Rubella Syndrome

About 10 to 15 per cent of infants born of mothers infected with rubella virus during the first and second trimesters of pregnancy develop the congenital rubella syndrome. The characteristic clinical features of this syndrome include microcephaly, congenital heart disease, cataracts, hepatosplenomegaly, lymphadenopathy, and failure to thrive.

Despite the presence of high titers of IgM neutralizing antibodies against rubella (see Chapter 21), the infants may continue to excrete the virus for as long as 3 years after birth. On the other hand, serum IgG levels are often low and agammaglobulinemia is occasionally present. These immunoglobulin abnormalities are associated with a variable incidence of defective humoral and cell-mediated immune responses.

Various explanations have been offered for the apparent paradox of persistent viral infection in the presence of specific antibody.[26] It has been postulated that infection persists because the intracellular virus is inaccessible to circulating antibody, and, thus, active infection terminates only upon the death of the last infected cell. It has also been possible to isolate rubella virus from the thymus and lymphoid tissue of affected infants. It is conceivable that a limited viral infection in the developing lymphoid system may produce the spectrum of cellular and humoral immunologic abnormalities which are found in these children. The hypothesis of specific cell-mediated immunologic tolerance in the presence of normal antibody formation, which has been postulated for subacute sclerosing panencephalitis (see Chapter 18), can thus be extended to the congenital rubella syndrome. However, if this concept were valid, one would expect the tolerance to be lifelong.

DRUGS

Corticosteroids, immunosuppressive agents, and cancer chemotherapeutic drugs may inhibit cell-mediated immunity and induce mild hypogammaglobulinemia. From a clinical standpoint, it has long been recognized that the protracted use of any of these agents is frequently associated with increased susceptibility to uncommon pathogens such as fungi, *Pneumocystis carinii,* and *Toxoplasma gondii.*

OVERWHELMING POSTSPLENECTOMY INFECTION IN CHILDHOOD

Children under the age of 4 years who have undergone splenectomy are unusually susceptible to a fulminating septicemia which is often fatal within 12 to 18 hours after the onset of symptoms.[7] Clinically, the signs and symptoms are those of overwhelming bacteremia and may consist of high fever, sore throat, headache, vomiting, convulsions, and coma. The organisms most frequently identified in blood cultures obtained from this group of patients are pneumococci and meningococci. This syndrome is most likely to occur when splenectomy is performed for one of the histiocytoses, inborn errors of metabolism, hepatitis with portal hypertension, thalassemia major, and Wiskott-Aldrich syndrome.

The pathogenesis of this unusual syndrome is uncertain, but it is known that the spleen acts as an efficient bacterial filter, and is important in the synthesis of antibodies and opsonins. For example, pneumococcal infection is a frequent complication of sickle cell anemia when repeated splenic infarcts lead to a deficiency of pneumococcal opsonins.[29] Similarly, overwhelming sepsis is often associated with hereditary splenic hypoplasia.[16]

DISORDERS OF PHAGOCYTOSIS

Phagocytic cells are of two types: (1) those which are present in the circulation such as polymorphonuclear leukocytes and monocytes; and (2) those which are present in the tissues such as macrophages and the other cells of the reticuloendothelial system. The primary function of the phagocytes is the digestion of foreign particles, foreign macromolecules, and damaged cells. In addition, recent experiments suggest that the macrophages may also play an important role in the processing of antigens and in the subsequent transfer of information to antibody producing cells. Furthermore, it is believed that the macrophages may be one of the cells responsible for target cell destruction in cell-mediated immune responses (see Chapter 1).

The initial phase of phagocytosis involves contact between the foreign particle and the surface of the phagocytic cell. It is at this stage that serum opsonins, such as antibodies, complement, and other poorly characterized serum factors may be of importance in facilitating the entry of foreign matter into the cell. The foreign material is subsequently brought into the cell within a vacuole (phagosome) formed by the interiorization of the cell membrane. After phagocytosis occurs, the phagosome generally fuses with the lysosomes, which then discharge their granules. The ingested material may undergo digestion during this latter phase of the phagocytic process, or it may continue to survive within the cell (e.g., the tubercle bacillus).

The disorders of phagocytosis may be divided into: (1) those which are based on a deficiency of phagocytic cells; and (2) those which are based on a deficiency of circulating opsonins.

DISORDERS OF PHAGOCYTIC CELLS

Chronic (Fatal) Granulomatous Disease of Childhood

Chronic granulomatous disease is a lethal, inherited disorder characterized by a history of recurrent infections, and by the presence of septic granulomatous lesions in the cervical lymph nodes, skin, lungs, and bone.[11]

Pathology. The granulomatous lesions are comparable to what one would expect with *M. tuberculosis* infection, rather than with the type of organisms usually cultured from the affected areas. The characteristic lesions consist of lymphocytic-histiocytic infiltration and Langhans' giant cells which surround areas of central necrosis. In addition, frankly purulent areas may be found in association with the granulomatous reactions. An interesting, but unexplained, finding is the accumulation of lipochrome pigment in the fixed macrophages of the lymphoid tissue.

Immunology. The usual parameters of humoral and cell-mediated immunity are normal in children with chronic granulomatous disease. Plasma cells are present in the tissues, and the serum immunoglobulin levels are normal or increased. Other relevant normal findings include a normal Rebuck skin window inflammatory cycle, normal clearing of particulate matter from the circulation by the cells of the reticuloendothelial system and normal serum complement levels.

The basic functional defect appears to reside primarily in the polymorphonuclear leukocytes and monocytes of the peripheral blood. The leukocytes of patients with chronic granulomatous disease seem to ingest bacteria normally. However, once ingested, certain species of bacteria such as staphylococci and gram-negative organisms survive for a much longer period of time than in normal leukocytes. In the majority of cases, there is a marked deficiency of vacuolization and lysosomal lysis (degranulation) on microscopic examination of leukocyte-bacteria preparations in vitro. However, a variant of chronic granulomatous disease has been described in which the patient's leukocytes display defective bacterial activity in the presence of normal degranulation.

There is also a consistent metabolic defect demonstrable in the leukocytes obtained from patients with chronic granulomatous disease. Normal phagocytosis is characterized metabolically by: (1) a marked increase in oxygen consumption; (2) an increase in the amount of glucose metabolized via the hexose monophosphate pathway; and (3) the formation of hydrogen peroxide. These metabolic changes do not occur when leukocytes from patients with chronic granulomatous disease are incubated with latex particles. Thus, the suggestion that hydrogen peroxide may function in an intracellular bactericidal, viricidal, and fungicidal system provides a possible explanation for the increased susceptibility to infection associated with this syndrome. The nitro-blue tetrazolium test (NBT) is used clinically to detect the defective intracellular respiration which leads to the deficiency of hydrogen peroxide.[3]

A tentative explanation for the selectivity of the bactericidal defect is provided by the observation that organisms which generate hydrogen peroxide intracellularly are killed by leukocytes from patients with chronic granulomatous disease. Apparently, their own metabolism compensates for the defective production of hydrogen peroxide by chronic granulomatous disease cells. Currently available data concerning enzyme abnormalities in chronic granulomatous disease, when considered together with the various patterns of inheritance, would suggest that the syndrome may be caused by more than a single enzyme defect.[3a]

Clinical Manifestations.   The vast majority of cases occur in male children in a genetic pattern compatible with an X-linked mode of inheritance. The carrier state can be detected in the mothers by quantitative measurements of the bactericidal capacity of their leukocytes, and by the NBT test. Family studies of a few female patients with chronic granulomatous disease have provided evidence that the syndrome may occasionally be transmitted as an autosomal recessive disorder.

The disease is characterized by recurrent infections with *Staphylococcus pyogenes,* and with organisms of low virulence such as coliform bacteria, *Serratia marcescens,* nocardia, and aspergillus. The pulmonary lesions may consist of: (1) extensive infiltrations which may be diffuse, miliary, or lobar in distribution; (2) cavitation; and (3) marked hilar lymphadenopathy. Other frequent clinical findings are liver abscesses, hepatosplenomegaly, pericarditis, draining cervical adenitis, and *S. marcescens* osteomyelitis. The prognosis is poor, and most patients do not reach adult life. The disorder can be diagnosed during the neonatal period since the polymorphonuclear leukocytes of normal newborn infants display normal phagocytosis and normal NBT reduction.

Job's syndrome, a condition characterized by repeated cutaneous staphylococcal abcesses in female infants, is considered to be an additional variant of chronic granulomatous disease.

Treatment. Active infections should be treated with appropriate antibiotics. However, the prophylactic use of antibiotics in an attempt to reduce the severity or frequency of infection does not appear to be effective in most instances.

Chediak-Higashi Syndrome

The Chediak-Higashi syndrome is characterized by the presence of abnormally large cytoplasmic granules (organelles) in a variety of cells, by increased susceptibility to infection, by pigmentary changes, and by pancytopenia.

Pathology. The basic structural abnormality is most easily detected by light microscopy in the polymorphonuclear leukocytes, but it can also be found in lymphocytes, monocytes, renal tubular cells, neurons, Schwann cells, melanocytes, the epidermis, and erythroid precursors.[8]

Under the electron microscope, the abnormal cytoplasmic granules are large, are surrounded by a single layer membrane, and appear to be undergoing degeneration. Histochemical studies demonstrate that these granules have an enzyme content similar to lysosomes, and, indeed, they probably are lysosomes. It is possible that the release of lysosomal enzymes may produce extensive tissue damage. In keeping with this hypothesis is the observation that the terminal pathologic event in the Chediak-Higashi syndrome is the widespread destruction of the normal architecture of affected tissues. In addition, there is frequently extensive infiltration of the tissues by immature lymphoid cells and histiocytes.

The presence of abnormally large melanin granules and cytoplasmic granules within the neurons provides the most likely explanation for the pigmentary changes and for the neuropathy which are frequently associated with the disease.

Immunology. To date, there is no generally accepted explanation for the increased susceptibility of patients with the Chediak-Higashi syndrome to infection. Cell-mediated and humoral immune responses are normal; the leukocytes ingest particles normally, and have normal bactericidal capacity.

It is of interest that comparable clinical and morphologic abnormalities have been demonstrated in inbred strains of Aleutian mink. These same animals are susceptible to the virus-induced Aleutian mink disease which is characterized by muscle wasting, leukopenia, vasculitis, plasmacytosis, hypergammaglobulinemia, and the presence of a serum anti-γ-globulin factor.

Clinical Manifestations.   The disease is inherited as an autosomal recessive disorder. Pseudo-albinism, manifested by pigmentary changes affecting the skin, hair, uveal tract, and ocular fundi, is a common presenting feature. For example, the children have lighter skin than their parents, and hair which is pale grey or brunet with streaks of grey. Photophobia and a horizontal nystagmus are frequent findings in the early stages of the disease. The increased susceptibility to infection often leads to pyodermas, ulcerations of the oral mucosa, and fevers of unknown origin. Less commonly, there may be lymphadenopathy, hepatomegaly and jaundice.

Individuals with the Chediak-Higashi syndrome invariably succumb within the first few years of life to an illness characterized by fever, pancytopenia, hepatosplenomegaly, lymphadenopathy, central nervous system disease and peripheral neuropathies. Hemorrhage or overwhelming infection are the usual immediate causes of death. Many of the features of this terminal illness are suggestive of those found in the malignant lymphomas (see Chapter 12).

The syndrome is diagnosed with relative ease by the finding of typical large neutrophil granules on the peripheral blood smear. The genetic defect and the heterozygous carrier state can be readily demonstrated in skin fibroblast cultures. These findings can be confirmed by electron microscopic studies. Other laboratory findings are unremarkable except for the pancytopenia which occurs during the terminal phases of the disease.

Treatment.   Infections should be treated with suitable antibiotics. Temporary remissions have been reported following splenectomy, and following the administration of cytotoxic drugs. However, it should be noted that the fulminant terminal phase may occasionally remit spontaneously.

Neutropenia

Neutropenia due to any cause may lead to deficient phagocytosis (see Chapter 9).

DEFICIENCY OF OPSONINS

Sporadic reports have appeared noting the association between a postulated deficiency of opsonins and a predisposition to infection. An opsonin is most simply defined as a serum factor which facilitates phagocytosis.

For example, patients with sickle cell anemia often show an increased susceptibility to pneumococcal infection. There is evidence to suggest that the splenic infarcts which are a common feature of this disease lead to an acquired deficiency of a non-antibody pneumococcal opsonin which is produced in the spleen.[29]

Another example of a possible opsonin deficiency is provided by some patients with mucocutaneous candidiasis which is not associated with a well defined immunologic deficiency syndrome. It is known that the in vitro clumping of *Candida* organisms can be induced by a nonantibody opsonin found in normal sera, and recently it has been found that the sera of certain patients with mucocutaneous candidiasis contain in IgG inhibitor directed against this *Candida* clumping factor.[6] However, it should be noted that mucocutaneous candidiasis may also be associated with impaired cell-mediated immunity, isolated IgA deficiency, or deficient phagocytosis due to myeloperoxidase deficiency. It has been postulated that the deficiency in cell-mediated immunity in this disorder is due either to the specific failure of lymphocytes to divide on exposure to antigen or to their failure to produce MIF (see Chapter 1). "Transfer factor" has been used successfully in the treatment of deficient cell-mediated immune responses.

Defective mobilization of polymorphonuclear leukocytes, possibly due to inadequate opsonic activity, has been described in diabetes, after alcohol ingestion, and in most infants with birth weights of less than 1925 gm. In addition, there have been case reports of a familial type of opsonin deficiency due to the presence of nonfunctioning C5.[21]

The most common clinical manifestations of opsonin deficiency include repeated local and systemic infections with gram-negative organisms or coagulase-positive staphylococci, and a tendency to eczematous dermatoses.

DISORDERS OF THE COMPLEMENT SYSTEM

Several genetically determined deficiencies of complement components (see Chapter 1) have been described (see Table 11-3). An autosomally inherited deficiency of C2 is associated with a marked reduction in the in vitro serum bactericidal activity and in the serum capacity for immune adherence. However, there is no clinical evidence of immune deficiency in this group of patients. Similarly, C4 deficiency has been reported, but does not appear to be associated with clinical symptoms. Deficiency of C1 esterase inhibitor, an autosomal dominant disorder, produces the characteristic signs and symptoms of hereditary angioedema (see Chapter 5). C1q deficiency occurs in various disorders associated with decreased IgG synthesis such as agammaglobulinemia, the lymphopenic forms of hypogammaglobulinemia, and multiple myeloma. The significance of this finding in relation to clinical sus-

TABLE 11-3. Disorders of the Complement System*

Inherited Deficiencies of Complement Components

C2 and C4 deficiency (no clinical symptoms)
C1 esterase inhibitor deficiency (hereditary angioedema, periodic disease)
C1q deficiency (associated with decreased IgG synthesis)
C5 deficiency (associated with impaired phagocytosis)
C3 deficiency (susceptibility to pyogenic infections)

Acquired Deficiencies of Complement Components

Increased utilization
    Antigen-antibody complexes (e.g., SLE, acute glomerulonephritis, S.B.E., cryoglobulinemia)
    Fixation to tissues (e.g., AIHA, chronic glomerulonephritis, joint effusions of rheumatoid arthritis)
Decreased synthesis
    Proliferative glomerulonephritis
    Systemic lupus erythematosus
    Liver disease
Increased breakdown
    Proteolytic enzyme breakdown of C3 in some forms of glomerulonephritis
Miscellaneous
    Myasthenia gravis
    Allograft rejection

Elevated Serum Complement Levels

Inflammatory Disorders

---

*Modified from Schur, P. H., and Austen, K. F. *Ann. Rev. Med.* *19*:1, 1968.

ceptibility to infection is yet to be established.[24] On the other hand, abnormalities of C3 in newborn infants have been described in association with an increased susceptibility to pyogenic infections.[1] The resulting clinical syndrome is readily reversed with infusions of fresh plasma.

The levels of serum complement are reduced in several clinical syndromes of immunologic interest including systemic lupus erythematosus, acute and chronic glomerulonephritis, cryoglobulinemia, subacute bacterial endocarditis, autoimmune hemolytic anemias, myasthenia gravis, and allograft rejection (see Chapters 6–10, 14, and 19). In general, the reduction in whole serum complement levels (hemolytic complement titers) reflects reduction of C3 or C4 levels due to the utilization of complement in antigen-antibody reactions. There is evidence that decreased synthesis of complement may occur in some patients with systemic lupus erythematosus or in the progressive form of proliferative glomerulonephritis in childhood, and that proteolytic enzyme breakdown of C3 may occur in some patients with acute poststreptococcal glomerulonephritis[27] (see Chapter 6).

Elevated levels of serum complement are found in a wide variety of inflammatory conditions. The mechanism which underlies this elevation is poorly understood.

REFERENCES

1. Alper, C. A., Abramson, N., Johnson, R. B., Jr., Jandl, J. H., and Rosen, F. S. Increased susceptibility to infection associated with complement-mediated functions and of the third component of complement (C3). *New Eng. Med.* *282*:349, 1970.

1a. August, C. S., Levey, R. H., Berkel, A. I., Rosen, F. S. and Kay, H. E. M. Establishment of immunological competence in a child with congenital thymic aplasia by a graft of fetal thymus. *Lancet 1*:1080, 1970.

2. Bach, F., Albertini, R. J., Joo, P., Anderson, J. L., and Bortin, M. M. Bone marrow transplantation in a patient with the Wiskott-Aldrich syndrome. *Lancet* *2*:1364, 1968.

3. Baehner, R. L., and Nathan, D. G. Quantitative nitro-blue tetrazolium test in chronic granulomatous disease. *New Eng. J. Med. 278*:971, 1968.

3a. Baehner, R. L., Nathan, D. G., and Karnovsky, M. L. Correlation of metabolic defects in leukocytes of patients with chronic granulomatous disease. *J. Clin. Invest. 49*:865, 1970.

4. Baldini, M. G. Platelet defect in Wiskott-Aldrich syndrome. *New Eng. J. Med. 281*:107, 1969.

5. Boder, E., and Sedgewick, R. P. Ataxia telangiectasia, a familial syndrome of progressive cerebellar ataxia, oculocutaneous telangiectasia and frequent pulmonary infection. *Pediatrics 21*:52, 1958.

6. Chilgren, R. A., Hong, R., and Quie, P. G. Human serum interactions with *Candida Albicans. J. Immun. 101*:129, 1968.

7. Diamond, L. K. Splenectomy in childhood and the hazard of overwhelming infection. *Pediatrics 43*:886, 1969.

8. Douglas, S. D., Blume, R. S., and Wolff, S. M. Fine structural studies of leukocytes from patients and heterozygotes with the Chediak-Higashi syndrome. *Blood 33*:527, 1969.

9. Fireman, P., Friday, G., and Kumate, J. Effect of measles vaccine on immunologic responsiveness. *Pediatrics 43*:264, 1969.

10. Gatti, R. A., Meuwissen, H. J., Allen, H. D., Hong, R., and Good, R. A. Immunological reconstitution of sex-linked lymphopenic immunological deficiency. *Lancet 2*:1366, 1968.

11. Good, R. A., Quie, P. G., Windhorst, D. B., Page, A. R., Rodey, G. E., White, J., Wolfson, J. J., and Holmes, B. H. Fatal (chronic) granulomatous disease of childhood. A hereditary defect of leukocyte function. *Seminars Hemat.* 5:215, 1968.

12. Gryboski, J. D., Self, T. W., Clemett, A., and Herscovic, T. Selective immunoglobulin A deficiency and intestinal nodular lymphoid hyperplasia: Correction of diarrhea with antibiotics and plasma. *Pediatrics 42:*833, 1968.

13. Hobbs, J. R. Immune imbalance in dysgammaglobulinemia type IV. *Lancet 1:*110, 1968.

14. Hong, R., Gatti, R., Rathburn, J. C., and Good, R. A. Thymic hypoplasia and thyroid dysfunction. *New Eng. J. Med. 282:*470, 1970.

15. Hoyer, J. R., Cooper, M. D., Gabrielson, A. E., and Good, R. A. Lymphopenic forms of congenital immunologic deficiency diseases. *Medicine 47:*201, 1968.

16. Kevy, S. V., Tefft, M., Vawter, G. F., and Rosen, F. S. Hereditary splenic hypoplasia. *Pediatrics 42:*752, 1968.

17. Kretschmer, R., August, C. S., Rosen, F. S., and Janeway, C. A. Recurrent infections, episodic lymphopenia and impaired cellular immunity. Further observations on "immunologic amnesia" in two siblings. *New Eng. J. Med. 281:*285, 1969.

18. Kretschmer, R., Say, G., Brown, D., and Rosen, F. S. Congenital aplasia of the thymus gland (DiGeorge's syndrome). *New Eng. J. Med. 279:*1295, 1968.

18a. Lux, S. E., Johnston, R. B., August, C. S., Say, G., Penchaszadek, V. B., Rosen, F. S., and McKusick, V. Chronic neutropenia and abnormal cellular immunity in cartilage-hair hypoplasia. *New Eng. J. Med. 282:*321, 1970.

19. Mandl, M. A. J., Watson, J. I., and Rose, B. Wiskott-Aldrich syndrome. Immunopathologic mechanisms and long term survival. *Ann. Intern. Med. 68:*1050, 1968.

20. Medical Research Council Working-party Summary Report. Hypogammaglobulinemia in the United Kingdom. *Lancet 1:*163, 1969.

20a. Miller, M. E., Mellman, W. J., Kohn, G., and Deitz, W. J., Jr. Depressed immunoglobulin G in newborn infants with Down's syndrome. *J. Pediat. 75:*996 1969.

21. Miller, M. E., and Nilsson, V. R. Complement dysfunction with deficient phagocytosis. Enhancement by serum. *New Eng. J. Med. 282:*354, 1970.

21a. Rivat, L., Ropartz, C., Burtin, P., and Cruchaud, A. Genetic control of deficiencies in γG sub-class observed among families with hypogammaglobulinemia. *Nature 225:*1136, 1970.

22. Rosen, F. S. The lymphocyte and thymus gland—congenital and hereditary abnormalities. *New Eng. J. Med. 279:*643, 1968.

23. Schmid, J. R., Kiely, J. M., Harrison, E. G., Bayrd, E. D., and Pease, G. L. Thymoma associated with pure red cell agenesis. *Cancer 18:*216, 1965.

24. Schur, P. H., and Austen, K. F. Complement in human disease. *Ann. Rev. Med. 19:*1, 1968.

24a. Seeger, R. C., Amman, A. J., Good, R. A., and Hong, R. Progressive lymphoid system deterioration. A new familial lymphopenic immunological deficiency disease. *Clin. Exp. Immunol.* 6:169, 1970.

25. Seligmann, M., Fudenberg, H. H., and Good, R. A. A proposed classification of primary immunologic deficiencies. *Amer. J. Med.* 45:817, 1968.

26. Simons, M. J. Congenital rubella: An immunological paradox. *Lancet* 2:1275, 1968.

27. Spitzer, R. E., Vallota, E. H., Forristal, J., Sudora, E., Stitzel, A., Davis, N. C., and West, C. D. Serum C3 lytic system in patients with glomerulonephritis. *Science* 164:436, 1969.

28. Strober, W., Wochner, R. D., Carbone, P. P., and Waldmann, T. A. Intestinal lymphangiectasia: A protein-losing enteropathy with hypogammaglobulinemia, lymphocytopenia, and impaired homograft rejection. *J. Clin. Invest.* 46:1643, 1967.

29. Winkelstein, J. A., and Drachman, R. H. Deficiency of pneumococcal serum opsonizing activity in sickle cell disease. *New Eng. J. Med.* 279:459, 1968.

30. Wochner, R. D., Drews, G., Strober, W., and Waldmann, J. A. Accelerated breakdown of immunoglobulin G (IgG) in myotonic dystrophy: A hereditary error of immunoglobulin catabolism. *J. Clin. Invest.* 45:321, 1966.

12

Clinical Immunology of the Lymphoreticular System

SAMUEL O. FREEDMAN

In the previous chapter it was noted that certain congenital immune deficiency states are associated with a high incidence of malignant lymphoproliferative diseases, autoimmune diseases, and an increased susceptibility to infection. Conversely, patients with Hodgkin's disease, lymphoma, and leukemia often display marked immunologic abnormalities, an increased incidence of autoimmune disorders, and a predisposition to develop second primary neoplasms. These observations have led to the hypothesis that individuals with lymphoproliferative diseases have an underlying disorder of the immune system which results in deficient host resistance to exogenous and endogenous allergens, microbial pathogens, and carcinogens.[22] The question of which is the primary disease, the lymphoproliferative process or the immunologic deficiency state, remains unanswered for the present.

When one considers other abnormalities of the lymphoreticular system, there is a striking parallelism between the pattern of immunologic deficiency and the granulomatous lesions which occur in Hodgkin's disease and in

372

sarcoidosis. Similarly, lepromatous leprosy and infectious mononucleosis represent additional forms of lymphoproliferative disease which are associated with immunologic abnormalities. It is for these reasons that Hodgkin's disease, lymphoma, leukemia, sarcoidosis, leprosy, and infectious mononucleosis will be considered together in a single chapter. (Burkitt's lymphoma is discussed in Chapter 13, and Waldenstrom's macroglobulinemia in Chapter 10.)

HODGKIN'S DISEASE, LYMPHOMA, AND LEUKEMIA

There are probably few other examples in medicine of terminology which is more inconsistent and confusing than that used to describe the group of tumors loosely designated as malignant lymphomas. For reasons which will become obvious in the ensuing discussion, it is esential to distinguish between Hodgkin's disease (a lymphogranulomatous process) and the malignant lymphoproliferative disorders such as chronic lymphocytic leukemia, lymphosarcoma, Waldenstrom's macroglobulinemia, and reticulum cell sarcoma.

PATHOLOGY

Hodgkin's Disease

Grossly, the lymph nodes in Hodgkin's disease are enlarged and may be either firm or soft in consistency. The most constant histologic change is an increase in the size and number of reticulum cells (many of which appear abnormal), and the presence of Sternberg-Reed cells. The Sternberg-Reed cells are of uncertain origin, vary from 15 to 45 μ in diameter, and can be identified by characteristic multiple or multilobate nuclei. The nuclei usually contain large, prominent nucleoli that have a pronounced affinity for acid dyes. Occasionally, these cells may be similar to multinucleate Langhans' giant cells or to foreign body giant cells.

Lymphoid tissues involved by Hodgkin's disease may exhibit many other histologic alterations including proliferation or depletion of lymphocytes, hyperplasia of fibroblasts and endothelial cells, and a variable infiltration with eosinophils, neutrophils and plasma cells. These other cellular constituents often outnumber the reticulum cells and Sternberg-Reed cells, appear morphologically normal, and are thought to represent an inflammatory response of the involved tissue to the fundamental changes of Hodgkin's disease. Thus, the term Hodgkin's granuloma is frequently used to describe the reactive, chronic inflammatory changes seen in the classic form of the disease.

Because defective lymphocyte function has been suggested as the cause of the immunologic abnormalities in Hodgkin's disease, the histologic classification proposed by Lukes and Butler and modified by Rye would appear to be the most useful for the purposes of the present discussion.[18] According to this scheme, the lesions of Hodgkin's disease may be divided into those cases in which there is: (1) lymphocyte predominance; (2) mixed cellularity; (3) lymphocyte depletion due to reticular proliferation or diffuse fibrosis; and (4) nodular sclerosis characterized by bands of densely packed collagenous tissue separating the cellular portions of the lymph node.

Chronic Lymphocytic Leukemia, Lymphosarcoma, and Reticulum Cell Sarcoma

Compared to Hodgkin's disease, the morphologic changes in chronic lymphocytic leukemia, lymphosarcoma, and reticulum cell sarcoma are considerably less complex. Lymph node biopsy in lymphosarcoma and chronic lymphatic leukemia shows destruction of the normal architecture of the lymph node and its replacement with highly packed primitive lymphocytes. In reticulum cell sarcoma, the predominant cell is three to four times larger than the malignant lymphocytes and there is abundant pale staining cytoplasm.

IMMUNOLOGY

The nature of the immunologic abnormalities which occur in Hodgkin's disease, lymphoma, and chronic lymphocytic leukemia will be considered next because they provide information which has been extremely valuable in formulating current theories regarding the etiology and pathogenesis of the lymphoid malignancies (see Table 12-1).

Cell-Mediated Immunity

The characteristic immunologic defect in Hodgkin's disease is manifested by a marked impairment of cell-mediated immunity (see Tables 22-7 and 12-1). The anergy demonstrated in many patients with Hodgkin's disease has been attributed to the abnormal lymphocyte function which occurs during the course of the disease, and to the marked lymphopenia which may develop in advanced cases (Fig. 12-1). Not infrequently, patients with Hodgkin's disease will continue to display manifestations of cell-mediated hypersensitivity to antigens encountered before the onset of their disease, but are unable to react to new antigens. It is also possible that the deficiency in cell-mediated immunity detected in some patients with Hodgkin's disease

TABLE 12-1. Summary of Typical Findings in Some Common Lymphoreticular
Disorders

	Chronic lymphatic leukemia	Infectious mononucleosis	Hodgkin's disease	Sarcoidosis
Pathology	Lymphoproliferative	Lymphoproliferative	Lymphogranulomatous	Lymphogranulomatous
Lymphocytosis	Frequent	Frequent	Unusual	Unusual
Impaired delayed hypersensitivity	Minimal	Never	Severe	Severe
Immunoglobulins	Frequently decreased	Occasionally increased	Variable	Frequently increased
Impaired antibody synthesis	Frequent	Unusual	Occasional	Unusual
Heterophile antibodies	Never	Frequent	Unusual	Never
Viral and fungal infections	Occasional	Unusual	Frequent and severe	Unusual
Pyogenic infections	Frequent and severe	Unusual	Occasional	Occasional
Hypercalcemia	Unusual	Never	Frequent	Frequent

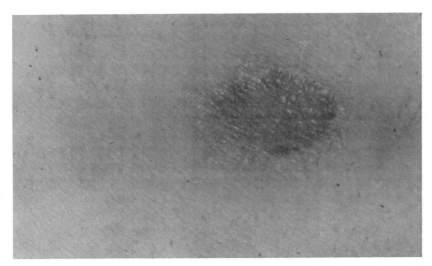

FIG. 12-1. Skin allograft completely viable after 11 months in a patient with Hodgkin's disease.

is due to the administration of chemotherapeutic agents with immunosuppressive properties.

In favor of the concept of impaired lymphocyte function is the observation that the in vitro lymphoid response to phytohemagglutinin is markedly impaired in Hodgkin's disease.[30] Furthermore, it has been shown that the passive transfer of delayed-type hypersensitivity to patients with Hodgkin's disease is extremely difficult to accomplish.[24] This inability to accept passive cellular transfer using suspensions of peripheral blood lymphocytes lends further strength to the argument that the lymphoid system in Hodgkin's disease is somehow unable to participate in the events leading to cell-mediated immunity.

On the other hand, the peripheral blood lymphocytes in Hodgkin's disease appear to be more active than normal lymphocytes. The peripheral blood changes in Hodgkin's disease are characterized by: (1) an increase in the number of lymphoid cells which actively synthesize DNA; (2) an increase in number of medium sized lymphoid cells with basophilic cytoplasm; and (3) the occasional presence of plasma cells.[5] These changes are similar to those found in conditions of known antigenic stimulation such as in infectious diseases, after immunization, and in systemic lupus erythematosus. However, in Hodgkin's disease the nature of the putative antigen is entirely unknown.

In contrast to Hodgkin's disease, the manifestations of delayed-type hypersensitivity are relatively normal in chronic lymphocytic leukemia, lymphosarcoma, or reticulum cell sarcoma unless the patient is profoundly debilitated or has received drugs with immunosuppressive properties. There is, however, evidence for impaired lymphocyte transformation on exposure to phytohemagglutinin in patients with chronic lymphocytic leukemia. This impaired transformation is not related to detectable abnormalities of cell-mediated hypersensitivity.[30]

Immunoglobulins

Abnormalities of immunoglobulins or other serum proteins are not a prominent feature of Hodgkin's disease. The most characteristic pattern for serum proteins found in advanced Hodgkin's disease is hypoalbuminemia, particularly when there is liver involvement, and an elevation of the α-globulin fractions. The levels of IgG are usually normal or slightly elevated, whereas the levels of IgA and IgM are often reduced or at the lower levels of normal.[11] When it occurs, the hypergammaglobulinemia of Hodgkin's disease may be monoclonal or polyclonal in nature. Significant hypogammaglobulinemia is rare in Hodgkin's disease.

On the other hand, immunoglobulin abnormalities are relatively common in chronic lymphocytic leukemia, lymphosarcoma, and reticulum cell sarcoma. About 75 per cent of patients with chronic lymphocytic leukemia display significant hypogammaglobulinemia during the course of the disease. A single immunoglobulin class or any combination of immunoglobulins may be involved in this deficiency. Hypoalbuminemia and α-globulin elevvations are less common than in Hodgkin's disease, but may appear in the advanced stages. Hypogammaglobulinemia occurs less frequently in lymphosarcoma or reticulum cell sarcoma than in chronic lymphocytic leukemia.

On the other hand, monoclonal IgM peaks occur in approximately 4 per cent of patients with chronic lymphatic leukemia or lymphosarcoma,[23a] and there is an increased excretion of urinary light chains in approximately 25 per cent of patients with all forms of leukemia or lymphoma.[17a] The significance of these findings is not clear at the present time.

Resistance to Infection

It is well known that systemic infections are more common in patients with lymphoma and leukemia than in patients with other forms of cancer. Furthermore, there is an interesting and highly significant distinction between the *types* of infection seen in Hodgkin's disease compared to those found in chronic lymphatic leukemia, lymphosarcoma, ·or reticulum cell sarcoma.

For example, the incidence of granulomatous infections in patients with Hodgkin's disease is significantly higher than in individuals with other systemic diseases of comparable severity. The frequency of active pulmonary tuberculosis in Hodgkin's disease is reported to be approximately 5 per cent, and the frequency of cryptococcosis is approximately 8 per cent.[16] Similar but less striking relationships have been reported between Hodgkin's disease and histoplasmosis or a variety of other fungal infections. In addition, there appears to be an increased susceptibility to viral infections in Hodgkin's disease (Fig. 12-2). In one study, it was found that 13 per cent of the infectious episodes in Hodgkin's disease were due to viral diseases, however only 1 per cent were due to viral disease in lymphosarcoma.[22]

By contrast, pyogenic infections due to bacterial organisms are not a prominent feature of Hodgkin's disease, whereas they do occur with relatively high frequency in acute and chronic lymphatic leukemia.

Patients with Hodgkin's disease are usually capable of producing a normal antibody response to injected antigens and have normal levels of circulating antibodies to frequently encountered viral and bacterial antigens. An important exception to this generalization is the observation that patients with Hodgkin's disease frequently fail to form circulating antibodies on exposure to adenoviruses.[23]

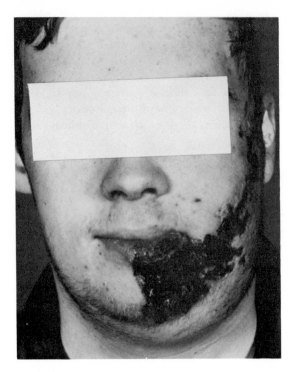

FIG. 12-2. Severe herpes zoster in a patient with Hodgkin's disease.

Autoimmune Diseases

There is an increased incidence of collagen-vascular diseases and autoimmune hemolytic anemias in patients with Hodgkin's disease and other lymphoreticular malignancies. The frequency of diffuse collagen-vascular diseases in normal individuals or in patients with solid tumors is approximately 0.5 per cent, whereas the frequency in patients with Hodgkin's disease and lymphoreticular malignancies is approximately 2 per cent.[21] Although detailed prevalence studies have not been carried out, it is also of interest that Sjögren's syndrome is frequently followed by reticulum cell sarcoma, and that Hashimoto's disease may be followed by malignant lymphoma of the thyroid.

Second Primary Neoplasms

Many experienced clinicians have observed that second primary neoplasms occur with increased frequency in chronic lymphatic leukemia, reticulum cell sarcoma, and lymphosarcoma. In one well controlled study, the incidence of second primary neoplasms in chronic lymphatic leukemia was 15 per cent, compared to 5 per cent in acute leukemia, 6 per cent in chronic granulocytic leukemia, and 3 per cent in the remainder of the patients studied.[12]

ETIOLOGY AND PATHOGENESIS
Viral Infection

Viral etiologies are now well established for numerous animal tumors including Rous sarcoma, Shope papilloma, chicken leukosis, mouse polyoma, and mammary carcinoma of mice. In more recent studies of viral oncology, a strain of NZB/Bl mice were observed to develop malignant lymphomas in 20 per cent of cases. Spleen cells from the mice with lymphoma were found to contain virus-like particles. Furthermore, when cell-free extracts from the spleens of NZB/Bl mice with lymphomas were injected into neonatal Swiss mice, 3 of 28 developed malignant lymphomas and all developed autoimmune manifestations.[20] It is of interest that related strains of inbred New Zealand mice develop thymic abnormalities, spontaneous hemolytic anemias, antinuclear antibodies, and glomerulonephritis (see Chapter 8), and it is conceivable that viral elements may be responsible for both neoplasia and autoimmune phenomena in these animals. In addition, there is an obvious analogy between this experimental model and the association between human collagen-vascular disease and malignant lymphoma discussed previously.

Transient depression of cell-mediated immune responses may occur during the course of viral infections, particularly those which follow the administration of live attenuated poliovirus vaccine or measles virus vaccine[7] (see Chapter 11). Because the pattern of immunologic deficiency is almost identical to that seen in Hodgkin's disease, these observations have been interpreted as indirect evidence in favor of a viral etiology for Hodgkin's disease. The observation that patients with Hodgkin's disease frequently fail to produce circulating antibodies against adenoviruses is of potential significance because certain strains of this group of respiratory pathogens are known to be oncogenic in rodents, and because Hodgkin's disease is often first detected in lymph nodes draining the respiratory tract. The possible inductive role of viruses in Burkitt's lymphoma is discussed in detail in Chapter 13.

Radiation

There appears to be little doubt that individuals exposed to relatively high doses of radiation demonstrate an increased frequency of leukemia and lymphoma. Most of the evidence for this relationship comes from epidemiologic studies on population groups exposed to elevated radiation dose levels. These studies have shown that the incidence of leukemia and lymphomas is significantly higher than normal in radiologists, individuals exposed to radioisotopes, atomic bomb casualties, infants who received thymic irradiation, and adults given therapeutic radiation for rheumatoid spondylitis.[17] At relatively low levels of radiation exposure, such as occur during diagnostic x-ray studies in adults or during prenatal exposure to radiation, a cause and effect relationship between radiation and leukemogenesis is much more difficult to substantiate.

Genetically Determined Immune Deficiency

A genetic basis for lymphomas and leukemias is suggested by an increased prevalence of these diseases in identical twins and in the immediate relatives of affected patients. Furthermore, there are a number of hereditary diseases associated with immunologic deficiency (e.g., primary agammaglobulinemia, ataxia telangiectasia, Wiskott-Aldrich syndrome, and Chediak-Higashi syndrome) in which there is an increased prevalence of lymphoproliferative malignancies (see Chapter 11). An increased prevalence of lymphoproliferative disorders and other neoplasms has also been described in hereditary diseases associated with chromosomal aberrations such as Down's syndrome (Mongolism) and Klinefelter's syndrome. The occurrence of autoantibodies in Down's syndrome is discussed in Chapter 15.

An interesting genetic concept has been proposed to explain the immunologic abnormalities observed in Hodgkin's disease, chronic lymphatic leukemia, and lymphosarcoma.[22] According to this hypothesis, the patient with a lymphoproliferative disease is an individual whose immune protective mechanisms against environmental carcinogens such as viruses, drugs, and radiation is defective. A genetic or constitutional basis for this defect is suggested by the frequent association between lymphoid malignancies and: (1) congenital immunologic deficiency states; or (2) a variety of autoimmune diseases.

The Kaplan-Smithers hypothesis[29] which states that Hodgkin's disease is a special form of a graft-versus-host reaction is essentially the same concept presented in different terminology. The marked lymphoid depletion seen in some patients with Hodgkin's disease is comparable to that which occurs in advanced graft-versus-host reactions (see Chapter 14).

However, it must be emphasized that the immunologic abnormalities observed in patients with lymphoid malignancies are usually seen late in the course of the disease. During the early stages, little or no immune disturbance can be detected. On the other hand, it is certainly possible that the relatively insensitive methods currently employed may fail to detect early abnormalities. At present, it seems fair to state that there is no direct evidence for an antecedent immune deficiency that is responsible for most lymphoid malignancies, but the hypothesis has intriguing possibilities.

CLINICAL MANIFESTATIONS

Hodgkin's Disease

Common presenting signs and symptoms are regional unilateral lympha-denopathy, especially of the cervical nodes, or respiratory difficulty if the mediastinal nodes are involved early in the disease. As the disease process advances, there may be hepatosplenomegaly and constitutional symptoms such as fever, night sweats, pruritus, excessive fatigue, and weight loss. Superior vena cava obstruction and pleural effusions are not infrequent complications during the late stages of the disease. In addition, there may be direct invasion of the pulmonary parenchyma by Hodgkin's tissue. The susceptibility of patients with Hodgkin's disease to granulomatous and viral infections has already been discussed.

Laboratory findings in advanced Hodgkin's disease include a marked anemia, which is often hemolytic in type, cryoglobulinemia, lymphopenia, and eosinophilia. Osteolytic lesions may occasionally be seen in x-rays of the vertebral bodies, and hypercalcemia is reported to occur in a significant number of patients.

The specific diagnosis is made by demonstration of a characteristic his-tologic picture on biopsy of involved lymphoid tissues. Bone marrow examination is usually not helpful, except in rare cases where there is extensive involvement of bone marrow.

Chronic Lymphatic Leukemia

The disease occurs primarily in middle and late adult life; it is rare in persons under the age of 20 years. The onset is usually gradual and the first signs may be painless enlargement of lymph nodes in the neck, axilla, or groin. Enlarged mediastinal lymph nodes may cause pressure symptoms such as tracheal compression or respiratory difficulty. Splenic enlargement, involvement of the skin, gastrointestinal symptoms, severe anemia, fever, and debility are all relatively common clinical features. The increased susceptibility to pyogenic infections in chronic lymphatic leukemia is primarily due to the hypogammaglobulinemia which occurs in about 30 per cent of patients with the disease.

The most significant laboratory finding is lymphocytosis in the peripheral blood. Eventually, the white blood count may range between 50,000 and 250,000/cu mm of which 90 per cent or more are mature lymphocytes with little variation in appearance. Severe anemia, which is often hemolytic, occurs in about one-third of patients.

Bone marrow examination usually reveals a marked predominance of small lymphocytes, but may occasionally be normal in the early stages of the disease. Even the most experienced pathologist may sometimes have difficulty in distinguishing between chronic lymphatic leukemia and lymphosarcoma on lymph node biopsy.

Lymphosarcoma and Reticulum Cell Sarcoma

Lymphosarcoma may arise in any lymphoid tissue, but the most common initial manifestation is painless, unilateral lymphadenopathy in the cervical region. Less commonly, nasopharyngeal, mediastinal, or intra-abdominal lymph nodes may be the first to be affected. The liver or spleen is enlarged in about one-third of patients. Later clinical features may include involvement of the skin, gastrointestinal tract, the nervous system and bones, as well as systemic symptoms such as fever, weight loss, and general debility. The diagnosis is made by finding the characteristic histologic picture of lymphosarcoma on lymph node biopsy.

Reticulum cell sarcoma clinically resembles lymphosarcoma in most respects except that the lymph nodes tend to be hard, tender, and fixed to the underlying tissues. There is less tendency to splenic or hepatic enlargement, or to involvement of the mediastinal lymph nodes. The diagnosis is made by lymph node biopsy.

TREATMENT

An understanding of the basic principles of treatment in Hodgkin's disease and the lymphoreticular malignancies is essential to the evaluation of the immunologic capacity of the patient, because both radiation and cancer chemotherapeutic drugs profoundly affect the immune response.

The clinical staging of Hodgkin's disease based on the degree of anatomic involvement has led, in recent years, to a much more optimistic approach to the treatment of malignant lymphoma (see Table 12-2). Furthermore, the increased use of lymphangiographic studies has improved the staging of Hodgkin's disease to the point where it is of primary therapeutic importance.

Radiotherapy is the treatment of choice in early Hodgkin's disease. Approximately 75 to 90 per cent of patients with stage I or stage II-A disease are reported to be free of disease for 5 years after aggressive radiotherapy. Whether extended irradiation has a role in the treatment of more advanced Hodgkin's disease is being evaluated in long-term studies. The clinical staging and indications for aggressive radiotherapy are not as well defined in lymphosarcoma and reticulum cell sarcoma.

TABLE 12-2. Clinical Staging of Hodgkin's Disease

Stage I. Disease limited to one anatomic group of lymph nodes
Stage II. Disease involving two or more groups of lymph nodes on the same side of the diaphragm
Stage III. Disease on both sides of the diaphragm, but confined to the lymph nodes and spleen
Stage IV. Disease involving both lymph nodes and extranodal sites
Each stage may be subdivided into A (no constitutional symptoms), or B (with constitutional symptoms: e.g., fever, night sweats, pruritus, or weight loss)

At present, systemic therapy with cytotoxic (and immunosuppressive) drugs is the treatment of choice for disseminated disease. This class of drugs may be used singly, in combination, or sequentially, but an optimum treatment plan must be developed for each individual patient. The major agents of established value in the lymphoreticular diseases are outlined in Table 12-3.

In chronic lymphatic leukemia there is great variability in the course of the disease. Since it may remain asymptomatic for many years, a large number of clinicians tend to withhold therapy until symptoms appear or there is other evidence of disease progression. When chemotherapy is indicated, chlorambucil or cyclophosphamide are the most commonly used cytotoxic agents. If remission occurs following a successful course of chemotherapy, the disease may remain quiescent for months or years without maintenance therapy.

Corticosteroids have a limited but useful role in the management of Hodgkin's disease, lymphomas, and chronic lymphatic leukemia. Most commonly, they are reserved for the autoimmune hemolytic anemia or thrombocytopenia which often accompanies the primary disease process. However, in patients who require symptomatic relief, but are unable to tolerate other drugs, due to toxic side-effects, corticosteroids occasionally provide dramatic but temporary improvement.

Supportive measures such as red cell and platelet transfusions, antibiotics, and control of hyperuricemia and hypercalcemia are important adjuncts to the therapy of these disorders.

TABLE 12-3. Chemotherapeutic Agents for the Treatment of Hodgkin's Disease, Lymphomas, and Chronic Lymphocytic Leukemia

Drug	Indication	Route and usual dose	Side-effects
Nitrogen mustard	Hodgkin's disease	0.4 mg/kg, I. V., single dose or in 2 to 4 single doses	Nausea, vomiting, bone marrow depression
Chlorambucil	Hodgkin's disease, lymphosarcoma, chronic lymphatic leukemia	0.1 to 0.2 mg/kg, P.O. daily	Bone marrow depression
Cyclophosphamide	As above plus reticulum cell sarcoma	8 to 15 mg/kg, I.V., weekly or 50 to 200 mg/day, P.O.	Nausea, vomiting, alopecia, bone marrow depression, hemorrhagic cystitis
Vinblastine	Hodgkin's disease, lymphosarcoma, reticulum cell sarcoma	0.1 to 0.3 mg/kg, I.V., weekly	Bone marrow depression, alopecia, neuropathy, paralytic ileus
Vincristine	Lymphosarcoma, reticulum cell sarcoma	0.01 to 0.075 mg/kg, I.V., weekly	Neuropathy, muscle weakness, alopecia, bone marrow depression
Prednisone	See text	10 to 100 mg/day, P.O.	Fluid and salt retention, diabetes, peptic ulcer, osteoporosis, Cushingoid facies, susceptibility to infections

DRUG-INDUCED PSEUDOLYMPHOMA

Lymphadenopathy may occur in association with the administration of a variety of drugs including hydantoin and its analogues, para-aminosalicylic acid, iron dextran, phenylbutazone, and meprobamate. In fact, the term "pseudolymphoma" has been used to describe a syndrome of lymphadenopathy, fever, morbilliform rash, arthralgias, hepatosplenomegaly, and eosinophilia which may appear following drug administration. The lymphadenopathy disappears promptly with the cessation of drug therapy, but recurs if the drug is reintroduced. The histologic picture may superficially resemble lymphoma, but malignant lymphoid cells are not seen in lymph node biopsies.

In contrast to this benign, reversible condition induced by a variety of drugs, it has recently become apparent that not all patients with hydantoin-induced lymphadenopathy experience regression after withdrawal of the drug. A significant number of patients with "pseudolymphoma" attributed to diphenylhydantoin subsequently progress to a fatal disease histologically indistinguishable from malignant lymphoma.[8] There is no evidence that the hydantoins cause a malignant change directly, but it is possible that they may unmask underlying lymphomas through their lymphostimulatory activity.

SARCOIDOSIS

Sarcoidosis is a granulomatous disease of unknown etiology with characteristic lesions occurring throughout the body. The mediastinal lymph nodes, peripheral lymph nodes, skin, and eyes are most commonly affected, but almost any organ may be involved. The many parallelisms which exist between Hodgkin's disease and sarcoidosis are striking, despite the fact that their etiologies and pathogenesis may be quite different. Both are characterized by granulomatous lesions, predominant involvement of lymph nodes, and a marked diminution of delayed hypersensitivity reactions (see Table 12-1).

PATHOLOGY

The characteristic lesion of sarcoidosis resembles that of any other epithelioid cell granuloma in a nonnecrotic stage and often cannot be distinguished histologically from tuberculosis, berylliosis, leprosy, brucellosis, or histoplasmosis. In addition, local "sarcoid reactions" may occur in regional lymph nodes draining a carcinoma, or in an area of chronic local infection.

In the early stages of the disease, the usual histologic picture in a lymph node biopsy consists of epithelioid cells surrounded by a small zone of lymphocytes, plasma cells, and Langhans' giant cells. Giant cells containing laminated calcific Schaumann bodies or stellate "asteroid" bodies are frequent, but neither of these inclusions is pathognomonic of sarcoidosis. The sarcoid nodules may appear in clusters or may coalesce to form larger complexes. Eventually, there is marked fibrosis with almost complete disappearance of inflammatory cells. Some central fibrinoid necrosis may occur, but caseation is unusual.

In the more advanced stages, there may be proliferation of fibroblasts with the deposition of dense collagenous fibers between the epithelioid cells. In the lung, it is this collagenous tissue which may eventually lead to fibrosing alveolitis (see Chapter 4).

ETIOLOGY

The etiology of sarcoidosis remains a mystery. Previous enthusiasm over inhaled pine pollen or *Mycobacterium tuberculosis* as possible causes of sarcoidosis has diminished considerably in recent years. Instead, there has been increasing interest in the possible role of anonymous mycobacteria as a causal agent in sarcoidosis. The evidence for this hypothesis is indirect, but suggestive. Scotochromogenic mycobacteria have been cultured from lymph nodes in patients with sarcoidosis,[1] but the possibility that these organisms are a form of coexistent infection rather than causal agents is a very real one. In keeping with this latter suggestion, it has been noted that scotochromogenic mycobacteria may occasionally produce nonspecific acute or subacute lymphadenitis in children. Serologic studies using the technique of double diffusion in agar gel revealed that the sera of 80 per cent of patients with sarcoidosis demonstrated significant reactions to mycobacterial antigens compared to an incidence of 25 per cent in the normal population.[2]

The fact that sarcoidosis is fairly common in northern Europe, eastern United States, Australia, and New Zealand, but rare in other parts of the world would suggest a specific external inciting agent. Epidemiologic studies in the City of New York demonstrated that the prevalence of sarcoidosis in the black population is approximately 10 times that of the white population. This finding would suggest that a genetic predisposition may also be of importance in determining susceptibility to the disease.

The possible role of immune phenomenon in the pathogenesis of sarcoidosis is suggested by the increased incidence of hypersensitivity syndromes such as erythema nodosum, uveitis, and arthritis in this disease.

IMMUNOLOGY

Cell-Mediated Immunity

Patients with sarcoidosis show a marked diminution in the manifestations of cell-mediated immunity[3] (see Tables 12-1 and 22-7). Intradermal skin tests with tuberculin or its derivatives are negative in more than 90 per cent of patients with sarcoidosis. Furthermore, individuals known to be tuberculin positive lose their skin reactivity following the development of sarcoidosis, but may occasionally regain it after regression of the disease. In contrast to Hodgkin's disease, patients with sarcoidosis are able to accept the passive cellular transfer of tuberculin sensitivity. Studies on homograft rejection or lymphocyte transformation in sarcoidosis have not been reported in detail.

Immunoglobulins

Polyclonal hypergammaglobulinemia, with increase in one or more of the immunoglobulin classes, is observed to a varying degree in patients with sarcoidosis.[1a] The immunoglobulins tend to be increased most frequently in patients with advanced disease or in patients with liver involvement. An increased incidence of positive tests for rheumatoid factor (10 per cent), antinuclear antibodies (5 per cent), and biologic false-positive serologic tests for syphilis (see Chapter 21) are found in patients with sarcoidosis, but these changes are not always related to immunoglobulin abnormalities.

Resistance to Infection

Unlike Hodgkin's disease, there is very little evidence for significant impairment of resistance to infection in sarcoidosis. However, a slightly increased prevalence of tuberculosis, histoplasmosis, and cryptococcosis has been reported in association with sarcoidosis. In the case of tuberculosis, it is not clear whether the frequent association of pulmonary tuberculosis and sarcoidosis is related to the fact that sarcoidosis is much more prevalent in certain economically deprived populations.

The circulating antibody response to viral and bacterial antigens, and the levels of serum properdin are normal in sarcoidosis. One interesting observation is that patients with sarcoidosis fail to produce antibodies against mycobacteriophages.[19] It has been suggested that this deficiency may permit the rapid destruction of anonymous mycobacteria by mycobacteriophages, thus making it extremely difficult to identify anonymous mycobacteria in the lesions of sarcoidosis. The validity of this rather complex hypothesis remains to be established.

The Kviem Reaction

The Kviem test consists of the intracutaneous injection of a heat sterilized suspension of splenic or lymph node tissues obtained from sarcoid patients. A papulonodular lesion which contains epithelioid tubercles and reaches its maximum development at the site of injection in 4 to 6 weeks is considered to constitute a positive test. Histologic examination of a skin biopsy taken from the injection site is required for positive diagnosis.

Optimistic reports continue to appear concerning the specificity of the Kviem reaction in the diagnosis of sarcoidosis, but there are several practical considerations which severely limit the usefulness of the test as a diagnostic procedure. A stable, standardized test material is still not commercially available. While excellent antigens have been prepared in several research laboratories, the same workers have not been able to produce additional batches of equal potency and specificity.[15] Some progress has been made towards purifying the active components of the Kviem reagent, but the product remains crude and unstandardized.

Using the best material available, it would appear that about 75 per cent of patients with active sarcoidosis of recent onset have positive Kviem reactions. The incidence of false-positive Kviem reactions in patients without sarcoidosis is negligible. However, the percentage of positive reactions in patients with disease of longer duration is significantly reduced. The test is most likely to be positive in patients with erythema nodosum, and least likely to be positive in patients with lymph node involvement or in patients on steroid therapy. An additional problem with sarcoid reactions induced by the Kviem antigen is that, in weak reactions, the histologic interpretation is somewhat difficult and is of equivocal diagnostic significance.

CLINICAL MANIFESTATIONS

Sarcoidosis is a chronic, relatively benign disease which may involve almost any organ in the body. Although the disease occurs primarily in adults, there is increasing evidence to suggest that sarcoidosis is not uncommon in children between the ages of 8 and 14 years.[28]

Although the clinical manifestations of sarcoidosis are extremely varied, a significant number of patients first present with one of five characteristic and well-defined syndromes: (1) isolated hilar lymphadenopathy; (2) erythema nodosum; (3) pulmonary fibrosis; (4) uveoparotid fever; or (5) hypercalcemia.

The hilar lymphadenopathy which occurs as a common manifestation of sarcoidosis may produce cough and dyspnea due to compression of pulmonary structures, or may be asymptomatic and discovered only on routine chest x-ray. Typical skin lesions include erythema nodosum, and nodules or plaque-like lesions which characteristically involve the face, ears, nose, and extensor surfaces of the extremities. Pulmonary fibrosis may result in severe and incapacitating dyspnea during the course of advanced sarcoidosis.

"Uveoparotid fever" consists of firm, painless enlargement of salivary and lacrimal glands as well as variable involvement of the eye with evidence of conjunctivitis, iritis, corneal and vitreous opacities, and retinitis. In some patients with more advanced disease, there may be hypercalcemia with or without evidence of nephrocalcinosis, palpable peripheral lymph nodes, polyarthritis, hepatosplenomegaly, phalangeal bone cysts, central nervous system lesions, peripheral neuropathy, and chronic myopathy which may occasionally involve the myocardium. Constitutional symptoms such as fever, weight loss and general debility may or may not be present.

At the time of diagnosis, a subdivision into subacute and chronic sarcoidosis based on the estimated duration of disease is often useful in determining prognosis and subsequent management. Patients in the *subacute* stage are estimated to have had their disease for less than 2 years and are usually discovered in the presymptomatic phase by means of a routine chest x-ray or by an episode of erythema nodosum. Most frequently, they are less than 30 years of age, have bilateral hilar lymphadenopathy on chest x-ray, a positive Kviem test, and a negative tuberculin reaction. The lesions are usually transient, and this group of patients has a good prognosis, with spontaneous recovery occurring in the majority of cases.

In the *chronic* stages, the disease is estimated to have been present for more than 2 years and there is usually evidence of extrathoracic organ involvement. This group of patients tends to be over 30 years of age. The tuberculin test remains negative, but Kviem reactivity may be lost. The prognosis is less favorable in these patients and symptomatic therapy is often required.

Death attributable to sarcoidosis occurs in about 10 per cent of chronic cases, and is usually the result of pulmonary insufficiency and cor pulmonale.

DIAGNOSIS

As noted previously, the major diagnostic application of the Kviem test is in patients with early or subacute disease, or in patients with erythema nodosum. Provided a potent antigen is available, the procedure is most useful in out-patients, and often eliminates the need to hospitalize the patient for organ biopsy.

In patients with chronic sarcoidosis, the Kviem reaction is positive in only about 20 per cent of cases.[15] In this situation, organ biopsy provides a much higher yield of positive results than an attempt to induce a cutaneous sarcoid nodule by means of Kviem antigen. The most productive sites for biopsy are cutaneous lesions and palpable lymph nodes. If there are no palpable lymph nodes, scalene biopsy, mediastinoscopy, or liver biopsy may be attempted in order to obtain a histologic diagnosis. Aspiration needle biopsy of the liver is reported to demonstrate characteristic granulomatas in 70 per cent of patients with hilar lymphadenopathy as the sole pulmonary manifestation. In patients with x-ray evidence of parenchymal lung involvement, lung biopsy may be preferable. All biopsy specimens should be cultured for acid-fast bacilli and fungi. In addition, those showing granulomatous lesions with routine stains should receive special stains for acid-fast bacilli and fungi.

The finding of hypergammaglobulinemia and hypercalcemia in some patients with sarcoidosis has already been discussed. Hyperuricemia is reported to occur in about 20 per cent of patients with this disorder.

TREATMENT

About two-thirds of patients with sarcoidosis require no treatment because the symptoms are seldom incapacitating, and because spontaneous remissions occur in a large proportion of cases. However, prompt treatment with systemic corticosteroids is mandatory if the function of a vital organ is threatened. The most common indications for corticosteroid therapy are ocular disease which imperils vision, diffuse pulmonary fibrosis, disabling arthritis, severe central nervous system lesions, myocardial lesions, hypersplenism, and persistent hypercalcemia with renal damage. The usual initial dose of prednisone is 20 to 30 mg, daily in divided doses until suppression of acute symptoms occurs. Maintenance therapy with prednisone in daily doses of 5 to 10 mg for as long as 9 to 12 months may be required in patients with widely disseminated or progressive lesions.

LEPROSY

Although not a common disease in North America or Europe, the lepromatous form of leprosy bears many immunlogic similarities to Hodgkin's disease and sarcoidosis.[27]

Lepromatous leprosy is characterized pathologically by diffuse granulomatous infiltrations of the skin, mucous membranes, and nervous system. These changes are generally associated with anergy to cutaneous allergens which usually induce delayed-type hypersensitivity in normal individuals.[31] In addition, there is evidence of impaired lymphocyte transformation in some patients with the disease. On the other hand, it is sometimes possible to obtain partial reversal of cutaneous anergy to tuberculin, histoplasmin, and lepromin in lepromatous patients by means of leukocyte transfer from patients sensitive to these allergens.[25] After treatment, delayed hypersensitivity responses may become more normal.

Levels of IgG and IgA immunoglobulins tend to be increased in lepromatous leprosy, whereas IgM levels are usually normal. The ability to develop circulating antibodies remains normal and there is no evidence of impaired phagocytosis.

INFECTIOUS MONONUCLEOSIS

Infectious mononucleosis is a benign, transient disease of presumed viral origin characterized by a striking lymphocytosis, lymphadenopathy, and the presence of large numbers of atypical lymphocytes in the peripheral circulation. Other typical features include the presence of heterophile antibodies, numerous other heteroantibodies and autoantibodies, and a frequent increase in serum immunoglobulin levels.

PATHOLOGY

Because infectious mononucleosis is almost always a benign, self-limited condition, the most significant morphologic changes are those described in peripheral blood smears. On light microscopy, the abnormal or "atypical lymphocytes" found in infectious mononucleosis are larger than normal adult lymphocytes, stain more darkly, and frequently show vacuolization of the cytoplasm. Another characteristic finding is the "ballerina skirt" appearance of the cytoplasm which presumably occurs due to indentation of the cell margins of the abnormal cells by erythrocytes and other formed elements of the blood. However, none of these changes are specific for infectious mononucleosis, and may appear in normal individuals or in patients with a wide variety of infectious diseases, particularly those of viral etiology.

Examination of histologic sections of enlarged lymph nodes in infectious mononucleosis usually reveals considerable variation in structure—a feature which is not common in lymphatic leukemia. Typical microscopic findings may include (1) scattered "atypical" lymphocytes similar to those found in the peripheral blood; (2) small groups of large cells with basophilic cytoplasm and clear nuclei; and (3) extensive proliferation of macrophages throughout the node. Hyperplasia of reticulum cells or marked lymphocytic proliferation may occasionally lead to difficulty in distinguishing between infectious mononucleosis and Hodgkin's disease or lymphosarcoma. However, the presence of atypical lymphoid elements in the same section is in favor of a diagnosis of infectious mononucleosis.

ETIOLOGY

An infectious etiology for infectious mononucleosis has long been postulated on the basis of epidemiologic data. The increased prevalence of infectious mononucleosis among young people living under relatively crowded conditions (e.g., boarding schools, colleges, and military camps) constitutes the major evidence for this hypothesis. However, in the past, there has been virtually no direct or even indirect evidence to implicate a causative agent in infectious mononucleosis.

Recently, it has been observed that significant titers of anti-EB virus antibodies (Epstein-Barr virus, herpes-like virus, or HLV) can be detected in the sera of patients with infectious mononucleosis by the techniques of immunofluorescence or complement-fixation.[13] The EB virus is similar to the herpes-like organism that has been detected by electron microscopy in cell lines derived from Burkitt's lymphoma (see Chapter 13), leukemic tissues, or buffy coats obtained from normal individuals or patients with a variety of other illnesses.

Despite the rather ubiquitous occurrence of the EB virus, there are certain observations which strengthen the possible causal relationship between EB virus and infectious mononucleosis. In patients with well-defined infectious mononucleosis, there is an excellent correlation between the presence of EB virus antibodies and heterophile antibodies. Furthermore, EB virus antibodies have been detected in patients who present with the clinical features of infectious mononucleosis but have a negative heterophile test. This latter observation would suggest that at least some "seronegative" patients have true infectious mononucleosis.

Of particular interest is a prospective study of infectious mononucleosis carried out among university students.[6] Of the students who had no EB virus antibody at the time of admission, 14 per cent subsequently contracted infectious mononucleosis within the next four years. On the other hand, none of the freshmen with EB virus antibodies developed infectious mononucleosis. All of the students with infectious mononucleosis demonstrated significant titers of EB virus antibodies and heterophile antibodies in their sera during the course of the illness.

In most of the reported investigations, EB virus antibodies tend to appear slightly later than the heterophile antibodies, but may persist for years after the heterophile antibodies have disappeared.

Nevertheless, a certain amount of caution is required in the interpretation of essentially serologic data. EB virus antigen has been demonstrated by immunofluorescence in long-term leukocyte cultures obtained from patients with infectious mononucleosis and virus particles have been observed by electron microscopy in the same preparation.[4] However, the virus has still not been isolated from patients with infectious mononucleosis, and virus particles have not been identified by electron microscopy in freshly isolated leukocytes. Furthermore, it has been reported that significant titers of EB virus antibody have been found in heterophile negative patients with the typical clinical and laboratory findings of infectious hepatitis.[10] It is conceivable that EB virus may represent a latent or "passenger" virus which is activated by the disease processes of infectious mononucleosis. The recent demonstration of antibodies to EB virus in patients with sarcoidosis constitutes an interesting, but unexplained, observation.

A number of other viral agents have been suggested as possible causes of heterophile-positive infectious mononucleosis, but the evidence is less convincing than for the EB virus. For example, sera from patients with infectious mononucleosis have been shown to agglutinate Hep-2 cells infected with Newcastle disease virus in tissue culture and to form precipitin bands in agar gel against Newcastle disease virus preparations. It is unlikely that there is significant antigenic cross-reactivity between the herpes-like viruses discussed above and Newcastle disease virus. The HLV are DNA containing organisms, whereas NDV belongs to the myxovirus group of RNA viruses.

IMMUNOLOGY

Heterophile Antibodies

The presence of heterophile antibodies has been used for many years as a nonspecific diagnostic test for infectious mononucleosis. Heterophile antibodies which agglutinate xenogeneic red blood cells (e.g., sheep, ox, beef) appear in about 90 per cent of patients with the typical clinical and laboratory findings of infectious mononucleosis, but may also appear in normal patients or in patients with other disease processes. However, in patients without infectious mononucleosis, the heteroagglutinins for sheep red blood cells can be removed completely by absorption with guinea pig or horse kidney preparations. In infectious mononucleosis, differential absorption will not lower the heterophile antibody titer.

A heterophile titer of at least 128 to 256 is considered in most laboratories to be necessary for the positive diagnosis of infectious mononucleosis. The more recently developed formalized horse cell spot test would appear to give comparable results to the classic Davidsohn differential absorption test, and is used in many clinics as a rapid diagnostic screening procedure.

Other Antibodies

A wide variety of circulating antibodies has been described in infectious mononucleosis, but their significance in the etiology or pathogenesis of the disease remains obscure. Elevated α-2 globulins and increased serum IgM levels are often observed during the acute phase of the disease. Despite the fact that the classic heterophile antibody considered to be diagnostic of infectious mononucleosis belongs to the IgM class of immunoglobulins, there appears to be no significant correlation between serum IgM levels and heterophile antibody titers.

Other antibodies which have been described in infectious mononucleosis include antinuclear antibodies, cryoglobulins of mixed IgG and IgM composition, cold agglutinins with anti-i specificity which are predominantly of the IgM type, rheumatoid factor, and a variety of IgM heteroantibodies directed against bacterial antigens such as proteus OX-19, salmonella, and streptococcus MG. Autoimmune hemolytic anemia of the cold agglutinin type (see Chapter 9) occurs to a varying degree in about 25 per cent of patients with infectious mononucleosis.

Cellular Immunology

Long-term lymphocyte suspension cultures can be established with relative ease from the peripheral blood of patients with infectious mononucleosis.[4] Circulating lymphocytes with a potential for long-term in vitro proliferation have also been described in patients with a variety of lymphoproliferative disorders such as lymphocytic leukemia, Hodgkin's disease, and lymphosarcoma. In healthy individuals, the establishment of such cell lines is feasible, but generally requires large quantities of blood with multiple simultaneous cultures. There is no evidence that cell lines derived from patients with heterophile-positive, infectious mononucleosis produce heterophile antibodies, heteroagglutinins, or hemolytic antibodies, despite the fact that immunoglobulin synthesis is normal.[9]

Two recent observations are of particular interest with respect to a possible relationship between infectious mononucleosis and Hodgkin's disease: (1) cells resembling Sternberg-Reed cells have been observed in biopsy material from serologically proved cases of infectious mononucleosis; and (2) a single patient with serologically proved infectious mononucleosis and an EB virus titer of 1:640 developed Hodgkin's disease 6 months after the onset of his original symptoms.[5a]

CLINICAL MANIFESTATIONS

The clinical features of infectious mononucleosis vary considerably among patients, but a typical patient may show signs of fever, generalized malaise, discrete, moderately enlarged lymph nodes (particularly in the posterior cervical chain), and splenomegaly. A sore throat with pharyngeal inflammation, tonsillar enlargement, and exudative tonsillitis is an extremely common finding. Another frequent manifestation of infectious mononucleosis is hepatitis with hepatomegaly, nausea, and occasional jaundice.

Other less common signs and symptoms include a macular or maculopapular skin eruption, ocular edema, CNS involvement with headache and neck stiffness, Guillain-Barre syndrome, Bell's palsy, pulmonary involvement with chest pain and cough, and myocardial involvement with tachycardia and arrhythmias.

Abnormal laboratory findings include the atypical lymphocytes and the heterophile antibodies which have been described previously. In addition, abnormalities of liver function, as measured by enzyme determinations such as alkaline phosphatase and serum glutamic-oxaloacetic transaminase (SGOT), are frequently observed. The serum bilirubin may occasionally be elevated and hyperuricemia is found in about 20 per cent of cases.

In the average uncomplicated case, the fever disappears spontaneously in about 10 days, but lymphadenopathy and splenomegaly may persist for as long as 4 weeks. Recurrences or protracted illness (as long as 3 months) are not uncommon, and the heterophile antibody titer may remain elevated for 4 to 6 months. Spontaneous rupture of the spleen, or rupture due to excessive palpation is an uncommon, but serious complication.

TREATMENT

There is no specific therapy for infectious mononucleosis. In severely ill patients, dramatic relief may occur occasionally following the administration of systemic corticosteroids (e.g., prednisone, 40 to 60 mg, daily in divided doses) for 5 to 10 days.

LYMPHOPROLIFERATIVE SYNDROMES RESEMBLING INFECTIOUS MONONUCLEOSIS

ACUTE INFECTIOUS LYMPHOCYTOSIS

The term acute infectious lymphocytosis is sometimes used to describe a syndrome which has certain broad similarities to infectious mononucleosis. The syndrome is characterized by an increased number of normal appearing small lymphocytes in the peripheral blood and occasionally in the bone marrow. The white blood cell count may range from 20,000 to 100,000, and eosinophilia may also be present. The syndrome usually occurs in children as a mild transient illness which is manifested by signs and symptoms of upper respiratory tract infection, abdominal pain, diarrhea, and, less commonly, by meningoencephalitis or morbilliform rash. Splenomegaly and lymphadenopathy occur infrequently.

Patients with acute infectious lymphocytosis have neither heterophile nor EB virus antibodies in their serum. However, in one outbreak, there was considerable evidence to suggest a causal relationship between acute infectious lymphocytosis and an enterovirus resembling the Coxsackie A subgroup.[14] Increased titers of neutralizing antibodies against this enterovirus were found in patients with the syndrome, and the virus was isolated from 20 per cent of the patients' stool specimens.

CYTOMEGALOVIRUS MONONUCLEOSIS

Cytomegalovirus infection in immunologically competent adults may be an occasional cause of a syndrome resembling heterophile-negative infectious mononucelosis.[26] Cytomegalovirus mononucleosis usually presents with fever, myalgia, headache, and cough. Occasionally, there is a transient morbilliform rash, but there is usually no pharyngitis, lymphadenopathy or hepatosplenomegaly.

The patients may develop a leukocytosis of 15,000 to 20,000/mm³ with 60 to 80 per cent lymphocytes in the differential count. In contrast to acute infectious lymphocytosis, the majority of the lymphocytes are of the atypical type similar to those seen in infectious mononucleosis. Complement-fixing antibodies against cytomegalovirus may be demonstrated in the sera of patients with this syndrome, and cytomegalovirus may be cultured from their urine and saliva. The significance of cytomegalovirus infection in opportunistic pulmonary infections is discussed in Chapter 4.

OTHER CAUSES

Other possible causes of syndromes resembling heterophile-negative infectious mononucleosis include mumps, acute infections with adenoviruses, and *Toxoplasma gondii*.

REFERENCES

1. Berger, H. W., Zaldivar, C., and Chusid, L. Anonymous mycobacteria in the etiology of sarcoidosis. *Ann. Intern. Med.* 68:872, 1968.

1a. Buckley, C. E., III, and Dorsey, F. A. A comparison of serum immuno-globulin concentrations in sarcoidosis and tuberculosis. *Ann. Inter. Med. 72:*37, 1970.

2. Chapman, J. S., and Speight, M. Further studies of mycobacterial antibodies in the sera of sarcoidosis. *Acta Med. Scand. 176* (suppl. 425):61, 1964.

3. Chase, M. W. Delayed-type hypersensitivity and the immunology of Hodgkin's disease with a parallel examination of sarcoidosis. *Cancer Res. 26:*1097, 1966.

4. Chessin, L. N., Glade, P. R., Kassel, J. A. Moses, H. L., Herberman, R. B., and Hirshaut, Y. The circulating lymphocyte—Its role in infectious mononucleosis. *Ann. Intern. Med. 69:*333, 1968.

5. Crowther, D., Fairley, G. H., and Sewell, R. L. Significance of the changes in circulating lymphoid cells in Hodgkin's disease. *Brit. Med. J. 2:*473, 1969.

5a. England, J. M., III. Infectious mononucleosis followed by Hodgkin's disease. *Lancet 1:*948, 1970.

6. Evans, A. S., Neiderman, J. C., and McCollum, R. W. Seroepidemiologic studies of infectious mononucleosis with EB virus. *New Eng. J. Med. 279:*1121, 1968.

7. Fireman, P., Friday, G., and Kumate, J. Effect of measles vaccine on immunologic responsiveness. *Pediatrics 43:*264, 1969.

8. Gams, R. A., Neal, J. A., Conrad, F. G. Hydantoin-induced pseudo-pseudolymphoma. *Ann. Intern. Med. 69:*3, 1968.

9. Glade, P. R., and Chessin, L. N. Infectious mononucleosis: Immunoglobulin synthesis by cell lines. *J. Clin. Invest. 47:*2391, 1968.

10. Glade, P. R., Hirshaut, Y., Douglas, S. D., and Hirshhorn, K. Lymphoid suspension cultures from patients with viral hepatitis. *Lancet 2:*1273, 1968.

11. Goldman, J. M., and Hobbs, J. R. The immunoglobulins in Hodgkin's disease. *Immunology 13:*421, 1967.

12. Gunz, F. W., and Angus, H. B. Leukemia and cancer in the same patient. *Cancer 18:*145, 1965.

13. Henle, G., Henle, W., and Diehl, V. Relation of Burkitt's tumor-associated herpes-type virus to infectious mononucleosis. *Proc. Nat. Acad. Sci. U.S.A. 59:*94, 1968.

14. Horwitz, M. S., and Moore, G. T. Acute infectious lymphocytosis: An etiologic and epidemiologic study of an outbreak. *New Eng. J. Med. 279:*399, 1968.

15. Israel, H. L. The diagnosis of sarcoidosis. *Ann. Intern. Med. 68:*1323, 1968.

16. Kelly, W. D., and Good, R. A. "Immunologic Deficiency in Hodgkin's Disease," in Bergsma, D. (ed.), *Immunologic Deficiency Diseases in Man,* New York, The National Foundation, 1968, p. 349.

17. Latourette, H. B. Induction of lymphoma and leukemia by diagnostic and therapeutic irradiation. *Radiol. Clin. N. Amer. 6:*57, 1968.

17a. Lindstrom, F. D., Williams, R. C., Jr., and Theogides, A. Urinary light chain excretion in leukaemia and lymphoma. *Clin. Exp. Immun. 5:*83, 1969.

18. Lukes, R. J., and Butler, J. J. The pathology and nomenclature of Hodgkin's disease. *Cancer Res. 26:*1063, 1966.

19. Mankiewicz, E., and Beland, J. The role of mycobacteriophages and of cortisone in experimental tuberculosis and sarcoidosis. *Amer. Rev. Resp. Dis. 89:*707, 1964.

20. Mellors, R., and Huang, C. Y. Immunopathology of NMZ/Bl mice: VI. Virus separable from spleen and pathogenic for Swiss mice. *J. Exp. Med. 126:*53, 1967.

21. Miller, D. G. The association of immune disease and malignant lymphoma. *Ann. Intern. Med. 66:*507, 1967.

22. Miller, D. G. The immunologic capability of patients with lymphoma. *Cancer Res. 28:*1275, 1968.

23. Millian, S. J., Miller, D. G., and Schaeffer, N. Viral complement-fixing antibody in patients with Hodgkin's disease, lymphosarcoma, reticulum cell sarcoma and chronic lymphocytic leukemia. *Cancer 18:*677, 1965.

23a. Moore, D. F., Migliore, P. J., Shulenberger, C. C., and Alexinian, R. Monoclonal macroglobulinemia in malignant lymphoma. *Ann. Intern. Med. 72:*43, 1970.

24. Muftuoglu, A. U., and Balkur, S. Passive transfer of tuberculin sensitivity to patients with Hodgkin's disease. *New Eng. J. Med. 277:*126, 1968.

25. Paradisi, E., deBonaparte, Y. P., and Morgenfeld, M. C. Response in two groups of anergic patients to the transfer of leukocytes from sensitive donors. *New Eng. J. Med. 280:*859, 1969.

26. Rifkind, D. Cytomegalovirus Mononucleosis. *Ann. Intern. Med. 69:*842, 1968.

27. Sheagren, J. N., Block, J. B., Trautman, J. R., and Wolff, S. M. Immunologic reactivity in patients with leprosy. *Ann. Intern. Med. 70:*295, 1969.

28. Siltzbach, L. E., and Greenberg, G. M. Childhood sarcoidosis—A study of 18 patients. *New Eng. J. Med. 279:*23, 1968.

29. Smithers, D. W. Hodgkin's disease II. *Brit. Med. J. 2:*337, 1967.

30. Trubowitz, S., Masek, B., and Del Rosario, A. D. Lymphocyte response to phytohemagglutinin in Hodgkin's disease, lymphatic leukemia, and lymphosarcoma. *Cancer 19:*2019, 1967.

31. Turk, J. L., and Waters, M. F. R. Cell-mediated immunity in patients with leprosy. *Lancet 2:*243, 1969.

13

Human Cancer Immunology

PHIL GOLD

The possible role of immunologic factors in determining host resistance to cancer has been extensively investigated over the past decade.[9] There is now convincing evidence that tumor-specific transplantation antigens (TSTA) may occur in rodent tumors induced by a variety of chemical carcinogens or oncogenic viruses. In general, different tumors induced by the same virus show extensive antigenic cross-reactivity, whereas the antigens of chemically-induced tumors are usually individually distinctive. If the TSTA are similar to normal transplantation antigens, they are probably lipid-protein-polysaccharide complexes in which the protein component is the most likely determinant group (see Chapter 14). Hence, the cross-reactivity between the TSTA of virus-induced tumors would suggest the incorporation and persistence of viral genetic material within the tumor cells.

Despite the modifications of host immune reactivity which may be caused by chemical carcinogens or oncogenic viruses, an animal bearing a freshly induced tumor is able to direct an immune response against the TSTA of the proliferating cancer cells. The available experimental evidence would suggest that cell-mediated immune reactions are probably more important than humoral antibodies in determining defense mechanisms against individual animal tumors.[2]

Since most experimental tumors are quite capable of killing their hosts, the existence of TSTA in a growing tumor in no way assures its rejection. Conversely, the lack of demonstrable tumor rejection on the part of the host does not necessarily indicate that the tumor lacks TSTA. The immunologic rejection of animal tumors requires specific stimulation of the host's immune system against tumor antigens, but this stimulation must take place before the induction or transplantation of the experimental tumor. Thus, it would appear that the TSTA are only weakly antigenic, and evoke a correspondingly weak immune response.

In humans, the supposition that there may be a comparable immune reaction of the host against his own tumor has inevitably led to a search for tumor-specific antigens in human neoplastic tissues. To state conclusively that patients with malignant disease are capable of reacting against tumor antigens would require a definitive answer to several questions: (1) Is there any evidence that human tumors contain antigenic components not present in normal tissues? (2) Can human tumor-specific antigens be distinguished experimentally from species-specific or individual-specific antigens? (3) Are these antigenic components capable of evoking an immunologic response in the human host of origin? (4) What is the effect, if any, of the immunologic response to tumor-specific antigens on the course of human cancer?

In this chapter, an attempt will be made to answer these questions with particular reference to those human tumors which have been investigated from an immunologic point of view.

CARCINOEMBRYONIC ANTIGEN OF THE HUMAN DIGESTIVE SYSTEM

A major difficulty in the antigenic analysis of human tumors is the lack of suitable normal control tissue for comparison with the tumor tissue under investigation. Unlike comparable animal experiments where normal tissues from syngeneic donors are readily available, human studies have been handicapped by a failure to distinguish between tumor-specific antigens and individual-specific antigens.

Human colonic cancer was utilized for studies on human digestive system antigens because this tumor almost never extends intramurally for more than 6 to 7 cm on either side of the lesion visible on gross examination.[10,11] Normal and neoplastic colonic tissues can be obtained from the same donor at the time of operation, thus eliminating confusion between tumor-specific and individual-specific antigens.

Rabbit antisera prepared against extracts of human colonic cancer were absorbed with an excess of normal colonic tissue obtained from the same donor. Using the technique of double diffusion in agar gel, it was then possible to demonstrate that human adenocarcinomata arising from the entodermally derived digestive system epithelium (rectum, colon, stomach, esophagus, liver, and pancreas) contained an identical tumor-specific antigen. A similar constituent was found in embryonic and fetal gut, pancreas, and liver during the first two trimesters of gestation. Because this antigenic component could not be detected in any other normal, diseased, or neoplastic tissues, it was named the carcinoembryonic antigen (CEA) of the human digestive system.

It is possible that the CEA may represent a cellular constituent which is repressed during the course of differentiation of the normal digestive system epithelium and which reappears in the corresponding malignant cells by a process of reversion to a more primitive state (derepressive-dedifferentiation).

Additional studies indicated that the CEA was a protein-polysaccharide complex of a consistent amino acid and carbohydrate composition, and was probably located close to the cell surface as determined by immuno-fluorescent staining techniques (Fig. 13-1). By means of ultrastructural techniques, it was possible to localize the antigenic material to the glycocalyx which surrounds the cell membrane (Fig. 13-2).[12]

Recently, a radioimmunoassay has been developed which is capable of detecting minute quantities of CEA liberated from bowel cancers into the circulation (see Table 13-1).[27] This technique appears to hold considerable promise as a diagnostic procedure for the early detection of cancer of the colon, and furthermore, it may prove to be of value in determining the prognosis of established lesions. For example, a strongly positive test may indicate a large tumor mass or metastatic spread of the primary tumor. In those cases where the serum concentration of CEA (see Table 13-1) falls to an undetectable level following surgery, the reappearance of antigen in the serum after several months would suggest a recurrence of tumor growth.

Some patients with proven primary gastrointestinal cancers, as well as pregnant women, were found to have circulating antibodies against the CEA by the hemagglutination technique (Table 13-2), but there was no correlation between the presence of antibodies and the clinical course of the neoplastic disease.[8] The spontaneously occurring anti-CEA antibodies in cancer patients and pregnant women were found to be predominantly macroglobulin in nature. Although the hemagglutination technique is biased

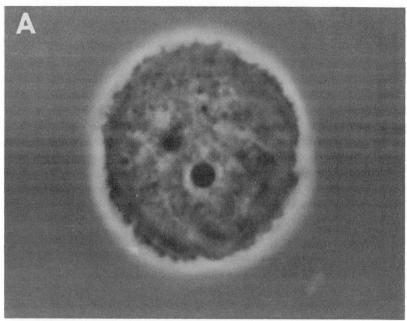

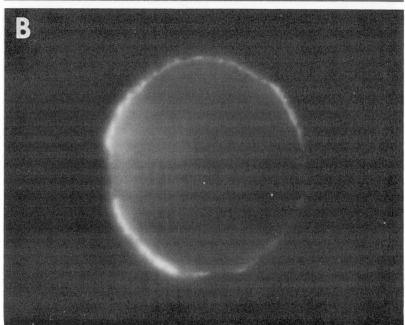

FIG. 13-1. Explanted cell of a colonic cancer reacted with fluorescein-conjugated anti-CEA antiserum. *A*, Phase contrast microscopy. *B*, Same cell observed by fluorescence microscopy, demonstrating "ring" or "beaded necklace" pattern of antigen localization to the cell surface. (Original magnification X 1250.)

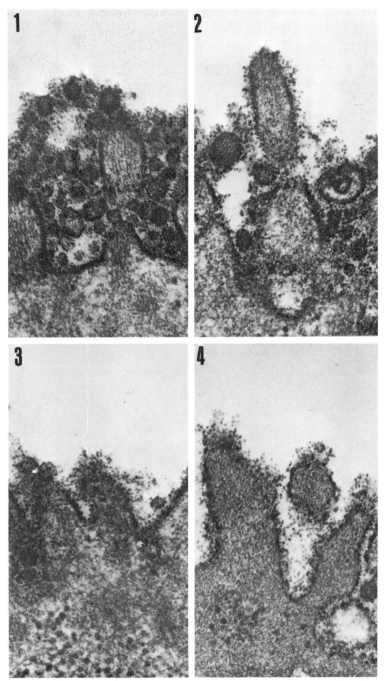

FIG. 13-2. Four areas of colonic cancer tissue reacted with ferritin-conjugated anti-CEA antiserum. Plasma membranes, outlined by Ruthenium Red, remain unlabeled. Ferritin is localized to glycocalyceal areas. (Electron photomicrograph X 100,000.)

TABLE 13-1. Circulating CEA as Measured by Radioimmunoassay

Subjects	Number tested	Number with detectable serum CEA	Serum concentration (ng/ml)
Normal subjects	28	0	—
Patients with colonic and rectal cancer			
Pre-operative	11	10	3–320
Post-operative			
No residual tumor	26	0	—
Residual, recurrent, or			
metastatic tumor*	23	23	8 to greater than 320
Patients with cancers of other digestive organs	32	3	2–160
Noncancerous diseases of the digestive system	20	0	—
Nonenteric cancer, and other miscellaneous			
diseases	36	0	—
Pregnant women	23	0	—

   * In general, the greater the quantity of tumor tissue, the higher the serum concentration of CEA.

TABLE 13-2. Circulating Anti-CEA Antibodies as Measured by Passive Hemagglutination

Subjects	Number tested	Number of positive reactions
Normals	14	0
Nonmetastatic digestive system cancer	30	25
Metastatic digestive system cancer	18	0
Noncancerous digestive system disease	32	2
Nondigestive system cancer	13	0
Miscellaneous noncancerous, nonenteric diseases	20	0
Normal pregnancies	18	11
Postpartum (1–7 days)	4	4
Spontaneous abortions	8	5

toward the detection of IgM antibodies, the apparent lack of effect of the maternal antibodies on the fetus may possibly be explained by their inability to cross the placenta.

It is also of interest that the anti-CEA antibodies were never detected after tumor dissemination had occurred. Because the CEA is a component of the tumor cell surface, the possibility exists that the antigen in a large mass of tumor might adsorb circulating anti-CEA antibodies if they were able to gain access to the tumor tissue. On the other hand, the demonstration of circulating CEA in the sera of patients with digestive system cancers suggests that circulating antigen-antibody complexes might be formed. In the latter event, it would not be possible to detect free antibody in the circulation.

The biologic significance of the anti-CEA antibodies is not completely clear at the present time, although several tentative conclusions may be reached. The implication is that these antibodies are either not protective to the host, or that they exist in insufficient quantity to produce a detectable cytolytic effect. It is also conceivable that they may be responsible for tumor growth enhancement by coating tumor cells with antibody globulin and thus protecting them from the cytolytic effects of cellular immune mechanisms. In addition, the anti-CEA antibodies might cause tumor enhancement by a negative feedback mechanism which results in a central suppression of the immune response. The relative importance of circulating antibodies and cellular immunity in determining host resistance to the growth of digestive system tumors is unknown at present.

Other investigators have described digestive system antigens which appear to be qualitatively different from the CEA.[18] These other digestive system antigens are not tumor-specific because they are found in normal tissues as well as in digestive system tumors. However, there is often a significant difference in the concentration of these tumor-associated digestive system antigens between normal and tumor tissues.

ALPHA₁-FETOPROTEINS IN PRIMARY HEPATOMA

An additional relationship between embryonic and tumor antigens was suggested by the observation that certain chemically induced mouse hepatomas synthesized an α_1-globulin lacking in normal adult mouse organs, but present in the tissues and sera of embryonic and neonatal mice.[1] The α_1-globulin associated with mouse hepatomas was also detected in the tissues of noncancerous mice during the process of liver regeneration after partial hepatectomy.

A similar α_1-globulin component was subsequently found in the sera of patients suffering from primary hepatomas. This substance, which has been named α_1-fetoprotein, is absent from normal adult human serum. Currently available evidence would suggest that the detection of α_1-fetoprotein in human sera by the technique of double diffusion in agar gel constitutes a useful diagnostic test for the detection of human primary hepatomas.[3] However, it should be noted that positive results are obtained with this technique in a small percentage of patients with other liver diseases, and in approximately 10 per cent of patients with teratoblastomas.[6] Serum α_1-fetoprotein can be detected in the sera of about 50 per cent of Caucasians with primary hepatomas and, depending on geographic location, in up to 80 per cent of non-Caucasians with primary hepatomas.

Recently, fetoprotein has been detected in the sera of 5 out of 10 pyridoxine-deficient baboons, but there was no evidence that the liver cells in these animals had undergone malignant transformation. This observation would suggest that pyridoxine deficiency is capable of inducing derepressive dedifferentiation in primate liver cells without a concomitant malignant change, or that α_1-fetoprotein synthesis may precede morphologic evidence of tumor transformation.

From the studies on CEA and on α_1-fetoproteins, it would appear that antigenic reversion during malignant transformation in human tissues is probably not an uncommon occurrence. In this context, the term "archiplasm," implying the reappearance of an early or old tissue component, would serve as a better synonym for cancer than the term neoplasm. The function of these primitive components in some forms of human cancer remains essentially unknown.

FUNCTIONAL REVERSION IN OTHER HUMAN CANCER TISSUES

A ferroprotein of hepatic origin, the α_2H globulin, is present in fetal organs and sera, but is not found in normal human serum 2 months after birth. This ferritin-like protein has, however, been detected by the technique of radioimmunodiffusion in the sera of approximately 80 per cent of children with a variety of tumors. However, approximately 10 per cent of sera from children with benign diseases were positive as well.[4] Similarly, a fetal sulphoglycoprotein has been identified in the gastric juice of 96 per cent of patients with carcinoma of the stomach, but was also found in 12 per cent of patients with other gastric diseases.[12a]

The ectopic production of these substances by cancerous tissues may well be considered as loss of specialization which may or may not be followed by redifferentiation along abnormal lines. The production of α_1-fetoproteins by testicular teratoblastomas, already noted, may well be an example of this type of phenomenon. Moreover, the inappropriate production and secretion of hormones by other malignant tumors is well recognized.

Recently, an alkaline phosphatase isoenzyme (Regan isoenzyme) has been identified in the sera of approximately 5 per cent of patients with various malignant tumors. This isoenzyme is biochemically and immunologically indistinguishable from placental alkaline phosphatase, and has been detected in both tumor tissue and in malignant effusion fluids. Measurement of this material is claimed to be useful in monitoring progression or regression of tumor, in identifying a source of serum alkaline phosphatase elevation, and in identifying malignant effusions.[25]

LYMPHOPROLIFERATIVE AND MYELOPROLIFERATIVE DISORDERS

BURKITT'S LYMPHOMA

In 1958, Burkitt described a tumor syndrome in African children which has subsequently been observed, but much more sporadically, in other parts of the world. The tumor manifests a peculiar predilection for growth in the jaw and facial bones, and many remain localized to the face. However, in most patients, there is widespread disease which runs its fatal course in a few months.

Histologically, the lesion has been identified as a malignant lymphoma, and, as such, has been of great interest to cancer chemotherapists because of its relative sensitivity to alkylating agents. Treatment with short, intensive courses of cyclophosphamide (e.g., 40 mg/kg, intravenously, repeated if necessary) has induced long-term remissions in approximately 20 per cent of cases, and a number of such patients are said to have been cured.

Epidemiologic studies indicate that the etiology of Burkitt's tumor is intimately related to an arthropod-borne infectious agent. This conclusion has been strengthened by the close association of endemic malaria with the geographic distribution of Burkitt's tumor. It has, in fact, been recently suggested that persistent immunologic stimulation by malarial infection and the concomitant lymphoreticular hyperplasia may be an important factor in the development of Burkitt's lymphoma.[24]

Electron microscopic examination of continuous cell cultures of Burkitt origin has now provided convincing evidence that a small proportion of most cell lines harbor virus particles indistinguishable from the herpes group of DNA viruses.[15] For convenience, this agent is referred to as EB (Epstein-Barr) virus, after the EB-1 line of Burkitt cells from which it was first isolated. (See section on infectious mononucleosis in Chapter 12 for further comments on EB virus.)

Great controversy still exists regarding the relationship between Burkitt's tumor, so-called conventional childhood lymphosarcoma, and acute leukemia in children. Nevertheless, if the EB virus could be established as a causative agent in Burkitt's tumor, it would provide the first example of a proven human oncogenic virus. The findings in Burkitt's lymphoma are of particular interest because herpes-like virus particles have been observed in a number of continuous suspension cultures of blast-type cells derived from lymph nodes, bone marrow, or buffy coats of patients with leukemia and other malignancies. However, similar viral particles have also been seen in cells cultured from patients with nonmalignant diseases as well as from peripheral leukocytes of healthy donors.

These observations have led some workers to caution that the EB virus may merely be a passenger in the type of culture examined.[15] Members of the herpes-group of DNA viruses frequently persist in patients who have recovered from illnesses induced by these agents. The virus may be subsequently reactivated as the result of various stimuli such as immunosuppressive therapy and debilitating diseases. Furthermore, it is possible that the EB virus may simply represent a common contaminant of long-term leukocyte cultures.

There is a great deal of experimental data available concerning the immunologic response to virus-induced tumors in animals. For this reason, an attempt has been made to obtain similar data in patients with Burkitt's lymphoma. Studies employing the technique of indirect membrane fluorescence indicate that the plasma membrane of the Burkitt cell may contain tumor-specific antigens capable of inducing an antibody response in the human host.[16] Furthermore, the sera from a significant number of patients demonstrate cross-reactions with lines of Burkitt cells other than their own, suggesting the presence of the same tumor-specific antigens in tumors of different individuals. These observations are entirely analogous to those which have been made with virus-induced animal tumors. It has also been found that leukocytes obtained from patients with infectious mononucleosis possess plasma membrane antigens which are indistinguishable by the immunofluorescent technique from those found in Burkitt's lymphoma cells.[17]

However, cautious interpretation of the available data is necessary. Further evidence from other laboratories, employing different techniques, will obviously be essential to the understanding of the exact etiology of Burkitt's lymphoma and the host-tumor interactions which occur in this condition.

The unusual susceptibility of Burkitt's lymphoma to cancer chemotherapeutic agents would suggest that the immunologic response may be of importance in host resistance. This contention is supported by the recent demonstration that certain patients with Burkitt's lymphoma demonstrate delayed type hypersensitivity reactions to antigens extracted from autologous tumor cells.[7] Positive skin responses were almost invariably limited to individuals who experienced significant clinical remissions after treatment. Moreover, the development of delayed type hypersensitivity was associated with more sustained clinical improvement than was found in patients where a comparable response was not observed.

In the light of the foregcing considerations, it is conceivable that the destruction of a relatively small number of malignant cells by appropriate chemotherapy may be sufficient to tip the balance in favor of tumor destruction by the host's own immunologic mechanisms.

OTHER LYMPHOPROLIFERATIVE AND MYELOPROLIFERATIVE DISORDERS

Several reports in recent years have suggested that human leukemic cells contain specific antigens which distinguish them qualitatively from their normal counterparts. Experiments utilizing the mixed lymphocyte reaction (see Chapter 14) demonstrated that human leukemic cells, appropriately stored, had a mitogenic effect on autologous lymphocytes obtained during remission. Moreover, mitomycin C-inactivated leukemic cells from a monozygotic twin with leukemia produced significant stimulation of lymphocytes obtained from the other healthy twin.

In these studies, it was apparent that mitogenic stimulation in mixed lymphocyte culture was the result of differences between HL-A transplantation antigens in the two groups of lymphocytes. In the two situations described above, an HL-A difference should not have existed unless a neoantigen associated with the HL-A system arose during the process of leukemic transformation. It is, therefore, particularly interesting that a recent study revealed a distinct correlation between the development of leukemia and certain patterns of the HL-A transplantation antigen system.[28] However, other workers have been unable to confirm these results.

The effect of Hodgkin's disease, lymphosarcoma, and chronic lymphatic leukemia on the immunologic system is discussed in Chapter 12; thymoma is discussed in Chapter 11; and multiple myeloma in Chapter 10.

ACCIDENTAL TUMOR TRANSPLANTATION

A number of accidental tumor allografts have taken place during transplantation of cadaveric kidneys from patients with metastatic cancer to recipients suffering from chronic renal disease. The immunologic significance of accidental tumor transplantation is best illustrated by comparing two reported patients in whom the transplanted tumor was a bronchogenic carcinoma.[20,29] In both instances, the recipients developed metastatic cancer from the renal source several months after successful kidney transplantation. Both patients had received immunosuppressive therapy in order to prevent renal graft rejection.

One patient died of widespread metastases 5 months after the graft. In the other patient, cessation of immunosuppressive therapy resulted in rejection of the kidney, but there was no immediate rejection of tumor tissue. However, when the rejected kidney, containing a large mass of tumor tissue, was removed, the residual metastatic cancer gradually disappeared. Furthermore, there was no evidence of tumor reappearance when a second successful kidney transplant was performed 9 months later, and the patient was placed on a full program of immunosuppression. Thus, complete destruction of the allografted cancer tissue would appear to have been accomplished by the host's immune system during a relatively brief period of normal function, once the mass of tumor tissue had been reduced.

The clinical situation described above is analogous to that found in experimental animal tumor systems where immunity has been induced. As described earlier, the state of tumor immunity only becomes apparent if the immunologic system is given a "head-start" on the tumor growth. In the case of the allografted tumor just considered, this advantage was presumably achieved by resecting a large proportion of the total tumor mass.

CHORIOCARCINOMA

A host-tumor relationship similar to that described for accidental tumor transplantation has been observed in women with choriocarcinomas. Choriocarcinoma is the term given to a malignant growth which develops in the uterus most commonly after a hydatidiform mole, but which may occasionally occur following any type of pregnancy. It is characterized by neoplastic proliferation of retained chorionic elements that invade the uterine wall and undergo metastases to remote organs. The interval between the primary pregnancy and clinical evidence of choriocarcinoma is usually about 4 to 6 months, but may vary from days to years.

The tumor arises from the chorionic membrane of the placenta and, therefore, contains components of both maternal and paternal origin. Because of the presence of paternal antigens, the tumor is, in fact, an allograft. Since choriocarcinomas are associated with a high fatality rate, this form of malignancy provides an excellent example of a human tumor which contains transplantation antigens foreign to the host, but which is not necessarily rejected. On the other hand, a number of regressions of metastatic choriocarcinoma have been reported following removal of the primary tumor. Furthermore, it is now well established that choriocarcinomas are very sensitive to cancer chemotherapeutic agents such as methotrexate, 25 mg/day for 5 days. With chemotherapy, the 5-year survival rate now probably exceeds 50 per cent. It is conceivable that both primary tumor removal and chemotherapy temporarily alter the tumor-host relationship in favor of the host so that an effective immune response promotes tumor regression.

Of particular immunologic interest is a case report of a single patient with metastatic choriocarcinoma which failed to regress on chemotherapy.[5] Apparent cure was achieved when the patient was immunized with her husband's leukocytes and was given antiserum prepared in rabbits against her husband's seminal fluid.

NEUROBLASTOMA

The immunologic response to neuroblastomas in children has been a subject of investigation because of the unusually high incidence of spontaneous regression reported with these tumors. Furthermore, neuroblastomas frequently regress when treated by methods considered to be insufficient for eradicating other tumors.

The colony-inhibition technique has proved to be particularly valuable for the detection of both humoral and cell-mediated immune reactions against the tumor-specific antigens of a variety of experimental and human tumor cell systems.[13] In a group of patients with neuroblastoma, the test was performed by exposing neuroblastoma cells in culture to the patient's own lymphocytes or to the lymphocytes of other patients with neuroblastomas. It was found that the growth of tumor cells was inhibited by autologous lymphocytes and by lymphocytes from other patients with neuroblastomas, but not by control lymphocytes.[14]

Another interesting finding was the observation that lymphocytes from the mothers of children with neuroblastomas inhibited neuroblastoma cells in culture regardless of whether the explanted tumor cells were obtained from the mother's own child or from other children. There are at least two possible explanations for these results: (1) neuroblastomas are induced by a virus which infects both mothers and children; or (2) the mothers are immunized during pregnancy against antigens from the fetal tumors.

SARCOMAS

Antibodies against a common antigen present in human osteosarcomas were detected by an immunofluorescence technique in the sera of nine patients with osteosarcoma.[22] Identical antibodies were found in the sera of 100 per cent of the patients' family members, 89 per cent of the patients' close contacts, and 25 per cent of randomly selected blood bank donors. In addition, the active sera frequently demonstrated immunologic cross-reactivity with sarcomas of other types, especially liposarcomas, fibrosarcomas, and chondrosarcomas.

The significance of these findings in relation to the etiology of human sarcomas in general, and osteosarcoma in particular, remains to be established. A genetic basis for osteosarcoma has been suggested by some workers because of the unusual familial incidence of this tumor. For example, there have been case reports of several siblings in the same family who developed osteosarcomas. In addition, these tumors may appear simultaneously at different sites in the same individual.

On the other hand, the finding of common tumor antibodies in patient contacts and the spontaneous appearance of multiple lesions is more in keeping with a viral etiology than a genetic basis for osteosarcoma. The validity of the viral hypothesis is reinforced by a number of observations. For example, a virus has been isolated from mice that induces lesions similar to osteosarcomas, and it has been shown that hamsters develop a low incidence of osteosarcomas following the injection of extracts of human osteosarcomas. Furthermore, it has been demonstrated that cell-free extracts from an osteosarcoma cell line: (1) induced antigenic and morphologic transformation of normal human embryo fibroblasts in tissue culture; and (2) induced the development of leukemias in mice. Electron microscopic examination of a tissue culture line of a human liposarcoma revealed type C virus particles, similar to avian and murine sarcoma viruses. Moreover, type A virus particles have been found in thin sections of tissues obtained from a human chondrosarcoma. The exact etiologic relationship between viral agents and the development of human sarcomas will undoubtedly be further clarified in the future.

MALIGNANT MELANOMA

Indirect evidence has accumulated from a number of sources that patients with malignant melanoma may develop an immune response against the growing tumor. For example, this malignant growth is one which occasionally undergoes spontaneous regression and may remain localized for long periods before dissemination. Moreover, even in patients with widespread disease, some metastatic deposits may regress while new ones appear and others continue to grow.

A number of studies, employing techniques such as immunofluorescence and cytotoxicity, have revealed that the sera of patients with melanoma often contain antibodies against their own tumor cells. Furthermore, certain of these antisera may demonstrate cross-reactivity with melanoma cell preparations from other patients with the same condition. It was found that melanoma patients produce two types of antibodies. One of these is active against cell surface components and is specific for the host's own tumor. The other reacts with cytoplasmic constituents present in most melanoma cell lines and presumably accounts for the cross-reactivity between sera.

In a report of 103 melanoma patients, it was found that over one-third of all of the sera studied had antibodies to autologous melanoma cells.[19] As in the case of the anti-CEA antibodies previously considered, the melanoma autoantibodies were virtually confined to patients in whom the disease had remained localized and had not undergone metastatic dissemination. In over 80 per cent of patients in whom serial studies were done, the autoantibodies disappeared as the disease became widespread.

CANCER CHEMOTHERAPY AND THE IMMUNE RESPONSE

The armamentarium of the cancer chemotherapist consists of seven classes of chemicals. These include alkylating agents, purine analogues, folic acid antagonists, halogenated pyrimidines, the vinca alkaloids, the corticosteroids and other hormones, and antibiotics (e.g., the actinomycin series). With few exceptions, the members of each class of drugs have a profound effect on the immune response. In animals, it has been demonstrated that these drugs are capable of inducing: (1) suppression of both humoral and cellular immune mechanisms; (2) specific immunologic tolerance to a variety of foreign antigens; (3) inhibition of transplantation immunity; and (4) enhancement of tumor growth. Thus, the terms immunosuppressive and anticancer in reference to this category of drugs are obviously interchangeable, and the choice of terms is entirely dependent on the situation in which they are employed. Much of what has been said regarding cancer chemotherapeutic agents may be equally well applied to radiation therapy.

Some workers have suggested that it is paradoxical, if not illogical, to employ immunosuppressive agents in cancer patients whose disease might possibly be due to a defect in immune resistance. On the other hand, it is somewhat difficult to reconcile this point of view with the demonstrated clinical effectiveness of chemotherapeutic agents in many forms of human cancer. Furthermore, as noted previously, anticancer drugs may even act additively with immunologic responses in such conditions as Burkitt's lymphoma and choriocarcinoma. Thus, before far reaching conclusions are drawn regarding the contraindications for using immunosuppressive drugs in cancer patients, a number of other factors must be considered.

Immunosuppressive anticancer agents are most effective in inhibiting a primary immune response, but are far less efficient in diminishing pre-existing levels of immunity. Since the tumor is always present for some time prior to the onset of chemotherapy, the primary immune response, if evoked at all, is presumably well established. It should also be remembered that there is a balance between the immunosuppressive and anticancer effects of the chemotherapeutic agents. Under these circumstances, a purely adverse immunosuppressive action should occur only if the tumor were completely insensitive to the drug, if drug resistance developed during ther-apy, or if the dosage and schedule of administration were inadequate for a significant anticancer effect. It should be noted as well that a few anti-cancer agents, such as uracil mustard, probably do not inhibit antibody synthesis when given in therapeutic doses.

IMMUNOPROPHYLAXIS AND IMMUNOTHERAPY OF HUMAN CANCER

At present, the immunoprophylaxis of human cancer is primarily of theo-retic interest. The lack of precise knowledge regarding the etiologic factors precludes even exploratory studies in this direction. Should a causative agent for any form of malignancy be conclusively demonstrated, it would take many years to determine the proper antigenic preparation for immuni-zation, the optimal time and route of administration, and the ultimate effectiveness of the prophylactic procedure employed. Consideration will, therefore, be limited to the more realistic, though poorly explored, area of immunotherapy in cancer patients.

Curative immunotherapy consists of either stimulating the patient's own immune responses, or providing him with preformed antibodies or immuno-logically competent cells. At present, the immunotherapy of cancer is in its earliest stages, but the few examples quoted below will serve to illustrate some of the approaches that may eventually prove to be of therapeutic value.

ACTIVE IMMUNOTHERAPY

Nonspecific systemic stimulation of immune responsiveness has been at-tempted in patients with lymphomas and leukemias by frequent and massive scarifications with BCG.[21] Local nonspecific stimulation of cell-mediated immune responsiveness has been accomplished by sensitization and subse-quent local challenge with simple chemical haptens such as dinitrofluorobenzene (DNFB).[15a] Lasting involution of malignant and premalignant skin lesions has been obtained by this method, and the immunity transferred to nonsensitized patients by means of peripheral blood leukocytes. Whether it will be possible to obtain comparable results with other tumors requires further investigation.

Active, specific immunotherapy has also been attempted in leukemic patients by the administration of formalin fixed, irradiated, or otherwise modified, leukemic cells. Although the results obtained by both types of procedures have been mildly encouraging, no significant conclusions of efficacy can be reached.

An entirely different approach to active immunotherapy has resulted from the observation that the antigenicity of tumor cells can be enhanced by coupling them to rabbit γ-globulin with bis-diazotized benzidine. Results in patients injected with autologous tumor cells complexed to γ-globulin were encouraging and suggest that both humoral and cellular immunity resulted.

It is apparent from most of these studies that if active immunotherapy is to be successful, it must be undertaken when there is minimal cancerous tissue in the host (e.g., during remission in leukemia, or following surgical resection of a tumor), and at a time when the patient's immune mechanisms are functioning adequately.

PASSIVE AND ADOPTIVE IMMUNIZATION

The results of passive serotherapy have, for the most part, been disappointing. In the majority of instances antisera produced in animals immunized with human tumors were employed. Not only were the malignant lesions not significantly impaired, but associated problems of soluble antigen-antibody complex diseases, and possible immunologic enhancement of tumor growth, were observed.

Other methods of passive immunization which have been attempted include the parenteral administration of peripheral blood lymphocytes and lymph node cells obtained from a pig previously immunized with the patient's own malignant cells;[26] and the injection of splenic cells obtained from rabbits immunized with autologous tumor cells into the pleural cavity of a patient with lymphosarcoma who had a malignant pleural effusion.[21] A related but somewhat different approach has been employed in patients with malignant melanoma.[23] Pairs of melanoma patients were immunized to each other's tumors by subcutaneous transplants of malignant cells. A subsequent exchange of white cells appeared to produce some evidence of clinical improvement in approximately one-third of patients.

BONE MARROW GRAFTS

Human bone marrow grafts following whole body irradiation at maximum tolerated doses have been attempted in patients with leukemia.[21] The majority of these patients succumbed shortly after transplantation to fulminating graft-versus-host reactions (secondary syndrome). In the few survivors, there was suggestive clinical evidence of remission and prolonged survival due to the treatment. In order to avoid the high incidence of fatal secondary syndrome, transfusions of human leukocytes have been carried out in non-irradiated leukemic patients. In these patients, the severity of the graft-versus-host reaction can be reduced by varying the dose of leukocytes and by the careful application of histocompatibility matching techniques similar to those employed in other forms of human transplantation (see Chapter 14). The early results of these investigations have been encouraging, but further well-controlled studies are needed.

THE FUTURE OF IMMUNOTHERAPY

Immunotherapy in human cancer is obviously in its infancy. The methods described are certainly not the only ones which could be employed and any combination of techniques would not be mutually exclusive. It must, however, be remembered that cancer immunotherapy is based on the assumption that the tumors involved contain specific components and that these antigens are capable of evoking an immune reaction on the part of the host which inhibits tumor growth. Although the evidence presented in this chapter indicates that some progress has been made towards establishing the validity of these assumptions, absolute proof is lacking. Furthermore, the ultimate test of any theory regarding the immunotherapy of human cancer requires human experimentation. Every precaution should be taken to ensure that even the patient with terminal cancer is not subjected to any form of manipulation which is potentially more hazardous than his already fatal disease.

REFERENCES

1. Abelev, G. I. Production of embryonal serum-globulin by hepatomas: Review of experimental and clinical data. *Cancer Res. 28:*1344, 1968.

2. Alexander, P., and Fairley, G. H. Cellular resistance to tumours. *Brit. Med. Bull. 23:*86, 1967.

3. Alpert, M. E., Uriel, J., and Nechaud, B. de. Alpha₁ fetoglobulin in the diagnosis of human hepatoma. *New Eng. J. Med. 278:*984, 1968.

4. Buffe, D., Rimbaut, C., Lemerle, J., Schweisguth, O., and Burtin, P. Présence d'une ferroprotéine d'origine tissulaire, l'α_2H dans le sérum des enfants porteurs de tumeurs. *Int. J. Cancer* 5:85, 1970.

5. Cinader, B., Hayley, M. A., Rider, W. E., and Warick, O. H. Immunotherapy of a patient with choriocarcinoma. *Canad. Med. Assoc. J.* 84:306, 1961.

6. Editorial. Fetoproteins. *Lancet* 1:397, 1970.

7. Fass, L., Herberman, R. B., Ziegler, J. Delayed cutaneous hypersensitivity reactions to autologous reactions of Burkitt-lymphoma cells. *New Eng. J. Med.* 282:776, 1970.

8. Gold, P. Circulating antibodies against carcinoembryonic antigens of the human digestive system. *Cancer* 20:1663, 1967.

9. Gold, P. The role of immunology in human cancer research. *Can. Med. Assoc. J.* 103:1043, 1970.

10. Gold, P., and Freedman, S. O. Demonstration of tumor-specific antigens in human colonic carcinomata by immunological tolerance and absorption techniques. *J. Exp. Med.* 121:439, 1965.

11. Gold, P., and Freedman, S. O. Specific carcinoembryonic antigens of the human digestive system. *J. Exp. Med.* 122:467, 1965.

12. Gold, P., Krupey, J., and Ansari, H. Position of the carcinoembryonic antigen of the human digestive system in the ultrastructure of the tumor cell surface. *J. Nat. Cancer Inst.* 45:219, 1970.

12a. Häkkinen, I., and Viikari, S. Occurrence of fetal sulphoglycoprotein antigen in the gastric juice of patients with gastric diseases. *Ann. Surg.* 169:277, 1969.

13. Hellström, I., Hellström, K. E., Pierce, G. E., and Bill, A. H. Demonstration of cell-bound and humoral immunity against neuroblastoma cells. *Proc. U.S. Nat. Acad. Sci.* 60:1231, 1968.

14. Hellström, K. E., and Hellström, I. Immunologic defences against cancer. *Hosp. Pract.* 5:45, 1970.

15. Henle, W. Evidence for viruses in acute leukemia and Burkitt's tumor. *Cancer* 21:580, 1968.

15a. Klein, E. Hypersensitivity reactions at tumor sites. *Cancer Res.* 29:2351, 1969.

16. Klein, G., Klein, E., and Clifford, P. Host defences in leukemia and Burkitt's tumor. *Cancer* 21:587, 1968.

17. Klein, G., Pearson, G., Henle, G., Henle, W., Diehl, V., and Niederman, J. C. Relationship between Epstein-Barr viral and cell membrane immunofluorescence in Burkitt tumor cells. *J. Exp. Med.* 128:1021, 1968.

18. Kleist, S. von, and Burtin, P. On the specificity of autoantibodies present in colon cancer patients. *Immunology* 10:507, 1967.

19. Lewis, M. G., Ikonopisov, R. L., Nairn, R. C., Phillips, T. M., Fairley, G. H., Bodenham, D. G., and Alexander, P. Tumour-specific antibodies in human malignant melanoma and their relationship to the extent of the disease. *Brit. Med. J.* 2:547, 1969.

20. Martin, D. C., Rubini, M., and Rosen, V. J. Cadaveric renal homotransplantation with inadvertent transplantation of carcinoma. *J.A.M.A. 192:*752, 1965.

21. Mathé, G. The immunological approach to the treatment of cancer. *Ann. Roy. Coll. Surg. Engl. 41:*93, 1967.

22. Morton, D. L., Malmgren, R. A., Hall, W. T., and Schidlovsky, G. Immunologic and virus studies with human sarcomas. *Surgery 66:*152, 1969.

23. Nadler, S. H., and Moore, G. E. Clinical immunologic study of malignant disease: Response to tumor transplants and transfer of leukocytes. *Ann. Surg. 164:*482, 1966.

24. O'Connor, G. T. Persistent immunologic stimulation as a factor in oncogenesis, with special references to Burkitt's tumor. *Amer. J. Med. 48:*279, 1970.

25. Stohlbach, L. L., Krant, M. J., and Fishman, W. H. Ectopic production of an alkaline phosphatase isoenzyme in patients with cancer. *New Eng. J. Med. 281:*757, 1969.

26. Symes, M. O., Ridell, A. G., Immelman, E. J., and Terblanche, J. Immunologically competent cells in the treatment of malignant disease. *Lancet 1:*1054, 1968.

27. Thomson, D. M. P., Krupey, J., Freedman, S. O., and Gold, P. The radioimmunoassay of circulating carcinoembryonic antigen of the human digestive system. *Proc. U.S. Nat. Acad. Sci. 64:*161, 1969.

28. Walford, R. L., Finkelstein, S., Neerhout, R., Konrad, T. P., and Shanbrom, E. Acute childhood leukemia in relation to the HL-A human transplantation genes. *Nature 225:*461, 1970.

29. Wilson, E. R., Hager, E. B., Hampers, C. L., Carson, J. M., Merrill, J. P., and Murray, J. E. Immunologic rejection of human cancer transplanted with a renal allograft. *New Eng. J. Med. 278:*479, 1968.

14

Organ Transplantation

PHIL GOLD

IMMUNOBIOLOGY OF TRANSPLANTATION

The potential value of organ transplantation has intrigued man since the writings of Greek mythology. Only in recent years, however, have the cooperative efforts of laboratory scientists and clinicians made the transplantation of human organs a practical, though still imperfect, therapeutic procedure. Unfortunately, the solutions to many of the problems related to performing successful human allografts have not kept pace with the technical advances in transplantation surgery. Although these difficulties include techniques of tissue preservation, the morals and methods of tissue procurement, and the means of public information, the discussion in this chapter will be confined to the problem of allograft rejection. The most recent terminology used to describe the phenomena of transplantation immunology is summarized in Table 14-1.

THE NATURE OF THE REJECTION PROCESS

The central problem in transplantation consists of the well established observation that tissues exchanged between virtually any two vertebrates that are not of an identical genetic constitution are rejected, whereas tissues exchanged between syngeneic animals or identical human twins survive for an indefinite period of time. The rate and violence of rejection is dependent on a variety of factors. However, in general, the major determinant in this reaction is the genetic disparity between the two individuals involved.

TABLE 14-1. Current Transplantation Terminology

Term	Definition
Autograft	Tissue transplanted from one site to another in the same individual (*Adjective:* Autologous)
Isograft	Tissue transplanted between genetically identical individuals (*Adjectives:* Isogeneic—monozygotic twins; Syngeneic —members of an inbred animal strain)
Allograft	Tissue transplanted between genetically dissimilar individuals of the same species (*Adjective:* Allogeneic)
Xenograft	Tissue transplanted between individuals of different species (*Adjective:* Xenogeneic)
Allostatic	Grafts which are intended to serve a temporary or mechanical function after transplantation so that continued viability of the tissue is not required
Allovital	Grafts which are intended to perform continued full, normal, metabolic function after transplantation
Orthotopic	The placement of a graft in the anatomic position normally occupied by such tissue
Heterotopic	The placement of a graft in an anatomic location not normally occupied by such tissue
Adoptive Immunity	Specific, permanent immunity conferred upon a previously unsensitized individual by the administration of immunologically competent and committed cells from a previously sensitized donor
First-set phenomenon	The chronology and events leading to graft rejection following initial exposure of a recipient to the tissue of a donor
Second-set phenomenon	The chronology and events leading to graft rejection following subsequent exposure of the recipient to tissue of the same donor

Although each species and organ may manifest quantitatively variable characteristics, a number of general conclusions may be drawn from transplantation studies in animals[29]: (*1*) the rejection phenomenon is not an innate response, but requires a latent period from the time of grafting in order to be "learned" by the recipient; (*2*) in skin transplants vascularization of the graft appears to facilitate the rejection mechanism; (*3*) at its peak, the rejection crisis involves the participation of lymphatic and blood vessels, inflammatory cells, and humoral factors; and (*4*) depending on the degree of genetic diversity, initial allografts between mammals are usually rejected within a two-week period.

EVIDENCE FOR AN IMMUNE MECHANISM IN ALLOGRAFT REJECTION

Chronology

The requirement of a preceding period of contact between graft and host and the augmentation of the rejection process by neovascularization or by surgical vascular anastamosis would be in keeping with the concept of host sensitization by antigenic constituents of the graft. The vascular union between graft and recipient probably permits the entry of soluble antigenic components, or breakdown products of the allograft, into the immunologically competent tissues of the host. However, it appears to be of greater importance that the vascular connections allow the antigen-reactive or antigen-processing cells of the host to gain access to the grafted tissue.

Although first-set rejection time for an ordinary allograft may be as long as 2 weeks, second-set rejection usually requires less than half of this time and is far more explosive. This latter type of reaction is not dissimilar from the antibody response observed in animals during initial and subsequent exposures to the same antigenic preparations.

The hypersensitivity associated with allograft rejection, like that seen in all other forms of immunologic hypersensitivity, is a systemic rather than a local event. Thus, following first-set rejection of a skin graft at one site, the application of a second piece of skin at a distant site or the transplantation of another organ between the same donor and recipient will lead to a second-set phenomenon. It is noteworthy, however, that specific reactivity appears first as a local immunologic process in regional lymph nodes. Only later does the more readily demonstrable state of generalized hypersensitivity appear.

Specificity of the Reaction

Like all immune reactions, the second-set phenomenon shows an exquisite specificity for the individual antigenic preparation. After first-set rejection, the events following the application of a second allograft in the same recipient is dependent upon the genetic similarity between the original and subsequent donors. The greater the disparity between donors, the closer will the rejection of the second graft approach a first-set phenomenon. On the other hand, if the same donor is used, a fully developed second-set phenomenon will be observed.

Effect of Immunosuppressive Procedures

Studies dealing with the effect of manipulation of the immune response on the survival of tissue allografts add further support to the concept of an immunologic mechanism in graft rejection. It has been demonstrated that a variety of immunosuppressive procedures, including neonatal thymectomy, lymphatic ablation, irradiation, and the administration of chemotherapeutic agents may lead to a prolongation of graft survival.

Immunologic Tolerance

The phenomenon of acquired immunologic tolerance is critically important to the understanding of graft rejection mechanisms.[13] The exposure of perinatal animals of a number of species to a variety of antigenic stimuli not only fails to elicit an immunologic response, but, under suitable conditions, renders the animal incapable of such reactivity when challenged with the same antigenic material during adult life. Of particular relevance to the present discussion is the demonstration that embryonic mice injected with viable allogenic cells will accept skin allografts from the same donor, or animals syngeneic to the donor, during adult life. Moreover, the administration of lymph node or spleen cells from normal adult animals, syngeneic to the tolerant host, leads to a breaking of tolerance and first-set rejection of the original skin graft. If the lymphoid cell donor has previously rejected a similar allograft, then a second-set phenomenon is observed in the once tolerant host. The state of tolerance, like that of immunity, is specific and does not extend to donors of strains other than the original donor strain.

Circulating Antibodies

The development of the rejection process is associated with the appearance of circulating antibodies against components of the transplanted tissue. These antibodies may be detected by a number of serologic procedures. The techniques most commonly employed are the cytoagglutination of donor cells or the demonstration of cytotoxicity against donor cells.

Immunologic Enhancement

Immunologic enhancement may be defined as the successful establishment, or delayed rejection, of an allograft as a consequence of the presence of specific humoral antigraft antibodies in the host. Although occasionally demonstrable following normal tissue allografts,[14b] this state has been observed most frequently during certain tumor transplanation studies.[6] At present, the underlying mechanism is incompletely understood. Humoral antibodies with enhancing properties are technically more difficult to demonstrate during the rejection of normal tissue allografts than are cytoagglutinins or cytotoxic antibodies.

NATURE OF THE IMMUNE REACTION IN GRAFT REJECTION

The accumulated evidence outlined in the previous section leaves little doubt that the major determinants in graft rejection are of immunologic origin. There remains the question of whether cell-mediated or humoral immunity is directly responsible for the rejection process. Although a clear distinction between these two classic forms of immune responsiveness no longer pertains (see Chapter 1), the weight of evidence suggests that cell-mediated immunity is of primary significance in graft rejection. Furthermore, it appears that the small lymphocyte, originating from either one or a number of different areas of the body, is of major importance in both the afferent and efferent limbs of the immune rejection mechanism.

Histology

Indirect evidence for cell-mediation is obtained from the histology of tissues undergoing rejection. A characteristic finding is the presence of leukocytic inflammatory cells of recipient origin in the vicinity of the graft. The predominant cell form is mononuclear with the majority resembling the small lymphocyte. The cellular morphology is, however, far from uniform. For example, small lymphocytes which appear to be identical under the light microscope may show definite ultrastructural variation by electron microscopy. In addition, macrophages and polymorphonuclear leukocytes are not infrequent, and an occasional plasma cell may be seen.

Vascular changes leading to complete obstruction of blood vessels may be observed. Although these vascular abnormalities may be related to functional impairment, as in the case of transplanted human kidneys, they are usually relatively late manifestations of the first-set phenomenon.

Cell Transfer Studies

Allograft sensitivity may be transferred to a normal adult animal by lymphoid cells from a previously sensitized member of the same inbred strain.[8] Application of a tissue graft from the same strain as that used to sensitize the lymphoid cell donor will lead to a second-set phenomenon in the adoptively sensitized host. In the great majority of studies reported, a similar transfer of allograft sensitivity could not be achieved by the use of serum from an actively sensitized animal.

Graft-Versus-Host Reaction

The ability of lymphoid cells to react against foreign tissues is clearly demonstrated in the graft-versus-host (GVH) reaction. This phenomenon is observed when an animal is injected with immunocompetent allogeneic cells against which it is incapable of mounting an immune response. Generally, the host in a GVH reaction is either a neonatal animal with an immature immune system, or an adult animal whose immune system has been impaired by disease, irradiation, or chemotherapeutic agents. In the neonatal animal, where lymphoid cells are frequently used as the antigen for the induction of tolerance, the GVH reaction is denoted by the term *runt disease*. The condition is characterized by failure to thrive, generalized wasting, severe diarrhea, alopecia, dermatitis, hepatosplenomegaly, and thymicolymphatic atrophy. Death frequently occurs after a variable period of time. In adult animals, where the clinicopathologic manifestations are quite similar, the process is sometimes referred to as *secondary syndrome*.

Tissue Culture Studies

In vitro conditions for demonstrating the cytolytic capacity of lymphocytes have been established. It has been shown in tissue culture studies, where complement and all other detectable serum factors have been omitted, that target cell destruction can be accomplished by specifically sensitized lymphocytes.

Transplantation in Millipore Chambers

Experiments have been performed in which allogeneic tissue has been transplanted within Millipore chambers. Grafts carried out in this manner demonstrate unusually prolonged or indefinite survival, even in a previously sensitized host. Since Millipore chambers are impermeable to cells, these observations imply that graft survival is favored by the exclusion of host cells from the transplanted tissue. On the other hand, humoral antibodies may gain access to the graft, indicating that these components alone may be incapable of evoking the rejection process.

Intradermal Reactions

Following allograft rejection, the intradermal injection of the sensitized host with cells or cell extracts of donor origin leads to a typical delayed-type skin reaction characteristic of cell-mediated hypersensitivity (*direct reaction*). In addition, the intradermal injection of the donor with lymphoid cells of the sensitized recipient provokes an identical cutaneous response (*transfer reaction*). No comparable phenomenon of either the immediate or delayed-type is observed when the sensitized host's serum is employed for intradermal testing.

Transplantation in Neonatal Lambs

Fetal and neonatal lambs possess virtually no γ-globulin in their circulation. Nevertheless, skin allografts applied to fetal lambs during gestation are rejected in a manner identical to that seen in adult sheep. This observation would suggest that, in this experimental model, immunoglobulins are of negligible importance in the rejection process.

Macrophage Inhibition

It has been found that the incubation of sensitized lymphocytes with specific antigen leads to the release of a humoral factor capable of inhibiting the migration of normal macrophages. The production of the macrophage Migration Inhibition Factor (MIF) is directly related to the ability of the lymphocyte donor to develop the usual cutaneous manifestations of delayed hypersensitivity in response to an intradermal injection of the specific antigen. However, the production of MIF is independent of the humoral immune status of the animal against the antigen in question (see Chapter 1). It is, therefore, of possible significance that lymphocytes obtained from animals after graft rejection, and incubated with donor cell preparations, release MIF.[2]

Role of Humoral Antibodies

Consideration of the preceding data strongly favors a cell-mediated immune process in allograft rejection. However, a number of arguments have been put forward which suggest that the complete spectrum of events which occurs during rejection may well involve humoral antibodies in some fashion. It has long been known that the application of a second skin allograft from the same donor within a few days of complete first-set rejection leads to a peculiar and violent accelerated response described as the white-graft reaction. The transplanted skin remains pallid upon the recipient bed, and never acquires a blood supply before becoming necrotic. The histopathologic picture is one of vascular obstruction and ischemia without the intervention of inflammatory cells. If the mechanism of graft rejection is accepted as being immunologic, then the white-graft reaction strongly implies a process mediated by humoral antibodies.

The evidence from Millipore chamber experiments, initially used as a major argument against humoral antibody participation in allograft rejection, is now less convincing. It has been found that humoral antibodies and complement enter Millipore chambers only with difficulty. Furthermore, when an adequate concentration of these reactants is achieved within the chambers, some allogeneic cell preparations undergo cytolytic destruction.[29]

Studies employing rodent tumor systems have led to the suggestion of a dual nature for the immune rejection process. In some dissociated tumor cell systems, humoral antibodies alone are enough to achieve allograft rejection. In other dissociated tumor cell systems, humoral and cell-mediated immunity appear to operate synergistically. However, in solid tumor systems, as well as in some dissociated tumor cell systems, humoral antibodies appear to be ineffectual and cell-mediated immune reactions dependent on lymphocytes are of prime importance. It appears that both the inherent properties of a given tumor cell line as well as the state of association or dissociation of the cells determine the response to humoral antibody.[29a]

Although most attempts to passively transfer allograft sensitivity with serum have failed, a number of successes has been achieved. Allograft rejection has been potentiated in both rodents and birds by the administration of whole serum or immunoglobulin fractions from animals immunized with preparations of tissues obtained from the allograft donor strain. Moreover, it has recently been reported that the immunization of rabbits with Group A Type 12 streptococcal cell membranes can elicit serum antibodies which have the ability to cause the rapid rejection of skin allografts in guinea pigs.[27] It was observed that the intradermal injection of this antiserum resulted in a cutaneous response histologically similar to the Arthus reaction. In addition to emphasizing the probable cross-antigenicity of bacterial and mammalian cell components, these observations suggest that soluble antigen-antibody complexes may participate in the process of allograft rejection.

At present it is uncertain how humoral antibodies interact with the apparently dominant action of cell-mediated immunity to bring about allograft rejection. It is of interest that a number of investigators have demonstrated the existence of transfer-factors in immune reactivity.[21] Transfer-factors may be defined as substances produced by immunologically committed cells, which may then passively sensitize uncommitted cells in their immediate vicinity. The extent to which such factors may be involved in allograft rejection remains unknown. However, this type of interaction would allow a unification of both cellular and humoral antibody factors in the rejection process.

PROLONGATION OF GRAFT SURVIVAL

Privileged Sites

The implantation of allografts into certain anatomic sites has, in many instances, resulted in the indefinite survival of the tissue. Common to all of these sites are peculiarities of either the blood or lymphatic circulation. It is these peculiarities which lead to impairment of either the afferent or efferent limb of the immune circuit involved in rejection (see Chapter 1).

Privileged sites dependent, at least in part, upon the lack of a direct vascular supply include the anterior chamber of the eye, the substantia propria of the cornea, and the meninges of the brain. The unusual anatomy of the lymphatic drainage of the testes appears to be the major factor conferring privilege in this area. The curious condition of immunologic insulation is found in the cheek pouch of the hamster where the afferent, but not the efferent, limb of the rejection process is impaired. Comparable situations may be associated with prolonged allograft survival in the thymus and in the brain.

Privileged Tissues

Collagen is the only tissue which can be considered privileged in the sense that its inherent properties permit the prolonged survival of allografts, or even xenografts. The heavy mucopolysaccharide coat, or glycocalyx, of the chondrocyte has been implicated as the material which serves to occlude the transplantation antigens on the surface of the cell, rendering them nonantigenic. This rather simplistic explanation, however, leaves a great deal to be desired. At present, the exact mechanisms which permit cartilage to survive in a foreign host are largely unknown.

Impairment of the Immune Response

Decreased immune reactivity may result from various conditions, both natural and induced. Patients with any of the primary or secondary immunologic deficiency syndromes, particularly those associated with depression of cell-mediated immunity, may manifest prolonged allograft survival (see Chapters 11 and 12). Of greater practical importance are those situations in which depression of immune reactivity is brought about by specific treatment of the host with immunosuppressive agents. These procedures will be discussed in the section on immunosuppressive therapy.

TRANSPLANTATION ANTIGENS

Cellular Localization

Since allografts do not occur in nature, it is reasonable to expect that the cellular components referred to as transplantation antigens would have been discarded during phylogenetic development unless they performed a vital function in maintaining cellular integrity. Proposed, but unproven, functions include membrane transport as well as cell contact and recognition phenomena. Regardless of their natural functions, transplantation antigens are the components of the cell against which the allograft rejection process is directed. Since the recipient is tolerant to his own cellular components, the rejection response must be evoked by transplantation antigens present in the donor but absent in the host.

Transplantation antigens appear to be present in all cells, but vary in concentration from tissue to tissue. The ability of red blood cells to produce allograft sensitivity has been questioned. However, there now seems to be little doubt that the ABO group of antigens are strong transplantation antigens, and that certain transplantation antigens found in other tissues are present on erythrocytes in minute quantities.

The antigenic locale of greatest importance in evoking allograft rejection is associated with the surface membrane of the transplanted cell. Nevertheless, the transplantation antigens are probably represented on most intracellular membranous structures, and microsomal preparations have been quite effective in eliciting allograft sensitivity.

Genetics

The synthesis of the transplantation antigens is controlled by gene complexes, referred to as histocompatibility loci. These loci range in number from at least 4 to 15 or more in the various species of rodents which have been studied. Hence, transplantation antigens represent allotypic variations of cell surface components resulting from genetic histocompatibility differences.

The transplantation antigens of mice have been studied in greatest detail and have been the subject of a number of recent, comprehensive reviews.[11] An indispensible factor in the analysis of mouse transplantation genetics has been the ability to develop highly inbred strains within this species. A great deal of information has been obtained by observing the duration of allograft survival in donor-recipient pairs of different genetic diversities.

The information gained from these studies in mice has stimulated a comparable search for transplantation antigens, and their corresponding histocompatibility loci, in man. In the last few years, there has been a rapid clarification of the serology and genetics of the human transplantation antigen systems. In man there appears to be a single major genetic histocompatibility system called the HL-A locus.[35] This system is analogous to the strong H-2 histocompatibility locus in mice,[30] with the important exception that HL-A isoantigens have not as yet been detected on human erythrocytes.[29a]

The complex HL-A locus is found on a pair of autosomal chromosomes with no individual carrying more than two alleles. Heterozygotes who do have two alleles transmit one or the other, but never both, to each offspring. It has been found that groups of antigenic specificities (e.g., HL-A 1, HL-A 2, HL-A 3 and HL-A 9) are usually transmitted together so that their genetic determinants form an allelic series referred to as a sublocus.[29a] At least three, and probably more, such subloci exist.

The expression of the histocompatibility genes is codominant. Hence, each parental haplotype, or collection of HL-A antigens whose determining genes have been inherited as a group, is completely expressed. At least eight major and an undetermined number of minor antigenic specificities can result from the gene products of the HL-A system, composing the most potent determinants of human allograft rejection (see Table 1-9).

The HL-A directed transplantation antigens are well represented on the surface of circulating human leukocytes, and corresponding humoral alloantibodies may develop in multiparous women or in individuals who have received multiple blood transfusions (see Chapter 9). Minor loci, such as the Group 5 system and possibly the Group 9 system, are independent of the HL-A complex and direct the synthesis of relatively weak transplantation antigens or polymorphisms (see Chapter 1) unrelated to allograft sensitization.

The knowledge that in man, as in lower animals, most of the strong transplantation antigens belong to one complex system has permitted several investigators to make family studies of the frequency of alleles for the HL-A subloci as they occur in the general population. One such study revealed that the ten most commonly observed combinations of alleles occur with a frequency of 3 to 14 per cent.[37]

In 65 per cent of families, all four of the HL-A alleles of the parents were different. Under these circumstances there is no possibility of parent-child identity for HL-A directed histocompatibility antigens. However, the probability of identity between siblings is 1:4. In an additional 25 per cent of families, the parents shared one common allele, giving both a parent-child and a sibling-sibling probability of identity of 1:4. In the remaining 10 per cent of families, one of the parents was homozygous for one of the alleles, so that the parent-child and sibling-sibling probabilities of identity were 0 and 1:2, respectively. These observations are of great practical importance in the selection of living, first-degree relatives for human organ transplantation.

Physicochemical Properties

The numerous efforts made to isolate the various transplantation antigens in pure form have recently been summarized.[17] Such attempts have had two motivations. First, the availability of purified transplantation antigens would allow the preparation of specific antisera of high titer, which could be used in the serotyping of donor and host prior to organ transplantation. Secondly, it is conceivable that the administration of the appropriate purified transplantation antigens prior to grafting across the HL-A barrier might allow the induction of a state of either high-dose or low-dose immunologic tolerance.[14a]

The chemical composition of the transplantation antigens as they occur in situ is uncertain as these components are usually obtained only after rather violent treatment of cell membranes with detergents or proteolytic enzymes. However, there appears to be general agreement that the transplantation antigens are composed of varying quantities of lipid, protein, and carbohydrate. The larger the quantity of lipid in the molecule, the less likely it is to be soluble in aqueous solution. This observation has led to a rather arbitrary division of the transplantation antigens on the basis of their solubility characteristics. Although the carbohydrate, protein, and lipid moieties have each been thought to be present in the antigenic determinant groups of the transplantation antigens, it would now appear that the lipid fraction is of little importance in this respect and the major antigenic determinant is a protein component. If this is the case, the potentially enormous variation in amino acid sequences could readily account for the extensive polymorphism in transplantation antigens within species, and the lack of detectable cross-reactivity even between those species which are closely related.

ATTENUATION OF THE HUMAN ALLOGRAFT RESPONSE

Except in the case of monozygotic twins, there is no genetic homogeneity in the human population. Therefore, the rejection of allografts transferred between humans is virtually inevitable, and the attenuation of allograft rejection is dependent upon measures taken before and after the transplantation procedure. Prior to surgery, all available means are employed to select an organ donor whose major transplantation antigens are as similar as possible to those of the prospective recipient (Histocompatibility Testing). Following transplantation, every effort is made to suppress the immunologic mechanisms of the recipient which may lead to rejection of the allografted tissue (Immunosuppressive Therapy).

HISTOCOMPATIBILITY TESTING

Methods of selecting the best possible donor-recipient pairs for human organ transplantation may be divided on the basis of whether they are performed in vivo or in vitro. However, it is probably more useful to distinguish between methods designed to achieve *tissue matching* and those designed to achieve *tissue typing*. Matching studies attempt to estimate general transplantation antigenic similarities or differences between the donor and recipient. In tests of tissue typing, the emphasis is placed on determining the absolute content of transplantation antigens in the tissues of the individuals involved (see Table 14-2).

TABLE 14-2. Tests of Histocompatibility

Tissue Matching Tests[1]	Direct skin grafting[2] "Third man" test Normal lymphocyte transfer test Irradiated hamster test	Performed in vivo[3]
	Mixed leukocyte culture test[4]	Performed in vitro
Tissue Typing Tests[5]	Lymphocytotoxicity[6,7] Leukagglutination[6] Platelet complement fixation Antiglobulin consumption Mixed hemagglutination Immunoadherence Immunofluorescence	

[1] Determine sums of similarities or differences between individuals.
[2] Leads to sensitization of the prospective recipient.
[3] Lack capacity for fine discrimination in determining the best of a good group of donors.
[4] Particularly applicable when prospective donor is a first-degree relative.
[5] Determine transplantation antigens of the individual tested.
[6] Tests most commonly employed in human studies at the present time.
[7] Gaining prominence in clinical transplantation because of sensitivity and reproducibility.

In either case, the ideal histocompatibility test should include as many of the following features as possible:

1. It should exclude from any panel of donors those individuals whose organs would elicit a violent rejection response on the part of the recipient.

2. It should select the individual whose tissues would be tolerated for the longest period of time by the prospective recipient.

3. It should not lead to recipient sensitization to the donor's tissues.

4. It should have a high degree of discrimination in determining the best of a number of apparently good donors.

5. It should be independent of the state of health of the prospective donor and recipient.

6. It should be applicable to cadaver donors.

7. The results should be available within a few hours.

At present there is no test which completely fulfills all of these criteria, although a great deal of progress has been made in this direction.

In Vivo Matching Tests

The in vivo matching tests are inexpensive and do not require sophisticated apparatus. On the other hand, days or weeks are required before results are obtained, and discrimination is generally poor. Thus, only gross differences or similarities of *total* transplantation antigenicity between donor and recipient are determined. These tests do not serve to type the tissues of either the donor or the recipient for the transplantation antigens whose synthesis is directed by the HL-A histocompatibility locus. Four in vivo matching tests and a variety of modifications have been described, but they are now primarily of historic and theoretic interest.

Direct Skin Grafting.   This test is based on the transfer of small skin grafts from a panel of prospective donors to the prospective recipient. The most suitable donor would, under these circumstances, be the one whose skin graft survived the longest.

"Third Man" Test.   This test utilizes the second-set rejection phenomenon in a neutral individual, or "third man," who has rejected a primary skin graft from the potential recipient. The "third man" receives skin allografts from a panel of prospective donors in the expectation that the skin of the donor whose transplantation antigens most closely resemble those of the prospective recipient will be rejected in the most violent fashion.

Normal Lymphocyte Transfer (NLT) Test.   This test is performed by the intradermal injection of the peripheral blood lymphocytes from a prospective recipient as well as from two healthy unrelated volunteers into a panel of prospective organ donors. Skin reactions are usually observed at the injection sites after 24 to 48 hours (early or graft-versus-host reaction) and after 4 days (late or host-versus-graft reaction). Since the reactivity of the prospective recipient's lymphocytes against the tissues of the donor is in question, the early reaction is the one of major significance in this procedure. The immunologic nature of the NLT test remains uncertain at the present time.

Irradiated Hamster Test. This test is based on the observation that allogeneic lymphocytes injected intracutaneously into irradiated hamsters produce no detectable reaction. However, when lymphocytes from two different strains of hamsters are mixed and then injected intracutaneously into a third irradiated hamster, a delayed-type intracutaneous reaction is observed. Similarly, when the lymphocytes from two humans are mixed and injected into irradiated hamsters, the severity of the cutaneous reactivity appears to be related to the degree of genetic disparity between the individuals involved. Thus, the irradiated hamster test is a "two-way" test since it measures the activity of the lymphocytes of each individual against those of the other. By appropriate treatment of the lymphocytes from the prospective donor, however, it may be possible to determine the reactivity only of the recipient against the donor in a unidirectional fashion (see description of mixed leukocyte culture test). The irradiated hamster test has enjoyed a limited clinical application, and no definitive statement of its efficacy can presently be made.

In Vitro Tests for Histocompatibility

The demonstration that human allograft rejection is determined primarily by a single major histocompatibility locus, the HL-A system, has led to the development of several in vitro techniques for histocompatibility testing. Since there is only a single locus, each parent can contribute one of two alleles to an offspring regardless of the number of alleles in the population. Thus, a maximum of four different genotypes may be seen in the siblings of any one family. It is, therefore, of crucial importance that the method utilized in histocompatibility testing be able to discern the best possible tissue donor within a group of live first-degree relatives, when they are available.

The in vivo matching tests cannot discriminate among the more subtle differences in histocompatibility that are required for choosing the best blood-related donor. Since it is such minor disparities that may well decide the long-term results of allotransplantation, it is precisely on this account that such tests have failed. Although all of the in vitro histocompatibility tests are applicable to the selection of the best related donor, the one available in vitro matching test will be considered first.

In Vitro Matching Test (Mixed Leukocyte Culture).   It has been known for some time that lymphocytes exposed to the action of phytohemagglutinin (PHA) in vitro undergo a process of blast transformation which can be distinguished morphologically (see Chapter 1). It was subsequently observed that when the leukocytes of two normal individuals were mixed and placed in culture, the lymphocytes underwent a similar blast transformation. In addition the cells demonstrated an increased incorporation of tritiated-thymidine, indicating a rise in DNA synthesis. However, when the leukocytes of monozygotic twins were placed in mixed culture, this phenomenon was not observed. Extensive studies have revealed that the degree of blast transformation which lymphocytes show in mixed culture is directly related to the genetic disparity of the two individuals at the HL-A locus.[3]

Without modification, the mixed leukocyte culture is a "two-way" test which measures the response of the lymphocytes of each individual against those of the other. However, by pretreating the cells of one of the lymphocyte donors with mitomycin C, the treated cells are rendered incapable of undergoing transformation. Under these circumstances, the test becomes unidirectional and measures only the response of the untreated lymphocytes. For histocompatibility testing, it is the prospective donor's cells that are treated with mitomycin C, so that only the response of the recipient's lymphocytes is determined.

Although the chance of finding a close match between randomly chosen individuals in the population is small, the probability rises sharply when first-degree relatives are employed. It has been found that the mixed leukocyte culture method is extremely sensitive in determining even minor histocompatibility differences at the HL-A locus and, therefore, is most applicable when allotransplantation procedures are being considered between siblings or between parents and offspring.

In Vitro Typing Tests

Usually the organ of a live, first-degree relative is not available for allografting, and, thus, the mixed leukocyte culture test is of limited value. However, the dilemma of selecting a well-suited, live, unrelated or cadaver donor has been partially resolved through the use of serotyping for transplantation antigens.[35]

Principles of Serotyping for Histocompatibility Antigens.   Serotyping for histocompatibility antigens is, in fact, a modification of the "third man" test in which the serum of the "third man" is used for screening purposes. Individuals who have undergone multiple blood transfusions may serve as a source of antisera for histocompatibility typing, but the antibodies found in such sera are frequently polyvalent and difficult to specify for a particular transplantation antigen. In general, sera obtained from multiparous women have been of much greater value for detecting human histocompatibility antigens (see Chapter 9). Half of the fetal transplantation antigens are of maternal origin, and by chance alone the mother and father may share all but one or a few antigenic determinants. Therefore, in a small number of individuals, the maternal antibodies developed against fetal transplantation antigens may show a high degree of specificity.

A number of highly specific antiserum preparations have been developed in different laboratories. Such sera were used initially for the recognition of antigens associated with the HL-A histocompatibility system, and were only subsequently employed for clinical purposes. It seems probable that many of the sera which now appear to be monospecific will eventually be found to contain more than a single species of antibody.

Some antisera for histocompatibility testing have been prepared by the immunization of human volunteers or higher primates with leukocytes or subcellular fractions, or by the application of skin allografts. Such procedures will be of greater value when more highly purified preparations of transplantation antigens become available.

Lymphocytotoxicity and Leukoagglutination Tests.   Since the transplantation antigens directed by the HL-A locus are well represented on peripheral blood leukocytes, it has been these cells which have been used almost exclusively in histocompatibility typing tests (see Table 1-9).

In the lymphocytotoxicity test, the lymphocytes from either a prospective organ donor or recipient are divided into several aliquots. Each aliquot of cells is then incubated, in the presence of complement, with one of a panel of antisera known to be directed against specific components of the transplantation antigen system. Specific transplantation antigen-antibody interaction on the surface of the lymphocyte leads to cell injury which may be detected by a loss of the lymphocyte's capacity to exclude the entry of materials such as Trypan Blue dye.[35]

In the leukoagglutination test, similar methodology is employed, but complement is not required. A positive test is indicated by a clumping of leukocytes.[35]

At the present time, the technique of lymphocytotoxicity would appear to be gaining popularity in many laboratories on the basis of sensitivity, simplicity, and reproducibility. Other in vitro histocompatibility serotyping tests include platelet complement fixation, the antiglobulin consumption test, mixed hemagglutination, immunoadherence, and methods involving immunofluorescence.

The advent of serotyping for histocompatibility has undoubtedly been a major factor in the recent increase in success of certain organ allografts between unrelated donors. Under conditions where patients with irreparable organ damage may be kept alive by artificial means while awaiting transplantation, as in the case of chronic renal failure, a large prospective recipient pool will inevitably accumulate. At the same time, a prospective donor pool may also become available. Any attempt to employ matching tests, on the basis of random selection, to determine the best donor-recipient combinations would be an insurmountable task. However, the development of serotyping, in conjunction with computerization, now makes this undertaking feasible, at least on a local scale.

The rapid technical advances being made in tissue preservation techniques may also permit prolonged organ storage to become a reality in the foreseeable future.[1] It would be possible to utilize organ banks only if detailed information were available concerning the transplantation antigens of both the stored organs and the patients awaiting an organ allograft.

Erythrocyte Antigens in Histocompatibility

With the exception of blood or bone marrow transfusions, only the ABO and P blood group antigens appear to be of importance in determining histocompatibility. Of these, the ABO system is by far the more important. The A and B blood group antigens are present not only on red blood cells, but on all tissues except those of the central nervous system. Skin and renal allografts performed across the ABO barrier frequently result in accelerated rejection. This response is even more pronounced if the recipient has been previously sensitized to the incompatible erythrocyte antigen and, in this context, the A_2 subgroup of the A system (see Table 1-7) appears to be particularly immunogenic.

Despite the fact that the data remain somewhat inconclusive, there is evidence to suggest that transplantation between individuals differing at the P locus may also be detrimental to the survival of both skin and renal allografts. The role of other erythrocyte isoantigens cannot be completely evaluated because only limited studies have been performed.

IMMUNOSUPPRESSIVE THERAPY

The fact that immunosuppression alone is an effective means of inhibiting human allograft rejection is supported by the results of kidney transplant survival in the era prior to the advent of adequate methods of histocompatibility testing. Although inferior to recent results, the success achieved far exceeded the expected rate of good random matching between donor and recipient. At the present time, there are several methods of immuno-suppression available to the clinician which may be used individually, sequentially, or simultaneously.

Irradiation Therapy

Whole Body Irradiation. Whole body irradiation was employed about a decade ago for the impairment of the immune response against allografts in humans but this procedure is no longer widely used. A dose of 200 to 600 rads of whole body irradiation produces temporary, severe pancyto-penia, and usually leads to a marked increase in susceptibility to infection. Although whole body irradiation in this range may be of value where there is a close genetic relationship between donor and recipient, it is doubt-ful whether the possible benefits are justified by the risk to the recipient.

Local Irradiation. Irradiation of the recipient graft bed prior to kidney transplantation in an attempt to destroy local lymphoid tissue has not been very effective in abrogating the rejection phenomenon. By contrast, irradia-tion of the graft itself, either in the immediate postoperative period or during rejection crises, has sometimes been useful in prolonging renal allo-graft survival. The mechanism of action is probably one of local destruction of the active cellular elements immediately involved in the rejection process. It has been found that this form of treatment may also hasten the "healing in" of a fresh renal graft. Since radiation nephritis occurs at local renal doses of about 1500 rads or more, 900 rads is usually the total maximum dose employed.

Extracorporeal Irradiation. Irradiation of the lymph by the implantation of radioactive isotopes into the area of the thoracic duct has been attempted only in animals. However, the irradiation of blood flowing through an arteriovenous shunt has been utilized in man in an attempt to diminish the mass of circulating lymphocytes which could take part in allograft rejection.[16] Since this technique has seldom, if ever, been employed in the absence of any other form of therapy, its efficacy is difficult to assess at present.

Immunosuppressive Drug Therapy

General Principles. The ultimate aim of immunosuppressive drug therapy in transplantation is the permanent deletion of immunologic responsiveness against a given set of antigens. Immunologic tolerance of both simple and complex antigens has been achieved in adult animals of a number of species by the use of immunosuppressive agents such as 6-mercaptopurine, cyclophosphamide, and amethopterin given at the time of antigen administration. Immunologic tolerance, therefore, is not a phenomenon restricted to the neonatal period.

Numerous immunosuppressive agents belonging to a variety of drug classes which include corticosteroids, purine analogs, folic acid antagonists, and alkylating agents have been used with varying degrees of success in attempts to inhibit animal allograft rejection. All of these agents may interfere with both the cell-mediated and humoral immune responses of the subject under treatment. Modifications of the immune response may occur at any one of the following stages in the process of allograft rejection: (*1*) interference with initial sensitization or with recognition of an antigen; (*2*) depression of cellular proliferation which is essential for the amplification of an immune response of either the cell-mediated or humoral type; (*3*) interference with the function of the immunologically competent, sensitized cell; or (*4*) blockade of the secondary mediators which produce damage following the interaction of antibody with tissue antigen. With these factors in mind, the immunosuppressive agents most commonly used in human organ transplantation will be considered[9] (Immunosuppressive drugs are also discussed in Chapter 6).

6-Mercaptopurine and Azathioprine.

Both 6-mercaptopurine and azathioprine inhibit the synthesis of the purine and pyrimidine components of DNA and RNA. Although azathioprine is catabolized to 6-mercaptopurine in the body, it has been suggested that the imidazolyl component of azathioprine may bind sulfhydryl groups and thereby exert an additional antimetabolic effect. Whether on this basis or not, azathioprine presently represents the single most effective agent available for the prevention of human allograft rejection.[29a] Both 6-mercaptopurine and azathioprine are given orally in doses of 1 to 5 mg/kg/day. The major side-effects include alopecia, anemia, leukopenia, hepatic toxicity, pancreatitis, esophagitis, and stomatitis.

Cyclophosphamide.

Cyclophosphamide is an alkylating agent of relatively low toxicity. Its mode of action as a potent immunosuppressive agent remains uncertain. Proposed, but unproven, mechanisms include cross-linking of DNA, blockade of the differentiation and/or division of immunologically competent cells, and a direct attack on the protein synthetic and enzymatic pathways of lymphoid tissues. Other body tissues are, of course, affected to greater or lesser extent.

Cyclophosphamide has not been widely used in human organ transplantation until recently, and optimum dosage schedules have not yet been established. The drug may be administered orally in doses of 2 to 8 mg/kg/day for relatively long periods of time, but when used to suppress the human allograft response it is more commonly given intravenously in large doses of 30 mg/kg or more, over relatively short periods of time. Side-effects include dizziness, nausea, vomiting, alopecia, mucosal ulceration, hepatotoxicity, and skin pigmentation.

Corticosteroids. Corticosteroids are known to be anti-inflammatory and to induce a lympholytic effect, but their mode of action in prolonging allograft survival remains largely unknown. High local concentration of cortisone may produce stabilization of cell and lysozomal membranes, and thus inhibits target cell damage by attacking lymphocytes. There is, however, no definite evidence for this effect.

Prednisone is the corticosteroid agent most frequently employed in human organ transplantation. When used to avert rejection, it is given orally in doses of 20 to 800 mg/day. The side-effects of prolonged corticosteroid therapy include severe pancreatitis, peptic ulceration, aseptic bone necrosis, hyperglycemia, withdrawal arthritis, Cushingoid features, cataract formation, hypertension, acne, and demineralization of bone.

Actinomycin C. Actinomycin C, an antibiotic, is a selective inhibitor of DNA-dependent messenger-RNA synthesis. Administered intravenously in doses of 4 to 8 μg/kg/day, the major side-effects of this agent are bone marrow depression, nausea, vomiting, and stomatitis.

Azaserine. Azaserine is an inhibitor of nucleotide synthesis. It is usually administered in a dose of 8 to 10 mg/day either intravenously or orally. The major side-effects of azaserine include delirium, coma, stomatitis, and jaundice.

Heterologous Antilymphocytic Antiserum (ALS)

Preparation. Immunization of one species of animals with lymphocytes or thymocytes of another leads to the production of heterologous antilymphocyte serum (ALS) or antithymocyte serum (ATS), respectively. Frequently, only the globulin fractions of the antisera (ALG or ATG) are employed clinically.

Investigations in animals with potent ALS preparations revealed a number of properties which include: (*1*) marked suppression of cell-mediated immunity as manifested by prolonged allograft survival; (*2*) a less marked immunosuppressive effect, or even an augmentation, of the humoral immune response; (3) a unique inhibition of second-set rejection in a previously sensitized subject; and (4) very low toxicity.[9]

Experience with ALS or ALG in man has been less favorable for a number of reasons. At present, there are no commercially available or standardized preparations of these materials. Hence, they are prepared by different investigators in different animals using human thymocytes or lymphocytes obtained by different methods. Both the route and, in particular, the duration of immunization appear to be critical factors in determining the immunosuppressive potency of ALS.

Because the immunization for ALS is performed with preparations of cells which seldom approach lymphocyte purity, a number of antibodies with specificities other than those directed against the lymphocyte are invariably obtained. These antibodies react with a variety of other circulating blood elements including erythrocytes, polymorphonuclear leukocytes, and platelets. Even when the contaminating specificities are absorbed from the antiserum, and only antilymphocytic activity remains, there can be no certainty of the potency of the preparation in prolonging allograft survival. In fact, it has been established that there is no relationship whatever between the lymphocytotoxic and immunosuppressive properties of ALS.

Mechanism of Action. Several different theories have been proposed to explain the mechanism of ALS action which include: (1) the nonspecific (sterile) transformation of lymphocytes so that they cannot respond to other antigens; (2) a specific (fertile) activation of lymphocytes in which the lymphocytes are forced to respond to the ALS and are thus diverted from a reaction against any other foreign protein; (3) a "blind-folding" effect of the lymphocyte coated with ALS antibodies; and (4) a selective depletion of a certain population of immunologically reactive cells such as those associated with the theoretic thymic-dependent system; and (5) a primary action on macrophages and other phagocytic cells of the reticuloendothelial system.[29b] At the moment, there is no evidence that any of these hypotheses will satisfactorily explain the mode of action of ALS.

Problems Associated with the Use of ALS in Human Organ Transplantation. Until recently there has been no way of assessing even the potential activity of ALS other than by its clinical administration. This difficulty has been partially overcome by the introduction of two methods of ALS testing which appear promising. The first utilizes the fact that higher primates share the HL-A histocompatibility locus with man. Thus, antihuman ALS may be tested by its ability to prolong skin or kidney allografts in monkeys and baboons.[5]

Perhaps of even greater significance is the description of a new in vitro procedure. It has been shown that potent ALS inhibits the usual rosette formation by sheep erythrocytes which occurs when they are incubated with specifically sensitized lymphocytes. This observation suggests that the sites against which ALS acts are those present on immunologically active cells, although it is unlikely that these sites are immunoglobulin in nature.[4]

The clinical efficacy of ALS in prolonging organ allografts in man is difficult to evaluate because improved surgical techniques and improved methods of histocompatibility testing have been introduced at the same time. Furthermore, ALS has not been utilized as the only immunosuppressive agent in any human allograft procedures. Although it has been shown that allograft rejection may be impeded with less vigorous use of other immunosuppressive agents when ALS is employed, it is uncertain what effect ALS would have if given alone.

Since ALS apparently fails to significantly inhibit humoral antibody formation, any form of rejection having a prominent humoral component may be completely unaffected. This may be the case in hyperacute renal allograft rejection which will be discussed later in this chapter.

Following prolonged ALS therapy, rising titers of anti-ALS antibodies appear. Thus, the effectiveness of ALS treatment probably decreases with time.

Occasional anaphylactic reactions have been observed following the administration of ALS, and urticaria may develop at the site of injection (see Chapter 2). The occurrence of clinical glomerulonephritis due specifically to ALS therapy has not been reported.[9] However, in several patients who have received ALS, immunofluorescent studies of renal biopsies have revealed a pattern consistent with the deposition of antigen-antibody complexes on the glomerular basement membrane. In others, a linear fluorescent pattern of anti-GBM antibody deposition suggests that cross-reacting antibody molecules have not been absorbed out of the ALS by the connective tissue at the site of ALS injection (see Chapter 6).

Dosage Schedules. The dosage schedule of ALS in man has varied from patient to patient and from group to group. On the average, when ALG is employed, individuals may receive doses of 1 to 5 ml per injection depending on the weight of the patient, the antileukocyte titer of the preparation, and the protein content of the preparation. Injections are given intramuscularly, and may begin 3 to 5 days before surgery. Injections are usually continued daily for approximately $2\frac{1}{2}$ weeks and are then reduced to every other day for 2 weeks, twice a week for 2 months, and once a week for a final month. The result is a treatment program of approximately 4 months.

Other investigators have suggested giving much higher doses of ALS or ALG for short periods of time in a more intensive fashion. The objective is to deplete the long-lived lymphocyte population thoroughly and rapidly. This approach might result in a much more profound and protracted immunosuppressive effect, and might also reduce the problems associated with the development of circulating antibodies to ALS.

Thoracic Duct Drainage

This method consists of the cannulation of the thoracic duct and the removal of several liters of thoracic duct lymph per day from the allograft recipient. The draining material may contain more than 10^9 lymphocytes per liter. The lymph may be centrifuged, the lymphocytes removed, and the supernatant reinfused into the recipient. On a prolonged basis, this procedure becomes rather cumbersome, and even short-term drainage has resulted in some infectious complications. Nevertheless, a definite immunosuppressive effect of thoracic duct drainage was reported in a group of patients who had undergone renal transplantation.[36]

General Complications of Immunosuppressive Therapy

Infection.   Irradiation and the immunosuppressive agents, with the possible exceptions of ALS and the corticosteroids, carry the inherent danger of nonspecific cell destruction. However, the major complication of immunosuppressive therapy is an increased susceptibility to infections caused by opportunistic agents such as *Pneumocystis carinii*, cytomegalovirus, *Pseudomonas,* and a wide variety of fungi (see Chapter 4). The reason may be that the immunosuppressive agents have a lesser effect in impairing the more firmly established immunity to common pathogenic microorganisms.

The lung appears to be the organ of predilection for these infectious agents, and the infections have a higher incidence in patients who require larger doses of immunosuppressive agents. The transplant lung syndrome has been described as one characterized by a marked alveolar-capillary diffusion block and diffuse infiltrations throughout the lung parenchyma. It has been suggested that this condition may have an immunologic basis. For example, it is conceivable that patients who receive kidney transplants may subsequently develop anti-GBM antibodies which lead to pulmonary damage by a mechanism similar to that postulated for Goodpasture's syndrome (see Chapter 6). However, the majority of patients who develop this complication are found to have either viral or *P. carinii* infection at autopsy.

The pathogenetic importance of cytomegalovirus infection has not been established since this organism is found at intervals in the urine of most patients following transplantation, even when they are otherwise in apparently good health. It is possible that immunosuppressive therapy permits the development of a latent cytomegalovirus infection, or alternatively, primary cytomegalovirus infection may follow immunosuppression. It is also of interest that patients dying after renal allografts are frequently found to have cytomegalovirus in the pancreas.

Another organ system frequently infected following transplantation of the kidney is the urinary tract itself. In a similar fashion, infections of the liver have followed hepatic transplantation in man. Other infectious syndromes which may follow immunosuppressive therapy include peritonitis, septic arthritis, meningitis, cholangitis, gastroenteritis, epididymitis, and disseminated bacteremias, fungemias or viremias.

Lymphoreticular Malignancy. Recently, a disturbing, but not totally unexpected, complication of immunosuppressive therapy has been described. To date, at least 12 patients receiving immunosuppressive therapy have been reported to have developed lymphoreticular malignancies such as lymphosarcoma and reticulum cell sarcoma.[9,25] The tumors have arisen in the liver, brain, and thorax. All patients had received azathioprine and prednisone, and several had also received ALG.

Considering the number of patients who have received allografts and subsequent immunosuppressive therapy, the number of individuals who have developed lymphoreticular tumors, especially reticulum cell sarcoma, is far higher than can be explained by chance alone.[20a] However, the underlying mechanism remains speculative. It is possible that the normal immune system serves as a surveillance mechanism for the elimination of cells which undergo malignant transformation, thereby avoiding the development of large tumors. If this were the case, tumors of all types, rather than those of the lymphoreticular system only, should occur. Recent evidence would suggest that this is, indeed, the situation.

A second possibility is related to the fact that the immunosuppressive agents primarily affect the lymphoreticular elements in the body. It is conceivable that they either induce mutations in certain lymphoreticular cells, or that they stimulate the primitive elements of this system to develop a high rate of mitosis in order to maintain a constant number of lymphoreticular elements within the body. It may be this abnormal stimulation which leads to the subsequent development of lymphoreticular malignancies.

SPECIFIC ORGAN TRANSPLANTATION IN MAN

KIDNEY TRANSPLANTATION

The transplantation of a normal, functioning, human kidney to a patient suffering from chronic renal failure has served as the prototype situation for human organ transplantation. More renal allografts have been performed than the sum of all other human organ allovital transplants combined. For this reason, more is known about the factors involved in renal allograft survival than about any other human organ.

Factors Contributing to the Relative Success of Human Renal Allografts

It has been suggested that the nature, composition, or location of the renal transplantation antigens are, for some unknown reason, less likely to evoke an immune response than those of certain other organ systems. Conversely, it has been proposed that the kidney serves as a source of a large, continuous, intravenous infusion of transplantation antigens into the recipient. On this latter basis, a state of high-dose tolerance to renal tissue might be achieved. As a consequence of either of these two possibilities, the immunologic rejection of foreign renal tissue, may be easier to control with the available methods of immunosuppression.

Since the kidneys are paired organs, it has been possible to utilize live, first-degree relatives as organ donors. Even when relatives have not been available, the use of live donors is still possible because of the pairing of the organs.

There can be no question that the success of human kidney transplantation has been markedly enhanced by the development and perfection of the methods of hemodialysis. Hemodialysis has permitted patients with chronic renal failure to be kept alive until an adequate donor can be found. Moreover, if a first allograft should fail, hemodialysis may be reinstituted until a second suitable donor is obtained.

Recipient Selection

Because the outcome of renal transplantation remains uncertain, this procedure should obviously be restricted to patients who are clearly in the terminal phase of renal failure. As a corollary of this requirement, there should be an absence of any features indicating reversibility of the condition which might occur if the patient were maintained on either conservative medical management, or a short period of hemodialysis. On the other hand, the renal failure should not be due to active progressive glomerulonephritis since, if quiescence of this process is not obtained prior to transplantation, the same pathology will almost invariably affect the transplanted kidney. Similarly, the renal failure should not be part of a generalized disease which only incidentally affects the kidney. This latter consideration, for example, would be of importance in certain forms of vasculitis or systemic lupus erythematosus (see Chapter 8). It is, however, of interest to consider that following renal transplantation for these conditions, immunosuppressive therapy would both impede rejection and possibly improve the underlying condition.

Diabetes should be considered as a relative contraindication to renal transplantation. However, in the absence of diffuse vascular disease, transplantation may still be undertaken despite the requirement for corticosteroid therapy.

Severe cerebrovascular or coronary artery disease secondary to renal hypertension should not be present in the potential recipient, and pancytopenia or malnutrition secondary to chronic uremia should be eliminated by an adequate preoperative course of hemodialysis. Any sign of infection should be treated by adequate antibiotic therapy prior to the institution of immunosuppressive therapy. Otherwise, the development of disseminated infection and septicemia will almost certainly supervene. Since the heterotopic transplantation of human kidneys utilizes the iliofemoral vasculature, occlusive disease of the blood vessels in this area precludes transplantation.

The age of the patient is of some importance. In this regard, the physiologic rather than the chronologic age must be considered. The only factor precluding kidney transplantation to a very young child is the relative sizes of the vessels used in the surgical anastomosis.

The lower urinary outflow tract should be normal. In this context, it should be remembered that uremia per se may impair the dynamics of bladder movements and may simulate a neurogenic bladder. These abnormalities usually disappear with adequate hemodialysis. Furthermore, transplantation in the presence of lower urinary tract disease has been performed after the construction of an ileal conduit prior to transplantation.

Any evidence of peptic ulceration must be considered at least a relative contraindication because large doses of corticosteroids may be required. If a severe ulcer diathesis is present, it may be necessary to perform a gastrectomy prior to transplantation.

Donor Selection

Whenever possible, and the situation is obviously quite rare, a monozygotic twin should be employed. In the majority of instances, when this is not possible, a first-degree relative who shows the closest possible histocompatibility with the potential recipient should be chosen as the organ donor. Other, carefully typed, live volunteers have been used as donors quite successfully and have included: (*1*) recipients' spouses; (*2*) unrelated volunteer subjects; and (*3*) patients undergoing nephrectomy of a normal kidney for reasons such as the presence of ureteral lesions or the use of a ureter for the drainage of spinal fluid in hydrocephalus.

Living donors should, of course, be carefully screened with regard to their own renal function. Normal anatomic configuration of the kidneys and the lower urinary tract must be assured by appropriate radiologic examinations, including aortograms to assess the renal arterial supply. Since 20 per cent of normal individuals have multiple renal arteries and since such arteries are end arteries, this common anomaly may lead to problems at surgery which will result in at least partial kidney necrosis.

The risk in a young adult volunteer following nephrectomy is negligible. At the time of writing, over 1700 nephrectomies have been performed for the purpose of kidney donation.[1a] A few rare complications have occurred, and one donor died during hospitalization for nephrectomy.[29a]

In centers where there has been a reluctance to employ live donors, or in situations where no suitable living donor has been available, cadaver kidneys have been transplanted. The criteria for establishing death of the donor vary from group to group, but usually include the absence of respiration and heart beat, and a flat electrocardiogram and electroencephalogram. When there is a prolonged agonal period, histocompatibility typing and an assessment of renal function may be performed prior to death.

The kidney should be removed and transplanted as soon after death as possible in order to avoid acute tubular necrosis. If transplantation must be delayed, the organ should be perfused and cooled. Kidneys kept in this fashion for 3 to 4 hours have functioned immediately after transplantation. In general, better results have been obtained with cadaver kidneys taken from individuals under 65 years of age. This finding is probably related to the greater prevalence of vascular pathology in the older age groups.

Procedure of Renal Transplantation

The recipient should be brought to the best possible metabolic state by dietary and other measures prior to transplantation. Hemodialysis, at intervals of 3 or 4 days may be continued for as long as necessary to bring the patient into biochemical balance. Infection must be eliminated by vigorous treatment with antibiotics. It should also be recognized that both iron and vitamin deficiency, particularly that of folic acid, may exist in patients maintained on long-term hemodialysis.

In some institutions elective bilateral nephrectomy is performed in all patients scheduled for transplantation. This operation eliminates the need for a possible subsequent surgical procedure while the patient is receiving immunosuppressive therapy. It also removes a potential or established site of infection and often facilitates the management of hypertension.

The psychologic preparation of the patient is obviously of great importance. If this preparation is overlooked, there may be severe postoperative emotional problems.

Human renal allografts are usually heterotopic, with the kidney being placed in either the right or left side of the pelvis. With living donors and surgery under optimum circumstances, the renal ischemia time is about 20 to 30 minutes and the production of urine is almost immediate. When cadaver kidneys are utilized, the physiologic condition of the organ is much more variable and renal function may be delayed for several days or even weeks because of the presence of acute tubular necrosis.

Functional Assessment of the Transplanted Kidney

Although it was originally believed that the denervated kidney transplanted between identical twins was deficient in its handling of sodium, renal isografts have subsequently been shown to be capable of completely normal function. Similar findings have been obtained in a number of patients with successful human kidney allografts. Under ideal circumstances, the following parameters of renal function have been observed to be within normal limits: blood urea nitrogen; serum creatinine and electrolytes; urinalysis; excretion of sodium, potassium, protein, and phenolsulfonphthalein; blood pH; urine cultures; clearances of creatinine, urea, paraaminohippuric acid, inulin, and radioactive ^{57}Co-vitamin B_{12}; intravenous pyelography; radio-renograms; radio-scintograms; responses to mannitol, salt loading, and salt restriction; antidiuretic hormone effect; and urine concentration and dilution tests.

The postoperative pattern in the first 24 to 48 hours after allotransplantation may vary from one of complete normality, as described above, to a total lack of renal function due to acute tubular necrosis in cadaver kidneys. Despite this wide variation, however, a rather characteristic functional pattern is observed in most patients. This is manifested first by the prompt excretion, either at the conclusion of the operation or shortly afterwards, of isotonic or slightly hypotonic urine. Usually the urine flow increases steadily over the ensuing few hours until a moderate to marked diuresis is apparent. Although initially depressed, the glomerular filtration rate and renal blood flow begin to rise until they approach or reach the normal range at varying times after the first 48 hours.

The postoperative diuresis characteristic of early allograft acceptance may serve as a useful prognostic sign and suggests an initially successful transplant. When good histocompatibility matching exists between a recipient and a live donor, the progressive increase in renal function occurs at the same rate and to the same degree in both individuals.

Pathophysiology of Renal Allograft Rejection

Except in the case of identical twins, a rejection crisis of greater or lesser violence and occurring at different intervals following transplantation is seen in the majority of patients receiving kidney allografts.

Hyperacute (or Immediate) Rejection. A hyperacute rejection of the transplanted kidney may occur within minutes to hours following the completion of the surgical anastomosis (see Chapter 6). Biopsies of acutely rejected kidneys taken within 1 hour after the completion of surgery have revealed the accumulation of large numbers of polymorphonuclear leukocytes within glomerular and peritubular capillaries, and immunofluorescence studies have demonstrated irregular accumulations of IgG in the same areas.

In one report, three recipients rejected five renal allografts within a few minutes to a few hours after their vascular anastomoses to the recipient.[33] When these kidneys were removed, they all showed the presence of cortical necrosis. The major vessels were patent, but the arterioles and glomeruli were the sites of fibrin deposition. There was little or no fixation of host immunoglobulin in the allografts, in contradistinction to the situation noted above. These findings were, therefore, characteristic of a generalized Shwartzman reaction (see Chapter 1).

Serologic studies in patients manifesting hyperacute renal allograft rejection demonstrated the presence of pre-existing antibodies against human histocompatibility antigens. The humoral antibodies which may initiate this reaction could well result from prior blood transfusions. Even if hyperacute rejection does not take place, there is a high correlation between the occurrence of these antibodies, a generally poor clinical course, and histologic evidence of obliterative vascular lesions in the transplanted kidney.[16a] Thus, many physicians refrain, insofar as possible, from giving transfusions to patients who may become candidates for kidney transplantation. Where such transfusions are absolutely necessary, washed red cells should be given, and all precautions should be taken to make certain that leukocytes have been removed from the blood preparations.

The pathogenesis of the Shwartzman type of hyperacute renal allograft rejection remains uncertain, but a number of possibilities have been suggested: (1) conditioning of the patient by the bacterial contamination and hemolysis that often accompany hemodialysis; (2) conditioning by immunosuppression; and (3) conditioning by the transplantation procedure itself. Some of the patients involved in this type of reaction show preformed lymphocytotoxic antibodies which may be an indication of predisposition to this phenomenon. High risk patients may, therefore, be recognized on occasion and should be treated prophylactically with anticoagulants.

Acute (or Early) Rejection. The more usual type of renal allograft rejection occurs between 3 to 14 days after transplantation, and may lead to irrevocable destruction of the kidney despite intensive immunosuppressive and supportive therapy. Even if the patient recovers from an acute rejection episode occurring within the first week after transplantation, the chances for the ultimate success of the allograft are far less than if the first rejection crisis had taken place at a later date.

The earlier the rejection appears (e.g., at 3 days), the more the damage seems to be confined to the intravascular area. Allograft biopsy has proved to be a most valuable procedure in the management of patients receiving renal allografts.[22] When performed during an early rejection crisis, the biopsy shows thrombi containing enmeshed polymorphonuclear leukocytes within the glomerular loops. Electron microscopic studies usually demonstrate the presence of fibrin, platelets, and polymorphonuclear leukocytes in the intravascular region, while immunofluorescence studies may reveal the deposition of IgG and C3 in the glomerular and peritubular vessels.

It is of interest that even when the amount of thrombosis within the capillary loops is severe and kidney function is depressed, the lesions may be reversible by the use of heparin therapy. These findings suggest that abnormalities of the coagulation system, triggered by immune mechanisms, may be of importance in early allograft rejection. The finding of fibrinogen degradation products in the urine during rejection crises lends support to the hypothesis that clotting factors may be activated during early allograft rejection. Furthermore, it has been observed that the urinary degradation products tend to disappear with effective immunosuppressive therapy.

If the early rejection crisis occurs closer to 7 days following transplantation, evidence of cell mediation becomes more apparent. There is infiltration of lymphoid cells and plasma cells in the interstitial spaces adjacent to the renal tubules. In addition, the lymphoid cells of recipient origin have a tendency to penetrate the tubular lumens where they are shed into the urine together with tubular cells. The presence of recipient lymphocytes and plasma cells suggest that allograft immunity is largely acquired subsequent to transplantation.

Chronic (or Late) Rejection. Completely effective immunosuppression is rarely if ever achieved, and renal biopsies of all long-term survivors show definite morphologic changes. There is, however, a lack of correlation between these changes and the immunologic mechanisms responsible for the structural alterations.

Graft persistence or repeated episodes of rejection crises lead to endothelial cell hypertrophy and proliferation, irregular thickening of the basement membranes, and a fusion of the epithelial foot processes. Mesangial cell proliferation is frequently found in the glomerular tuft. Even apparently normally functioning kidneys inevitably show fusion of glomerular epithelial foot processes and subepithelial deposits on the basement membranes.

Morphologic features characteristic of the late irreversible stage include marked glomerular endothelial proliferation as well as the accumulation of aggregated polymorphonuclear leukocytes and platelets which virtually occlude the vascular lumens. Immunofluorescent studies may reveal the deposition of IgG and C3 in the perivascular areas and in the areas of endothelial proliferation.

As the proliferation continues, the lumens of the arteriolar vessels become progressively narrower, and tubular atrophy may occur as a result of increasing ischemia or immunologic damage. Although absolute proof is lacking, it is possible that the nephrotic syndrome which sometimes occurs during the course of chronic allograft rejection may represent a specific immunologic attack upon the glomerular basement membrane.

Clinical Features of Hyperacute Rejection

Hyperacute rejection is frequently visualized in the operating room by prompt failure of perfusion of the cortical area after the vascular anastamosis has been performed. When hyperacute rejection occurs a few hours after surgery, it may be manifested by cessation of urinary flow after a short period of normal function. Early kidney biopsy is of great value in establishing the diagnosis.

Clinical Features of Acute Rejection

There is rarely any difficulty in recognizing a fully-developed rejection crisis. Of far greater importance is the detection of early signs and symptoms, since appropriate immunosuppressive therapy at this time may save the allograft. On the other hand, if rejection appears inevitable by the criteria to be discussed below, the transplant should be removed, hemodialysis reinstituted, and the patient prepared for retransplantation.

Oliguria. The hallmark of the acute rejection reaction is the onset of oliguria or anuria. This is almost always associated with fluid retention and weight gain. If the oliguria or anuria follows a preceding period of normal renal function, allograft rejection must be distinguished from cortical necrosis, arterial occlusion, venous thrombosis, ureteral obstruction, or obstruction of the urethral catheter with blood clots. The procedures of urethral catheter irrigation, arteriography, venography, cystoscopy, cystography, and ureteral catheterization may be utilized to help exclude these latter possibilities.

Although the oliguria may represent a decreased renal perfusion due to allograft rejection, it may, of course, also represent a physiologic response due to decreased intravascular volume. Hence, in assessing oliguria at any time following transplantation it must be certain that the patient is in a state of fluid and electrolyte balance. When failure of renal function occurs, it is important that the use of azathioprine be discontinued since the kidney is the normal route of excretion for this material. Immunosuppression should be maintained with corticosteroid drugs.

A variety of radioisotopic methods for the determination of renal blood flow and glomerular filtration rate have been developed which offer the advantage of rapid analysis without urine collections. These are of particular value when accurate urine volume determinations are difficult to perform because of oliguria.

Renomegaly.   Renomegaly, or swelling of the transplanted kidney, associated with pain and tenderness is another excellent indication of allograft rejection. The pain, which is due to swelling of sufficient degree to stretch the surrounding tissues, may radiate down to the testicle on the side of the transplant.

Fever.   The development of fever, particularly in patients not receiving prophylactic steroids, is a nonspecific but very characteristic sign of rejection. Even steroids do not invariably suppress the febrile reaction, or fever may follow steroid withdrawal. It is important to note that fever of up to 103 to 106° F daily may occur for many days after transplantation, yet be unassociated with rejection or any other demonstrable renal pathology. A persistent low-grade fever may, however, indicate ultimate allograft failure. All of the usual causes of a febrile reaction, particularly the presence of infection, should be considered and excluded.

Hypertension.   Many renal allograft recipients are hypertensive as a result of their original renal disease. However, when adequate control of blood pressure has been achieved after transplantation, the reappearance of severe hypertension is highly suggestive of a rejection process.

Laboratory Findings.   The hematologic features of acute rejection are poly-morphonuclear leukocytosis and thrombocytopenia. Although a decrease in the platelet count occurs in many patients prior to the onset of clinical rejection, it should be noted that this finding may also be associated with drug toxicity in patients who receive immunosuppressive agents.

Any increase in the urinary sediment, whether due to erythrocytes, leuko-cytes, or casts may be a sign of impending rejection. Of particular sig-nificance with regard to the rejection process are: (1) large epithelioid cells with multiple intracytoplasmic inclusions; (2) small lymphocytes which may be associated with tubular epithelial cells to form casts; and (3) small darkly staining epithelial cells which tend to occur in small clusters (Type 1 epithelial cells). The functional significance of these cells remains unknown, although they have been found in the urine of patients with acute tubular necrosis. Employing the immune adherence technique, it has been shown that antibody-coated mononuclear cells may occasionally be present in the urinary sediment at the time of rejection.

The sudden appearance of proteinuria in a patient whose urine has previously been free of protein, or a sudden massive increase in urinary protein is suggestive of impending rejection. Although occasionally associ-ated with the nephrotic syndrome, the proteinuria seen during rejection is characteristically nonselective (see Chapter 6).

Other laboratory findings suggestive of rejection are a rising blood urea nitrogen, elevation of the serum creatinine, and a fall in creatinine clear-ance. Decreased renal perfusion results in very low urinary sodium concen-tration and a relatively high osmolality. Renal tubular acidosis has been described during rejection, but it is probably a side-effect of azathioprine therapy. Hypercalcemia due to secondary hyperparathyroidism may be asso-ciated with rejection and a decrease in the glomerular filtration rate.

Since kidney tissue is rich in a variety of enzymes, elevations in both serum and urinary levels of certain of these enzymes may be of value in assessing the rejection process. Elevations of serum lactic dehydrogenase, urinary lactic dehydrogenase, serum alkaline phosphatase, and urinary lysozyme have been described in association with rejection of renal transplants.

Renal Biopsy.   Open renal biopsy may be of assistance in making the differ-ential diagnosis between rejection and acute tubular necrosis, or may be of some value in assessing the degree and nature of rejection in patients whose renal function remains depressed despite intensive immunosuppressive therapy.[22] If fibrosis is observed without significant infiltration of lymphoid cells or acute vascular changes, this finding would indicate that permanent damage has been incurred which cannot respond to additional therapy.

However, if acute vascular and cellular changes are present, further immunosuppressive therapy may be indicated. Occasionally, the presence of an unsuspected bacterial nephritis may be detected on renal biopsy.

Immunologic Studies. Of the immunologic studies thus far described, alterations in the serum levels of C2, C3, and C4, appear to be the most promising in the clinical assessment of renal allograft recipients.[10] Serum levels of C2, C3, and C4 are usually elevated or normal at the onset of rejection, but may be reduced as a severe episode persists.

The formation of humoral antibodies against HL-A directed transplantation antigens has already been described. In addition, heterophile antibodies, which are not of the Forssman or Paul-Bunnell type, have been demonstrated in the sera of patients receiving renal allografts.[26] The function of the heterophile antibodies remains uncertain, but they may be of some importance as an early warning of impending rejection.

Clinical Features of Chronic Rejection

After a renal allograft has remained in place for several months, it may undergo two different forms of rejection. The first type is simply a delayed form of the acute rejection process. More commonly, however, the late or chronic rejection phenomenon is manifested by a gradual decline in renal function over a period of weeks or months. Not infrequently, episodic rejection crises occur which become increasingly resistant to immunosuppressive therapy.

The diagnosis of late rejection is primarily one of exclusion, and this process must be differentiated from pyelonephritis or ureteral obstruction. Not infrequently, late rejection is observed following the discontinuation of steroid therapy. However, recipients on steroid medication are not protected against this form of rejection, and may show gradual deterioration despite maintenance or even increasing doses of prednisone.

The clinical features associated with late rejection may include the reappearance of hypertension, tenderness over the allografted kidney, fluid retention, fever, general malaise, polyarthritis, and alopecia. In contrast to acute rejection crises, oliguria, low urine sodium, and high urine osmolality are infrequent findings in chronic rejection. The recurrence of glomerulonephritis in patients whose renal failure was initially caused by this disease (see Chapter 6), and the development of nephrotic syndrome may also form part of the picture of chronic rejection.

Renal arteriography performed during a late or chronic rejection process may reveal varying degrees of irregular narrowings in the secondary and tertiary renal arterial branches. Although these signs may be observed very early after transplantation, they are much more characteristic of the late and slowly progressive chronic rejection process. As in the case of the acute rejection crisis, patients with late rejection manifest abnormalities in serum complement levels. Instability, rather than the absolute values of C2, C3, and C4, appears to be of primary importance in diagnosing chronic rejection.

Increased immunosuppressive therapy usually fails to alter the course of the chronic rejection process. However, these patients occasionally stabilize with reduced renal function, and are said to be in a burned out stage of chronic rejection.

Specific Complications of Renal Transplantation

Post-Transplantation Glomerulonephritis. The recurrence of glomerulonephritis in transplanted kidneys is fully discussed in Chapter 6. It is of significance that the incidence of post-transplantation glomerulonephritis in allografted kidneys has been found to be somewhat higher in children than in adults.

Metabolic Changes.   In patients who have not been brought into adequate metabolic balance by hemodialysis prior to transplantation, there have been instances of massive diuresis and hypokalemia in the immediate post-operative period. This complication has occasionally led to severe dehydration, shock, and even death shortly after the transplantation procedure.

Secondary hyperparathyroidism is found in almost all patients with chronic renal failure, but parathyroid function usually returns to normal after successful renal allotransplantation. However, occasionally the parathyroid glands may become autonomous and parathyroidectomy may be necessary during the postoperative period. Hyperparathyroidism in the recipient may even lead to the presence of renal calculi in the transplanted kidney shortly after allografting. In children, significant bone disease associated with hyperparathyroidism is not usually reversed by renal transplantation. Therefore, skeletal changes and failure of normal growth are important causes of chronic invalidism in the young allograft recipient.

Pregnancy and Fertility.   Pelvic heterotopic transplantation of an allografted kidney in women has not been found to be a contraindication to childbirth. Although large doses of corticosteroids may have resulted in very occasional teratogenic effects, the action of azathioprine during human gestation has yet to be completely evaluated. However, at least four normal children have been born of mothers on immunosuppressive therapy and appear to be developing normally. Azathioprine and prednisone do not appear to have detrimental effects on spermatogenesis, and several male patients have fathered normal children while on immunosuppressive therapy.

Transmission of Other Diseases. The kidneys of donors dying of cancer should be used cautiously, if at all, for transplantation since a malignant tumor has been transmitted with the graft on at least six occasions. At least two of the recipients died of metastatic disease (see Chapter 13).

Other diseases which have been passed from donor to recipient include viral hepatitis, histoplasmosis, thrombocytopenic purpura, and delayed-type hypersensitivities. Viral hepatitis may also occur in renal allograft recipients as the result of the multiple hemodialyses and blood transfusions that are usually required by these patients.

Embolic Phenomena. Fat embolism has been described following kidney transplantation, but the underlying mechanism remains obscure. More readily understandable are the problems of lower limb and pelvic thrombo-embolism which are similar to those occurring after any form of urogenital surgery.

Clinical Results of Renal Transplantation

At present, kidneys for transplanation are obtained in approximately equal numbers from living donors and from cadavers. More than 5000 kidney transplants had been performed by April 1970,[29a] and, of these, 3645 had been reported from approximately 100 institutions to the Human Kidney Transplant Registry for the 7-year period ending January 1, 1970.[1a] The survival data for human renal allografts between live, related donor-recipient pairs at 1 and 2 years is summarized in Table 14-3. These figures represent a statistically significant improvement over those reported prior to 1966 when the cumulative survival time for nontwin sibling allografts was 63 per cent and 57 per cent survival at 1 and 2 years, respectively. Similar gains have been recorded for grafts from parental donors. Unfortunately, the registry data do not permit the ascertainment of the level of function of the surviving allografts.

The most impressive feature, however, continues to be the progressive improvement achieved with cadaver kidneys. Prior to 1966, only 32 per cent of cadaver organs were functioning at 1 year, and only 24 per cent were functioning at 2 years. Between January 1, 1966 and January 1, 1970, 50 per cent were functioning at 1 year and 40 per cent had survived 2 years.

There are, of course, wide variations in success between different centers. In some areas, the 1-year survival rate of allografts approaches 100 per

TABLE 14-3. Survival Data for Renal Allografts between Live, Related
Donor-Recipient Pairs (Accumulated Statistics from January 1,
1966, to January 1, 1970)[1a]

Donor group	Number of transplants	Survival (%) 1 Year	2 Years
Monozygotic twins	12	>90	*
Dizygotic twins	7	>90	*
Nontwin siblings	495	78	74
Parents	545	75	70

* Insufficient sample size for adequate statistical
analysis.

cent. As might be expected, the best results are associated with the largest
experience, the more extensive use of live related donors, the development
of sophisticated systems for histocompatibility typing, and the meticulous
supervision of immunosuppressive therapy. It is of interest that in one
of the largest and oldest series, 28 of 46 patients who received allografts
from blood-relatives between November, 1962, and March, 1964, were alive
at the time of a report in August, 1968.[31] By contrast, only 2 of the original
18 recipients who received organs from nonrelated donors were still alive.

Patient survival exceeds graft survival in many institutions because second, third, and even fourth transplants may succeed where previous allografts have failed. Under appropriate circumstances second transplants appear to function at least as well, or better than, the first transplant. Whether
the privilege enjoyed by a second transplant is based on immunologic
mechanisms remains uncertain at present. Nevertheless, it is quite possible
to provide the allograft recipient with a "second chance" provided that
adequate facilities exist for interim hemodialysis.

HEART TRANSPLANTATION

The first human heart allograft was reported through the news media
in December, 1967. Subsequent events generated an unprecedented degree
of interest which served to focus public attention on the ethics of human
organ transplantation in general, and of heart transplantation in particular.

The medical problems encountered in heart transplantation are somewhat different from those associated with renal allografts. Firstly, the heart is an unpaired organ so that only cadaver donors can be employed. Furthermore, unlike the situation in renal failure, where life can be maintained for an almost indefinite period by artificial means, the ability to prolong life in severe cardiac disease is often extremely limited. For both of these reasons prospective histocompatibility testing is of little value in cardiac allografts, and greater reliance must be placed on the use of immunosuppressive agents. It must also be remembered that even if heart transplantation were to become a feasible procedure, without the necessity of typing for transplantation antigens, the number of prospective donors is extremely small with respect to the number of potential recipients.

The suggestion that a transplanted heart might react differently from other transplanted tissues is based on the fact that the heart is a simpler functional unit than organs such as the kidney or liver. Although there is some evidence that muscle tissue may be quantitatively less antigenic than blood leukocytes, there is no evidence to support the concept that the heart is less vulnerable to rejection than other human allografts.[18]

In September, 1969 the American College of Surgeons—National Institutes of Health Organ Transplant Registry reported that 145 heart transplants had been performed in 143 patients. At that time, 29 of the recipients were alive, 20 had survived 6 months or more, and 8 had survived for more than one year.[29a] It remains uncertain whether the survival time of patients who are suitable candidates for heart allografts is significantly prolonged by the transplantation procedure. The general consensus appears to be that cardiac transplantation is an expensive experiment of unproven merit. On the other hand, there are those who contend that the first series of heart transplants were successful in the sense that they led to a concentrated effort that may result in valuable progress.

LUNG TRANSPLANTATION

As of April, 1970, at least twenty whole lung allografts, obtained from cadavers, and four lobar allografts, obtained from living donors, had been performed.[34] Although the usual survival time following lung transplantation has been from a few days to a few months at best,[7] the longest survivor lived for 11 months after operation.[29a]

The most serious problems which remain to be solved with regard to lung transplantation include: (1) the transplanted lung is particularly susceptible to infections; (2) the ability of lung to clear secretions is dependent, to some extent, on an intact nerve supply which is lost during the transplantation procedure; (3) unlike any other body organ, the lung has a double circulation which includes the necessity for the bronchial arteries to provide nutrition to parts of the left lung parenchyma; and (4) there is a latent period between the time of transplantation and the resumption of normal pulmonary function.

LIVER TRANSPLANTATION

The feasibility of hepatic allotransplantation has been established by experimental studies in which animals have been kept alive for protracted periods of time after complete hepatectomy and liver replacement. The problems of liver allotransplantation in man are, however, complicated by a number of specific problems peculiar to this organ.[32] Orthotopic transplantation of the liver is an extremely difficult technical procedure, and, although hetertopic procedures have been described for the implantation of auxiliary livers, none is ideal.

Since the liver is an unpaired organ, only cadaver donors can be employed. Because the human liver is extremely sensitive to ischemic damage, the major difficulty with human liver allotransplantation has been that of preserving adequate liver function between the time of donor death and the actual transplantation procedure.

There is very little available information concerning the immunology of liver allograft rejection. However, it has been reported that the migration of peripheral leukocytes in a patient who had received a liver transplant could be inhibited by incubation with fetal liver homogenate at a time when there was biochemical evidence of rejection.[14] A liver biopsy obtained at the same time showed liver cell necrosis and infiltration of lymphocytes and plasma cells in the portal tracts. Successful treatment of the rejection crisis with prednisone returned the migration index to normal. These observations would support the contention that liver allograft rejection in man is mediated by cellular immune mechanisms.

As of April, 1970, approximately 100 liver transplants had been performed in man. No recipient of a heterotopic graft survived beyond 7 weeks after operation, but at least three recipients of orthotopic grafts lived for more than 1 year.[29a] Despite the poor survival rate, the fact that recipients of human liver allografts could live for a year or more after operation is somewhat encouraging.

PANCREATIC TRANSPLANTATION

Five cases of pancreatic allotransplantation have been reported in detail.[19] All of the recipients were severe juvenile diabetics with vascular complications, nephropathy, and chronic renal failure. Since these patients were poor risks for chronic hemodialysis or for renal allotransplantation alone, the objective was to transplant a kidney and a pancreas from the same cadaver donor. The principal technique used was the transplantation of the entire pancreas with the attached duodenum into the recipient's iliac fossa. In the immediate postoperative period, there was evidence of adequate pancreatic function in four of the five patients. The longest survival of a human pancreatic transplant reported to date was 134 days.

INTESTINAL TRANSPLANTATION

Preliminary animal experiments with the allotransplantation of small bowel components in dogs have been encouraging. In humans, the major indication for small bowel transplantation would be in patients with massive bowel destruction due to infarction or volvulus, or in children with intestinal atresia. At the time of writing, one such operation had been performed and the patient died 14 hours postoperatively.[19]

CORNEAL AND SCLERAL TRANSPLANTS

The human cornea holds a unique position in the history and biology of human transplantation. As indicated previously, the cornea enjoys a privileged existence on the surface of the eye because, under normal circumstances, it is an avascular tissue. The preservation of corneal tissue is relatively simple, and viable corneas can be obtained several hours after death. Corneas may be stored in tissue banks and can be shipped for long distances without deterioration. Furthermore, immunosuppressive therapy is not required in order to avoid rejection. Thus, corneal transplantation has been a well established clinical procedure for many years.[12]

Surprisingly little is known about the immunology of corneal transplantation, but it has been established that the cornea contains tissue antigens as well as antigens of serum proteins. The most important isoantigens appear to be intracellular, concentrated in the epithelial layer, and closely related to erythrocyte antigens. High titers of circulating anticorneal antibodies have been detected 5 to 20 days after surgery, but these appear to be more closely related to the development of iridocyclitis (see Chapter 17) than to graft failure.

Similarly, a high incidence of success has been achieved with scleral allografts without the use of immunosuppressive agents. The sclera, like the cornea, may therefore be considered as a privileged site, although little is known of the immune response which occurs following the allotransplantation of scleral tissue in humans.

It should be noted that in both corneal and scleral allografts, the transplanted tissue may serve both allostatic and allovital functions. Most of the available evidence indicates that successful corneal allografts are associated with the continued viability of the transplanted tissue. Nevertheless, it remains possible that, under certain circumstances, the donor tissue may function as an architecturally intact superstructure which is gradually replaced by normal recipient tissue.

BONE AND CARTILAGE TRANSPLANTATION

It has been known for half a century that human bone could be transplanted successfully. Studies performed in both man and experimental animals have demonstrated that a bone allograft behaves in much the same fashion as other allografted tissues. The transplanted cells are destroyed within 1 to 2 weeks by the various mechanisms of immune rejection. However, the dead skeleton of the transplanted bone still retains some osteogenetic inductive capacity. Thus, the dead allograft is slowly recolonized by host blood vessels, and the transplanted bone is slowly removed and replaced by new bone of host origin. From these observations, it would appear that transplanted bone functions in an allostatic rather than in an allovital capacity.

Unlike bone transplants, transplanted cartilage functions as an allovital graft. As noted previously, chondrocytes are the only mammalian cells which can be allogeneically transplanted without provoking an immune response. For example, sex chromatin studies have revealed that donor cells remain in place for many years after grafting. Since cartilage allografts behave as autografts, no immunosuppression is required. At present cartilage allografts are used in clinical practice primarily for the reconstructive surgery of the nose, ears, and skull defects.

The use of osteochondral allografts to resurface joints has been an area of active investigation over a long period of time. Allografts of this type have been performed successfully in experimental animals, but only when the underlying metaphysis did not exceed 2 to 3 mm in thickness.[15] When the supporting shell of underlying bone was thicker, the bony layer underwent absorption and collapse. Although similar transplants have not as yet been reported in man, it is possible that they may play an important part in providing functioning, resurfaced joints in the future.

SKIN TRANSPLANTATION

The history of the study of rejection of skin allografts is, in a sense, the history of transplantation itself. The intralymphatic situation of the skin allograft, the peculiarities of its vascular attachment to the host, and the highly antigenic properties of the epidermis have made the skin allograft the most exacting test of human histocompatibility. For exactly the same reasons, attempts at the allogeneic transplantation of skin between humans have almost invariably failed. In fact, the failure to reject a skin allograft has become an important criterion for the assessment of immunologic deficiency states. It seems rather ironic that the organ which has been of such aid to the investigator in the field of transplantation will, in all probability, be the last tissue to be successfully allotransplanted.

At present, the function of the skin transplant appears to be limited to fulfilling an allostatic role in situations where large areas of skin have been denuded by extensive burns, ulcerated infections, or impaired vascular supply.

SPLEEN TRANSPLANTATION

Recent interest in splenic allotransplantation has been generated by the suggestion that the spleen may be a source of antihemophilic globulin (AHF, factor VIII). The evidence for this hypothesis has come primarily from studies in dogs with hemophilia where splenic transplantation has occasionally returned AHF levels to normal, or close to normal, levels. At the time of writing, a single heterotopic splenic transplant for hemophilia had been performed in man.[24] The allograft was removed on the fourth postoperative day because of rupture of the transplanted spleen.

There are a number of factors which mitigate against further attempts at splenic allotransplantation for human hemophilia. Because it is uncertain whether the human spleen is the major site of AHF production, the risks of surgery and immunosuppression probably are not justified by the potential benefits. Moreover, AHF concentrates are more widely available and are more potent than they have been in the past.

THYMIC TRANSPLANTATION

The use of thymic allografts in the treatment of immunologic deficiency states is discussed in Chapter 11.

BONE MARROW TRANSPLANTATION

The use of bone marrow allografts in the treatment of leukemia[20] is discussed in Chapter 13. Other potential applications for bone marrow grafts are in patients with bone marrow aplasia, in individuals accidentally exposed to massive doses of irradiation, or in the treatment of certain primary immunologic deficiency syndromes (see Chapter 11).

REFERENCES

1. Abbott, W. M., and Sell, K. W. Organ preservation in transplantation. *Transplantation Proc. 1:*781, 1969.

1a. Advisory Committee of the Human Transplant Registry. Eighth report of the human kidney transplant registry. *Transplantation* (In press).

2. Al-Askari, S., David, J. R., Lawrence, H. S., and Thomas, L. In vitro studies on homograft sensitivity. *Nature 205:*916, 1965.

3. Bach, F. H. Transplantation: Problems of histocompatibility testing. *Science 159:*1196, 1968.

4. Bach, J. F., Dardenne, M., Dormont, J., and Antoine, B. A new in vitro test evaluating anti-lymphocyte serum potency. *Transplantation Proc. 1:*403, 1969.

5. Balner, H., Dersjant, H., and van Bekkum, D. W. Studies in immunosuppression. Methods to evaluate anti-human lymphocyte sera. *Transplantation Proc. 1:*629, 1969.

6. Batchelor, J. R. The use of enhancement in studying tumor antigens. *Cancer Res. 28:*1410, 1968.

7. Blumenstock, D. A., Otte, H. P., Grosjean, O. B., Mulder, M. A. Transplantation of the lung. *Transplantation Proc. 1:*223, 1969.

8. Brent, L., and Medawar, P. B. Cellular immunity and the homograft reaction. *Brit. Med. Bull. 23:*55, 1967.

9. Carpenter, C. B., and Merrill, J. P. Modification of renal allograft rejection in man. *Arch. Intern. Med. 123:*501, 1969.

10. Carpenter, C. B., Ruddy, S., Shehadeh, I. H., Merrill, J. P., Austen, K. F., Müller-Eberhard, H. J. Metabolism of radiolabelled C'3 and C'4 in human renal allograft recipients. Transplantation *Proc. 1:*279, 1969.

11. Davies, D. A. L. "Transplantation Antigens," in *Human Transplantation,* ed. by Rapaport, F. T., and Dausset, J. New York, Grune and Stratton, 1968, p. 618.

12. D'Amico, R. A. "Ophthalmologic Aspects of Transplantation," in *Human Transplantation,* ed. by Rapaport, F. T., and Dausset, J., New York, Grune and Stratton, 1968, p. 332.

13. Dresser, D. W., and Mitchison, N. A. The mechanism of immunological paralysis. *Adv. Immun. 8:*129, 1968.

14. Eddleston, A. L. W. F., Williams, R., and Calne, R. Y. Cellular immune response during rejection of a liver transplant in man. *Nature 222:*674, 1969.

14a. Fahey, J. L., Mann, D. L., Asofsky, R. and Rogentine, G. N. Recent progress in human transplantation immunology. *Ann. Intern. Med. 71:*1177, 1969.

14b. French, M. E., and Batchelor, J. R. Immunologic enhancement of rat kidney grafts. *Lancet 2:*1103, 1969.

15. Gibson, T. Cartilage and bone transplantation. *Transplantation Proc. 1:*246, 1969.

16. Hume, D. M., and Wolf, J. Modification of renal homograft rejection by irradiation. *Transplantation 5:*1174, 1967.

16a. Jeannet, M., Pinn, V. W., Flax, M. H., Winn, H. J., and Russell, P. S. Humoral antibodies in renal allotransplantation in man. *New Eng. J. Med. 282:*112, 1970.

17. Kahan, B. D., and Reisfield, R. A. Transplantation antigens. *Science 164:*514, 1969.

18. Kantrowitz, A., and Haller, J. D. (eds.) Symposium on heart transplantation. *Amer. J. Cardiol. 22:*761, 1968.

19. Lillehei, R. C., Idezuki, Y., Kelly, W. D., Najarian, J. S., Merkel, F. K., and Goetz, F. C. Transplantation of the intestine and pancreas. *Transplantation Proc. 1:*230, 1969.

20. Mathé, G., Amiel, J. L., Schwarzenberg, L., Schneider, M., Cattan, A., Schlumberger, Y. R., Nouza, K., and Hrask, Y. Bone marrow transplantation in man. *Transplantation Proc. 1:*16, 1969.

20a. McKhann, C. F. Primary malignancy in patients undergoing immunosuppression for renal transplantation. *Transplantation 8:*209, 1969.

21. Meuwissen, H. J., Stutman, O., and Good, R. A. Functions of the lymphocytes. *Seminars Hemat. 6:*28, 1969.

22. Millard, P. R., Herbertson, B. M., and Evans, D. B. Renal biopsy in clinical management of transplantation. *Lancet 1:*113, 1970.

23. Nora, J. J., Cooley, D. A., Fernbach, D. J., Rochelle, D. G., Milam, J. D., Montgomery, J. R., Leachman, R. D., Butler, W. T., Rossen, R. D., Bloodwell, R. D., Hallman, G. L., and Trentin, J. J. Rejection of the transplanted heart. *New Eng. J. Med. 280:*1079, 1969.

24. Peacock, E. E., Jr., Webster, W. P., Penick, G. D., Madden, J. W., and Hutchin, P. Transplantation of the spleen. *Transplantation Proc. 1:*239, 1969.

25. Penn, I., Hammond, W., Brettschneider, L., and Starzl, T. E. Malignant lymphomas in transplantation patients. *Transplantation Proc. 1:*106, 1969.

26. Rapaport, F. T., Kano, K., and Milgrom, F. Heterophile antibodies in human transplantation. *J. Clin. Invest. 47:*633, 1968.

27. Rapaport, F. T., Markowitz, A. S., and McClusky, R. T. The bacterial induction of homograft sensitivity. III. Effects of group A streptococcal membrane antisera. *J. Exp. Med. 129:*623, 1969.

28. Russell, P. S. Kidney transplantation. *Amer. J. Med. 44:*776, 1968.

29. Russell, P. S., and Monaco, A. P. The biology of tissue transplantation. *New Eng. J. Med. 271:*502, 553, 610, 664, 718, 1964.

29a. Russell, P. S., and Winn, H. J. Transplantation. *New Eng. J. Med. 282:*786, 848, 896, 1970.

29b. Sheagren, J. N., Edelin, J. B., Barth, R. F., and Malmgren, R. A. Reticuloendothelial blockade produced by antilymphocytic serum. *Lancet 2:*297, 1969.

30. Snell, G. D., and Stimpfling, J. H. *Genetics of Tissue Transplantation, Biology of the Laboratory Mouse,* 2nd ed., New York, Blakiston, 1966, pp. 457–491.

31. Starzl, T. E., Brettschneider, L., Martin, A. J., Groth, C. G., Blanchard, H., Smith, G. V., and Penn. I. Organ transplantation, past and present. *Surg. Clin. N. Amer.* 48:817, 1968.

32. Starzl, T. E., Brettschneider, L., Penn, I., Bell, P., Growth, C. G., Blanchard, H., Kashiwagi, N., and Putnam, C. W. Orthotopic liver transplantation in man. *Transplantation Proc.* 1:216, 1969.

33. Starzl, T. E., Lerner, R. A., Dixon, F. J., Growth, C. G., Brettschneider, L., and Terasaki, P. I. Shwartzman reaction after human renal homotransplantation. *New Eng. J. Med.* 278:642, 1968.

34. Stevens, P. M., Johnson, P. C., Bell, R. L., Beall, A. C. and Jenkins, D. E. Regional ventilation and perfusion after lung transplantation in patients with emphysema. *New Eng. J. Med.* 282:245, 1970.

35. Terasaki, P. I., and Singal, D. P. Human histocompatibility antigens of leukocytes. *Ann. Rev. Med.* 20:175, 1969.

36. Tilney, N. L., Atkinson, J. C., and Murray, J. E. The immunosuppressive effect of thoracic duct drainage in human kidney transplantation. *Ann. Intern. Med.* 72:59, 1970.

37. Van Rood, J. J., and Eernisse, J. G. The detection of transplantation antigens in leukocytes. *Seminars Hemat.* 5:187, 1968.

15

Clinical Immunology of the Endocrine System

SAMUEL O. FREEDMAN

THYROID DISEASE

During the past 15 years, there has been intense interest in the association between disorders of the thyroid gland and immunologic abnormalities. The detection of thyroid autoantibodies in a significant proportion of patients with Hashimoto's thyroiditis (lymphadenoid goiter), primary atrophic hypothyroidism (spontaneous myxedema), and Graves' disease (diffuse goiter with hyperthyroidism), has given rise to the hypothesis that they are all variants of the same condition and should be grouped together under the term "autoimmune thyroiditis." The finding that long-acting thyroid stimulator (LATS) has all of the physicochemical properties of an IgG immunoglobulin has lent further strength to the autoimmune theory. The validity of these concepts will be examined critically in the discussion which follows.

Hashimoto's Thyroiditis

The term Hashimoto's disease is not used by all pathologists with precisely the same meaning, but there appears to be general agreement that it constitutes a distinct entity, and can usually be distinguished from other forms of thyroiditis due to bacterial or viral infection, radiation, or trauma. On gross examination, the thyroid gland may be enlarged, uniformly and bilaterally, to several times its normal size. The consistency varies from hard to rubbery, and there is a slight nodularity of the surface. Generally accepted microscopic findings include: (1) a reduction in the size of thyroid follicles which contain little or no colloid; (2) diffuse infiltration by lymphocytes and plasma cells with the formation of lymphoid follicles containing germinal centers; (3) characteristic large thyroid epithelial cells, with abundant eosinophilic cytoplasm, lining the thyroid vesicles (Askanazy cells); and (4) a variable degree of connective tissue infiltration and fibrosis. The larger size of the gland is due to the increase in lymphoid, epithelial, and fibrous tissues, but the relative amounts of each of these components varies considerably among specimens.

Primary Atrophic Hypothyroidism

Some pathologists and immunologists consider this condition to be an atrophic variant or an end stage of Hashimoto's thyroiditis. On gross examination, the thyroid gland is usually small or normal in size and firm in consistency. Microscopic examination shows replacement of follicles by dense connective tissue, extensive lymphocytic infiltration, and pronounced epithelial destruction. The overall picture is that of sclerosis and atrophy of the thyroid parenchyma.

Graves' Disease

In thyrotoxicosis due to diffuse thyroid hyperplasia, the thyroid gland is enlarged, highly vascular, and has a characteristic meaty appearance. On microscopic examination, the characteristic changes are present throughout the gland. The epithelial cells which line the follicles are tall and columnar, and may produce papillary infoldings into the follicular lumina. The colloid is decreased in amount and tends to be vacuolated around the periphery of the follicles. Accumulation of lymphocytes, often with distinct germinal centers, in the intrafollicular spaces is often a prominent feature.

IMMUNOLOGY

Types of Thyroid Antibodies

The original serologic studies in thyroid disorders were undertaken about 1955 in an attempt to explain the elevated γ-globulin levels which were found in the sera of some patients with Hashimoto's disease. Since then, a variety of antibodies directed against thyroid constituents or associated with clinical thyroid disease have been demonstrated in human sera (see Table 15-1). The characteristics of these antibodies will be described in this section. An attempt will then be made to correlate their incidence with the clinical manifestations of various thyroid disorders.

Antibodies to Thyroglobulin. Antibodies to thyroglobulin were first detected by double diffusion in agar gel in patients with Hashimoto's thyroiditis. Because of its simplicity, this technique remains useful for the detection of large amounts of antibody, but more refined methods are required when lesser quantities of antibody are present. More sensitive and semiquantitative methods for detecting antibodies to thyroglobulin include the tanned sheep cell hemagglutination test,[14] and immunofluorescent staining of thyroglobulin in thyroid follicles.[7] Thyroglobulin antibodies are predominantly IgG, but IgA antibodies may account for up to 20 per cent of the total antigen binding capacity; IgM antibodies to thyroglobulin are virtually nonexistent.[33]

Antibodies to the Second Component of Colloid (CA2). A small percentage of patients with Hashimoto's thyroiditis who have raised serum γ-globulin levels have no demonstrable antibodies to thyroglobulin. Instead, their sera react with a colloid antigen distinct from thyroglobulin in that it does not contain iodine. These CA2 antibodies may be detected by diffuse immunofluorescent staining of colloid which is not inhibited by thyroglobulin, and is quite dissimilar from the flocculated pattern of colloid staining obtained with antithyroglobulin antibodies.[2]

Thyroid Cytoplasmic (Microsomal) Antibodies. These antibodies are directed against cytoplasmic components of the thyroid epithelial cells. Ultracentrifugation studies would suggest that the antigen is primarily localized to the microsomal fraction of the cell. Cytoplasmic antibodies can be demonstrated by complement fixation methods,[29] by immunofluorescence techniques, by a cytotoxic effect on thyroid epithelial cells in tissue culture, and by the mixed hemabsorption test. The latter two methods are techni-

TABLE 15-1. Types of Human Thyroid Antibodies

Antigen	Diffusion in agar gel	Complement-fixation	Hemagglu-tination	Immunofluo-rescence	Cytotoxicity	Mixed hemabsorption	Bioassay
				Common methods of detection			
Thyroglobulin	+		+	Colloid (flocculated)			
CA2		+		Colloid (diffuse)			
Cytoplasmic				Cytoplasm	+	+	
LATS							+

cally complex and not suitable for general use except in specialized research laboratories. It is generally agreed that thyroid cytoplasmic antibodies belong predominantly to the IgG class of immunoglobulins.[32]

Long-acting Thyroid Stimulator (LATS). An abnormally long-acting thyroid stimulator which appears to originate in the cells of the reticuloendothelial system is found in the sera of 50 to 80 per cent of thyrotoxic patients.[22] It has been suggested that this substance may be one of the factors responsible for hyperplasia of epithelial cells and excessive production of thyroid hormone in certain patients with thyrotoxicosis. LATS has many of the properties of an antibody rather than those of an ordinary hormone substance (e.g., it is associated with the IgG fraction of serum and its activity is destroyed by splitting the heavy and light chains of IgG). Furthermore, lymphocytes isolated from the peripheral blood of patients with LATS, and stimulated by the addition of phytohemagglutinin, can synthesize LATS in vitro.

Incidence and Diagnostic Significance of Thyroid Antibodies in Thyroid Disease

The measurement of microsomal antibodies by the complement-fixation technique and thyroglobulin antibodies by the tanned cell hemagglutination technique are probably the most useful tests for clinical purposes. Both methods provide quantitative results and can be performed by a competent laboratory technician without special training. Immunofluorescent studies may provide additional information in patients where serologic testing is negative or inconclusive.

The incidence of thyroid antibodies in patients with thyroid disease and in normal control subjects is summarized in Table 15-2. It will be noted that elevated levels of microsomal and thyroglobulin antibodies occur in an incidence significantly greater than in normal control subjects in three major types of thyroid disorders: Hashimoto's thyroiditis, primary hypothyroidism, and Graves' disease. A slightly increased incidence of thyroid antibodies in low titer has also been reported in adenomatous goiter, granulomatous thyroiditis (de Quervain's disease), and carcinoma of the thyroid,[1] but thyroid antibodies are rarely of diagnostic significance in these conditions.

In interpreting the results of thyroid antibody determinations, two additional factors should be kept in mind. The first is that the incidence of thyroid antibodies in normal subjects tends to increase with age and is higher in females than males.[12] The second is that high titers of thyroid antibodies have been reported in patients with pernicious anemia, Addison's disease, myasthenia gravis, liver disease, various collagen-vascular disorders, diabetes mellitus, and chromosomal abnormalities.

TABLE 15-2. Percentage of Thyroid Antibodies in Thyroid Disease

	Microsomal antibodies*	Thyroglobulin antibodies†	Total with thyroid antibodies	LATS‡
Hashimoto's thyroiditis	89	78	98	—
Graves' disease	37	35	53	80
Primary hypothyroidism	57	52	75	—
Normal controls	15	17	26	—

* Complement fixation titer greater than 1:4.
† Tanned cell hemagglutination titer greater than 1:25.
‡ McKenzie assay using concentrated serum (Carneiro, L., Dorrington, K. J., and Munro, D. S. *Clin. Sci. 31:*215, 1966.) (Table adapted from Irvine, W. J., *Practitioner 199:*180, 1967.)

Hashimoto's Disease.   The major clinical application of thyroid antibody determinations is in the diagnosis of Hashimoto's thyroiditis. As noted in Table 15-2, a significant elevation of thyroid antibodies occurs in 80 to 90 per cent of patients with Hashimoto's thyroiditis. An additional test procedure which does not depend on thyroid function is particularly useful in this disorder because most patients are metabolically normal during the early stages of the disease. If Hashimoto's thyroiditis is suspected on clinical grounds, the diagnosis is strongly supported by a tanned cell titer for thyroglobulin antibodies of 1:2500 or greater, or a complement-fixation titer for cytoplasmic antibodies of 1:32 or greater.[17] Nevertheless, because false-positive antibody tests are relatively common, the diagnosis should be confirmed histologically by a needle biopsy of the enlarged gland.

Primary Atrophic Hypothyroidism.   In hypothyroidism, thyroid antibodies are not diagnostic in themselves, but may be helpful in distinguishing primary hypothyroidism from secondary hypothyroidism due to pituitary failure.

Graves' Disease.   In patients with hypothyroidism, the titer of thyroid antibodies shows no significant correlation with the severity of the disease or the response to treatment with radioactive iodine. However, it has been suggested that thyroid antibodies may be of value as a guide to the risk of hypothyroidism in patients undergoing subtotal thyroidectomy for thyrotoxicosis. It has been stated that in the presence of high titers of complement-fixing antibodies (1:32 or greater), the incidence of hypothyroidism during the first year is significantly increased from 8 per cent to 25 per cent,[12] but this observation requires further study and confirmation. There appears to be no correlation between titers of thyroid antibodies and the development of hypothyroidism following other forms of treatment.

LATS is found almost exclusively in patients with thyrotoxicosis or in patients who have recovered from thyrotoxicosis. The highest incidence and titers of LATS tend to occur in patients who have large goiters or pretibial myxedema. The association between exophthalmus and LATS is obscure, but recent evidence would suggest that no direct cause and effect relationship exists.[23]

Subacute Thyroiditis. Low, but significant titers of thyroid antibodies have been demonstrated in patients recovering from subacute thyroiditis.[35] About 50 per cent of these patients also had rising titers to one of several viral antibodies, suggesting that the thyroid antibodies appeared as a consequence of virus-induced tissue damage in the thyroid gland.

Genetic Factors in Thyroid Immunity

Several statistical, clinical, and experimental observations support the hypothesis that hereditary factors may play an important role in the pathogenesis of "autoimmune thyroiditis."

An interesting animal model exists. A strain of white leghorn chickens has been described in which genetically determined thyroiditis appears spontaneously and is accompanied by circulating thyroglobulin antibodies, histologic damage to the thyroid gland, and decrease in serum thyroxin levels.[11]

In human, familial studies of patients with autoimmune thyroid disease demonstrate the existence of thyroid disease and/or thyroid antibodies in approximately 50 per cent of siblings, and almost invariably in one or other parent of the affected individual.[16] Studies of monozygotic twins with thyroiditis or Hashimoto's thyroiditis reveal a high degree of concordance with respect to clinical disease, circulating thyroid antibodies, and LATS. These correlations would point to a common underlying immunologic defect. The pattern of inheritance in familial and twin studies is suggestive of a dominant autosomal gene with incomplete gene expression.

There have been numerous reports of the occurrence of other autoantibodies in patients with Hashimoto's thyroiditis. However, most of these studies are difficult to interpret because organ-specific antibodies are found in a significant proportion of normal individuals. Unless a large number of patients are studied with rigid statistical controls, observations on hospitalized patients are subject to considerable selective bias. Despite these difficulties, there appears to be little doubt that there is a significant correlation between thyroid antibodies and gastric parietal cell antibodies in patients with "autoimmune thyroiditis" or pernicious anemia or both conditions (see Chapter 9). This well documented association of autoantibodies and disease states would suggest a predisposition for both types of disorders to occur in the same individual.

Another interesting observation is the frequently reported association between thyroid antibodies and the chromosome anomalies which occur in diseases such as ovarian dysgenesis (Turner's syndrome), and Down's syndrome (mongolism).[13] It appears that patients with chromosomal aberrations have an increased tendency to develop thyroid autoimmunity, but the reason for such an association is not clear.

Pathogenesis of Autoimmune Thyroiditis

Early workers in the field of "autoimmune thyroiditis" suggested that thyroglobulin is normally confined to the thyroid follicles so that immunologically competent cells do not encounter the "secluded antigen" during fetal life and, therefore, fail to develop tolerance towards it. According to this theory, subsequent injury to the thyroid gland due to infection or other forms of injury causes "leakage" of antigen, production of cytotoxic thyroid antibodies, and ultimately results in autoimmune tissue damage in the thyroid gland.

This theory is no longer tenable for a variety of reasons. Sophisticated studies using a radioimmunoassay technique provide evidence for the presence of minute amounts of circulating thyroglobulin in 60 per cent or normal individuals.[30] Studies in monkeys and rats indicate that thyroglobulin appears to reach the circulation by way of the lymphatics. Clearly, these observations mitigate against the theory that thyroglobulin is a "secluded antigen." Also against the "leakage" theory of thyroglobulin antibody formation is the observation that thyroid antibodies are rarely detected in patients without thyroid disease whose thyroid has been exposed to radiation or surgery.

Experimental thyroiditis accompanied by circulating thyroglobulin antibodies can be produced in animals with relative ease by the injection of autologous, homologous, or heterologous thyroid tissue emulsified in Freund's adjuvant. However, in most experimental systems, there is little or no correlation between the titers of thyroid antibody and the presence of experimental thyroiditis. This finding suggests that circulating antibody is not primarily responsible for in vivo tissue damage despite the fact that a cytotoxic effect is demonstrable in tissue culture preparations. On the other hand, experimental thyroiditis has recently been passively transferred in rabbits by means of serum obtained from animals actively immunized with thyroglobulin.[25]

Experimental thyroiditis can be passively transferred with lymphocytes, and the presence of experimental thyroiditis appears to correlate fairly well with delayed skin reactions to thyroid antigens.[24] These latter observations might lead to the conclusion that cell-mediated hypersensitivity may be of major importance in the development of experimental thyroiditis. Unfortunately, quantitative estimations of cell-mediated hypersensitivity to tissue antigens are extremely difficult in humans with currently available techniques. It should also be noted that many of the early experiments on the role of cell-mediated hypersensitivity in experimental thyroiditis have been criticized by recent reviewers in the light of current knowledge.[34]

The structural similarities between LATS and IgG raises the interesting question as to whether this substance functions as an antibody directed against thyroid antigens. The present evidence is insufficient to either confirm or refute this hypothesis. Although it is true that LATS activity can be demonstrated in the sera of rabbits immunized with thyroid tissue, attempts to demonstrate an immunologic reaction between LATS and human thyroid tissue by fluorescent antibody techniques have produced equivocal results.[13a] Several investigators have reported that LATS activity is neutralized by thyroid microsomal fractions, but other workers have been unable to reproduce their findings with consistency.[28] Furthermore, clinical studies have failed to reveal any correlation between LATS, thyroglobulin, and microsomal antibodies.[4]

In summary, it seems reasonable to conclude that "autoimmune thyroiditis" is probably a familial disorder. Additional environmental or hormonal factors such as emotional stress, iodine deficiency, viral infections, puberty, and pregnancy may act on genetically predisposed individuals to produce clinical thyroid disease.

CLINICAL MANIFESTATIONS

Hashimoto's Thyroiditis

Hashimoto's thyroiditis is most common in middle-aged women. The principal clinical feature is that of marked enlargement of the thyroid gland which is usually insidious, but progressive, in onset. Despite considerable thyroid enlargement, pressure symptoms are rarely present, and signs of thyroid dysfunction are infrequent in the early stages. It is postulated, but difficult to prove, that a significant number of patients with Hashimoto's thyroiditis will eventually progress over a period of years to overt clinical myxedema.

Graves' Disease

The classic form of Graves' disease has its highest incidence in women between the ages of 20 and 40 years, but may occur in either sex and in almost any age group. The characteristic symptoms of weakness, sweating, weight loss, nervousness, heat intolerance, diarrhea, palpitations, and dyspnea are well known. The physical findings may include diffuse or nodular thyroid enlargement, fine tremor of the hands, warm moist skin, tachycardia with or without atrial fibrillation, evidence of congestive heart failure, muscle wasting, lymphadenopathy and splenomegaly, and mental changes ranging from delirium to severe depression. Exophthalmos with its associated signs and symptoms may be a prominent feature or completely absent. A minority of patients demonstrate a peculiar form of bilateral, localized, nonpitting edema over the tibia and dorsum of the foot known as pretibial myxedema.

Primary Atrophic Hypothyroidism

The principal symptoms of hypothyroidism consist of weakness, fatigue, cold intolerance, constipation, menorrhagia or amenorrhea, weight gain, hoarse voice, anginal pain, and poor memory. Common physical findings include characteristic puffiness of the face and eyelids, pallor, thinning of the outer margins of the eyebrows, thick tongue, coarse dry skin and brittle hair, slow speech, delayed return of deep tendon reflexes, bradycardia, hypotension, signs of pleural and pericardial effusions, and a mental state ranging from coma or extreme lethargy to marked anxiety.

Laboratory Diagnosis of Thyroid Disorders

The serum levels of protein bound iodine (PBI) and thyroxin (T_4), the resin uptake of radioactive triiodothyronine (T_3), and the uptake of radioactive iodine (^{131}I) by the thyroid gland tend to be increased above normal levels in Graves' disease and decreased in primary atrophic hypothyroidism. The significance of thyroid antibodies in the diagnosis of thyroid disorders has been discussed previously in this chapter.

TREATMENT

Hashimoto's Thyroiditis

The most common form of treatment in Hashimoto's thyroiditis is replacement therapy with thyroxine, 0.2 to 0.3 mg/day, or desiccated thyroid 120 to 200 mg/day. The purpose is to correct or avoid the hypothyroidism which usually results from this disease.

The administration of corticosteroids sometimes produces a rapid reduction in the size and hardness of the gland, and a moderate decrease in the titers of thyroid antibodies. A typical dosage schedule might consist of prednisone, 60 mg/day, in divided doses for 10 days. Radiation therapy or partial thyroidectomy are rarely required in Hashimoto's thyroiditis.

Graves' Disease

The treatment of hyperthyroidism is primarily directed at halting the excessive secretion of thyroid hormone. The most commonly employed forms of therapy at present are the use of antithyroid agents (such as propylthiouracil) which block hormone synthesis, the administration of radioactive iodine (^{131}I), and subtotal thyroidectomy after suitable preparation.

Primary Atrophic Hypothyroidism

The major objective in the treatment of hypothyroidism is the replacement of thyroid hormone. Several preparations are available for this purpose including desiccated thyroid, sodium L-thyroxine, and sodium L-triiodothyronine. The recommended dosage for each of these preparations depends on the severity of the disease, and the presence or absence of cardiac complications.

PRIMARY ADRENAL ATROPHY (ADDISON'S DISEASE)

The term primary adrenal atrophy or Addison's disease is used to describe atrophic adrenal insufficiency which is not secondary to pituitary insufficiency.

Addison's disease is characterized by a chronic deficiency of adrenocortical hormones resulting from the irreversible destruction of the cortex of both adrenal glands. The extensive tissue destruction in the adrenal cortex may be secondary to tuberculosis, metastatic carcinoma, fungal disease, scleroderma, amyloidosis, or hemochromatosis; or it may be idiopathic. At present, the idiopathic type of primary adrenal atrophy is probably the most common, with tuberculosis accounting for the majority of the secondary causes.

PATHOLOGY

In primary adrenal atrophy of the idiopathic type, the adrenal glands are greatly reduced in size bilaterally. On microscopic examination, the adrenal cortex is markedly thinned with disappearance of most of the cortical cells. The remaining cortical cells tend to show irregular enlargement and dense cytoplasmic staining. These changes are accompanied by a diffuse infiltration with lymphocytes and plasma cells as well as a minimal increase in connective tissue. The microscopic picture is not entirely dissimilar from that seen in the thyroid gland in primary myxedema.

IMMUNOLOGY

The experimental observation that adrenalitis and circulating antibodies to adrenal tissue could be produced in rabbits by the injection of adrenal extracts homogenized in Freund's adjuvant[3] has lead to a search for circulating antibodies in human adrenal disease.

Antibodies specific for the cytoplasm of human adrenocortical cells have been detected by immunofluorescence and complement-fixation techniques in the sera of patients with idiopathic adrenal atrophy, but not in the sera of patients with tuberculous adrenalitis.[9] The incidence of adrenal-specific antibodies in patients with idiopathic adrenal atrophy is approximately 66 per cent for females and 33 per cent for males.

A second type of adrenal antibody, which occurs in about 5 per cent of patients with idiopathic adrenal atrophy, appears to react by the immunofluorescence technique with all types of cells producing steroid hormones (e.g., adrenocortical cells, testicular Leydig cells, hilus cells of the ovary and testis, theca interna and corpus luteal cells of the ovary, and cells of the placental trophoblast.[18]

Both the adrenal-specific antibody and the antibody which cross-reacts with other steroid producing cells have been found to be predominantly IgG. Current evidence is consistent with the view that the adrenal antigens, like thyroid and gastric antigens, are insoluble, microsomal lipoproteins.[15]

Inhibition of leukocyte migration with extracts of human fetal adrenal glands was reported in approximately 50 per cent of patients with primary adrenal atrophy, but no positive tests were obtained in patients with tuberculosis of the adrenal glands. A parallel study showed that adrenal extracts did not induce blast transformation in lymphocyte cultures as determined by ^{14}C thymidine incorporation.[26] No correlation was observed between the occurrence of anti-adrenal cell-mediated immunity, the duration or severity of illness, or the presence of circulating anti-adrenal antibodies. Thus, there is suggestive but not conclusive evidence for cell-mediated hypersensitivity in the pathogenesis of primary adrenal atrophy.

When patients with idiopathic adrenal insufficiency are investigated for evidence of other disease of possible immunologic significance, it is found that there is an unusually high incidence of thyroid disorders, pernicious anemia, hypoparathyroidism, and diabetes mellitus.[8] In addition, thyroid and gastric antibodies occur with a higher than normal frequency in patients with idiopathic adrenal insufficiency. On the other hand, there is no increased incidence of associated immunologic disorders or other organ-specific antibodies in patients with tuberculous adrenal insufficiency.

To date, there is no conclusive evidence that adrenal antibodies are of significance in the pathogenesis of primary adrenal atrophy. However, their presence may be of assistance in confirming a suspected diagnosis of primary adrenal atrophy. For diagnostic purposes, the immunofluorescence technique is of more value than the complement-fixation technique because it is considerably more sensitive.

CLINICAL MANIFESTATIONS

The most common presenting symptoms consist of profound weakness, easy fatiguability, anorexia, frequent episodes of nausea, vomiting, and diarrhea. On physical examination, there may be evidence of increased pigmentation of the skin which is most pronounced in the creases of the palms, recent scars, pressure areas, and nipples. Additional physical signs include hypotension with a small heart, hyperplasia of lymphoid tissues, and scanty axillary and pubic hair. Common laboratory abnormalities are: decreased levels of serum sodium and chloride, increased serum potassium, and decreased plasma corticoids, urinary 17-ketosteroids, and 17-hydroxy-corticoids. The white blood count usually shows a moderate neutropenia, lymphocytosis, and an eosinophil count over 300/cu mm.

TREATMENT

Most of the metabolic abnormalities of primary adrenal atrophy can be corrected by replacement therapy with hydrocortisone, 30 mg (or cortisone, 37.5 mg), given daily by mouth in divided doses. Most patients, however, do not obtain sufficient salt-retaining effect from these drugs and require extra dietary salt or supplementation with desoxycorticosterone acetate (DOCA), 2 mg, daily bucally, or fludrocortisone acetate, 0.1 to 0.25 mg, daily by mouth. The benefit produced by corticosteroids in primary adrenal atrophy seems to be entirely due to their replacement effect rather than due to an immunosuppressive action. At present, the bulk of the available evidence would suggest that the changes in the hormone secreting cells of the adrenal cortex are essentially irreversible.

SPERM ANTIBODIES

SPERM AGGLUTINATING ANTIBODIES IN MALES

It is now reasonably well established that the presence of sperm agglutinating antibodies in the seminal fluid may be one of the causes of male infertility.[31] It is postulated that these antibodies immobilize otherwise normal spermatozoa in the ejaculate, thus rendering them incapable of penetrating the mucous secretions of the cervix. Sperm antibodies may be detected by agglutination in vitro and by immunofluorescent methods. In most patients, they are present in the serum as well as in the seminal fluid, but not necessarily in parallel concentrations.

As a rule, the presence of sperm agglutinating antibodies is almost always associated with long-standing obstruction of the efferent seminiferous ducts. However, only about 25 per cent of patients with obstructed efferent ducts develop sperm antibodies. (Obstruction of the efferent seminiferous ducts occurs most commonly as the result of epididymitis, accidental ligation of the vas deferans during herniorrhaphy, or deliberate ligation of the vas deferans as a family limitation procedure.) It has been observed that obstruction leads to extravasation of sperm into the epididymis, which becomes infiltrated with macrophages, lymphocytes, and plasma cells. There may even be spermatozoa in the lymph vessels. It has, therefore, been suggested that some patients who resorb their own spermatozoa secondary to obstruction respond by the formation of autoantibodies.

The relationship between sperm antibodies and male infertility has been investigated by several groups interested in the subject. In one series, 3 per cent of 2000 infertile males had sperm agglutinating antibodies in a titer of 1:32 or higher, whereas no antibodies were found in any of 400 fertile males.[31] Semen analysis of the patients with sperm agglutinating antibodies showed normal sperm count and motility in one-third, oligospermia and subnormal motility in one-third, and aspermia in the remaining one-third. Testicular biopsies performed in patients with aspermia due to complete obstruction of the efferent ducts were normal, indicating that sperm antibodies are not capable of preventing spermatogenesis. Thus, the bulk of the evidence would suggest that sperm antibodies may be an occasional cause of male infertility.

Therapy with corticosteroids, or with testosterone-induced suppression of spermatogenesis has not proved successful to date.

SPERM AGGLUTINATING ANTIBODIES IN FEMALES

It is well known that prostitutes have a poor reproductive history and a high incidence of abortion. In a group of prostitutes studied for sperm agglutinating antibodies, the incidence of positive reactions was 73 per cent compared to 25 per cent in a group of unmarried women.[5] The route of sensitization following unprotected coitus would appear to result from sperm migration and absorption through the vagina, uterus, tubes, or peritoneum. On the other hand, prevention of exposure to semen in the same group of patients led to a fall in antibody titers after a period of several months. It was found that there was a relationship between sperm agglutinating antibody titers and infertility, but there was no correlation with the increased rate of spontaneous abortion. Tissue fixed serum antibodies were demonstrated by the immunofluorescence technique in the cervix and endometrial tissues of patients with high titers of circulating sperm antibodies.

These observations have led to the interesting hypothesis that sperm agglutinating antibodies in females may produce infertility by immobilizing spermatozoa in the cervical or endometrial secretions. Thus, sperm agglutinating antibodies may be conceivably be a cause of female as well as male infertility.

One interesting approach to the therapy of female infertility attributed to sperm agglutinating antibodies is to advise the use of condoms for a period of at least 3 months. The purpose is to prevent antigen exposure in the female. Preliminary results suggest that condom therapy results in a decrease in antibody titers in most female patients and a significant increase in the number of pregnancies after unrestricted intercourse is permitted.

ABNORMALITIES OF THE GONADS

PREMATURE OVARIAN FAILURE

In the preceding discussion of primary adrenal atrophy, it was noted that a small number of patients possess adrenal antibodies which cross-react with the steroid producing cells of the ovary (e.g., the hilus cells, the theca interna, and the corpus luteal cells). In one series, all of the Addisonian patients with antibodies directed against ovarian cells had either complete failure of menstruation or an early menopause.[19] Antibody reactive with ovarian tissue was absent in patients with tuberculous adrenal insufficiency, gonadal dysgenesis, other autoimmune disorders, and normal controls. It is possible, therefore, that ovarian antibodies may inactivate the hormone producing capacity of ovarian cells, thus interfering with normal cyclic variations in ovarian estrogen and progesterone production. However, considerable further investigation is required before this theory can be substantiated.

GONADAL DYSGENESIS

Antibodies to thyroid, gastric parietal cells, and antinuclear factors have been detected in a significant number of patients with gonadal dysgenesis (Turner's syndrome).[13] As noted previously in the section on the thyroid in this chapter, thyroid antibodies are frequently found in patients with Down's syndrome. On the other hand, autoantibodies have not been detected in Klinefelter's syndrome. The increased incidence of autoantibodies in patients with chromosomal aberrations has led some workers to speculate that parents with autoimmune disorders may be predisposed to produce chromosomally unbalanced offspring. However, the exact relationship between chromosome anomalies and organ-specific antibodies remains obscure at present.

HYPOPARATHYROIDISM

Antibodies against parathyroid cells have been detected by the indirect immunofluorescence technique in the sera of 38 per cent of patients with idiopathic hypoparathyroidism, 26 per cent of patients with primary adrenal atrophy, 12 per cent of patients with Hashimoto's thyroiditis, and 6 per cent of normal controls.[8] The antibodies belong to the IgG class of immunoglobulins, and react primarily with the oxyphil cells of both the normal human parathyroid gland and parathyroid adenomas.[20] A serum which reacted by immunofluorescence with oxyphil cells in the parathyroid gland also reacted positively with human gastric parietal cell cytoplasm and with steroid producing cells in the gonads, but did not cross-react with human thyroid cytoplasm, rat kidney tubules, or rat liver sections. The significance of these findings in the pathogenesis of idiopathic hypoparathyroidism in humans is not yet established.

IMMUNE RESPONSES TO EXOGENOUS HORMONES

Protein or peptide hormones of animal origin are foreign to the human host and are therefore capable of evoking an antibody response. Most immunologic reactions to hormone preparations appear to be due to the hormone itself, rather than to the numerous contaminants which appear in most commercial products.

INSULIN

Insulin is a polypeptide whose molecular structure is well known. Analyses of the amino acid sequence has shown that the primary structure of the insulin molecule differs only slightly from one species to another.[21] Nevertheless, the repeated injection of insulin from one animal species to another, or from animals into humans can give rise to antibody formation.[6] On the other hand, insulin antibodies have never been demonstrated in the sera of patients who have not received insulin.

Adverse immunologic responses to exogenous insulin may take the form of allergic reactions or insulin resistance. Allergic reactions to insulin are usually manifested by local or generalized urticaria following the initiation of insulin therapy. These reactions are presumably mediated by reagins, as most patients will demonstrate immediate wheal and flare reactions following the intradermal injection of 0.025 ml of crystalline insulin diluted to a concentration of 2 units/ml.

The management of allergic reactions to insulin may be of considerable importance because it is rarely possible to discontinue insulin therapy in diabetics who require this form of treatment. Most commercial insulin is prepared from both beef and pork pancreases, but some manufacturers are able to supply insulin which is chemically modified to render it less antigenic (sulfated insulin), or insulin prepared from a single animal species.

Fortunately, most urticarial reactions to injected insulin are relatively mild and transient. For this reason, it is often more practical to administer antihistamines during the initial phases of insulin treatment instead of changing to unfamiliar insulin preparations. Almost inevitably, "desensitization" will occur within a few days provided the daily insulin requirement is given in several small doses of crystalline zinc insulin at intervals of 4 to 6 hours. When the urticaria has disappeared, the patient may be switched to one of the longer-acting preparations, and the antihistamines discontinued.

Insulin resistance may be another manifestation of an immunologic reaction to insulin and, in fact, most cases of chronic insulin resistance appear to be immunogenic in origin. Insulin-binding antibodies can be demonstrated by radioimmunoassay techniques[6] in the sera of practically all patients who have received insulin for 3 months or more. However, it is only in the occasional patient that the amount of antibody produced is sufficiently large to inhibit hormone activity and cause clinically significant insulin resistance. Such patients may have insulin requirements in excess of 200 units/day. The insulin-binding antibodies appear to be physicochemically distinct from reagins. Thus, while insulin resistance and insulin allergy may occasionally occur in the same patient, the combination is relatively uncommon.

It is generally agreed that beef insulin is more antigenic for humans than pork insulin. About 50 per cent of patients resistant to the usual commercial mixtures of beef and pork insulin will show a significant decrease in insulin requirements if changed to pure pork insulin. Another approach to the problem of insulin resistance is a trial of a chemically modified insulin such as sulfated insulin.[27] The administration of prednisone or other corticosteroid hormones will often produce a marked amelioration of insulin resistance, but this form of therapy has its obvious disadvantages in diabetic patients. The mechanism by which corticosteroids reverse antibody mediated insulin resistance is not well understood. Another unexplained phenomenon is the occasional spontaneous disappearance of insulin resistant diabetes in patients who develop one of the collagen-vascular diseases.[10]

OTHER HORMONES

As might be expected from their protein or peptide structure, urticarial or anaphylactic reactions have been reported following the injection of corticotropin (ACTH), thyrotropin, other pituitary preparations, and parathyroid hormone (see Chapter 2). Resistance to corticotropin and gonadotropins has been reported in animals, and presumably occurs in some patients following their repeated administration.

REFERENCES

1. Anderson, J. W., McConahey, W. M., Alarcon-Segovia, D., Emslander, R. F., and Wakim, K. G. Diagnostic value of thyroid antibodies. *J. Clin. Endocr.* 27:937, 1967.

2. Balfour, B. M., Doniach, D., Roitt, I. M., and Couchman, K. G. Fluorescent antibody studies in human thyroiditis. Autoantibodies to an antigen of the thyroid colloid distinct from thyroglobulin. *Brit. J. Exp. Path.* 42:307, 1961.

3. Barnett, E. V., Dumonde, D. C., and Glynn, L. E. Induction of autoimmunity to adrenal gland. *Immunology* 6:382, 1963.

4. Beall, G. W., and Solomon, D. H. LATS and thyroid autoantibodies. *Clin. Exp. Immun.* 3:615, 1968.

5. Behrman, S. J. "The Immune Response and Infertility: Experimental Evidence," in *Progress in Infertility,* Boston, Little, Brown, 1968, p. 675.

6. Berson, S. A., and Yalow, R. S. Insulin in blood and insulin antibodies. *Amer. J. Med. 40:*676, 1966.

7. Beutner, E. H., and Witebsky, E. Studies on organ specificity. XIV Immuno-fluorescent studies of thyroid reactive autoantibodies in human sera. *J. Immun. 88:*462, 1962.

8. Blizzard, R. M., Chee, D., and Davis, W. The incidence of adrenal and other antibodies in the sera of patients with idiopathic adrenal insufficiency (Addison's disease). *Clin. Exp. Immun. 2:*19, 1967.

9. Blizzard, R. M., and Kyle, M. Studies of the adrenal antigens and antibodies in Addison's disease. *J. Clin. Invest. 42:*1653, 1967.

10. Bruce, D. H., Bernard, W., and Blackard, W. G. Spontaneous disappearance of insulin-resistant diabetes mellitus in a patient with a collagen disease. A case report, with review of the literature for conditions associated with insulin resistance. *Amer. J. Med. 48:*268, 1970.

11. Cole, R. K., Kite, J. H., Jr., and Witebsky, E. Hereditary autoimmune thy-roiditis in fowl. *Science 160:*1357, 1968.

12. Dingle, P. R., Ferguson, A., Horn, D. B., Tubman, J., and Hall, R. The incidence of thyroglobulin antibodies and thyroid enlargement in a general practice in north-east England. *Clin. Exp. Immun. 1:*277, 1966.

13. Doniach, D., Roitt, I. M., and Polani, P. E. Thyroid antibodies and sex chromosome anomalies. *Proc. Roy. Soc. Med. 61:*278, 1968.

13a. Fedder, G., and Feltkamp, T. E. W. Failure to detect long-acting thyroid stimulator with the immunofluorescence technique. *Clin. Exp. Immun. 6:*167, 1970.

14. Fulthorpe, A. J., Roitt, I. M., Doniach, D., and Couchman, K. A stable sheep cell preparation for detecting thyroglobulin auto-antibodies and its clinical applications. *J. Clin. Path. 14:*654, 1961.

15. Goudie, R. B., McDonald, E., Anderson, J. R., and Gray, K. Immunological features of idiopathic Addison's disease: Characterization of the adrenocortical anti-gens. *Clin. Exp. Immun. 3:*119, 1968.

16. Hall, R., and Stanbury, J. B. Familial studies of autoimmune thyroiditis. *Clin. Exp. Immun. 2:*719, 1967.

17. Irvine, W. J. Auto-immunity and endocrine disorders. *Practitioner 199:*180, 1966.

18. Irvine, W. J., Chan, M. W., and Scarth, L. The further characterization of autoantibodies reactive with extra-adrenal steroid-producing cells in patients with adrenal disorders. *Clin. Exp. Immun. 4:*489, 1969.

19. Irvine, W. J., Chan, M. W., Scarth, L., Kolb, F. O., Hartog, M., Bayliss, R. I. S., and Drury, M. I. Immunological aspects of premature ovarian failure associated with idiopathic Addison's disease. *Lancet 2:*883, 1968.

20. Irvine, W. J., and Scarth, L. Antibody to the oxyphil cells of the human parathyroid in idiopathic hypoparathyroidism. *Clin. Exp. Immun. 4:*505, 1969.

21. Kitabachi, A. E. The biological and immunological properties of pork and beef insulin, proinsulin and connecting peptides. *J. Clin. Invest. 49:*979, 1970.

22. McKenzie, J. M. Humoral factors in the pathogenesis of Graves' disease. *Physiol. Rev. 48:*252, 1968.

23. McKenzie, J. M., and McCullagh, E. P. Observations against a causal relationship between the long-acting thyroid stimulator and ophthalmopathy in Graves' disease. *J. Clin. Endocr. 28:*1177, 1968.

24. McMaster, R. B., Lerner, E. M., and Exum, E. D. The relationship of delayed hypersensitivities and circulating antibody to experimental thyroiditis in inbred guinea pigs. *J. Exp. Med. 113:*611, 1961.

25. Nakamura, R. M. and Weigle, W. O. Transfer of experimental autoimmune thyroiditis by serum from thyroidectomized donors. *J. Exp. Med. 130:*263, 1969.

26. Nerup, J. and Bendixen, G. Anti-adrenal cellular hypersensitivity in Addison's disease. II. Correlation with clinical and serological findings. *Clin. Exp. Immun. 5:*341, 1969.

27. Moloney, P. J., Aprile, M. A., and Wilson, S. Sulfated insulin for treatment of insulin resistant diabetics. *J. New Drugs 4:*258, 1964.

28. Ochi, Y., and DeGroot, L. J. Long acting thyroid stimulator of Graves' disease. *New Eng. J. Med. 278:*719, 1968.

29. Roitt, I. M., Ling, N. R., Doniach, D., and Couchman, K. G. The Cytoplasmic autoantigen of the human thyroid. I. Immunological and biochemical characteristics. *Immunology 7:*375, 1964.

30. Roitt, I. M., and Torrigiani, G. Identification and estimation of undegraded thyroglobulin in human serum. *Endocrinology 81:*421, 1967.

31. Rumke, P. Sperm-agglutinating autoantibodies in relation to male infertility. *Proc. Roy. Soc. Med. 61:*275, 1968.

32. Torrigiani, G., and Roitt, I. M. Sedimentation characteristics of human thyroid autoantibodies. *Immunology 6:*73, 1963.

33. Torrigiani, G., Roitt, I. M., and Doniach, D. Quantitative distribution of human thyroglobulin antibodies in different immunoglobulin classes. *Clin. Exp. Immun. 3:*621, 1968.

34. Turk, J. L. *Delayed Hypersensitivity,* New York, Wiley, 1967, pp. 219–221.

35. Volpe, R., Row, V. V., and Ezrin, C. Circulating viral and thyroid antibodies in subacute thyroiditis. *J. Clin. Endocr. 27:*1275, 1968.

16

Clinical Immunology of the Digestive System

SAMUEL O. FREEDMAN

ALIMENTARY AND GASTROINTESTINAL ALLERGY

TRUE GASTROINTESTINAL ALLERGY

"Gastrointestinal allergy is a diagnosis frequently entertained, occasionally evaluated, and rarely established."[11] This statement made 20 years ago is probably equally valid today. The term gastrointestinal allergy, as commonly used, refers to sensitization of the gastrointestinal tract as a shock organ. Alimentary allergy, on the other hand, refers to a hypersensitivity response in other organs triggered by food allergens.

Although there is little doubt that ingested foods may precipitate *acute* attacks of asthma, rhinitis, or urticaria on a hypersensitivity basis, the occurrence of reagin-mediated hypersensitivity reactions confined solely to the gastrointestinal tract is much more difficult to document. That such reactions may occur is suggested by the fact that gastrointestinal symptoms such as vomiting, diarrhea, and abdominal cramps may occasionally be associated with acute anaphylactic reactions or acute asthma provoked by food substances. The pathophysiologic mechanisms in the gastrointestinal tract are similar to those of the immediate type of allergic reaction in other organs and consist of edema, spasm of smooth muscle, and increased secretion of mucus.

485

Unfortunately, the diagnosis of gastrointestinal allergy is made much more frequently on the basis of clinical impressions instead of properly controlled clinical studies. Because no suitable diagnostic tests exist at present, the diagnosis of gastrointestinal allergy still rests on the clinical documentation of symptoms after *repeated* challenges with the suspected food following periods when that food is completely removed from the patient's diet. In addition, all of the conditions which may mimic gastrointestinal allergy should be excluded by appropriate investigations. An approach such as this is preferable to the arbitrary and permanent elimination of an important nutrient from the patient's diet on the basis of a positive skin test or the presence of circulating antibodies against food antigens.

CONDITIONS WHICH MIMIC GASTROINTESTINAL ALLERGY

Hypersensitivity reactions of the gut to specific ingested food are difficult to substantiate because the symptoms claimed to be characteristic are highly variable and may occur in a wide range of non-immunologic gastrointestinal disorders. Furthermore, testing procedures used to establish the diagnosis such as skin tests, elimination diets, and the detection of circulating antibodies to food substances are of limited reliability and reproducibility. Nevertheless, there are a number of gastrointestinal conditions which may be associated with antibodies to food or may improve on elimination of certain foods from the diet. It should be noted, however, that the presence of circulating antibodies to foods, or the reversal of symptoms on withdrawal of foods, does not necessarily imply a hypersensitivity mechanism. Some of the conditions which may mimic true alimentary or gastrointestinal allergy or may be associated with circulating antibodies to food substances will be reviewed in the section which follows.

Lactose Intolerance Syndrome

Chronic diarrhea in infants has been described as the result of a deficiency of disaccharidases or sugar splitting enzymes. Of particular importance to the present discussion is the congenital absence of lactase which digests lactose, the major sugar of breast milk or cow's milk. If unrecognized, the clinical course of infants with this disorder may be progressively downhill, due to severe diarrhea, dehydration, malnutrition, and electrolyte disturbances, and may ultimately result in the death of the infant. However, if milk is eliminated from the diet, the diarrhea ceases. Conversely, if milk is reintroduced, the symptoms promptly recur.

More recently, it has been recognized that a similar syndrome may occur in adults. It has been estimated that milk intolerance characterized by abdominal bloating, cramps, flatulence, and diarrhea, 1 to 4 hours after the ingestion of one or two glasses of milk, occurs in approximately 5 per cent of the adult Caucasian population and in approximately 70 per cent of adult Negroes and Orientals.[10] In the majority of these individuals the enzyme lactase is deficient, and their symptoms can be reproduced by the administration of milk or lactose. The amount of lactose necessary to produce symptoms in adults varies considerably, but 50 gm, the amount present in a quart of milk, will almost invariably provoke discomfort in affected individuals. However, the adult with primary lactase deficiency who drinks little or no milk will not have symptoms.

The acquired adult type of milk intolerance most commonly appears in the late teens or early twenties and is usually idiopathic. If the symptoms of milk intolerance appear for the first time after the third decade, underlying gastrointestinal disease must be considered in the differential diagnosis. Some of the secondary causes of lactose malabsorption in adults include: the adult forms of celiac disease and malabsorption syndrome, extensive small bowel resections, infectious diarrhea, ulcerative colitis, and regional enteritis. The intestinal symptoms are presumably due to the formation of lactic acid, acetic acid, and gas within the gastrointestinal lumen by the action of the gut bacteria on undigested lactose. The stools are usually watery and have a sour odor.

Typical laboratory findings consist of stools with an acid pH, and an impaired lactose tolerance test in the presence of a normal glucose tolerance test. Patients with lactase deficiency almost invariably have characteristic symptoms following the ingestion of lactose during the test. However, an abnormal lactose tolerance test does not distinguish between primary and secondary lactase deficiency. A flat curve should, therefore, be followed by a d-xylose absorption test as a general measure of small intestinal integrity. A jejunal biopsy for the quantitative assay of lactase may be necessary to confirm the diagnosis, and is often essential for the exclusion of underlying mucosal disorders.

Rising titers of hemagglutinating antibodies to whole milk have been described in some infants with lactase deficiency and milk intolerance,[24b] but milk antibodies are apparently absent in the sera of most adults with the lactose intolerance syndrome.[1] This peculiar tendency of children under the age of 3 years to develop circulating antibodies to food antigens has been observed in a wide variety of intestinal disorders and is not specific for the lactose intolerance syndrome. The most likely explanation is that there is an increased absorption of whole milk proteins due to diminished proteolysis or because the intestinal mucosa is damaged.

The treatment consists of the removal of milk and unfermented milk products from the patient's diet. Fermented cheese, yogurt, and buttermilk do not contain lactose and may be substituted for milk in adults. Infants and children may be placed on a lactose free formula such as Nutramigen.

Allergic Gastroenteropathy

A type of protein-losing enteropathy thought to be due to gastrointestinal allergy was described in six children aged 3 to 10 years.[26] These patients had diarrhea, vomiting, hypoalbuminemia, hypogammaglobulinemia, periorbital edema, iron deficiency anemia, and peripheral blood eosinophilia associated with other atopic manifestations such as atopic dermatitis, bronchial asthma, and rhinitis. In some of these patients it was demonstrated that the feeding of milk increased both the clinical symptoms and the enteric loss of protein, whereas the removal of milk from the diet appeared to reverse the entire process.

Other common causes of protein-losing enteropathy in children were excluded by detailed investigations. Mucosal biopsies were normal except for marked infiltration of the lamina propria by eosinophilis in three cases. Precipitins to whole milk were demonstrated in the sera of three patients, but the possible role of these antibodies in the pathogenesis of the disease process is not established.

There is some evidence that patients with allergic protein-losing gastroenteropathy who do not respond to a milk-free diet may be improved by the systemic administration of corticosteroids.

A somewhat similar syndrome of infancy has been described in which circulating antibodies to cow's milk were associated with gastrointestinal blood loss of up to 21 ml/day, iron-deficiency anemia, hypoproteinemia, and peripheral edema.[29] Removal of milk from the diet resulted in the reversal of the blood loss. In neither of these two syndromes is there any direct evidence that the underlying defect in the gastrointestinal mucosa is the result of antibody-mediated tissue damage.

Protein-losing gastroenteropathy associated with intestinal lymphangiectasia may also occur in patients with immunologic deficiency syndromes (see Chapter 11).

Cot Death

Infants who die unexpectedly and mysteriously (cot death) constitute yet another group of patients in which milk hypersensitivity has been invoked as a possible etiologic factor.[21] There appears little doubt that this syndrome occurs in bottle-fed infants, that sera of such infants contain high titers of hemagglutinating antibodies to cow's milk proteins, and that regurgitated cow's milk may be found in the lung parenchyma after death. As a result of these observations, it has been claimed that death occurs as the result of an anaphylactic reaction in the lung to cow's milk protein, but there is no direct proof of this hypothesis. Other workers have shown that there is no significant difference between titers of serum antibodies to cow's milk protein in the sera of infants dying suddenly and unexpectedly and in control infants. Furthermore, anaphylactic reactions are not usually mediated by antibodies which can be detected by the hemagglutination technique (see Chapter 2).

Wiskott-Aldrich Syndrome

There is a high incidence of circulating antibodies to cow's milk in the sera of patients with the Wiskott-Aldrich syndrome, but their significance is not clear (see Chapter 11).

Gluten-Induced Enteropathy

Most children with celiac disease and many adults with nontropical sprue (adult celiac disease, idiopathic steatorrhea, or gluten enteropathy) improve dramatically when wheat, barley, and rye flour are excluded from their diets. Detailed investigations have shown that the characteristic signs and symptoms of diarrhea, weight loss, and failure to absorb essential vitamins and minerals are due to the inability of these patients to tolerate dietary gluten (a constituent of cereal flours). More specifically, it appears to be gliadin (the ethyl-alcohol soluble component of gluten) which is responsible for the absorptive and morphologic abnormalities seen in this disease.

Circulating antibodies to gliadin have been demonstrated by a variety of techniques in the sera of patients with gluten-induced enteropathy. However, variations in the antigens studied and the antibody assays employed preclude an accurate assessment of the incidence of such antibodies, and there is no apparent correlation between the severity of the disease and antibody titers. Furthermore, it has been shown by several groups of investigators that there is a high incidence of antibodies to other dietary proteins, particularly cow's milk, in patients with gluten-induced enteropathy.[15] Precipitins to gliadin and to cows' milk proteins have been demonstrated in the stools of patients with celiac disease giving rise to the suggestion that the polypeptides of gluten or milk may elicit the production of IgA antibodies within the gut.[12]

There is now convincing evidence that the gut is capable of local antibody production to viral and bacterial antigens.[3] However, immunofluorescent studies in celiac disease have failed to provide conclusive evidence that gliadin-specific antibodies are synthesized by the immunocytes of the small bowel. To date the only significant abnormal immunologic findings in gluten-induced enteropathy are the presence of an isolated IgM deficiency in about two-thirds of patients,[2] and an increase in the proportion of IgG- and IgM-containing cells in the jejunal mucosa.[25] Otherwise, the immunopathology of gluten-induced enteropathy remains obscure, as does the relationship between this interesting disease process and circulating or coproantibodies to dietary proteins.[4]

The diagnosis of gluten-induced enteropathy depends on the combined demonstration of the absence or blunting of villi in a jejunal biopsy and clinical improvement on a gluten-free diet. Increased amounts of fat in the stools, impaired absorption of d-xylose, and characteristic radiographic features of segmenting and clumping in the bowel occur in most patients, but are not essential to the diagnosis.

Specific treatment consists of providing the patient with a gluten-free diet which results in varying degrees of improvement in individual patients.

Hereditary Angioedema

Although it is not a true hypersensitivity phenomenon, hereditary angio-edema due to an inherited deficiency of C1 esterase inhibitor may produce symptoms which mimic gastrointestinal allergy (see Chapter 5).

ULCERATIVE COLITIS

Many investigative approaches have been made to the pathogenesis of non-specific ulcerative colitis. For example, repeated attempts over the years to implicate a specific causative microorganism have been entirely unsuccessful. Psychiatric studies have confirmed the widely held clinical impression that psychosomatic factors are of importance in precipitating acute exacerbations, but there is no general agreement concerning a psychiatric "common denominator" in ulcerative colitis patients.

More recently, the possible role of immune mechanisms in the etiology of ulcerative colitis has been suggested on the basis of presumptive evidence from clinical and laboratory studies. This evidence includes the nature of the inflammatory reaction in the colon, the occurrence of antibodies to colonic constituents, the association with thymomas, the response to corticosteroid treatment, and the coexistence of other presumed hypersensitivity phenomena such as erythema nodosum, urticaria, uveitis, chronic active liver disease, primary biliary cirrhosis, and arthritis in some patients with ulcerative colitis.

PATHOLOGY

The pathologic process is that of acute, nonspecific inflammation which is most common in the rectosigmoid region, but may involve any portion of the colon or terminal ileum. The characteristic findings at surgery or on sigmoidoscopic examination are multiple, irregular, superficial ulcerations. Repeated attacks may eventually lead to the appearance of polypoid structures and neoplastic changes. On microscopic examination, the inflammatory process rarely extends beyond the mucosa and submucosa. Other characteristic features include ulceration of a variable degree with surrounding polymorphonuclear leukocytes, infiltration of the lamina propria with large amounts of plasma cells and eosinophils, and damage to the colonic basement membrane. Less commonly, there may be a vasculitis of the colonic mucosa. The pathologic process is rarely segmental, there is little tendency to fibrosis, and there is no granulomatous reaction.

IMMUNOLOGY

Sera from patients with ulcerative colitis demonstrate an increased incidence of antibodies against colonic antigens by a variety of immunologic techniques.[16] However, these antibody titers do not correlate with the clinical status of the patient, and they may be elevated in a small but significant percentage of normal individuals. The colonic antigens employed in most of these studies were derived from normal colonic mucosa and are mucopolysaccharide in nature. The antibodies directed against colonic antigens are predominantly IgM, but may be found to a lesser extent in the IgG components. (See Chapter 13 for discussion of colonic antibodies in carcinoma of the colon.)

It has been demonstrated that the colon antigens of man cross-react by most immunologic methods with colon antigens from rabbits and rats, thus indicating a lack of species specificity.[20] Of greater interest is the observation that human colonic antigens cross-react with a type-specific lipopolysaccharide derived from *E. coli* 014.[17] In addition to the type-specific O antigen, the relatively crude lipopolysaccharide extracts used in these experiments contain large amounts of heterogeneic antigens known to be present in most species of the family Enterobacteriacea (e.g., *Escherichia, Salmonella,* and *Shigella*). It has thus been suggested that the tissue damage in ulcerative colitis might be related to the production of antibodies against the normal intestinal flora. Such a situation could be considered analogous to the hypothesis that the cardiac lesions of rheumatic fever result from the demonstrated cross-reactivity between group A streptococci and human heart muscle (see Chapter 7).

Several groups of investigators have attempted to show by immunofluorescent and other techniques that anticolonic or antibacterial antibodies may be produced locally in the gastrointestinal mucosa of patients with ulcerative colitis. To date, these experiments have produced equivocal findings. Similarly, there is only fragmentary evidence for the in vivo binding of immunoglobulins or the local deposition of complement in the colonic epithelium of patients with ulcerative colitis.

It has been suggested for many years that hypersensitivity to cow's milk may be of importance in the etiology of ulcerative colitis. There appears to be little doubt in the minds of many experienced clinical gastroenterologists that a small percentage of patients with ulcerative colitis improve dramatically on withdrawal of milk from their diet and relapse on its reintroduction. An increased titer of hemagglutinating antibodies to cow's milk has been reported to occur in ulcerative colitis, but the titers did not decrease with clinical improvement following withdrawal of milk.[30] Unfortunately, there are very few well controlled studies which attempt to correlate lactose intolerance or antibodies to cow's milk with the presence of ulcerative lesions in the colon or terminal ileum. Clearly, more work needs to be done in this area before any definite conclusions can be reached.

The occasional, but unexplained, association between thymoma, ulcerative colitis, and hypogammaglobulinemia has given rise to further speculation that immune mechanisms may be of significance in ulcerative colitis.[14]

The evidence discussed in the preceding paragraphs leads to the tentative conclusion that tissue damage in ulcerative colitis is not dependent on circulating antibodies. There has, therefore, been a search for possible cellular immune mechanisms which may be of importance. For example, it was shown that lymphocytes obtained from patients with ulcerative colitis had a cytotoxic effect on human fetal colonic cells maintained in tissue culture, whereas sera from the same patients had no effect.[23] On the other hand, attempts to induce blastogenic transformation in explanted lymphocytes obtained from patients with ulcerative colitis have not been successful with either colon antigens or lipopolysaccharide extracts from E. coli.[9]

In summary, there is little conclusive experimental evidence at present that immune mechanisms are directly involved in the etiology of ulcerative colitis. It is conceivable that an immune response might be initiated by infection with a bacterial strain which cross-reacts with colonic antigens, but much further work needs to be done before this theory can be fully substantiated.[28]

CLINICAL MANIFESTATIONS

The clinical pattern of chronic, nonspecific ulcerative colitis may vary from a mild increase in the frequency of bowel movements to an acute and fulminating disease with severe diarrhea and prostration. There may be up to 30–40 bowel movements daily with blood and mucus in the stools, usually accompanied by crampy lower abdominal pain. In some patients, constipation may occur instead of, or alternating with, diarrhea. Other symptoms may include rectal tenesmus, anal incontinence, anorexia, dyspepsia, malaise, fever, and weight loss. There is a marked tendency to spontaneous exacerbations and remissions.

On physical examination, there may be mild abdominal tenderness and distension. Inspection of the rectal area may reveal evidence of pruritus ani, fissures, fistulas, and abscesses. Sigmoidoscopic examination is abnormal in over 90 per cent of patients with ulcerative colitis. Changes in the mucosa may range from mild hyperemia and petechiae to severe ulceration and polypoid changes in patients with advanced lesions. Radiographic changes may be confined to one area of the colon or terminal ileum, or they may be generalized. Common radiographic changes include hypermotility of the colon, decreased size of the colon and its lumen, pseudopolyps, and the loss of haustral markings. The stools contain blood and pus, but no pathogenic organisms.

The complications of nonspecific ulcerative colitis include hypochromic, microcytic anemia due to blood loss, hypoproteinemia, acute hemorrhage, perforation, pericolic abscesses, stricture, toxic megacolon, and malignant degeneration. The immunologic aspects of carcinoma of the colon are discussed in more detail in Chapter 13.

TREATMENT

Because the nature of the disease is poorly understood, treatment is, of necessity, empiric. During the acute phase, bed rest, sedation, and a low-residue diet are almost mandatory. A minority of patients may show considerable improvement following the elimination of milk products from the diet.

Despite the uncertain pathogenesis, the judicious use of corticosteroids and sulfonamides provides adequate control of symptoms in the majority of cases. A sulfonamide preparation such as salicylazosulfapyridine, 2 to 8 gm, daily, is often effective in mild cases as the sole form of drug therapy. In more severe or refractory cases, prednisone may be given by mouth in doses of 20 to 80 mg daily, or, alternatively, hydrocortisone retention enemas (100 mg/2 oz. of vegetable oil) may be prescribed in an attempt to reduce the systemic side-effects of corticosteroids. Preliminary reports on the use of azathioprine in the treatment of ulcerative colitis are encouraging but should be interpreted with caution in a disease which is prone to spontaneous remission.

Total colectomy with ileostomy may be indicated if medical therapy is not successful after an adequate trial. The usual indications for emergency surgery in ulcerative colitis are severe hemorrhage or perforation. Elective surgery may occasionally be the treatment of choice in unremitting disease or in children who have stunted growth or sexual immaturity as a consequence of chronic ulcerative colitis.

GRANULOMATOUS ILEOCOLITIS

Granulomatous ileocolitis is a predominantly inflammatory disease of unknown etiology which usually involves the small intestine (regional enteritis, Crohn's disease), but less commonly may affect the large bowel (granulomatous colitis). In the colon, the pathologic changes of ulcerative colitis are primarily those of a mucosal disease, whereas the lesions of granulomatous colitis extend transmurally. However, in the colon, there is often considerable clinical, radiologic, and pathologic overlap between the two disorders. One clinical difference of prognostic significance is the much lower incidence of carcinoma of the colon in granulomatous colitis than in ulcerative colitis.

There is very little data to suggest that immunologic factors may be of importance in the pathogenesis of granulomatous ileocolitis except that the disease often improves on corticosteroid therapy, and preliminary trials with azathioprine have been encouraging. Because of the close similarity between the focal granulomas seen histologically in granulomatous ileocolitis and those seen in sarcoidosis, a recent report of a 50 per cent incidence of positive Kviem reactions in patients with regional ileitis is of considerable interest.[20a] It is conceivable that there may be an etiologic agent common to the two diseases, or the abnormal tissues may share a common antigen.

CHRONIC ACTIVE LIVER DISEASE

An immunologic basis has been postulated for the chronic hepatitis that progresses unrelentingly for months or years in the absence of an obvious causative agent or triggering event.[5] The term chronic active hepatitis has been used by many authors to describe this condition,[8] but until the responsible etiologic factors are understood more completely the classification of disease entities such as chronic active hepatitis, lupoid hepatitis, subacute hepatitis, active juvenile cirrhosis, and plasma-cell hepatitis will remain confusing. At present, the more general term "chronic active liver disease" seems the most appropriate form of nomenclature.[7] Lupoid hepatitis probably represents a variant of chronic active liver disease which is associated with a positive LE-cell test, or positive tests for antinuclear antibodies.

It has been suggested that chronic active liver disease occurs as the result of liver damage initially caused by the hepatitis virus, and that prepetuation of the disease is due to an immunologic response to antigens released from the damaged liver cells.[19] Alternatively, one could postulate the existence of a persistent "slow virus" in the liver parenchyma. However, in many patients with chronic active liver disease, there is no previous history of either hepatitis or jaundice, and the etiology remains obscure. Some cases of chronic active liver disease become quiescent, but others apparently progress to the "cryptogenic" form of cirrhosis.[5] The term "cryptogenic" cirrhosis will be used to describe postnecrotic cirrhosis which occurs in the absence of a previous history suggestive of viral hepatitis.

PATHOLOGY

Characteristic microscopic findings on biopsy consist of a variable degree of liver cell necrosis which is associated with infiltration of the portal tracts by plasma cells and lymphocytes. At times, the percentage of plasma cells may be as high as 40 per cent, but this feature is not essential for the pathologic diagnosis. Proliferation of bile ducts may occur in some patients. The destruction of hepatic parenchyma may eventually lead to a variable degree of fibrosis, collapse of reticulum, and nodular regeneration of the type usually associated with postnecrotic cirrhosis. Thus, a biopsy specimen obtained in a fully developed case of chronic active liver disease may show accumulation of lymphoid aggregates and plasma cells superimposed on the morphologic features of postnecrotic cirrhosis.

IMMUNOLOGY

The most consistent finding of possible immunologic significance in chronic active liver disease is the marked increase in total serum globulin which occurs in the majority of patients. The serum γ-globulin is almost always in excess of 2 gm/100 ml and may occasionally rise to a level as high as 5 to 6 gm/100 ml (Fig. 16-1). The bulk of the increase in γ-globulin is in the IgG components, and monoclonal (M) peaks are occasionally detected on cellulose acetate electrophoresis. Immunoglobulin abnormalities

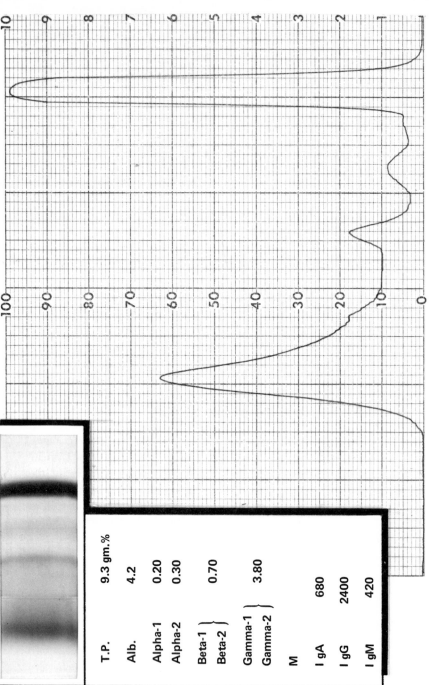

T.P.	9.3 gm.%
Alb.	4.2
Alpha-1	0.20
Alpha-2	0.30
Beta-1 ⎱ Beta-2 ⎰	0.70
Gamma-1 ⎱ Gamma-2 ⎰	3.80
M	
I gA	680
I gG	2400
I gM	420

FIG. 16-1. Characteristic immunoglobulin profile of a patient with chronic active liver disease. Note the marked hypergamma-globulinemia and increase in IgG.

of this magnitude are not common in Laennec's cirrhosis, post-hepatitic cirrhosis, or in normal individuals. In addition to the positive LE-cell phenomena and antinuclear antibodies found in patients with lupoid hepatitis, positive sheep cell agglutination tests for rheumatoid factor occur in a significant number of patients.

It is these observations which have led several groups of investigators to postulate an immunologic basis for chronic active liver disease and have led to a search for other antibodies.[19] Complement-fixing antibodies against cytoplasmic liver antigens can be demonstrated in the sera of many patients with chronic active hepatitis (autoimmune complement-fixation test, AICF). However, this test is also positive with cytoplasmic constituents obtained from a variety of other human and animal tissues. The AICF test is thus nonspecific and is positive in numerous other disease processes with immunologic features such as systemic lupus erythematosus without hepatic involvement and primary biliary cirrhosis. The antigenic constituents which react in the AICF test have been identified as microsomes or mitochondria.

Using immunofluorescence techniques, it has been shown that the sera of approximately 70 per cent of patients with chronic active liver disease contain antinuclear, smooth muscle, mitochondrial, and bile canalicular antibodies.[27] The antinuclear antibodies may be of the "diffuse," "speckled," or "nucleolar" varieties (see Chapter 8). The antibodies to smooth muscle are of particular interest because they are found in approximately 60 per cent of patients with chronic active liver disease. However, like the antibodies detected by the AICF test, the smooth muscle antibodies are neither organ-specific nor species-specific. They will react by the immunofluorescence technique against a variety of human and rat smooth muscle tissues. The antibodies to bile canaliculi are of little diagnostic value as they are also detected in 75 per cent of patients with primary biliary cirrhosis and 65 per cent of patients with viral hepatitis. The mitochondrial antibodies are discussed in more detail in the section on primary biliary cirrhosis.

TABLE 16-1. Incidence of Immunofluorescent Antibodies in the Sera of Patients with Chronic Liver Disease

Antibody	Chronic active hepatitis (%)	Primary biliary cirrhosis (%)	Cryptogenic cirrhosis (%)
Antinuclear	80	45	38
Smooth muscle	60	45	30
Mitochondrial	25	90	25

The incidence of antibodies found by the immunofluorescence technique in chronic active liver disease, biliary cirrhosis, and cryptogenic cirrhosis is summarized in Table 16-1. The fact that the same spectrum of antibodies is found in all three conditions has led to the hypothesis that a single immune process, of unknown mechanism, may eventually lead to chronic active liver disease, biliary cirrhosis, or cryptogenic cirrhosis, depending on the relative degree of involvement of liver cells or bile canaliculi.[5] Serum antibodies are not consistently demonstrable in any other form of chronic liver disease.

CLINICAL MANIFESTATIONS

The clinical syndrome occurs most commonly in young women and is characterized by recurrent fever, jaundice, and malaise. In some patients, the primary clinical manifestations are associated with or even preceded by arthralgias, amenorrhea, pericarditis, pleuritis, ulcerative colitis, and skin rashes.

Laboratory findings include the positive tests for antinuclear and immunofluorescent antibodies already described, and marked hypergammaglobulinemia. In addition, there is laboratory evidence of severe hepatocellular liver damage manifested by elevated levels of serum glutamic oxalacetic transaminase (SGOT), hyperbilirubinemia, and bromsulfpthalein retention. The occasional patient may have a positive Coombs' test, a positive STS (see Chapter 21), or a positive test for rheumatoid factor.

Chronic active liver disease may cause mild protracted disability or it may progress to death within a period of years or months. Exact figures regarding prognosis are difficult to obtain because of disagreement regarding nomenclature, and the introduction of newer treatment methods. Before the introduction of corticosteroids, approximately 50 per cent of patients died of liver failure within 5 years of the onset of the disease.

TREATMENT

The single most effective form of treatment is the administration of systemic corticosteroids such as prednisone in doses of 20 to 40 mg daily. Preliminary reports suggest that azathioprine in doses of 1.5 to 2 mg/kg of body weight per day, or 6-mercaptopurine in doses of 2.5 to 5 mg/kg of body weight per day, may produce clinical and laboratory improvement in some patients and may reduce, but not permanently eliminate, the need for corticosteroid drugs. General supportive measures include adequate rest, vitamin supplements, and avoidance of alcohol and all other primary hepatotoxic agents.

PRIMARY BILIARY CIRRHOSIS

Primary biliary cirrhosis (chronic intrahepatic obstructive jaundice) is one of the less common forms of intrahepatic cholestasis. The disease is of unknown cause, tends to occur almost exclusively in women, and may occasionally be associated with ulcerative colitis. The occurrence of antibodies against liver constituents in this disease has led to the suggestion that immunologic mechanisms may be involved in its pathogenesis.

PATHOLOGY

The initial histologic change in primary biliary cirrhosis is a chronic granulomatous reaction surrounding and involving the small bile ducts, which eventually results in their complete destruction. At the same time, the portal areas may become heavily infiltrated with lymphocytes, plasma cells, and occasionally with eosinophils. Electron microscopic studies indicate that the fundamental disease process is not hepatocellular, but is related to bile duct abnormalities. Thus, the jaundice which occurs in the early stages of the disease may be, in part, due to leakage of conjugated bilirubin from damaged bile ducts into the circulation. Eventually, there is tissue proliferation in the interlobular spaces, fibrosis of the entire portal triad, and the characteristic pathologic picture of septal cirrhosis.

IMMUNOLOGY

Studies employing the techniques of complement-fixation and immuno-fluorescence have demonstrated a high incidence of circulating antibodies against both cytoplasmic constituents and bile canaliculi in patients with primary biliary cirrhosis.[22] Mitochondrial antibodies, detected by the immunofluorescence technique, are found in the sera of approximately 90 per cent of patients with primary biliary cirrhosis, and it has been suggested that their presence may constitute a valuable diagnostic test. However, the degree of overlap of mitochondrial, smooth muscle, and antinuclear antibodies in chronic active hepatitis, primary biliary cirrhosis, and cryptogenic cirrhosis has already been discussed in the section on chronic active hepatitis (see Table 16-1). In addition, the mitochondrial antibodies lack both organ and species specificity as they may be detected using unfixed sections of rat liver, rat kidney, monkey stomachs, or monkey submaxillary glands.

Impairment of the normal mechanisms of delayed hypersensitivity, as measured by induction of allergic contact dermatitis to dinitrochlorobenzene and lymphocyte transformation, is noted in about 50 per cent of patients with biliary cirrhosis.[6] It has been suggested that these findings are the result of a granulomatous process which may extend beyond the liver.

CLINICAL MANIFESTATIONS

Characteristic clinical findings in primary biliary cirrhosis include pruritus, the insidious onset of jaundice, marked hepatomegaly, and dark urine, all of which usually progress over a number of years to terminal liver failure. The laboratory findings are essentially those of an obstructive type of jaundice with high levels of serum alkaline phosphatase, cholesterol, and phospholipids. Patients with primary biliary cirrhosis frequently develop xanthomas of the skin which are believed to be secondary to the elevated levels of serum lipids, rather than to a primary disturbance in lipid metabolism.

TREATMENT

The only treatment in primary biliary cirrhosis is supportive therapy. The major objectives are to maintain adequate nutrition with vitamin supplements and to attempt to relieve itching with cholestyramine resin, 4 gm, three times a day, which binds bile salts in the gut. Antihistamines, soothing lotions, and baths may occasionally provide symptomatic relief of severe pruritus. The role of corticosteroids in the treatment of primary biliary cirrhosis is not clearly established.

HEPATITIS-ASSOCIATED (AUSTRALIA) ANTIGEN

Hepatitis-associated antigen (HAA), a particle approximately 20 mμ in diameter with an electron microscopic appearance compatible with that of a virus, has been detected in the sera of approximately 70 per cent of patients with post-transfusion hepatitis, in approximately 30 per cent of patients with infectious hepatitis, and in approximately 25 per cent of patients with chronic active hepatitis.[1a] Of the tests currently available for hepatitis antigen, the micro-Ouchterlony technique is probably the simplest to perform, but the complement-fixation test is the most sensitive. Hepatitis antigen often appears in the plasma before the signs and symptoms of acute hepatitis, and, in about 7 per cent of patients remains present for an indefinite period after recovery.[24a] It was originally called the Australia antigen because it was first identified in an Australian aborigine and was thought to represent a solely inherited trait.

Additional evidence linking the hepatitis antigen to a hepatitis virus is the observation that the particles can be isolated from the blood by density gradient sedimentation,[32] and the addition of anti-HAA antiserum results in their agglutination. Furthermore, the liver cells of patients with hepatitis antigen in their blood demonstrate fluorescent granules in or near the nuclei when treated with fluorescent anti-HAA antiserum. However, since several outbreaks of infectious hepatitis with a short incubation period have not been associated with the hepatitis antigen, it appears likely that hepatitis can be caused by more than one group of viruses.

It is of considerable interest that hepatitis antigen also occurs in association with Down's syndrome in institutionalized patients, leukemia, Hodgkin's disease, lepromatous leprosy, chronic renal dialysis, open heart surgery, and in a small percentage of apparently normal blood donors (see Table 16-2). Although jaundice is rare in these groups of patients, there is usually biochemical and histologic evidence of chronic hepatitis. The occurrence of immunologic deficiency states in association with Down's syndrome, leukemia, Hodgkin's disease, and lepromatous leprosy is discussed in Chapters 11 and 12. Thus, it seems reasonable to postulate that either immune deficiency or multiple transfusions (e.g., in chronic dialysis patients), or both (e.g., in leukemia patients) predisposes to infection with hepatitis virus. A minority of multiply transfused hemophiliacs develop anti-HAA antibodies and serve as a source of antisera.

TABLE 16-2. Conditions Associated with HAA

Disorder	Frequency of antigen (%)
Post-transfusion hepatitis	70
Infectious hepatitis	30
Chronic active liver disease	25
Down's syndrome (in institutions)	30
Lepromatous leprosy	20
Leukemia	10
Hodgkin's disease	4
Chronic renal dialysis	50
North American blood donors	0.1–0.5
Normal individuals in Southeast Asia	4–20

Genetic factors may also be of importance in determining susceptibility to hepatitis virus. The Australia antigen occurs in 4 to 20 per cent of individuals living in the tropics or in Southeast Asia in the absence of detectable liver disease. Genetic studies in these areas indicate that susceptibility to the Australia antigen is inherited as a simple autosomal recessive trait. However, the exact relationship between the infectious and genetic etiologies of this trait remains to be established.

At present the detection of hepatitis antigen in the blood serves as a valuable diagnostic procedure for identifying patients with serum hepatitis, and for excluding blood donors who are potential carriers of serum hepatitis. It is of interest that five patients with cirrhosis complicated by hepatoma had positive tests for serum HAA.[24] Two of these patients also had positive tests for α_1-fetoprotein (see Chapter 13).

OTHER SERUM PROTEIN ABNORMALITIES IN LIVER DISEASE

The hypergammaglobulinemia which sometimes occurs in Laennec's cirrhosis is discussed in Chapter 10; the immunoglobulin abnormalities which occur in chronic liver diseases are summarized in Table 22-5; and the significance of α_1-fetoprotein in the diagnosis of hepatoma is discussed in Chapter 13.

LIVER INJURY DUE TO DRUG HYPERSENSITIVITY

In discussing the subject of drug-induced liver injury, it is often difficult to distinguish clearly between drugs which are direct hepatotoxins, drugs which produce liver damage due to a metabolic abnormality of the host, and drugs which produce liver damage due to hypersensitivity mechanisms. Generally accepted criteria for liver injury due to drug hypersensitivity include: (*1*) a relatively fixed sensitization period of 1 to 4 weeks of exposure to the drug before symptoms appear, or a history of previous exposure; (*2*) prompt recurrence of hepatic dysfunction on re-administration of small doses of the drug; and (*3*) a high incidence of associated drug fever, rash, urticaria, lymphadenopathy, and peripheral blood eosinophilia.[31]

If these criteria are accepted, the best examples of commonly used drugs which produce jaundice on a hypersensitivity basis are para-aminosalicyclic acid (PAS), chlorpromazine, halothane anesthesia,[13] and perhaps iproniazid and its homologues. Hypersensitivity mechanisms have been suggested for liver damage caused by many other drugs, but the evidence is at best circumstantial and limited to a relatively small number of case reports.

The pathologic lesions in the liver may consist of extensive hepatocellular degeneration (e.g., iproniazid), or marked cholestasis characterized by intra-lobular bile stasis and infiltration of the portal triads with mononuclear and eosinophilic inflammatory cells (e.g., chlorpromazine).

The signs and symptoms of hepatitis due to drug hypersensitivity vary with the causative agent. If hepatocellular damage predominates, the clinical and laboratory picture resembles acute viral hepatitis. In the cholestatic type of drug-induced hepatitis, the clinical features may resemble extrahepatic biliary obstruction so closely that laparotomy may be necessary to establish the diagnosis. The coexistence of other manifestations of hypersensitivity such as fever, arthralgias, skin rashes, lymphadenopathy, and eosinophilia may provide presumptive evidence in favor of hepatitis due to drug hypersensitivity.

Treatment consists of prompt withdrawal of the suspected drug.

ATROPHIC GASTRITIS

The possible role of immunity in the pathogenesis of atrophic gastritis and pernicious anemia is discussed in detail in Chapter 9.

IMMUNOLOGIC DISORDERS WITH GASTROINTESTINAL MANIFESTATIONS

The association between immunoglobulin abnormalities and gastrointestinal disease which occurs in disorders such as hypogammaglobulinemia, nodular lymphoid hyperplasia of the small intestine, isolated IgA deficiency, and thymoma is discussed in Chapter 11.

APHTHOUS STOMATITIS

The etiology of aphthous stomatitis (canker sores) is unknown. Viral agents and hypersensitivity mechanisms have been suggested as possible causes, but there is no direct evidence for either of these hypotheses. Experimental studies have shown that homogenates of fetal oral mucosa will stimulate lymphocyte transformation in cultures of leukocytes obtained from patients with recurrent oral ulceration.[18] These observations would suggest that cellular immune mechanisms may be of importance in the pathogenesis of aphthous stomatitis.

REFERENCES

1. Bayless, T. M., Partin, J. S., and Rosensweig, N. S. Absence of milk antibodies in milk intolerance in adults. *J.A.M.A. 201:*50, 1967.

1a. Blumberg, B. S., Sutnick, A. I., and London, W. T. Australia antigen as a hepatitis virus. Variation in host response. *Amer. J. Med. 48:*1, 1970.

2. Brown, D. L., Cooper, A. G., and Hepner, G. W. IgM metabolism in coeliac disease. *Lancet 1:*858, 1969.

3. Bull, D. M., and Tomasi, T. B. Deficiency of immunoglobulin as an intestinal disease. *Gasteroenterology 54:*313, 1968.

4. Davis, S. D., Bierman, C. W., Pierson, W. E., Maas, C. W., and Ianetta, A. Clinical nonspecificity of coproantibodies in diarrheal stools. *New Eng. J. Med. 282:*612, 1970.

5. Doniach, D., Walker, J. G., Roitt, I. M., and Berg, P. A. "Autoallergic hepatitis." *New Eng. J. Med. 282:*86, 1970.

6. Fox, R. A., James, D. G., Scheuer, P. J., Sharma, O., and Sherlock, S. Impaired delayed hypersensitivity in primary biliary cirrhosis. *Lancet 1:*959, 1969.

7. Geall, M. G., Schoenfield, L. J., and Summerskill, W. H. J. Classification and treatment of chronic active liver disease. *Gasteroenterology 55:*724, 1968.

8. Gelzayd, E. A., and Kirsner, J. B. Immunologic aspects of chronic active hepatitis in young people: A critical review of the recent literature. *Amer. J. Med. Sci. 253:*98, 1967.

9. Hinz, C. F., Jr., Perlmann, P., and Hammarstrom, S. Reactivity in-vitro of lymphocytes from patients with ulcerative colitis. *J. Lab. Clin. Med. 70:*752, 1967.

10. Huang, S. S., and Bayless, T. M. Milk and lactose intolerance in healthy Orientals. *Science 160:*83, 1968.

11. Ingelfinger, F. J., Lowell, F. C., and Franklin, W. Gastro-intestinal allergy. *New Eng. J. Med. 241:*303, 1949.

12. Katz, J., Kantor, F. S., and Herskovic, T. Intestinal antibodies to wheat fractions in celiac disease. *Ann. Intern. Med., 69:*1149, 1968.

13. Klion, F. M., Schaffner, F., and Popper, H. Hepatitis after exposure to halothane. *Ann. Intern. Med. 71:*467, 1969.

14. Kirk, B. W., and Freedman, S. O. Hypogammaglobulinemia, thymoma, and ulcerative colitis. *Canad. Med. Assoc. J. 96:*1272, 1967.

15. Kivel, R. M., Kearns, D. H., and Leibowitz, D. Significance of antibodies to dietary proteins in the serums of patients with nontropical sprue. *New Eng. J. Med., 271:*769, 1964.

16. Lagercrantz, R., Hammarstrom, S., Perlmann, P., and Gustafsson, B. E. Immunologic studies in ulcerative colitis. III. Incidence of antibodies to colon-antigen in ulcerative colitis and other gastrointestinal diseases. *Clin. Exp. Immun. 1:*263, 1966.

17. Lagercrantz, R., Hammarstrom, S., Perlmann, P., and Gustafsson, B. E. Im-

munological studies in ulcerative colitis. IV. Origin of autoantibodies. *J. Exp. Med.* *128*:1339, 1968.

18. Lehner, T. Stimulation of lymphocyte transformation by tissue homogenates in recurrent oral ulceration. *Immunology 13*:159, 1967.

19. MacKay, I. R., and Whittingham, S. "Auto-immune" chronic hepatitis. *Postgrad. Med. 41*:72, 1967.

20. McGiven, H. R., Ghose, T., and Nairn, R. C. Autoantibodies in ulcerative colitis. *Brit. Med. J. 2*:19, 1967.

20a. Mitchell, D. N., Cannon, P., Dyer, N. H., Hinson, K. F. W., and Willoughby, J. M. T. The Kveim test in Crohn's disease. *Lancet 1*:571, 1969.

21. Parish, W. E., Richards, C. B., France, N. E., and Coombs, R. R. A. Further investigations on the hypothesis that some cases of cot-death are due to a modified anaphylactic reaction to cow's milk. *Int. Arch. Allerg. 24*:215, 1964.

22. Paronetto, F., Schaffner, F., and Popper, H. Antibodies to cytoplasmic antigens in primary biliary cirrhosis and chronic active hepatitis. *J. Lab. Clin. Med. 69*:969, 1967.

23. Perlmann, P., and Broberger, O. In-vitro studies of ulcerative colitis. II. Cytotoxic action of white blood cells from patients on human foetal colon cells. *J. Exp. Med. 117*:717, 1963.

24. Sherlock, S., Fox, R. A., Niazi, S. P., and Schuer, P. J. The association of chronic liver disease and primary liver cell cancer with Australia (hepatitis) associated antigen. *Lancet 2*:609, 1970.

24a. Shulman, N. R., Hirschman, R. J., and Barker, L. F. Viral hepatitis. *Ann. Inter. Med. 72*:256, 1970.

24b. Silver, H., and Douglas, D. M. Milk intolerance in infancy. *Arch. Dis. Child. 43*:17, 1968.

25. Soltoft, J. Immunoglobulin-containing cells in non-tropical sprue. *Clin. Exp. Immun. 6*:413, 1970.

26. Waldmann, T. A., Wochner, R. D., Laster, L., and Gordon, R. S. Allergic gastroenteropathy. A cause of excessive gastrointestinal protein loss. *New Eng. J. Med. 276*:761, 1967.

27. Walker, G., and Doniach, D. Antibodies and immunoglobulins in liver disease. *Gut 9*:266, 1968.

28. Watson, D. W. Immune responses and the gut. *Gastroenterology 56*:944, 1969.

29. Wilson, J. F., Heiner, D. C., and Lahey, M. E. Milk induced gastrointestinal bleeding in infants with hypochromic microcytic anemia. *J.A.M.A. 189*:122, 1964.

30. Wright, R., and Truelove, S. C. Circulating antibodies to dietary proteins in ulcerative colitis. *Brit. Med. J. 2*:138, 1965.

31. Zimmerman, H. J. Toxic hepatopathy. *Amer. J. Gastroent. 49*:39, 1968.

32. Zuckerman, A. J., Taylor, P. E., and Bird, R. G. Review: Antigens and viruses in acute hepatitis. *Clin. Exp. Immun. 7*:439, 1970.

17

Clinical Immunology of the Eye

SAMUEL O. FREEDMAN

ENDOGENOUS UVEITIS

In recent years, considerable attention has been focused on possible immunologic factors in the pathogenesis of uveitis. The term uveitis, as commonly employed, refers to any inflammatory process which involves one or more components of the uveal tract (iris, ciliary body, and choroid). The term *anterior uveitis* is used to denote inflammation of the iris alone (iritis) or inflammation of the iris and ciliary body (iridocyclitis). Inflammation of the choroid usually involves the retina as well, and, therefore, the terms *posterior uveitis* and chorioretinitis are often used interchangeably (Table 17-1).

Exogenous uveitis occurs as the result of the direct introduction of a microorganism into the eye secondary to surgery, traumatic injury, or corneal ulceration. The resultant inflammatory process is characterized by suppuration and by the involvement of other ocular tissues in addition to the uveal tract. *Endogenous uveitis,* on the other hand, is usually nonsuppurative, even though it may be associated in some instances with organisms lodged in the vitreous or retina. The origin of these organisms is from within the body rather than from external sources. Hypersensitivity to infectious

506

agents and autoimmune mechanisms have been postulated as possible causes of nonsuppurative, endogenous uveitis, although the etiology is essentially unknown in many cases. (Suppurative endogenous uveitis may occasionally occur as the result of blood-borne dissemination of pyogenic organisms, or direct invasion of the optic nerve during meningitis.)

TABLE 17-1. Methods of
Classifying
Uveitis

Anatomic
    Anterior
        Iritis
        Iridocyclitis
    Posterior
        Choroiditis
        Chorioretinitis

Source of Microorganisms
    Exogenous
        Surgery
        Trauma
        Corneal Ulceration
    Endogenous
        Nonsuppurative
        Suppurative

Pathologic
    Granulomatous
    Nongranulomatous

It has been suggested that endogenous, nonsuppurative uveitis may be further divided into granulomatous and nongranulomatous uveitis on the basis of characteristic clinical and pathologic findings.[29] Under this scheme of classification, granulomatous uveitis is said to result from actual invasion of the uveal tract by nonpyogenic organisms, whereas nongranulomatous uveitis is said to be due to a hypersensitivity reaction to organisms lodged in tissues elsewhere in the body.

Because the distinction between granulomatous and nongranulomatous uveitis is based primarily on pathologic findings, this form of classification is of limited value in clinical practice. For instance, it is frequently possible to distinguish granulomatous from nongranulomatous uveitis when only the anterior segment of the eye is affected. However, the clinical separation between these two forms of endogenous uveitis becomes much less certain when the posterior segment is involved. Coexisting anterior segment disease may make it impossible or extremely difficult to perform an adequate examination of the retina. Furthermore, the occasional patient with a nongranulomatous anterior uveitis may develop granulomatous lesions at a later date. For these reasons, a simple subdivision into anterior and posterior uveitis appears to be more satisfactory for clinical purposes.

PATHOLOGY

Granulomatous Uveitis

The essential pathologic feature is that of granulomatous inflammation characterized by the presence of large mononuclear wandering cells which eventually become epitheloid.[9] Giant cells derived from the epithelioid cells may aggregate into large nodules resembling tubercles. In addition, there may be necrosis of adjacent structures, accumulation of lymphocytes and plasma cells, and fibrosis of the involved areas during the chronic stages. Recurrent or persistent disease may lead to eventual destruction and disorganization of the eye.

Nongranulomatous Uveitis

The pathologic picture in the acute phase consists of capillary dilatation with an out-pouring of polymorphonuclear leukocytes.[9] These are then rapidly replaced by lymphocytes, plasma cells, and large macrophages. The end result is pin-point areas of necrosis, atrophy, or fibrosis. Repeated episodes may lead to complete functional disorganization of the involved portions of the eye.

IMMUNOLOGY

Precipitins against human uveal pigment were demonstrated in the sera of approximately 65 per cent of patients with endogenous uveitis.[3] These autoantibodies are more frequent in patients with bilateral disease, with severe disease, and with long duration of symptoms. However, they are not correlated with any specific disease entity and occur with equal frequency in exogenous uveitis. Their significance in the pathogenesis of uveitis is, therefore, far from clear. It is more than likely that these "autoantibodies" are the result, rather than the cause, of damage to the uveal tract.

Other workers have reported on the occurrence of anti-DNA antibodies in about 25 per cent of patients with uveitis due to presumed infective causes.[6] The meaning of this observation is not understood at the present time.

In experimental animals, anterior segment disease has been produced after immunization and subsequent conjunctival challenge with a variety of antigens such as HSA, dextran, and keyhole limpet hemocyanin.[2] In another series of experiments, rhesus monkeys injected with monkey retinal tissues incorporated in Freund's adjuvant developed ocular lesions similar to human chorioretinitis.[15] However, the pathogenesis of these animal lesions remains obscure, and it is very difficult to correlate experimental uveitis with its presumed human counterpart. Despite an impressive accumulation of indirect evidence which appears to implicate various microorganisms in the pathogenesis of human endogenous uveitis, there is very little information available on the exact mechanism of presumed immunologic tissue damage in the uveal tract.[1]

ETIOLOGY AND CLINICAL MANIFESTATIONS

Endogenous uveitis has been described in association with a number of infectious and noninfectious systemic diseases (Table 17-2). However, no cause and effect relationship has been established in most instances. The most important reason for the lack of precise information on etiology is that biopsies of the uveal tract during the course of acute uveitis carry the risk of damaging vision. If the eye is finally enucleated after months or years of disease, the changes are usually the pathologic sequelae of chronic inflammation and are of no assistance in establishing a precise etiologic diagnosis. Some of the more common associations between uveitis and systemic disease are described below.

Toxoplasmosis

There is little doubt that invasion of the uveal tract with *Toxoplasma gondii* may result in uveitis. The organisms have been demonstrated on many occasions in the retinae of patients with a posterior uveitis.[7] Because the pathologic changes appear to begin in the retina and involve the choroid secondarily, the term *Toxoplasma* retinochoroiditis is used in preference to chorioretinitis. The question which remains unanswered is whether posterior uveitis occurring in patients with serologic evidence of previous *Toxoplasma* infection can be attributed to active or latent infection with the organism, or whether it may be due to entirely unrelated causes.

TABLE 17-2. Etiology of Endogenous Uveitis

	Predominant lesion	
Suspected cause	Anterior uveitis	Posterior uveitis
Associated with Infectious Agents		
Toxoplasmosis		x
Histoplasmosis		x
Other fungi		x
Helminths		x
Tuberculosis		x
Syphilis	x	x
Brucellosis	x	
Cytomegalovirus infection		x
Associated with Systemic Diseases		
Sarcoidosis	x	
Juvenile rheumatoid arthritis	x	
Ankylosing spondylitis	x	
Ulcerative and granulomatous colitis	x	
Serum sickness	x	
Ocular Syndromes		
Vogt-Koyangi-Harada syndrome	x	x
Ocular herpes zoster or simplex	x	
Behçet's syndrome	x	

The problem is especially difficult because asymptomatic infections with *T. gondii* are common in the normal population. The Sabin-Feldman dye test for toxoplasmosis (see Chapter 21) has been reported to be positive in 85 per cent of adults in France and in 20 to 60 per cent of adults in the United States depending on the geographic location.[10] It is, therefore, quite conceivable that a positive serologic test may be a coincidental finding in a patient with uveitis due to unrelated causes. The titer of antibodies is not helpful in establishing a diagnosis because lesions typical of *Toxoplasma* chorioretinitis may develop in patients with low antibody titers, and many patients without retinal lesions have high antibody titers. It has been suggested that if the titer of antibodies is significantly higher in the aqueous humor than in the serum, the results are indicative of active toxoplasmosis.[10]

The characteristic eye lesions produced by demonstrated active infection with *T. gondii* consists of a focal exudation retinochoroiditis.[26] On fundus-copic examination, the retinal exudates may appear as one or more white opacifications, about 1 disc in diameter, which obliterate retinal vessels. The lesions may occur in any portion of the fundus and are usually associ-ated with inflammatory debris in the overlying vitreous (Fig. 17-1).

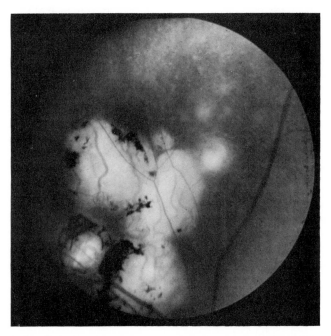

FIG. 17-1. Typical lesions in *Toxoplasma* retinochoroiditis. (Courtesy Dr. S. T. Adams, Montreal General Hospital.)

At present, the diagnosis of *Toxoplasma* retinochoroiditis should be enter-tained only in those patients who have a characteristic clinical picture as well as a positive Sabin-Feldman dye test. (A rising titer or a titer greater than 1:512 on a single determination is considered positive.) Con-versely, a negative test can be used to exclude the diagnosis of ocular toxoplasmosis. The complement-fixation test for toxoplasmosis may also be used as an exclusion procedure (see Chapter 21). A delayed type intra-dermal reaction to toxoplasmin is of only limited value as a diagnostic test because of the high incidence of *Toxoplasma* infection in the general population.

It must also be remembered that other organisms such as *Treponema pallidum, Mycobacterium tuberculosis, Aspergillus,* and *Coccidioides* have, in rare instances, been isolated from the retinas of patients with the focal exudative retinochoriditis said to be characteristic of ocular toxoplasmosis.[26]

Histoplasmosis

The evidence for active infection with *Histoplasma capsulatum* as an important cause of endogenous uveitis is much less convincing than in the case of toxoplasmosis. *Histoplasma* chorioretinitis has been suggested as a definite clinical entity because 93 per cent of patients with characteristic funduscopic findings had positive skin tests to histoplasmin compared with a rate of 25 per cent in the general population.[25] In another survey of 1417 persons in one endemic area, 1.6 per cent were found to have retinas suggestive of healed *Histoplasma* chorioretinitis. All of these patients had either a positive histoplasmin skin test or changes on chest radiographs compatible with presumed pulmonary histoplasmosis. These findings were interpreted as evidence of previous *Histoplasma* infection.[4]

However, it must be pointed out that *H. capsulatum* has never been isolated from the eye of a patient with endogenous uveitis, nor has it ever been demonstrated in histologic sections of ocular tissues in endogenous uveitis. Furthermore, a study of 134 patients with culturally or histologically proven systemic histoplasmosis failed to uncover a single case of *Histoplasma* uveitis.[20] It is, of course, possible that *Histoplasma* uveitis does not occur in the acute phase of histoplasmosis, but is a delayed consequence of the disease.

On funduscopic examination, the characteristic findings in presumed *Histoplasma* chorioretinitis consist of subretinal hemorrhages in the macular area, discrete choroidal lesions in the periphery, and a clear vitreous. The hemorrhagic lesions in the retina may, in some cases, lead to detachment of the retina in the macular region. It has been reported that injections of histoplasmin during the acute phase may increase the severity of the hemorrhagic lesions.[24] In healed lesions, scar tissue forms at the sites of the previous hemorrhages in the macular region.

Diagnostic procedures in suspected *Histoplasma* uveitis include serologic studies and histoplasmin skin tests. Of the several serologic procedures available, the titer of complement-fixing antibodies to the histoplasmin antigen appears to give the best correlation with clinical activity (see Chapter 21). However, it should be emphasized once again that a positive serologic test does not necessarily imply active infection. Skin testing with histoplasmin antigen is of limited value in endemic areas, but may be useful in other parts of the country. A negative skin test combined with negative serology and a normal chest radiograph effectively excludes histoplasmosis from the differential diagnosis.

Other Fungal Infections

Other pathogenic fungi which have been demonstrated as uncommon causes of uveitis include *Aspergillus, Blastomyces, Coccidioides immitis, Cryptococcus,* and *Mucor.*[18,24] The retinal findings are nonspecific in these patients and the diagnosis is usually made at autopsy or enucleation of the eye.

Helminthic Infections

The larvae of the dog and cat roundworm (*Toxocara canis*) are often widely disseminated throughout the body and may produce granulomatous lesions in almost any organ where they finally come to rest. Infestation with these parasites occurs most commonly in small children who have close contact with puppies.

The eye lesions usually involve the vitreous primarily, but there may be a uveal component to the inflammatory process in some patients. The typical appearance is that of a whitish inflammatory mass in the vitreous which may extend into the adjacent retina and choroid.[5] At times, it may be difficult to distinguish the lesions from a retinoblastoma. Less commonly, the larvae may produce isolated raised choroidal lesions without much involvement of the vitreous. The diagnosis is made solely by the visualization of larvae, which may or may not be moving, within the eye. If no larvae are seen, the diagnosis may be suspected on the basis of the findings outlined above, but cannot be confirmed. Similar lesions have been reported in onchocerciasis, cystocercosis, filariasis, and echinococcosis.[24,29]

Tuberculosis

The importance of the tubercle bacillus as a cause of endogenous uveitis has probably been greatly overemphasized in the past. Vigorous treatment of suspected tuberculous ocular lesions with antituberculous agents, including tuberculin desensitization, has usually failed to produce significant improvement. Furthermore, organisms have not been detected in chronic lesions. Nevertheless, *M. tuberculosis* has been isolated from the choroid and retinas of patients with disseminated tuberculosis.[21] Clinically, the tubercles appear as discrete, white choroidal exudates with blurred margins during the acute phase, and as areas of retinal scarring on recovery.

From the data available, it would appear that ocular tuberculosis occurs only in patients with active pulmonary tuberculosis, tuberculous meningitis, or other forms of active systemic tuberculous infection. There is no convincing evidence to suggest that tuberculosis is a cause of endogenous uveitis in patients in whom the sole manifestation of possible tuberculous infection is a positive tuberculin test.

Syphilis

A wide variety of ocular lesions such as posterior uveitis, anterior uveitis, and interstitial keratitis may occur in congenital syphilis. *Treponema pallidum* can be demonstrated in the majority of such lesions if a careful search is made. The choroidal lesions are nonspecific, but may occasionally be of the focal exudative type and, thus, may be confused with congenital toxoplasmosis. With the exception of the findings in congenital syphilis, there is nothing to suggest that the occurrence of a positive serologic test for syphilis and endogenous uveitis in the same patient implies a cause and effect relationship.

Brucellosis

Brucellosis has been reported as a rare cause of anterior uveitis.[12] However, as the diagnosis of chronic brucellosis is in itself difficult to establish, the possible relationship between brucellosis and endogenous uveitis is even more tenuous.

Cytomegalovirus Infection

Ocular lesions similar to those seen in toxoplasmosis have been reported in cytomegalovirus inclusion disease. The intranuclear inclusion bodies characteristic of the cytomegalovirus have been identified in the retinas of infants dying with the disease.[8]

Sarcoidosis

The association of endogenous uveitis with sarcoidosis is reported to occur in about 40 to 50 per cent of patients with the disease. When uveitis is present, the anterior segment of the uveal tract is more commonly involved than the posterior segment. Other ocular lesions which may occur during the course of sarcoidosis include vitreous opacities, optic neuritis, and lacrimal gland enlargement (see Chapter 12).[23]

Rheumatic Diseases

An association between anterior uveitis and certain rheumatic diseases has been described. In one series, approximately 10 per cent of cases of uveitis fell into this category.[13] Recurrent, acute, anterior uveitis is a frequent finding in juvenile rheumatoid arthritis and in young males with ankylosing spondylitis. In adult females, the joint symptoms associated with anterior uveitis are less specific consisting, for the most part, of an asymmetrical, nonankylosing, peripheral polyarthritis usually confined to the lower extremities. Rheumatoid factor is usually absent in all of these patients. The significance of the correlation between rheumatic diseases not associated with rheumatoid factor and anterior uveitis is not well understood.

Typical endogenous uveitis is not a common feature of classic rheumatoid arthritis occurring in adults. However, in some patients suffering from rheumatoid arthritis there may be episodes of recurrent scleritis with occasional extension of the inflammatory process to involve the anterior portion of the uveal tract. The usual ocular lesion in Reiter's syndrome is a conjunctivitis, but anterior uveitis may occur in rare instances.

Ulcerative and Granulomatous Colitis

Uveitis, which is almost always anterior, occurs in about 2 per cent of patients with ulcerative colitis, regional enteritis or related conditions.[14]

Serum Sickness

Uveitis and optic neuritis are occasional manifestations of the serum sickness which occurs following the administrations of large volumes of horse serum (see Chapter 2).

Vogt-Koyanagi-Harada Syndrome

The most consistent finding in this rare syndrome of unknown cause is an anterior uveitis. Other manifestations may include retinal detachment, posterior uveitis, alopecia, poliosis (premature whitening of the hair), vitiligo, and deafness.[19] Less commonly, there may also be headache, fever, and meningeal signs (uveoencephalitis).

Herpes Simplex and Herpes Zoster

Uveitis may occasionally occur in association with herpes zoster involving the nasociliary nerve and in association with herpes simplex infections of the cornea.

Behçet's Syndrome

Behçet's syndrome consists of uveitis, genital ulceration, and involvement of the central nervous system. The disease is common in the Near East, but rare in North America and Western Europe. The etiology is obscure, but a virus is suspected.

DIAGNOSIS

The investigation of a patient with endogenous uveitis involves consideration of all the diagnostic possibilities discussed in the preceding section. As the possible causes are multiple, there appears to be little justification for a standard "diagnostic work-up" applied indiscriminately to all patients with uveitis. The history and clinical picture should serve as a guide for the selection of suitable investigative procedures for individual patients.

The funduscopic examination is sufficiently characteristic in presumed ocular toxoplasmosis or histoplasmosis to direct subsequent investigation towards a search for confirmatory evidence of infection with these organisms. A chest radiograph is also indicated in suspected ocular histoplasmosis. It should, of course, be remembered that neither a positive delayed-type intradermal reaction or the demonstration of circulating antibodies provides conclusive evidence of active infection with *Histoplasma* or *Toxoplasma* organisms.

Where it appears indicated by the history and clinical picture, skin testing with blastomycin, coccidioidin, aspergillin, or tuberculin, or serologic testing for brucellosis or syphilis may provide additional evidence in support of the presumed clinical diagnosis. In patients whose uveitis primarily involves the anterior segment of the eye, a careful search should be made for evidence of systemic disease processes such as sarcoidosis, juvenile rheumatoid arthritis, ankylosing spondylitis, and ulcerative or granulomatous colitis (Table 17-2). Some of the more obscure causes of endogenous uveitis are usually diagnosed only at the time of enucleation or autopsy.

Even the most careful and detailed investigation will fail to uncover a suspected or presumed cause of endogenous uveitis in over 80 per cent of patients who present with this condition.

TREATMENT

As indicated in the preceding section on the immunology of endogenous uveitis, there is very little evidence that living microorganisms are actually present in the uveal tract in the majority of patients at the time when the inflammatory process is at its peak. It is much more likely that clinical uveitis occurs as a direct or indirect consequence of *previous* invasion by microorganisms or as a consequence of other systemic disease processes. Therefore, it would seem more logical to direct therapy towards the suppression of inflammation rather than towards the eradication of presumed infection which is probably no longer present.

Local and systemic corticosteroid therapy often appears to shorten the course of the disease, although no controlled studies have been reported. The corticosteroids presumably produce improvement through their anti-inflammatory action. It is also customary to include a mydriatic agent such as phenylephrine drops in the treatment plan in order to prevent the formation of posterior synechiae. Homatropine which is both mydriatic and cycloplegic often provides considerable comfort to the patient. Because of the danger of permanent blindness, the treatment of endogenous uveitis should only be attempted in consultation with an ophthalmologist who can evaluate daily changes in the appearance of the ocular tissues.

Various treatment plans have been suggested for endogenous uveitis of presumed specific origin. These include pyrimethamine and sulfadiazine for suspected ocular toxoplasmosis, and histoplasmin desensitization for presumed ocular histoplasmosis. The value of these forms of therapy is not firmly established, and thus corticosteroids remain the treatment of choice in both conditions.

The immunosuppressive agent 6-mercaptopurine has been reported to produce temporary improvement in uveitis in about 70 per cent of patients.[17] However, it must be remembered that permanent or temporary spontaneous remissions are common in uveitis. Therefore, it is impossible to form a firm opinion on the merits of any particular type of therapy in the absence of well controlled double-blind studies.

LENS-INDUCED UVEITIS

It has been known for many years that the lens antigens are similar in various mammalian species, but different in each animal from any other body tissue antigens.[11] It has been postulated that the liberation of lens material into the human eye following surgery or trauma may induce a sterile inflammatory reaction on a presumed hypersensitivity basis. Many terms have been employed in the literature to describe this condition, including lens-induced uveitis, phacoanaphylaxis, and endophthalmitis phacoanaphylactica.

PATHOLOGY

Histologic examination of eyes removed after the development of lens-induced uveitis characteristically reveals the accumulation of polymorphonuclear leukocytes and macrophages at the site of lens injury. More severe cases may display extensive damage to the uveal tract. The anterior uvea may be infiltrated with lymphoid and plasma cells, but the choroid is usually spared.

IMMUNOLOGY

Skin testing with bovine lens extract has been performed for many years in patients with suspected lens-induced uveitis. It is found that delayed-type intradermal reactions occur in the majority of patients with the characteristic clinical manifestations. However, the results of skin testing are not reproducible in the same patient; some patients with lens-induced uveitis have negative tests, and some normal patients show positive tests.

Circulating antilens antibodies have been demonstrated by the passive hemagglutination technique in the sera of patients with the clinical picture of traumatic lens-induced uveitis. In a group of 64 patients with leakage of lens protein into the eye during the course of cataract removal, 28 developed signs and symptoms of lens-induced uveitis and 14 developed circulating antilens antibodies during the postoperative period.[28] There was a definite correlation between the amount of lens material in the anterior chamber and the presence of antilens antibodies. Precipitin studies by the technique of double diffusion in agar gel demonstrated cross-reactivity between human lens antigen and human uveal antigen. This antigenic relationship provides a possible explanation for the appearance of uveitis following the release of lens protein into the eye.

In another study, low titers of complement-fixing antibodies to autologous lens protein were found in a significant proportion of patients with senile cataracts prior to surgery.[27] It is possible that the antigenic stimulation in this latter group of patients was provided by leakage of lens protein through a damaged lens capsule surrounding the mature cataract.

Despite the rather impressive evidence for an immunologic basis for lens-induced uveitis, it must be pointed out that the disease process has never been consistently reproduced in experimental animals.

CLINICAL MANIFESTATIONS

Following operative or traumatic rupture of the lens capsule, the clinical picture is essentially that of an anterior uveitis beginning within 1 to 10 days after rupture has taken place. The symptoms vary in severity from a mild iritis to a protracted and intense endophthalmitis. The opposite eye in a sensitized patient may occasionally develop a similar disease process if it contains a cataract. It has been estimated that of all the patients who suffer a disruption of the lens capsule, one-half will have no significant inflammatory reaction, one-quarter will develop lens-induced uveitis, and one-quarter have pre-existing ocular disease which makes a precise diagnosis exceedingly difficult.

TREATMENT

Removal of the lens or residual lens material is the obvious first principle of treatment. This usually results in a prompt clearing of the uveitis. The concomitant use of local and systemic corticosteroids may also be of benefit.

SYMPATHETIC OPHTHALMIA

Sympathetic ophthalmia is a bilateral inflammation of the entire uveal tract, almost invariably caused by a perforating wound that involves uveal tissue. The traumatized eye is usually referred to as the *exciting* eye and the other eye is called the *sympathizing* eye. In the majority of cases of sympathetic ophthalmia, the sympathizing eye begins to show changes between 2 weeks and 2 months following injury.

PATHOLOGY

On histologic examination, a prominent lymphocytic infiltration is visible in the posterior part of the choroid which, therefore, appears thickened.[16] There is also phagocytosis of uveal pigment by nests of epithelioid cells. Granulomatous changes may appear in the anterior portion of the uvea. If the process is allowed to continue for any period of time, the entire uveal tract is ultimately involved and destroyed.

IMMUNOLOGY

A possible immunologic basis for lesions of sympathetic ophthalmia is suggested by: (*1*) the latent period required for the development of lesions in the sympathizing eye; (*2*) the failure to isolate pathogenic organisms from the lesions; (*3*) the histopathologic picture; and (*4*) the dramatic response to steroids. It was demonstrated many years ago that some patients with sympathetic ophthalmia will develop delayed reactions to extracts of uveal pigment. However, circulating antibodies to uveal tissue have never been consistently demonstrated in sympathetic ophthalmia and the disease process has never been successfully reproduced in experimental animals.

It is conceivable that sympathetic ophthalmia is entirely a manifestation of cell-mediated immunity. Another puzzling feature is that uveal tissue is frequently damaged to a greater or lesser extent during the course of ocular surgery, but sympathetic ophthalmia rarely appears under these circumstances.

CLINICAL MANIFESTATIONS

The exciting eye is usually injected, easily irritated, and on examination shows the changes of a low-grade uveitis. When the sympathizing eye becomes involved, the patient may complain of photophobia and some diminution in vision. Eventually, a fulminant anterior and posterior uveitis develops in the sympathizing eye, a process that may persist until the globe becomes atrophic and all vision is lost. In other patients, the disease may be milder and may finally disappear, leaving the patient with varying degrees of visual loss. Funduscopic examination of the eye during the acute phase may show blurring of the disc margins, generalized retinal edema, and, occasionally, detachment of the retina.

TREATMENT

Because of the danger of bilateral blindness, the possibility of sympathetic ophthalmia should always be anticipated long before symptoms occur. Every patient in whom there is traumatized uveal tissue or a retained ocular foreign body should be observed closely. If the exciting eye is so obviously damaged that it can never again retain useful vision, it should be enucleated at the earliest possible opportunity. Once the opposite eye becomes involved, it may be too late to enucleate the exciting eye. In fact, once definite signs of sympathetic ophthalmia have appeared in the sympathizing eye, removal of the exciting eye may be inadvisable since the exciting eye may eventually have the better vision of the two.

Local and systemic treatment with corticosteroids is often beneficial.

ALLERGIC CONJUNCTIVITIS

Allergic conjunctivitis is probably the most common immunologic disorder which affects the ocular tissues. The conjunctivas are particularly susceptible to allergic reactions because the mucous membranes of the eye are easily reached by air-borne allergens and are frequently exposed to contact allergens such as drugs and cosmetics.

ETIOLOGY

Allergic Dermatoconjunctivitis

The conjunctivas may become involved together with the eyelids in a contact type of dermatoconjunctivitis. The immunologic mechanism is that of cell-mediated hypersensitivity analogous to that seen in allergic contact dermatitis (see Chapter 5). Topical ophthalmic preparations such as procaine and related local anesthetic agents, penicillin, neomycin, sulfonamides, and atropine are among the most common causative agents. Cosmetics, hair dyes, perfumes, soaps, shaving lotions, nail polish, and similar substances constitute some of the other possible causes of allergic dermatoconjunctivitis.

Atopic Conjunctivitis

An acute allergic conjunctivitis, mediated by reagins, is a common accompaniment of respiratory allergy due to pollens, molds, animal danders, and other inhalant allergens. Secondary infection, usually brought about by excessive rubbing of the eyes is a frequent complication of atopic conjunctivitis.

Vernal Conjunctivitis

This form of conjunctivitis tends to occur most commonly in male children during the spring and summer months. It is characterized by the appearance of large papules which may occur either on the undersurface of the upper lid or, less commonly, on the conjunctivas near the limbus. There is also a thick tenacious mucus discharge. Subjective symptoms consist of photophobia, lacrimation, and severe itching or burning. Because of its seasonal incidence, vernal conjunctivitis has been attributed to possible immunologic causes, but there is no convincing evidence to support this hypothesis.

Phlyctenular Keratoconjunctivitis

Phlyctenular keratoconjunctivitis consists of the formation of small, yellow nodules (which frequently ulcerate) in the cornea and conjunctiva. There is no direct evidence that this condition occurs as an allergic response to bacterial antigens, although there has been considerable speculation in this regard for many years.

Idiopathic Chronic Conjunctivitis

Many patients are referred for allergy consultation because of chronic symptoms of itching, burning, or tearing eyes. The intense inflammatory reaction seen in acute allergic conjunctivitis is usually absent in these patients, and there is nothing to suggest chronic inflammation or acute infection as the cause of symptoms. Some authors have suggested that hypersensitivity to staphylococcal toxins may be responsible for many such cases of low-grade chronic conjunctivitis or dermatoconjunctivitis.[22] The results of intradermal skin testing with staphylococcal toxoid or with attempts at desensitization with staphylococcal toxoid have been inconclusive. Therefore, it is preferable to refer to this vaguely defined but common condition as idiopathic chronic conjunctivitis or idiopathic chronic dermatoconjunctivitis.

Mucocutaneous Syndromes

Conjunctivitis may be a prominent feature of erythema multiforme exudativum (Stevens-Johnson syndrome), Reiter's syndrome, and Behçet's syndrome (see Chapter 5).

CLINICAL MANIFESTATIONS

Acute allergic conjunctivitis is usually characterized by bilateral itching, tearing, and redness of the conjunctivas, accompanied by a minimal mucoid discharge. The signs and symptoms of dermatoconjunctivitis of the contact type are similar, but there is also an acute or subacute dermatitis of the eyelids. The findings in vernal conjunctivitis and phlyctenular keratoconjunctivitis have been described previously.

TREATMENT

Symptomatic relief of allergic conjunctivitis may be provided by the administration of an oral antihistamine such as chlorpheniramine, 4 mg, four times a day. Antihistamine eye drops are considerably less effective and may occasionally produce secondary sensitization of the conjunctivas and eyelids. In more severe cases, corticosteroid ophthalmic drops may provide dramatic relief of symptoms. Corticosteroid eye drops are also indicated in the management of vernal conjunctivitis and phlyctenular keratoconjunctivitis. However, if there is any suspicion of ophthalmic herpes or corneal ulceration, corticosteroid eye drops should be avoided.

ALLERGIC DISORDERS OF THE EYELIDS

Allergic contact dermatitis, atopic dermatitis, or acute angioedema frequently involve the skin or mucous membranes of the eyelids (see Chapter 5). The diagnosis and management of these dermatologic conditions which may affect the eyelids is similar to that recommended for other areas of the body.

A common condition of the eyelids is a scaling dermatitis of the lid margins (blepharitis marginalis) due to seborrhea. Its association with other manifestations of seborrheic dermatitis elsewhere in the body is usually sufficient to distinguish this condition from the allergic disorders of the eyelids described above.

REFERENCES

1. Aronson, S. B. The uvea. *Arch. Ophthal. (Chicago) 79:*491, 1968.

2. Aronson, S. B., Martenet, A. C., Yamamoto, E. A., and Bedford, M. J. Mechanisms of the host response in the eye. II. Variations in ocular disease produced by several different antigens. *Arch. Ophthal. (Chicago) 76:*266, 1966.

3. Aronson, S. B., Schnellmann, D. C., and Yamamoto, E. A. Uveal auto-antibody in ocular disease. *J.A.M.A. 196:*225, 1966.

4. Asbury, T. The status of presumed ocular histoplasmosis. *Trans. Amer. Ophthal. Soc. 64:*371, 1966.

5. Ashton, N. Larval granulomatosis of the retina due to toxocara. *Brit. J. Ophthal. 44:*129, 1960.

6. Burns, R. M., Rheins, M. S., and Suie, T. Anti-DNA in the sera of patients with uveitis. *Arch. Ophthal. (Chicago) 77:*776, 1967.

7. Crawford, J. B. Toxoplasma chorioretinitis. *Arch. Ophthal. (Chicago) 76:*829, 1966.

8. Christensen, L., Beeman, H. W., and Allen, A. Cytomegalic inclusion disease. *Arch. Ophthal. (Chicago) 57:*90, 1957.

9. Coles, R. S. "Allergy of the Uvea," in *Ocular Allergy,* ed. by Theodore, T. H., and Schlossman, A., Baltimore, Williams and Wilkins, 1958, p. 324.

10. Desments, G. Definitive serological diagnosis of ocular toxoplasmosis. *Arch. Ophthal. (Chicago) 76:*839, 1966.

11. Halbert, S. P., Locatcher-Khorazo, D., Swick, L., Witmer, R., Seegal, B., and Fitzgerald, P. Homologous immunological studies of ocular lens. I. In vitro observation. *J. Exp. Med. 105:*439, 1957.

12. Hewson, G. E. Uveitis due to brucellosis. *Trans. Ophthal. Soc. U.K. 84:*297, 1964.

13. Kimura, S. J., Hogan, M. J., O'Connor, G. R., and Epstein, W. V. Uveitis and joint diseases. *Arch. Ophthal. (Chicago)* 77:309, 1967.

14. Korelitz, B. I., and Coles, R. S. Uveitis (iritis) associated with ulcerative and granulomatous colitis. *Gastroenterology 52:*78, 1967.

15. Lerner, E. M., II, Stone, S. H., Myers, R. E., and von Sallmann, L. Autoimmune chorioretinitis in rhesus monkeys. *Science 162:*561, 1968.

16. Lugossy, G. Clinical problems of auto-allergic ocular diseases. *Ophthalmologica 153:*93, 1967.

17. Newell, F. W., Krill, A. E., and Thomson, A. The treatment of uveitis with 6-mercaptopurine. *Amer. J. Ophthal. 62:*629, 1966.

18. Pettit, T. H., Learn, R. N., and Toos, R. Y. Intraocular coccidiomycosis. *Arch. Ophthal. (Chicago)* 77:655, 1967.

19. Seals, R. L., and Rise, E. N. Vogt-Koyanagi-Harada syndrome. *Arch. Otolaryng. (Chicago)* 86:85, 1967.

20. Spaeth, G. L. Absence of so-called histoplasma uveitis in 134 cases of proven histoplasmosis. *Arch. Ophthal. (Chicago)* 77:41, 1967.

21. Theobald, G. D. Acute tuberculous endophthalmitis: Report of a case. *Trans. Amer. Ophthal. Soc. 55:*325, 1957.

22. Theodore, F. H. The classification and treatment of allergies of the conjunctiva. *Amer. J. Ophthal. 36:*1689, 1953.

23. Uveoparotitis (Editorial) *Brit. Med. J. 2:*459, 1967.

24. Van Metre, T. E., Jr. Role of the allergist in diagnosis and management of patients with uveitis. *J.A.M.A. 195:*167, 1966.

25. Van Metre, T. E., Jr., and Maumenee, A. E. Specific ocular uveal lesions in patients with evidence of histoplasmosis. *Arch. Ophthal. (Chicago)* 71:314, 1964.

26. Van Metre, T. E., Jr., Knox, D. L., and Maumenee, A. E. The relation between toxoplasmosis and focal exudative retinochoroiditis. *Amer. J. Ophthal. 58:*6, 1964.

27. Vulchanor, V. H., Nikolov, L. S., and Kehayor, I. R. On the significance of phacoautoantibodies demonstrated in the sera of patients with senile cataract. *Immunology 12:*321, 1967.

28. Wirotsko, E., and Spalter, H. F. Lens-induced uveitis. *Arch. Ophthal. (Chicago)* 78:1, 1967.

29. Woods, A. C. *Endogenous Inflammations of the Uveal Tract,* Baltimore, Williams and Wilkins, 1961.

18

Clinical Immunology of the Nervous System

SAMUEL O. FREEDMAN

Immunization of animals with preparations of central nervous tissue emulsified in Freund's adjuvant will produce acute inflammatory and demyelinating lesions of the brain and spinal cord (experimental allergic encephalomyelitis or EAE). Similarly, immunization of animals with preparations of peripheral nervous tissue will lead to a peripheral neuropathy (experimental allergic neuritis or EAN).

Experimental studies have demonstrated that the antigen (encephalitogen) responsible for EAE is a highly basic, water-soluble protein of low molecular weight which is a constituent of myelin. The bulk of the available evidence points to the fact that EAE is a manifestation of delayed type or cell-mediated hypersensitivity. The lesions of EAE can be transferred between experimental animals by means of suspensions of lymph node cells, and there is an accumulation of perivascular lymphocytes in the CNS during the acute phase of EAE.

These observations have led to the suggestion that some human demyelinating diseases and some forms of human peripheral neuritis may be mediated by immunologic mechanisms. The evidence for and against the hypothesis that experimental allergic encephalomyelitis and experimental allergic

525

neuritis have their counterparts in human disease processes will be examined critically in this chapter.

POSTVACCINIAL AND POSTINFECTIOUS ENCEPHALITIS

Approximately one-third of cases diagnosed as encephalitis in North America follow vaccination with smallpox, rabies, and other vaccines or follow an acute infectious disease such as measles, German measles, chickenpox, smallpox, or mumps (Table 18-1). These forms of encephalitis should be distinguished from acute viral encephalitis due to actual invasion of central nervous tissue by the causative organism. The postvaccinial and postinfectious group of encephalitides are characterized by: (*1*) the appearance of encephalitis during the period when the acute infectious process is subsiding rather than during the acute phase of the illness; (*2*) characteristic pathologic findings in the central nervous system; and (*3*) failure to isolate the infectious agent from central nervous tissue.[1]

TABLE 18-1. Causes of Postvaccinial and Postinfectious Encephalitis

Postvaccinial
Smallpox vaccine
Rabies vaccine
Pertussis vaccine
Influenza vaccine
Yellow fever vaccine
Postinfectious
Measles
German measles
Chickenpox
Mumps
Smallpox

PATHOLOGY

The initial pathologic change is the infiltration of small vessel walls by mononuclear cells and by a smaller number of polymorphonuclear leukocytes. However, the outstanding pathologic feature is extensive perivascular demyelinization in the brain and spinal cord. The areas of demyelinization can be recognized in standard hematoxylin-eosin sections by the appearance of pale staining areas, but may be even more clearly distinguished by special myelin stains. Petechial hemorrhages due to necrotic changes in the small vessel walls are conspicuous in some specimens.

ETIOLOGY AND CLINICAL FEATURES

Smallpox Vaccination

The incidence of postvaccinial encephalitis following smallpox vaccination varies from 1:100,000 to 1:20,000 depending on the geographic location.[28] The frequency of this complication does not appear to be related to the source or to the antigenicity of the vaccine used. A similar illness may occur after smallpox itself.

The incubation period is usually between 8 and 15 days after vaccination, although it may be shorter after revaccination. Characteristic prodromal symptoms are headache, drowsiness, fever, and vomiting. These early symptoms may be followed by neck stiffness and convulsions. The fully developed clinical syndrome may include a flaccid paralysis of all four limbs indicating spinal cord involvement, and cerebral signs such as cranial nerve changes, stupor, and coma. Polyneuritis and mononeuritis may also occur in a small proportion of patients. The cerebrospinal fluid almost always demonstrates elevated protein levels and an increase in the number of lymphocytes.

With modern supportive treatment, the fatality rate is about 5 per cent and is usually caused by brain stem involvement. Recovery, when it occurs, is often surprisingly complete, although, in some cases, there may be subtle changes in personality or intellectual capacity for many years afterwards.

Rabies Vaccination

Since the introduction of duck embryo rabies vaccine, and the proved effectiveness of antirabies hyperimmune antiserum, encephalitis caused by the Semple type of rabies vaccine prepared from rabbit nervous tissue has become largely a disease of historic interest (see Chapter 21). Nevertheless, the condition is of considerable theoretic importance because of its etiologic and clinical similarity to EAE. The disease, like EAE, is presumably caused by the repeated injection of rabbit nervous tissue into a human recipient. However, one case has been reported following the use of duck embryo vaccine.[25]

The incidence of encephalomyelitis following vaccination with the Semple type vaccine ranges from 1:1000 to 1:4000 depending on the series reported. Clinical signs usually appear 4 to 15 days after beginning the course of vaccination injections. The first clinical sign may be local urticaria at one or more of the injection sites in the abdomen. Subsequently, there may be signs and symptoms similar to those described for smallpox encephalomyelitis. Increased CSF protein levels and an increase in the number of lymphocytes in the CSF are common findings. The fatality rate is approximately 10 per cent. About one-third of patients who recover have residual neurologic disorders, usually of a minor nature.

Other Vaccines

There have been occasional reports of neurologic complications following the administration of pertussis vaccine, polyvalent influenza vaccine, and yellow fever vaccine,[26] but these cases are extremely rare.

Rubeola (Measles)

Measles encephalitis is the most frequent and most serious of the postinfectious encephalitides. The incidence is approximately 1:1000, but is considerably lower in children under the age of 2 years. The time of onset is usually during the recovery period when the fever and rash are subsiding, but neurologic complications may occasionally antedate the appearance of rash by several days.

The clinical picture is variable but severe cases are typically dominated by convulsions and coma. Other characteristic neurologic features may include cranial nerve palsies, transverse myelitis and varying degrees of spastic or flaccid monoplegia, hemiplegia, or paraplegia. The CSF protein is increased in about 50 per cent of patients and there is an increase in lymphocytes in the CSF in about 40 per cent. The fatality rate is approximately 10 per cent. Of the survivors, about one-half are left with disabling sequelae such as hemiplegia, paraplegia, seizures, or intellectual impairment.

Rubella (German Measles)

The incidence of encephalomyelitis following *acquired* rubella is approximately 1:5000. The clinical findings are similar to those which occur with rubeola. On the other hand, the neurologic complications of *congenital* rubella are not dependent upon immunologic mechanisms. Following intrauterine infection, the virus can always be isolated from the brain as well as from other organs. The resultant cerebral anomalies such as microcephaly and mental retardation are the result of direct invasion of central nervous tissue by the rubella virus.

Varicella (Chickenpox)

Encephalomyelitis is a very rare complication of chickenpox, and no estimates of its true incidence are available.

Mumps

True encephalomyelitis following mumps is a rare occurrence with an estimated incidence of 1:6000. This complication must, however, be distinguished from mumps meningitis which occurs in about 10 per cent of patients. This latter condition is due to direct invasion of the meninges by mumps virus and is characterized by neck stiffness, headache, and drowsiness. About 50 per cent of patients with mumps, including those without meningeal signs, will show an increase in the number of lymphocytes in the CSF. Mumps meningitis, as distinguished from mumps encephalitis, is a benign condition. The only known residual disability attributable to mumps meningitis is the rare occurrence of unilateral nerve deafness.

IMMUNOLOGY

In postvaccinial encephalomyelitis due to rabies vaccine of the Semple type, the assumption is that the neurologic lesions are caused by hypersensitivity to rabbit spinal cord. Circulating antibodies to brain antigens and delayed type intradermal reactions to extracts of nervous tissue have been demonstrated in patients following rabies vaccination, but neither form of immune response has been found to correlate well with the severity of the encephalitis.[1] The evidence for an immunologic basis for other forms of postvaccinial and postinfectious encephalomyelitis is purely circumstantial (i.e., the lesions are similar to those seen in EAE, and the infectious agent cannot be isolated from the affected portions of the central nervous system). However, to date, there has been no convincing demonstration that either circulating antibodies or cell-mediated hypersensitivity are directly involved in the pathogenesis of the disease process.

TREATMENT

Beneficial results have been reported following the administration of corticosteroids or ACTH, but no controlled studies have been carried out. General supportive measures such as analgesics, anticonvulsant therapy, control of secondary infection with antibiotics, and management of fluid and electrolyte balance are indicated until the disease has run its course.

IDIOPATHIC POLYNEURITIS

Experimental allergic neuritis (EAN), produced in animals by immunization with peripheral nervous tissue, closely resembles idiopathic polyneuritis in humans. (Synonyms include Landry-Guillain-Barre syndrome, Landry's ascending paralysis, acute postinfectious neuritis, acute peripheral neuritis, and acute polyradiculitis.) Although no specific virus has been implicated in its pathogenesis, idiopathic polyneuritis frequently follows a mild upper respiratory or gastrointestinal infection, infectious hepatitis, or infectious mononucleosis. With the decline in the prevalence of poliomyelitis because of mass immunization programs, idiopathic polyneuritis is probably the most common cause of acute generalized paralytic disease in North America and Western Europe.[3]

Common features shared by idiopathic polyneuritis and EAN include a latent period of 6 to 14 days between the antecedent infection or inoculation of nervous tissue, a gradually ascending symmetrical polyneuropathy, a tendency to spontaneous remission, pathologic lesions occurring in the nerve roots and peripheral nerves, and lymphocytic infiltration in the liver, heart, and other internal organs. The suggestion has been made, therefore, that immunologic mechanisms may be of importance in the pathogenesis of certain forms of peripheral neuritis.

IMMUNOPATHOLOGY

Experimental studies have shown that the antigen in peripheral nervous tissue responsible for the production of EAN in animals is different from the antigen in central nervous tissue responsible for EAE.[27] It has also been demonstrated by immunofluorescent techniques that rabbit antihuman nerve antiserum combines only with the myelin of peripheral nerves and peripheral nerve roots in guinea pigs.[10] It does not combine with other peripheral nervous system components and does not combine with central nervous system myelin.

In humans, the pathologic findings in idiopathic polyneuritis are inconstant, but quite similar to those seen in EAN. The most characteristic findings consist of infiltration of the spinal ganglia and dorsal and ventral nerve roots with lymphocytes, plasma cells, and histiocytes. In addition, there is a variable degree of segmental demyelination and Wallerian degeneration of the nerve fibers. Evidence of low-grade perivascular inflammation may persist in some patients for years after the clinical symptoms have subsided.[3]

Immunologic studies have demonstrated the presence of complement-fixing antibodies against crude extracts of human nervous system tissues in the sera of 50 per cent of patients with idiopathic polyneuritis.[22] Antibodies were also found in a significant percentage of patients with collagen-vascular diseases (with and without neuropathy), as well as in patients with chronic neuropathies of uncertain etiology. Antibodies were uncommon or absent in multiple sclerosis, carcinomatous neuropathy, and diabetic neuropathy. No cause and effect relationship has been established between these complement-fixing antibodies and the etiology, course, or severity of the disease.

On the other hand, the recent observation that buffy coat cells from patients with idiopathic polyneuritis will, at times, destroy myelin in vitro,[2] and the prominence of lymphocytic infiltrations in pathologic sections of nervous tissue, would suggest that idiopathic polyneuritis in humans may be a manifestation of cell-mediated hypersensitivity. Furthermore, lymphocytes from patients with idiopathic polyneuritis were stimulated in culture by a peripheral nerve antigen of human origin, but not by a basic protein of central nervous system origin (encephalitogen).[17a] The knowledge that EAN has been passively transferred in animals by suspensions of lymphoid cells lends further support to the hypothesis that cell-mediated immunity may be of major importance in the pathogenesis of idiopathic polyneuritis.[4]

CLINICAL FEATURES

The most characteristic clinical manifestation of idiopathic polyneuritis is a severe and rapidly ascending polyneuropathy. Symptoms of muscular weakness and tingling paresthesias usually begin in the feet and legs and then, over a period of days, may progressively involve the trunk, arms, and cranial muscles. Common complications are paralysis of the intercostal muscles and diaphragm leading to respiratory paralysis, dysphagia, and inability to clear bronchial secretions. The deep tendon reflexes are diminished or absent, objective signs of sensory impairment may or may not be present, and the plantar reflexes are either flexor or absent. The CSF protein is elevated in the majority of cases, but the CSF cell count is increased in only a small number of patients with the disease.

There is, however, considerable disagreement among clinicians regarding precise criteria for the diagnosis of idiopathic polyneuritis. This confusion has arisen because of the wide variability in clinical manifestations and because it is rarely possible to establish a preceding infection in more than 50 per cent of cases. The following diagnostic criteria appear to be the most generally accepted: (1) the paresis should not be secondary to any systemic, toxic, or metabolic disorders known to be associated with neuropathy; (2) sensory involvement may occur, but should be less severe than motor impairment; (3) the cerebrospinal fluid should contain 10 leukocytes or less per cubic milliliter and 60 mg or more of protein per 100 ml.[15]

The fatality rate is approximately 5 per cent, with most fatalities occurring during the first 2 weeks of the illness. After 2 to 3 weeks have elapsed, the disease usually does not progress further. However, if peripheral nerves have degenerated, the recovery is slow and may require 6 to 18 months before regeneration is complete. Despite the serious nature of the disease, and the protracted recovery period, about 90 per cent of the survivors recover without significant sequelae.

TREATMENT

The treatment of idiopathic polyneuritis consists of prednisone, 40 to 60 mg, daily in divided doses, and general supportive measures. When indicated, assisted respiration, treatment of respiratory infection with antibiotics, support of the blood pressure with vasopressor agents, and careful control of fluid and electrolyte balance are of great value in increasing the number of survivors.

MULTIPLE SCLEROSIS

Multiple sclerosis is the most common and the most disabling of the demyelinating diseases. For this reason, considerable investigative effort in recent years has been directed towards elucidating its etiology and pathogenesis. The resemblance of the pathologic lesions to EAE and the long recognized demonstration of increased γ-globulin levels in the CSF in this disease have led many workers to postulate an immune mechanism.

PATHOLOGY

The most characteristic pathologic finding in gross specimens is the occurrence of yellowish-grey plaques on the cut surfaces of the brain and spinal cord. They occur most commonly in the long tracts of the spinal cord, around the ventricular system, and within the subcortical white matter and cerebellum. There are no lesions in the spinal ganglia or peripheral nerves. Small plaques may occur around CNS venules suggesting a possible perivascular origin of early lesions.

Microscopically, the lesions consist of areas of demyelination and gliosis. Significant damage to the axon fibers is uncommon in early lesions. Perivascular accumulation of lymphocytes and plasma cells may occur, but this is not an important feature in multiple sclerosis. In this latter respect, multiple sclerosis tends to differ from both EAE and EAN.

IMMUNOLOGY

Human encephalitogen has been shown to produce delayed-type skin reactions in guinea pigs with EAE,[5] but there is no direct evidence to suggest that multiple sclerosis is a disease of autosensitization to human central nervous system components. Antibodies to brain tissue demonstrable by conventional complement-fixation or precipitin techniques do not occur more frequently in patients with multiple sclerosis than in control patients.[21] Nevertheless, there is a considerable amount of indirect evidence that hypersensitivity mechanisms may be of primary importance in producing the lesions of multiple sclerosis. As will become apparent from the discussion which follows, the nature and origin of the antigen which triggers the immune response remains obscure.

Probably the most important single item of indirect evidence stems from the observation that 80 per cent of patients with multiple sclerosis show increased levels of IgG in the CSF in the presence of normal serum levels of IgG. It has been demonstrated that there is a positive correlation between the amount of IgG in plaques of demyelination and the concentration of IgG in the CSF.[29] This observation has led to the tentative conclusion that the increase in IgG in the CSF is a reflection of an excess of IgG in the brain and spinal cord. In another study, it was demonstrated that lymphocytes obtained from the CSF of a patient with multiple sclerosis, and maintained in tissue culture, were capable of synthesizing IgG and IgA in vitro.[9] Here again, the suggestion is that the immunoglobulins present in the CSF were derived, at least in part, from cells within the CNS. Immunochemical studies indicate that the composition of the IgG in the CSF in multiple sclerosis differs from the composition of the IgG in the patient's serum. In approximately 50 per cent of patients with multiple sclerosis and an elevated level of IgG in the CSF, there is an increased ratio of kappa to lambda light chains in the CSF compared to the patient's own serum or to CSF in other neurologic disorders.[19]

Another approach to the problem is that of cytotoxicity studies using mammalian central nervous tissue grown in tissue culture. Both sera and lymphocytes obtained from patients with multiple sclerosis were shown to be toxic for glial cells and myelin under the conditions of the experiment.[6,7] However, more recent studies using explants of rat cerebellum, as the test medium, demonstrated that myelotoxicity is not limited to samples of serum or CSF obtained from patients with multiple sclerosis, but is also observed in samples obtained from patients with viral encephalitis, motor neurone disease, and degenerative myelitis.[17,18] Thus, it is conceivable that myelo-toxicity of serum or CSF may occur as a consequence of myelin destruction rather than as a primary factor in its causation. The degree of myelotoxicity of CSF samples is, in general, correlated with the degree of increase in IgG.

The failure to consistently identify anti-encephalitogen antibody in multiple sclerosis[20] has led to a search for other antigenic stimuli. Numerous unsuccessful attempts have been made in the past to demonstrate an infective agent as the cause of multiple sclerosis. However, recent studies would suggest a possible relationship between a "slow virus" of the myxovirus group and demyelinating diseases. Infection with a "slow virus" is usually characterized by: (1) a long latent period lasting from several months the several years in which the virus presumably remains dormant; (2) a protracted, progressive, and afebrile clinical course; and (3) limitation of the infection to a single organ or organ system.

The most interesting evidence comes from studies on the pathogenesis of a rare neurologic disorder called subacute sclerosing panencephalitis (Dawson's disease, Van Bogaert's disease). The disease occurs in children and is characterized by slowly progressive mental deterioration, spastic paralysis, coma, and finally death due to intercurrent infection. Spontaneous remissions are common but, as in multiple sclerosis, there may be a relentless increase in symptoms over a period of months or years.

In microscopic sections of brain tissue obtained from patients with subacute sclerosing panencephalitis, there is a generalized inflammatory process which involves both the white and grey matter. Of particular interest are the demyelination and gliosis of white matter, and the pathognomic inclusion bodies which occur in this disease. Electron microscopic studies have demonstrated that these inclusion bodies are probably virus particles, and complete, infective measles virus has been recovered from the brain tissues of at least two patients with subacute sclerosing panencephalitis.[8,23]

At the same time, it has been shown that patients with subacute sclerosing panencephalitis have extremely high or rising titers of antibodies reactive with measles virus.[30] Of even greater interest is the observation that titers of antibodies to measles virus tend to be higher in the CSF and sera of patients with multiple sclerosis than in normal controls.[24]

It has recently been reported that biopsy material taken from the brain of a patient with Creutzfeldt-Jakob disease (spongiform encephalopathy) produced a fatal encephalopathy in a chimpanzee 13 months after inoculation.[14] Kuru, a neurologic disorder occurring in natives of New Guinea, has been transmitted in a similar manner to chimpanzees following an incubation period of 18 to 30 months.[13] Kuru also resembles multiple sclerosis in that it occurs only in particular geographic areas.

Certain neurologic disorders of sheep, such as scrapie and visna, provide additional examples of virus-induced diseases which bear many similarities to multiple sclerosis. The incubation period ranges from 6 months to several years and the diseases can be transmitted by means of a filterable agent. Pathologically, there are patchy areas of demyelination, degeneration of neurons, and variable inflammatory changes.

Because of the clinical and pathologic similarities between measles encephalitis, subacute sclerosing panencephalitis, scrapie, visna, and multiple sclerosis, it is possible that multiple sclerosis may be caused by active infection with a "slow virus." The lymphocytic choriomeningitis virus (LCM) infection which persists in "tolerant" mice (see Chapter 6) provides an intriguing experimental model for this concept. For example, it is possible that acute measles encephalitis is a "fast" form and subacute sclerosing panencephalitis is a "slow" form of the same disease process. However, despite repeated attempts by various workers, a viral agent has never been isolated from the central nervous system in multiple sclerosis.

Because both EAE and EAN appear to be manifestations of cell-mediated immunity, an extensive search has been made for evidence of cellular immune mechanisms in multiple sclerosis. In humans, there is preliminary data to suggest that a CNS tissue antigen will stimulate blastogenic transformation in tissue culture of peripheral blood lymphocytes obtained from patients with multiple sclerosis,[11] but these results have not been confirmed by other workers.[16] More convincing evidence for the role of cell-mediated hypersensitivity in multiple sclerosis must, of necessity, await the development of more precise and reproducible methods of measuring delayed-type hypersensitivity in man.

CLINICAL FEATURES

Multiple sclerosis is most common in the northern temperate zone; it tends to affect both sexes equally; and the commonest age of onset is between 20 and 40 years. From a clinical standpoint, the disease can be differentiated from other similar neurologic diseases by two characteristic features: (1) the neurologic lesions are widespread (hence the name multiple or disseminated sclerosis) and cannot be explained by a single anatomic lesion in the brain or spinal cord; and (2) the signs and symptoms are subject to repeated exacerbations and remissions over a period of years.

At the onset, minor visual disturbances, fleeting ocular palsies, minimal weakness, stiffness or fatiguability of a limb, and mild emotional disturbances may occur for months or years before the true diagnosis becomes apparent. As the disease progresses, common signs of multiple involvement of the central nervous system may include slurred speech, intention tremor, nystagmus, retrobulbar neuritis, incontinence, increased deep tendon reflexes, bilateral extensor plantar responses, and bitemporal pallor. Late in the course of the disease, there may be profound mental changes such as inappropriate euphoria or maniacal states, progressive disability due to paraplegia in flexion with contractures, and finally death caused by inter-current infection.

The average duration of life following onset is stated to be 10 to 15 years, but many patients may live much longer with varying degrees of disability. A number of patients may have a complete remission of signs and symptoms and it is only at autopsy that evidence of demyelination is found.

The only abnormal laboratory findings of significance are the increased levels of IgG in the CSF found in about 80 per cent of cases. There is a slight rise in the mononuclear cell count in the CSF in approximately 50 per cent of patients.

TREATMENT

There is no satisfactory form of specific therapy for multiple sclerosis. Rehabilitation, physical therapy, superficial psychotherapy, and prompt treatment of bed sores or urinary tract infection constitute the most important general supportive measures which may make the patient's life more comfortable during the course of a long and demoralizing illness. It has been suggested that corticosteroids may be of value in controlling acute exacerbations, or, when administered on a chronic basis, in reducing the frequency of relapses. However, because the disease is of such long duration, is subject to spontaneous exacerbations and remissions, and there is a wide variation in symptomatology between individuals, the effectiveness of any single form of treatment is difficult to evaluate in a controlled fashion.

HEADACHE

Many early workers in the field of clinical allergy reported that certain types of vascular headache were improved by the avoidance of specific food or inhalant substances. However, later, more carefully controlled studies by several groups of investigators have failed to provide convincing evidence for allergy as a cause of chronic, recurring headaches.[12] Two types of vascular headache have been said to be associated with allergic factors: classic migraine and cluster headaches.

CLASSIC MIGRAINE

Classic migraine headaches consist of recurrent episodes of headaches which vary considerably in intensity, frequency, and duration. Common clinical features include: unilateral onset; nausea and vomiting; associated sensory, motor, and mood disturbances; and a frequent familial occurrence. It is believed that cranial artery distension and dilatation occurs during the painful phase, but there is no permanent change in the involved vessels. At present, there appears to be little justification for allergic investigation or allergic management of patients with classic migraine headaches.

The headaches are best treated symptomatically with vasoconstricting agents such as ergotamine tartrate. A common dosage schedule is two 1-mg tablets given at the onset of symptoms and followed by 1 mg every 30 to 60 minutes until relief is obtained. No more than six tablets (6 mg) should be taken in a 24-hour period. Methysergide bimaleate in doses of 2 to 4 mg, three times daily, is often effective in the prophylaxis of severe recurrent vascular headaches such as migraine. However, the usefulness of this drug is limited by the rare occurrence of retroperitoneal fibrosis following long-term therapy.

CLUSTER HEADACHES

Cluster headaches consist of vascular headaches which are predominantly unilateral, and are usually associated with flushing, sweating, rhinorrhea, and increased lacrimation on the same side as the headache. Characteristically, the headaches are brief in duration, and usually occur in closely spaced groups separated by remissions. This type of headache has also been referred to as: Horton's headache, histamine cephalgia, and migrainous neuralgia. The bulk of the available evidence would suggest that cluster headaches, like classic migraine, are due to dilatation of extracranial arteries. Although the headaches, in certain susceptible individuals, can be reproduced by the subcutaneous injection of histamine, there is nothing to suggest that spontaneous cluster headaches are due to histamine release. Attempts at histamine desensitization or other forms of allergic management have been disappointing in the hands of most investigators. The treatment of choice is the judicious use of vasoconstricting agents similar to those employed in the treatment of migraine.

HEADACHE OF NASAL VASOMOTOR REACTION

Headache and nasal discomfort (tightness or burning) may result from congestion and edema of nasal or paranasal mucous membranes. The nasal congestion may be due to allergy, infection, or idiopathic vasomotor rhinitis. The headache is predominantly anterior in location and is mild or moderate in intensity. This type of headache is probably the only variety which may be associated with extrinsic allergic factors. The management is that of the underlying allergic rhinitis, infection, or vasomotor rhinitis (see Chapter 3).

COLLAGEN-VASCULAR DISEASES

Neurologic manifestations may occur during the course of collagen-vascular diseases such as systemic lupus erythematosus and polyarteritis nodosa (see Chapter 8).

PERNICIOUS ANEMIA

The neurologic complications of untreated pernicious anemia are described in Chapter 9.

REFERENCES

1. Anderson, J. R., Buchanan, W. W., and Goudie, R. B. *Autoimmunity, Clinical and Experimental.* Springfield, Illinois, Thomas, 1967, p. 246.

2. Arnason, B. G. W., Winkler, G. F., and Hadler, N. M. Cell-mediated demyelination of peripheral nerve in tissue culture. *Lab. Invest. 21:*1, 1969.

3. Asbury, A. K., Arnason, B. G., and Adams, R. D. The inflammatory lesion in idiopathic polyneuritis. Its role in pathogenesis. *Medicine 48:*173, 1969.

4. Astrom, K-E., and Waksman, B. H. The passive transfer of experimental allergic encephalomyelitis and neuritis with living lymphoid cells. *J. Path. Bact. 83:*89, 1962.

5. August, C. S., Kies, M. W., and Alvord, E. C., Jr. Delayed-type skin sensitivity to human encephalitogen in experimental allergic encephalomyelitis. *Nature 241:*1021, 1967.

6. Berg, O., and Kallen, B. Effect of mononuclear blood cells from multiple sclerosis patients on neuroglia in tissue culture. *J. Neuropath. Exp. Neurol. 23:*550, 1964.

7. Bornstein, M. B., and Appel, S. H. Tissue culture studies of demyelination. *Ann. N.Y. Acad. Sci. 122:*280, 1965.

8. Chen, T. T., Wanatabe, I., Zeman, W., and Mealey, J., Jr. Subacute sclerosing panencephalitis: Propagation of measles virus from brain biopsy in tissue culture. *Science 163:*1193, 1969.

9. Cohen, S., and Bannister, R. Immunoglobulin synthesis within the central nervous system in disseminated sclerosis. *Lancet 1*:366, 1967.

10. Field, E. J., Ridley, A., and Caspary, E. A. Specificity of human brain and nerve antibody as shown by fluorescence microscopy. *Brit. J. Exp. Path. 44*:631, 1963.

11. Fowler, I., Morris, C. E., and Whitely, T. Lymphocyte transformation in multiple sclerosis induced by cerebrospinal fluid. *New Eng. J. Med. 275*:1041, 1966.

12. Friedman, A. P. Differentiation between allergic and non-allergic headache. *New York J. Med. 62*:3105, 1962.

13. Gajdusek, D. C., Gibbs, C. J., Jr., and Alpers, M. Experimental transmission of a Kuru-like syndrome to chimpanzees. *Nature 209*:794, 1966.

14. Gibbs, C. J., Jr., Gajdusek, D. C., Asher, D. M., Alpers, M. P., Beck, E., Daniel, P. M., and Mathews, W. B. Creutzfeldt-Jakob disease (spongiform encephalopathy): Transmission to the chimpanzee. *Science 161*:388, 1968.

15. Hinman, R. C., and Magee, K. R. Guillain-Barre syndrome with slow progressive onset and persistent elevation of spinal fluid protein. *Ann. Intern. Med. 67*:1007, 1967.

16. Hughes, D., Caspary, E. A., and Field, E. J. Lymphocyte transformation induced by encephalitogenic factor in multiple sclerosis and other neurological diseases. *Lancet 2*:1205, 1968.

17. Hughes, D., and Field, E. J. Myelotoxicity of serum and spinal fluid in multiple sclerosis. A critical assessment. *Clin. Exp. Immun. 2*:295, 1967.

17a. Knowles, M., Saunders, M., Currie, S., Walton, J. N., and Field, E. J. Lymphocyte transformation in the Guillain-Barré syndrome. *Lancet 2*:1168, 1969.

18. Lamoureux, G., and Borduas, A. G.: Immune studies in multiple sclerosis. *Clin. Exp. Immun. 1*:363, 1966.

19. Link, H., and Zetteruall, O. Multiple sclerosis: disturbed lambda chain ratio of immunoglobulin G in cerebrospinal fluid. *Clin. Exp. Immun. 6*:435, 1970.

20. Lisak, R. P., Heinze, R. G., Falk, G. A., and Kies, M. W. Search for anti-encephalitogen antibody in human demyelinative diseases. *Neurology 18*:122, 1968.

21. McLeod, I., Ridley, A. R., Smith, C., and Field, E. J. Failure to demonstrate circulating antibody to alcoholic brain extracts in multiple sclerosis. *Brit. Med. J. 1*:1525, 1962.

22. Melnick, S. C. Thirty-eight cases of the Guillain-Barre syndrome. An immunological study. *Brit. Med. J. 1*:368, 1963.

23. Payne, F. E., Baublis, J. V., and Itabashi, H. H. Isolation of measles virus from cell cultures of brain from a patient with subacute sclerosing panencephalitis. *New Eng. J. Med. 281*:585, 1969.

24. Pette, E. Measles virus. A causative agent in multiple sclerosis? *Neurology 18*:168, 1968.

25. Prussin, G., and Katabi, G. Dorsolumbar myelitis following antirabies vaccination with duck embryo vaccine. *Ann. Intern. Med. 60*:114, 1964.

26. Scott, T. F. M. Postinfectious and vaccinial encephalitis. *Med. Clin. Amer.* *51*:701, 1967.

27. Sherwin, A. L., and Laviolette, R. An immunological comparison of central and peripheral nervous tissues. *Int. Arch. Allerg. 31*:152, 1967.

28. Spillane, J. D., and Wells, C. E. C. The neurology of Jennerian vaccination. A clinical account of the neurologic complications which occurred during the small-pox epidemic in South Wales in 1962. *Brain 87*:1, 1964.

29. Tourtellote, W. W., and Parker, J. A. Multiple sclerosis: Correlation between immunoglobulin-G in cerebrospinal fluid and brain. *Science 154*:1044, 1966.

30. Zeman, W., and Kolar, O. Reflections on the etiology and pathogenesis of subacute sclerosing panencephalitis. *Neurology 18*:1, 1968.

19

Clinical Immunology of Skeletal Muscle

SAMUEL O. FREEDMAN

MYASTHENIA GRAVIS

Myasthenia gravis is a disorder characterized by fluctuating weakness and fatiguability of skeletal muscle. The underlying physiologic defect appears to be a blockade of neuromuscular transmission in the region of the motor end-plate, but the precise nature of the biochemical or morphologic defect is not well understood. The defect at the neuromuscular junction might conceivably be the result of: (1) diminished acetylcholine production; (2) increased cholinesterase activity at the neuromuscular end-plate; or (3) an alteration in the structure of the end-plate.

A possible immunologic basis for myasthenia gravis is suggested by several observations: (1) the demonstration of circulating antibodies against both skeletal muscle components and the "myoid" cells of the thymic medulla in some myasthenic patients; (2) the association between myasthenia gravis and thymoma; (3) histologic changes in the germinal centers of the thymic medulla in many patients with myasthenia gravis; and (4) the frequent occurrence of other autoantibodies in myasthenic patients.

541

Physiopathology

There is a certain amount of circumstantial evidence to suggest that an unknown humoral substance may be responsible for the block in neuromuscular transmission in myasthenia gravis. In favor of this hypothesis is the observation that some infants born of myasthenic mothers suffer from neonatal myasthenia during the first 3 weeks of life.[17] The assumption is that a humoral blocking substance crosses the placenta. The finding that thymectomy sometimes produces a marked improvement in myasthenia gravis would suggest that the postulated humoral factor may be liberated from a diseased thymus. However, much further investigation is required to firmly establish the role of a neuromuscular blocking substance in the pathogenesis of myasthenia gravis.

Morphologic abnormalities in myasthenia gravis may occur in both the affected skeletal muscles and in the thymus gland. In the skeletal muscle, typical findings consist of simple atrophy of muscle fibers, nonspecific changes in the terminal branches of the motor nerve fibrils, and an inflammatory exudate consisting essentially of lymphocytic infiltration adjacent to normal and abnormal fibers (lymphorrhages).[6] Electron microscopic studies have failed to demonstrate a specific morphologic change that is directly related to the disturbance in neuromuscular transmission.[28]

The thymus gland in myasthenia gravis may show evidence of thymoma (10 per cent), diffuse hyperplasia of the thymic medulla (70 per cent), or no demonstrable change (20 per cent). The thymomas which occur in association with myasthenia gravis may be benign or malignant, and the histologic picture is quite variable.[21]

Normally, the thymus undergoes atrophy in adult life and is almost completely replaced by fatty tissue. The development of germinal centers, consisting almost entirely of lymphoid cells, in the majority of adult patients with myasthenia gravis is of particular interest. In this connection, it should be remembered that the thymus, unlike peripheral lymph node tissues, does not ordinarily respond to antigenic stimulation by forming germinal centers and plasma cells. Consequently, it has been suggested that the lymphoid changes in the thymic medulla in myasthenia gravis may represent a chronic inflammatory process analogous to that seen in the thyroid in autoimmune thyroiditis.[9] On the other hand, the morphologic changes in the thymus might represent an atypical response to antigenic stimulation similar to that occasionally found in animals following direct injection of antigen into the thymus.

On microscopic examination, numerous lymph follicles with germinal centers are seen in the medulla with resultant compression of the cortex.

In addition to epithelial and lymphoid components, "myoid" cells with histochemical properties similar to striated muscle have been described in normal adult and fetal thymuses.[5] It is these "myoid" cells which cross-react antigenically with striated muscle in immunofluorescence experiments. There is no evidence of an increase in the number of epithelial cells in the thymus gland, and there is no generalized lymphoid hyperplasia.

Although only 10 per cent of patients with myasthenia gravis have an associated thymoma, 30 per cent of patients with thymoma have myasthenic symptoms. It has been stated that more patients with thymoma die as a result of myasthenia gravis than as a result of recurrent or metastatic tumor.[21] Thymomas consisting of large, pale, epithelial cells are much more commonly associated with myasthenia gravis than are spindle cell thymomas.

IMMUNOLOGY

Antibodies directed against the I bands of striated muscle have been demonstrated by the immunofluorescence technique in the sera of about 20 per cent of patients with myasthenia gravis[24] (Fig. 19-1). However, the precise localization of immunofluorescence staining within the striated muscle cells remains somewhat controversial. Earlier investigators believed that serum autoantibodies in myasthenia gravis have a selective affinity for the A bands of striated muscle rather than for the I bands.[27] The serum antibodies demonstrable by immunofluorescence techniques have also been shown to cross-react with epithelial cells of the thymus.[18] Other workers have provided evidence that it may be the "myoid" cells which account for the bulk of the immunofluorescence in the thymus.[5]

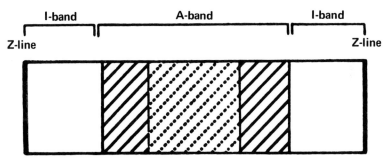

FIG. 19-1. Schematic representation of light microscope appearance of striated muscle.

Antimuscle antibodies may be demonstrated by hemagglutination[4] and complement-fixation[10] techniques in approximately 40 per cent of patients with myasthenia gravis. When myasthenia gravis is associated with a thymoma, antimuscle and antithymus antibodies are almost universally present. On the other hand, the incidence of antimuscle and antithymus antibodies in normal control subjects is less than 1 per cent.[18]

Studies employing the complement-fixation and immunofluorescence techniques have provided evidence that the antibody activity of myasthenic serum is localized in the IgG fraction.[14] Serum complement levels show considerable variation during the course of the disease, but tend to be low during acute exacerbations.[16] Other autoantibodies such as antinuclear factors, antithyroid antibodies, and antigastric antibodies all tend to occur in a significantly higher proportion of myasthenic patients than in normal control subjects.[18] Myasthenia gravis has been reported in association with thymoma and hypogammaglobulinemia,[26] as well as in association with marked hypergammaglobulinemia.[1] Recent in vitro studies have shown thymus tissue obtained from patients with myasthenia gravis synthesized twice as much immunoglobulin as normal thymus tissue.[22]

It is stated that myasthenia gravis is often improved by pregnancy and made worse by hyperthyroidism, but these observations are difficult to substantiate without adequately controlled studies. Nevertheless, a possible relationship between hyperthyroidism and myasthenia gravis is of considerable interest because of the postulated similarities between thyroiditis and thymitis.[9] In one large series of patients with myasthenia gravis, approximately 13 per cent had concomitant thyroid disease.[19] It is thus possible that at least some of the antithyroid antibodies found in the sera of patients with myasthenia may be due to coexisting diseases of the thyroid.

Despite the unquestioned existence of autoantibodies and other immunologic abnormalities in many patients with myasthenia gravis, it is very difficult to establish a correlation between antibodies and the pathogenesis of the disease or its clinical course. The antimuscle antibodies become fixed to the I bands of skeletal muscle rather than to the neuromuscular end-plate where the pathophysiologic defect is believed to occur.[13a] The impression that antibodies do not cause the disease is further strengthened by the observation that some patients with thymoma may have antimuscle and antithymus antibodies without clinical or laboratory evidence of myasthenia gravis.[13] Furthermore, when one studies the sera of infants born of myasthenic mothers, it is found that some infants may have antimuscle antibodies, but no neonatal myasthenia, whereas other infants have myasthenia but no antibodies.[17]

Clinical studies have failed to detect a statistically significant correlation between the levels of antimuscle antibodies, serum complement levels, and clinical status.[15] There is usually no decrease in antibody titers following the removal of a thymoma.

Thus, there is no direct or indirect evidence to support the contention that antimuscle and antithymic antibodies in human myasthenic patients possess neuromuscular blocking activity. At the present state of knowledge, the most plausible hypothesis is that the immunologic findings in myasthenia gravis result from chronic inflammatory changes in the thymus (thymitis); this is analogous to the thyroiditis which occurs in Hashimoto's disease.[9] Guinea pigs immunized with homologous thymus or muscle in Freund's complete adjuvant developed lymphocytic infiltrates in the thymic medulla and electromyographic evidence of a block in neuromuscular transmission similar to that found in human myasthenia gravis.

It is conceivable, but not proven, that the diseased thymus releases a humoral substance (not an antibody) which causes the neuromuscular block characteristic of myasthenia gravis. Evidence in favor of a nonantibody neuromuscular blocking substance of thymic origin comes from animal experiments in which guinea pigs were injected with extracts of bovine thymus.[7] If enough extract (thymin) was injected, the animals developed both myositis and myasthenic neuromuscular block. Furthermore, it has been demonstrated that neuromuscular transmission is increased in thymectomized mice, whereas it is decreased in animals receiving additional thymic tissue in the form of isografts.[8] This latter observation would suggest that thymin secreted by the normal thymus is an inhibitor of transmission at the neuromyal synapse.

However, if such a substance were released from the abnormal thymus in myasthenia gravis, complete remission should occur in all cases following thymectomy. The fact that thymectomy may result in minimal or no improvement in many patients has been attributed by the proponents of this theory to irreversible structural changes of the motor end-plates or muscle fibers.

CLINICAL MANIFESTATIONS

Myasthenia gravis is characterized by marked weakness and fatiguability of muscles, particularly those enervated by the bulbar nuclei (e.g., the muscles of the face, neck, tongue, throat, and eyes). However, if a sufficient number of patients are carefully studied, almost any muscle in the body may be affected. The disease tends to occur predominantly in young people. Although it is most common in women between the ages of 20 to 40 years, it may occur at any age from infancy to the ninth decade of life.

The most common initial manifestation is the rapid development of profound weakness on exercise of the affected muscles. Usually the signs and symptoms are multiple and may consist of any combination of: ptosis of the eyelids; ocular muscle paresis, strabismus and diplopia; a characteristic myasthenic facies devoid of wrinkles and with a "snarling smile;" difficulty in use and movements of the tongue; difficulty in chewing, swallowing, or speaking; weakness of the neck and jaw muscles; weakness of the muscles of respiration; weakness of the extremities; and, occasionally, a waddling gait. There are characteristically no sensory defects or reflex changes in myasthenia gravis.

If suspected on clinical grounds, the diagnosis may be confirmed in most cases by the rapid intravenous injection of edrophonium chloride, 2 to 10 mg. In myasthenia gravis, this drug will almost always produce a dramatic, but temporary, increase in muscle strength, usually lasting for about 1 minute. A similar temporary effect, of longer duration, may be obtained by the intravenous injection of neostigmine methylsulfate, 1.5 mg, together with atropine, 0.6 mg (to prevent parasympathomimetic side-effects of neostigmine). Both edrophonium and neostigmine possess anticholinesterase activity and thus serve to reactivate the neuromuscular junction.

The presence of circulating antimuscle or antithymus antibodies in a patient suspected of myasthenia gravis may provide supporting evidence in favor of the diagnosis. However, the relatively high incidence of negative antibody determinations in otherwise typical cases severely limits the usefulness of immunologic studies as an exclusion procedure. All patients with myasthenia gravis, and particularly those with circulating antimuscle antibodies, should have detailed radiologic studies of the neck and anterior thorax in an attempt to locate an underlying thymoma. Electromyographic studies in myasthenia gravis may show a decline in the amplitude of muscle action potential following rapidly repeated supramaximal stimulation of the peripheral nerve to the affected muscle.

TREATMENT AND PROGNOSIS

Pyridostigmine bromide, an analogue of neostigmine, is probably the most satisfactory drug with which to begin treatment in a newly discovered myasthenic patient. The usual dosage is 60 to 180 mg daily, at intervals spaced to provide maximum relief. Long-acting tablets of 180 mg are especially useful at bedtime. Other related anticholinesterase drugs which may be employed in the specific pharmacologic treatment of myasthenia gravis include neostigmine bromide, up to 180 mg per day in divided doses, and ambenonium chloride, 5 to 25 mg, four times daily. Therapy should always be carried out in consultation with a neurologist who is in a position to evaluate subtle changes in neuromuscular function as well as the potential hazards of overtreatment with potent anticholinesterase drugs.

The value of thymectomy in the treatment of myasthenia gravis is extremely difficult to assess in the absence of controlled studies. Furthermore, the disease is subject to spontaneous exacerbations and remissions. However, if the concept of "thymitis" is a valid one, and if a systemically acting humoral agent is indeed released from a diseased thymus gland, there exists a powerful argument for surgery in selected cases. Unfortunately, the presence or absence of antimuscle and antithymic antibodies is of no value in selecting patients for surgery. Clinically, it has been found that patients with pathologic evidence of "thymitis" improve most after thymectomy, whereas older patients whose thymuses show predominantly involution and atrophy usually obtain poor results.

At present, generally accepted criteria for thymectomy in myasthenia gravis are: (1) patients of either sex under the age of 40 years; (2) duration of disease of less than 5 years; and (3) poor control of symptoms with anticholinesterase medications.[20] Thymoma is usually an indication for surgery, but remission of myasthenia gravis rarely occurs as a result. In patients who are poor surgical risks, radiotherapy by supravoltage techniques may be utilized as a palliative measure.

The failure of thymectomy to produce improvement in many patients without thymoma may be attributed to: (1) the irreversible changes in the motor end-plate or striated muscle previously mentioned; or (2) to a failure to remove aberrant thymus tissue. Approximately 20 per cent of the population has aberrant thymus tissue which is usually located in the neck adjacent to the thyroid or inferior parathyroid glands. Residual thymus tissue or undetected metastases may also explain the occasional onset of myasthenia gravis weeks or months following thymectomy.

Radiotherapy may be the treatment of choice in patients with minor symptoms who do not respond well to anticholinesterase medication, or in patients over the age of 40. Preliminary reports suggest that encouraging results have been obtained with immunosuppressive and cytotoxic agents such as azathioprine and 6-mercaptopurine.

The prognosis is extremely variable. The illness usually develops over a few weeks and is then followed by periodic remissions and relapses, particularly during the first few years. Fatalities occur most often during the first 2 years, are usually due to respiratory paralysis, and are frequently precipitated or complicated by respiratory infection. If the disease has been present for 10 or more years, it usually runs a more benign course. If malignant thymoma is present, the prognosis is much less favorable due to direct invasion of adjacent organs or metastatic spread of the tumor.

POLYMYOSITIS

The term polymyositis is applied to a general class of primary myopathies in which muscular weakness is the major clinical manifestation. Some patients with typical pathologic lesions of polymyositis (degeneration of muscle fibers and infiltration with chronic inflammatory cells) also develop inflammatory dermal lesions which may be the predominant clinical feature. Hence, the term dermatomyositis appears frequently in the literature as a synonym for polymyositis. However, in the present discussion, dermatomyositis will be considered as a subgroup in the general category of disease entities known as polymyositis. The classification and prevalence of polymyositis syndromes is summarized in Table 19-1.

TABLE 19-1. Classification and Prevalence of Polymyositis Syndromes

Polymyositis (35%)

Subacute symmetric weakness of proximal limb and trunk muscles without dermatitis. Occurs almost exclusively in adults between 30 and 50 years of age.

Dermatomyositis (35%)

Polymyositis in association with inflammatory skin lesions. Twice as common in females, occasionally occurs in childhood, but is usually a disease of adults between 20 and 70 years of age.

Polymyositis or Dematomyositis with Collagen-Vascular Disease (10%)

Occurs in patients with rheumatoid arthritis, systemic lupus erythematosus, scleroderma, rheumatic fever, or Sjögren's syndrome. There is more muscular weakness and atrophy than can be accounted for by the underlying disease process.

Polymyositis or Dermatomyositis with Malignancy (20%)

Most frequently associated with carcinomas of the lung, breast, stomach, and female pelvic organs. Slightly more common in males, and more common over the age of 40 years. Dermal lesions appear in the majority of patients in this category.

A possible immunologic basis for polymyositis has been suggested because of the frequent relationship between polymyositis and other collagen-vascular diseases. There is also experimental evidence to link thymic lesions with polymyositis in animals.

PATHOLOGY

On microscopic examination, there is focal necrosis of muscle fibers, infiltration with chronic inflammatory cells which are often perivascular, interstitial fibrosis, considerable variation in the size of muscle fibers, and an occasional prominent nucleus in the small fibers which indicates that they are regenerating. Involvement of the skeletal muscles is common in other collagen-vascular diseases, but the histologic pattern is different. In systemic lupus erythematosus, rheumatoid arthritis, scleroderma, and rheumatic fever, interstitial inflammation is the predominant feature and there is only occasional damage to an isolated muscle fiber (Fig. 19-2). In polyarteritis nodosa, secondary changes in the muscle fibers may occasionally occur secondary to vasculitis, or to denervation. Thus, polymyositis may be differentiated from most primary myopathies by its inflammatory component, and, in most cases, from the collagen-vascular diseases by the presence of primary damage to muscle fibers. However, in some patients it may be extremely difficult to distinguish, on morphologic criteria alone, between primary polymyositis and that associated with collagen-vascular diseases.

IMMUNOLOGY

Positive tests for rheumatoid factor and/or antinuclear antibodies have been reported in about 25 per cent of patients with polymyositis, but it is not clear whether these patients had rheumatoid arthritis or systemic lupus erythematosus as the primary disease process. Diffuse hypergammaglobulinemia may occur in a significant number of patients. On the other hand, typical dermatomyositis is occasionally found in association with primary agammaglobulinemia in children. Attempts to demonstrate circulating antimuscle antibodies by the immunofluorescent technique failed to reveal a significant difference in incidence between polymyositis and other diffuse muscle wasting diseases.[23] It would thus appear that the presence of antimuscle antibodies in polymyositis represents a secondary or nonspecific phenomenon.

Of greater interest is the recent demonstration of a rising titer of complement-fixing antibodies to an extract of autogenous tumor in a patient with polymyositis and carcinoma.[2] Immunofluorescent studies in the same patient showed deposits of γ-globulin around the muscle bundles and upper cutis.

Despite the rather limited evidence for immunologic mechanisms in the pathogenesis of human polymyositis, the results of animal experimentation provide several provocative analogies. For instance, when guinea pigs were given injections of heterologous muscle mixed with Freund's adjuvant, they developed a generalized myositis similar to human polymyositis.[3] The production of severe myositis in guinea pigs by the injection of bovine thymus tissue, and the antigenic cross-reactivity between thymic "myoid" cells and skeletal muscle have been discussed previously in this chapter.

Further evidence for a possible relationship between the thymus gland and polymyositis comes from observations in a South African rodent, *Praomys (Mastomys) natalensis*.[25] Some of these animals develop spontaneous thymomas which are associated with polymyositis, myocarditis, and antimuscle antibodies as demonstrated by the immunofluorescence

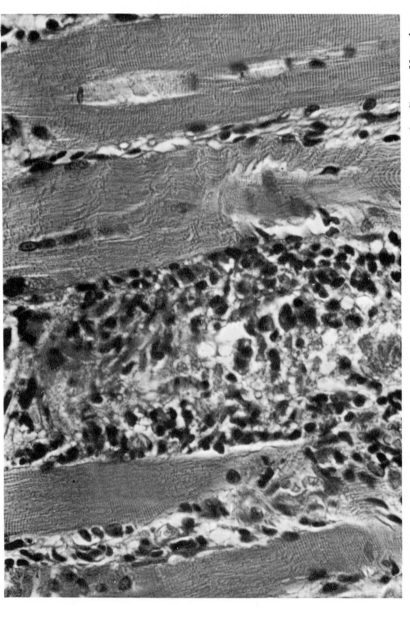

FIG. 19-2. Muscle biopsy from a patient with polymyositis associated with collagen vascular disease. Note the pronounced interstitial infiltration with inflammatory cells. (Original magnification × 500.)

technique. Thus, the Mastomys may serve as a useful model for studying the complex interrelationships between the thymus gland, antimuscle antibodies, polymyositis, and myasthenia gravis.

CLINICAL MANIFESTATIONS

Because of the widely varying patterns of disease in polymyositis (see Table 19-1), the signs and symptoms may vary from chronic weakness in the proximal muscles in childhood with complete spontaneous recovery, to the fulminating and rapidly fatal adult form of dermatomyositis. The most characteristic findings in the musculoskeletal system consist of proximal muscle weakness which usually involves the pelvic girdle and thigh muscles. Less commonly, there may be weakness of the laryngeal and posteropharyngeal muscles, shoulder girdle, and anterior neck muscles. Muscle pain, tenderness, and edema may occur in the more acute cases.

When there is dermal involvement, the typical skin eruption consists of dusky erythema and edema of the face, neck, shoulders, upper thorax, and proximal portions of the arms. Heliotrope suffusion of the upper eyelids, due to partial circulatory stasis in a large number of small telangiectatic vessels has been considered pathognomonic of the disease. Less commonly, there may be dusky red, erythematous patches on the knuckles, elbows, knees, and medial malleoli. Raynaud's phenomenon, dysphagia due to involvement of the esophagus, gastrointestinal hemorrhage, myocardial involvement, albuminuria, or pneumonitis have been reported in a small percentage of patients with typical polymyositis.

Polymyositis is sometimes difficult to differentiate on clinical grounds from progressive muscular dystrophy because proximal muscle weakness is a feature of both disorders. However, in polymyositis, the progression of the disease is usually much more rapid and the laryngeal, pharyngeal, and neck muscles are more commonly involved. Furthermore, polymyositis may begin at any age, whereas the muscular dystrophies rarely begin after the age of 30 years. The major problem in differential diagnosis occurs in childhood when it may be exceptionally difficult to distinguish between polymyositis and a rapidly advancing muscular dystrophy.

An interesting clinical variant is the "pseudomyasthenic" form of polymyositis in which the patient usually presents with a history more suggestive of myasthenia gravis than polymyositis. There is a dramatic response to intravenous edrophonium, but none to oral neostigmine or related anticholinesterase drugs. These patients almost invariably have polymyositis associated with a primary carcinoma of the bronchus, and thus provide another interesting link between myasthenia gravis and polymyositis.

There are several types of laboratory investigations which may be helpful in confirming the suspected diagnosis of polymyositis. Serum enzymes such as the serum creatinine phosphokinase (CPK), serum aldolase, serum glutamic oxalacetic transaminase (SGOT), and the serum glutamic pyruvic transaminase (SGPT) tend to be elevated during the acute stages of the disease. These enzymes are normally present within the muscle fibers, and are released into the circulation as a consequence of muscle fiber breakdown.

The characteristic electromyographic findings consist of complex polyphasic patterns of motor unit action potentials on voluntary activity. These EMG changes are most frequently observed in the proximal musculature of the upper and lower limbs. Conclusive evidence of polymyositis may or may not be obtained on biopsy of the involved muscles. A normal muscle biopsy, in the presence of gross muscle weakness and a characteristic clinical picture, is usually attributed to the uneven distribution of the lesions.

It is almost redundant to note that a careful search for underlying malignancy or an associated collagen-vascular disease should be made in all patients with the characteristic clinical and laboratory features of polymyositis.

TREATMENT AND PROGNOSIS

In adult patients with severe polymyositis, corticosteroids at relatively high dose levels constitute the only effective form of therapy. The usual initial dose in adults is prednisone, 40 to 80 mg, daily, reducing gradually over several months to a maintenance dose of 5 to 10 mg daily. It may be necessary to continue maintenance therapy for 2 to 3 years in order to obtain a complete remission of symptoms. Response to treatment may be monitored by serial determinations of serum enzyme levels. However, it should be noted that clinical improvement usually lags behind enzyme changes by 4 to 6 weeks. Premature reduction in dosage or cessation of treatment may be followed by a severe relapse, or relapse may occur spontaneously without obvious cause many years after the disease has been apparently quiescent. Fluorinated corticosteroids such as triamcinolone should not be used in the treatment of polymyositis since they can produce a primary myopathy in patients without muscle disease.

In polymyositis or dermatomyositis which is not associated with malignancy or collagen-vascular disease, complete remission with little residual weakness can be anticipated in about 50 per cent of patients, partial improvement in 25 per cent, considerable disability in 10 per cent, and death in 15 per cent. If the polymyositis or dermatomyositis is associated with malignancy or collagen-vascular disease, the prognosis is that of the underlying disorder. The removal or destruction of a malignant tumor may sometimes result in a dramatic improvement in the symptoms of polymyositis.

In children with dermatomyositis, the prognosis is considerably better than in adults, and complete, spontaneous recovery over a period of several months is not unusual. Therefore, if possible, it is probably best to withhold corticosteroids in children until the clinical course becomes apparent.

REFERENCES

1. Aach, R., and Kissane, J. (eds.) Clinicopathologic conference. The unusual association of myasthenia gravis and hypergammaglobulinemia. *Amer. J. Med. 45*:451, 1968.

2. Alexander, S., and Foreman, L. Dermatomyositis and carcinoma. A case report and immunological investigation. *Brit. J. Derm. 80*:86, 1968.

3. Dawkins, R. L. Experimental myositis associated with hypersensitivity to muscle. *J. Path. Bact. 90*:619, 1965.

4. Djanian, A. Y., Witebsky, E., and Beutner, E. H. Formalinized tanned cell hemagglutination test for demonstration of auto-antibodies in myasthenia gravis. *Proc. Soc. Exp. Biol. Med. 123*:80, 1966.

5. Feltkamp-Vroom, T. Myoid cells in human thymus. *Lancet 1*:1320, 1966.

6. Fenichel, G. M. Muscle lesions in myasthenia gravis. *Ann. N. Y. Acad. Sci. 135*:79, 1966.

7. Goldstein, G. The thymus and neuromuscular function. A substance in thymus which causes myositis and myasthenic neuromuscular block in guinea pigs. *Lancet 2*:119, 1968.

8. Goldstein, G., and Hoffman, W. W. Endocrine function of the thymus affecting neuromuscular transmission. *Clin. Exp. Immun. 4*:181, 1969.

9. Goldstein, G., Strauss, A. J. L., and Pickeral, S. Antigens in thymus and muscle effective in inducing autoimmune thymitis and the release of thymin. *Clin. Exp. Immun., 4*:3, 1969.

10. Grob, D., and Namba, T. Complement fixation by muscle nucleoprotein and serum of patients with myasthenia gravis and other diseases. *J. Clin. Invest. 42*:940, 1963.

11. Kakulas, B. A. Destruction of differentiated muscle cultures by sensitized lymphoid cells. *J. Path. Bact. 91*:495, 1966.

12. MacKay, I. R., Whittingham, S., Goldstein, G., Currie, T. T., and Hare, W. S. C. Myasthenia gravis: Serological and histological studies in relation to thymectomy. *Aust. Ann. Med. 17*:1, 1968.

13. McFarlin, D. E., Barlow, M., and Strauss, A. J. L. Antibodies to muscle and thymus in non-myasthenic patients with thymoma. Clinical evaluation. *New Eng. J. Med. 275*:1321, 1966.

13a. Namba, T., and Grob, D. Cholinesterase activity of motor end plate in human skeletal muscle. *J. Clin. Invest. 49*:936, 1970.

14. Namba, T., Himei, H., and Grob, D. Complement fixing and tissue binding serum globulins in patients with myasthenia gravis and their relation to muscle ribonucleoprotein. *J. Lab. Clin. Med. 70:*258, 1967.

15. Nastuk, W. L., Kessler, H. J., Grynbaum, A., Smith, M., and Herrmann, C. Immunological changes following thymectomy in myasthenia gravis. *Arch. Neurol. 15:*1, 1966.

16. Nastuk, W. L., Plescia, O. J., and Osserman, K. E. Changes in serum complement activity in patients with myasthenia gravis. *Proc. Soc. Exp. Biol. Med. 105:*177, 1960.

17. Oosterhuis, H. J. G. H., Feltkamp, T. E. W., and van der Geld, H. R. W. Muscle antibodies in myasthenic mothers and their babies. *Lancet 2:*1226, 1966.

18. Oosterhuis, H. J. G. H., van der Geld, H. R. W., and Feltkamp, T. E. W. Studies in myasthenia gravis. Part 2. The relation of some clinical and immunological data. *J. Neurol. Sci., 4:*417, 1967.

19. Osserman, K. E., Tsairis, P., and Weiner, L. E. Myasthenia gravis and thyroid disease: Clinical and immunological correlation. *J. Mount Sinai Hosp. N. Y. 34:*469, 1967.

20. Osserman, K. E. Thymectomy for myasthenia gravis. *Ann. Intern. Med. 69:*398, 1968.

21. Shields, 'T. W. The thymus gland. *Surg. Clin. N. Amer. 49:*61, 1969.

22. Smiley, J. D., Bradley, J., Daly, D., and Ziff, M. Immunoglobulin synthesis in-vitro by human thymus: Comparison of myasthenia gravis and normal thymus. *Clin. Exp. Immun. 4:*387, 1969.

23. Stern, G. M., Rose, A. L., and Jacobs, K. Circulating antibodies in polymyositis. *J. Neurol. Sci. 5:*181, 1967.

24. Strauss, A. J. L., and Kemp, P. G., Jr. Serum auto-antibodies in myasthenia gravis and thymoma: Selective affinity for I-bands of striated muscle as a guide to the identification of antigens. *J. Immun. 99:*945, 1967.

25. Strauss, A. J. L., Snell, K. C., Duntley, B. J., Soban, E. J., and Stewart, H. L. Spontaneous thymoma, polymyositis, and serum-autoantibodies to striated muscle in the rodent, subgenus *Praomys (Mastomys) Natalensis.* Similarities to thymoma with myasthenia gravis in man. *Lancet 1:*1126, 1968.

26. te Velde, K., Huber, J., and van der Slikke, L. B. Primary acquired hypogammaglobulinemia, myasthenia, and thymoma. *Ann. Intern. Med. 65:*554, 1966.

27. van der Geld, H., and Oosterhuis, H. J. G. H. Muscle and thymus antibodies in myasthenia gravis. *Vox Sang. 8:*196, 1963.

28. Woolf, A. L. Morphology of the myasthenic neuromuscular junction. *Ann. N. Y. Acad. Sci. 135:*35, 1966.

20

Drug Hypersensitivity

SAMUEL O. FREEDMAN

The clinical features, diagnosis, and treatment of the varied manifestations of drug hypersensitivity have been discussed in the appropriate chapters of this book which deal with the immunologic abnormalities of organ systems. No attempt will be made to repeat that information in this chapter on drug hypersensitivity.

Instead, the well established syndromes of drug hypersensitivity and the commonly used drugs which may evoke one or more of these syndromes are summarized in Table 20-1. Only those syndromes for which there is some direct or, at least, circumstantial evidence in favor of immunologic mechanisms are included in the table. For example, fever due to presumed drug hypersensitivity (drug fever) has not been listed as a separate entity because it usually accompanies other patterns of reaction such as serum sickness, vasculitis, or cutaneous eruptions. In those instances where fever occurs as the sole demonstrable manifestation of drug hypersensitivity, the immunologic mechanisms have not been well defined.

The table is primarily designed as a guide for identifying possible offenders when drugs are suspected as a cause of hypersensitivity syndromes, and is not intended to be a complete listing of all possible drug allergens.[12]

Central to any discussion of hypersensitivity reactions to drugs is the difficult question of how a drug becomes antigenic. The answer is not always readily available. However, judging from the low molecular weight of most of the drugs known to provoke hypersensitivity reactions, it seems

555

TABLE 20-1. Common Clinical Patterns of Drug Hypersensitivity

Drug	Urti-caria	Contact derma-titis	Morbil-liform erup-tions	Fixed drug erup-tions	Exfoli-ative derma-titis	Photosen-sitivity dermatitis	Bron-chial asthma	P.I.E. syn-drome	Auto-immune hemolytic anemia	Neutro-penia	Thrombo-cytopenia	Allergic vascu-litis	Serum sick-ness	Ne-phrop-athy	SLE syn-drome	Anaphy-laxis	Drug-induced liver injury
Acetazolamide	x										x						
Acetylsalicylic acid	x						x				x					x	
Alpha methyl dopa									x								
Aminopyrine and derivatives										x	x						
Antazoline									x		x						
Barbiturates			x	x	x							x					
Chlorpropamide	x					x											
Demethylchlortetracycline	x					x										x	
Griseofulvin	x												x	x			
Gold salts			x		x						x	x		x			
Halothane																	x
Hydantoins									x	x	x		x		x		
Hydralazine															x		
Iodides	x	x			x						x		x			x	
Iproniazid		x															x
Isoniazid			x						x								
Mercurials	x													x		x	
Neomycin		x															

Drug	1	2	3	4	5	6	7	8	9	10	11	12	13	14	15	16	17	18
Nitrofurantoin	x							x									x	
Para-aminosalicylic acid								x	x									x
Penicillins	x	x	x			x	x	x				x	x	x	x	x		
Phenolpthalein				x														
Phenacetin								x				x						
Phenindione									x					x				
Phenothiazines	x					x		x	x			x						x
Phenylbutazone					x				x	x					x			
Piperazine citrate												x						
Probenecid														x		x		
Procaine		x												x	x			
Quinidine	x							x	x	x	x							
Sedormid										x								
Stibophen								x			x							
Streptomycin		x	x									x			x			
Sulfonamides	x		x	x	x	x		x	x	x	x	x	x			x		
Tetracyclines	x										x						x	
Thiazides	x				x					x								
Thiouracils								x			x							
Tolbutamide					x				x	x				x				
Trimethadione														x	x			

reasonable to conclude that they must act as haptens (see Chapter 1). In this connection, it should be emphasized that only highly reactive drugs capable of forming irreversible covalent bonds in vivo with high molecular weight carriers are likely to function as haptens. In those instances where the drugs themselves do not possess this property, there is evidence to suggest that metabolic breakdown products of the drug probably form allergenic hapten-protein conjugates. Hypersensitivity reactions to large molecules such as foreign serums, vaccines, and other biologic materials are discussed in detail in Chapter 2 and will not be included in this chapter.

Four principles relating to drug hypersensitivity are worth remembering before entering into a detailed discussion of some of the possible mechanisms and the clinical patterns of drug hypersensitivity:

1. Not all adverse reactions to drugs are caused by antigen-antibody mechanisms. A simple classification of untoward drug reactions is listed in Table 20-2.

TABLE 20-2. Adverse Reactions to Drugs

Normal Response to Excessive Dosage (Drug Factor)
Exaggeration of normal pharmacologic effect (e.g., purpura due to coumarins)
Exaggeration of normal side-effects (e.g., tinnitus due to acetylsalicylic acid)

Abnormal Response to Usual Dosage (Host Factor)
Metabolic Abnormality (e.g., hemolytic anemia due to primaquine in patients with glucose-6-phosphatase deficiency)
Hypersensitivity (e.g., thrombocytopenic purpura due to quinidine, anaphylaxis due to penicillin)
Idiopathic (e.g., agranulocytosis due to phenylbutazone, many drug eruptions)

2. A single drug is often capable of inducing several different types of allergic drug reactions in different individuals, or in the same individual. For example, the various clinical types of hypersensitivity which have been attributed to penicillin are listed in Table 20-3.

3. The presence of circulating antibodies to drugs or their metabolic by-products does not necessarily mean that the patient will develop clinical symptoms following administration of the drug. For instance, most patients who receive penicillin develop hemagglutinins against the drug, regardless of whether they are allergic to it or not.

4. Because in vitro tests or skin tests are only occasionally of value in drug hypersensitivity, a knowledge of the drugs which commonly provoke a specific clinical syndrome is often the most satisfactory guide to etiologic diagnosis.

TABLE 20-3. Hypersensi-
Reactions to
Penicillin

Anaphylaxis
Serum sickness
Urticaria
Contact dermatitis
Maculopapular eruptions
Diffuse erythema
Hemolytic anemia
Interstitial nephritis
Acquired hemophilia

MECHANISMS OF DRUG HYPERSENSITIVITY

Although the mechanisms of hypersensitivity reactions to drugs are, in general, poorly understood, a few isolated instances in which the mode of antigen-antibody reaction is at least partially delineated will be described below. There is little doubt that other immunologic mechanisms may be of equal importance in other forms of drug hypersensitivity, but these have not, as yet, been described with the same degree of precision.

REAGIN-MEDIATED HYPERSENSITIVITY TO PENICILLIN

One of the best examples of reagin-mediated hypersensitivity due to drugs is provided by anaphylactic and urticarial reactions caused by benzylpenicillin (penicillin G). Penicillin itself does not appear to be capable of forming antigen-antibody conjugates, but it is known that at least three haptenic determinant groups are formed in vivo following the administration of benzylpenicillin.[6] The benzylpenicilloyl (BPO) group is considered to be the major antigenic determinant, since approximately 95 per cent of benzylpenicillin that reacts with tissue proteins forms BPO groups (Fig. 20-1). One of the minor haptenic groups is thought to be benzylpenamaldic acid, but the identity of the others is unknown.

Penicilloyl-polylysine, an artificial hapten, has been used extensively for the detection of reagins directed against BPO determinant groups. The results of extensive trials in humans indicate that 30 to 75 per cent of individuals reported to be sensitive to penicillin demonstrate positive wheal and flare reactions to this material.[8] The widely varying incidence of positive tests obtained by different investigators appears to depend largely on two factors: (1) the interval between the suspected penicillin reaction and the performance of the skin test; and (2) the type of reaction which occurred. With respect to the second consideration, it is of interest that many individuals who have had severe anaphylactic reactions to penicillin may show a positive wheal and flare reaction to penicillin itself, but not to penicylloyl-polylysine. It is therefore assumed that the anaphylactic reactions are due either to the minor determinant groups or to the protein contaminants which have been described in some penicillin preparations.[17]

IgG and IgM antibodies with BPO specificity have been detected by the highly sensitive hemagglutination technique in 100 per cent of patients

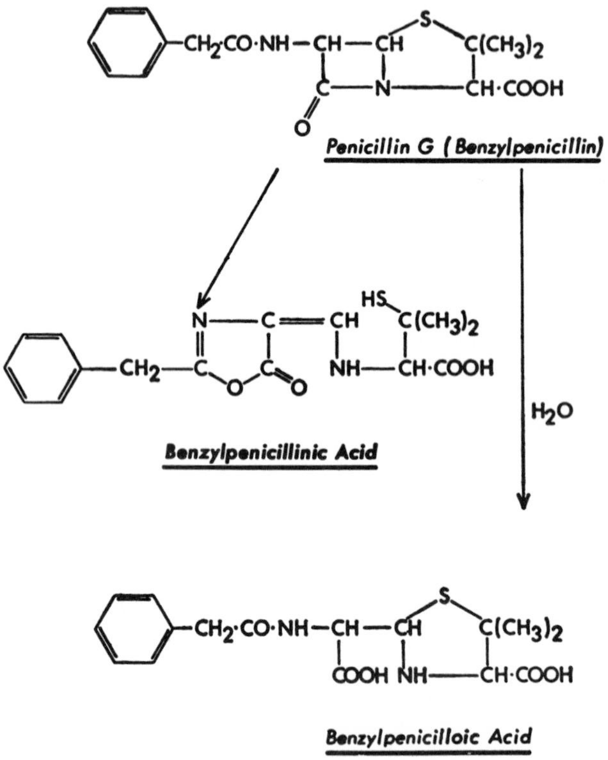

FIG. 20-1. Probable mechanism of degradation of benzyl-penicillin in vivo. The benzylpenicilloyl haptenic group is formed mainly from benzylpenicillenic acid, and benzyl-penamaldic acid is formed mainly from benzylpenicilloic acid.

who have had recent penicillin G therapy.[9] However, these antibodies appear to be of proven pathogenic significance in only the small minority of patients who develop penicillin-induced hemolytic anemias after high dosage penicillin therapy.

DRUG-INDUCED SENSITIZATION OF BLOOD CELLS

At least three different immune mechanisms are associated with drug-induced sensitization of peripheral blood cells: (1) the hapten type associated with positive anti-γ-globulin (Coombs') tests; (2) the "innocent bystander" type associated with positive anticomplement Coombs' tests; and (3) the α-methyl dopa type of autoimmune hemolytic anemia which is unlike the previous types in that the presence of the drug is not required for the development of a positive Coombs' test. (See Chapter 9 for a description of the Coombs' test.) The immunochemical characteristics and etiologic agents involved in the various types of hematologic drug reactions are summarized in Tables 20-4 and 20-5.

TABLE 20-4. Immunochemical Mechanisms in Drug-Induced Sensitization of Blood Cells

| Mechanism | Coombs' test | | Immunoglobulin class of antibody | Specificity of drug-induced antibody |
	anti-IgG-globulin	anti-C		
Hapten type	+	−	IgG	Drug
"Innocent bystander" type	−	+	IgG, IgM	Drug
Alpha methyl dopa type	+	−	IgG	Rh blood group antigens

Hapten Mechanism

Detectable quantities of penicillin are bound firmly to the erythrocyte membrane in patients receiving more than 5 million units of penicillin daily, usually by the intravenous route. The drug-erythrocyte complex probably acts as an antigen resulting in the formation of IgG antibodies with specificity for BPO determinant groups.[7] Following antigen-antibody interaction, the IgG antibodies become fixed to the cell surface and the direct Coombs' test for IgG becomes positive. Additional proof of the proposed mechanism is provided by the observation that antibodies eluted from the patient's cells will react only with erythrocytes previously sensitized with penicillin.

TABLE 20-5. Etiologic Agents in Drug-induced Sensitization of Blood Cells

Disease	Mechanism	Drugs
Hemolytic Anemia	Hapten type	Penicillin
	"Innocent bystander" type	Stibophen, acetophenetidin, para-aminosalicylic acid, isoniazid, sulfonamides, quinidine, antazoline, hydantoins
	Alpha methyl dopa type	Alpha methyl dopa, mefenamic acid.
Thrombocytopenia	"Innocent bystander" type	Sulfonamides, quinidine, sedormid, aminopyrine, stibophen, tolbutamide
Neutropenia	"Innocent bystander" type	Aminopyrine, phenylbutazone, hydantoins, sulfonamides, quinidine

"Innocent Bystander" Mechanism

This mechanism provides a possible explanation for the hemolytic anemias, neutropenia, or thrombocytopenia which are induced by chemically unrelated drugs. In these patients, cell injury can only be demonstrated in vitro by the interaction of normal peripheral blood cells, complement, the patient's serum, and the suspected drug. The best studied reactions in this group are the thrombocytopenias induced by sedormid and quinidine.[16]

The hypothesis which follows has been suggested as the immunologic basis for the drug-induced blood dyscrasias associated with positive anticomplement Coombs' tests. Following exposure to the drug, an antibody is produced which has a far greater affinity for the drug than for the cell membrane. The next step in the proposed immunologic reaction probably consists of the formation of free antigen-antibody complexes in the circulation. It is these drug-antibody complexes, rather than the drug itself, which have a high binding affinity for peripheral blood cells.

During the binding process, complement components become fixed and activated at the cell surface. Subsequently, the drug-antibody complex dissociates itself from the cell surface leaving complement behind, and the anticomplement Coombs' test becomes positive. In this fashion, a large number of cells can be injured by a small number of drug-antibody complexes.

Thus, serologic specificity is directed towards the drug rather than towards the cell type, but the drug is not demonstrable on the cell surface. In other words, the peripheral blood cells are injured as "innocent bystanders" of an immune reaction. This type of reaction provides a possible clinical example of the phenomenon of immune adherence (see Chapter 1).

It is not clear why certain cell types are selected for injury with the same or with different drugs. For example, quinidine can induce both a hemolytic anemia and thrombocytopenia, but usually not in the same patient. With quinidine, red cell injury is mediated by IgM immunoglobulins, and thrombocytopenia is mediated by IgG immunoglobulins.

Alpha Methyl Dopa Type Mechanism

It is now well established that 10 to 40 per cent of patients who receive α-methyl dopa for the treatment of hypertension develop a positive IgG Coombs' test.[1] The incidence of positive Coombs' tests is directly related to the dosage, but 6 to 12 months of therapy is usually required before the test becomes positive. It is also of interest that a lower, but nevertheless significant, number of hypertensive patients not treated with α-methyl dopa develop a positive Coombs' test.[3] In addition, it should be noted that hypertensive individuals, regardless of whether they are treated with α-methyl dopa have a higher incidence of antinuclear antibodies than normal individuals.[3a]

In α-methyl dopa-induced hemolytic anemia, the specificity of the antibodies is not directed toward the drug, but to Rh antigens on the erythrocyte surface. The latent period required before the positive Coombs' test appears, and the fact that the latent period is as long on the second exposure, is compatible with the thesis that the drug may act on the mechanism of formation of the erythrocyte membrane at some point during the maturation process. The resultant change in the composition of the cell surface might render it antigenic and thus stimulate antibody formation. The strong photochemical oxidative properties of α-methyl dopa and the relative ease with which it binds to protein, particularly IgG, make this an attractive hypothesis.[18]

Clinically, less than 1 per cent of patients with positive Coombs' tests who have received α-methyl dopa go on to develop a hemolytic anemia which is indistinguishable from autoimmune hemolytic anemia. The reason why so few patients develop a frankly hemolytic state is unclear, but may be related to differences in the physicochemical properties of the antibodies or to the number of antibody molecules which sensitize the erythrocytes.

An autoimmune hemolytic anemia similar to that produced by α-methyl dopa has recently been reported with mefenamic acid therapy.[14] The two drugs are chemically unrelated.

CELL-MEDIATED HYPERSENSITIVITY

The immunologic mechanisms which mediate allergic contact dermatitis have been discussed in Chapter 5. It is conceivable that some forms of systemic reactions to drugs may depend on cell-mediated hypersensitivity mechanisms, but there is no direct evidence to support this hypothesis. Attempts to correlate drug hypersensitivity with in vitro tests of cellular immunity such as lymphocyte transformation following antigen exposure have led to inconclusive results.[13]

ASPIRIN DISEASE

Acetylsalicylic acid may produce a variety of untoward reactions, such as urticaria, angioedema, various skin eruptions, and asthma, which are suggestive of a hypersensitivity process. However, in most instances, no immunologic basis has been found for these symptoms. In a few patients, circulating antibodies have been demonstrated against aspirin-protein conjugates, but other investigators have been unable to reproduce these results.

The commonest and most distressing adverse reaction to aspirin is referred to as "aspirin disease," and typically occurs in middle-aged patients with preexisting nasal polyps, peripheral blood eosinophilia, and intrinsic bronchial asthma. These patients develop asthmatic attacks of increasing severity following the ingestion of aspirin, but may take sodium salicylate with impunity. However, there have been a few case reports of similar reactions occurring with related drugs such as indomethacin, aminopyrine, and phenylbutazone.

Although this "disease" or intolerance to aspirin has many features suggestive of an allergic process, there is no substantial immunologic evidence for this supposition. The unique structure of aspirin and its ability to acetylate body constituents such as albumin suggests that the acetylation process itself may be important in the pathogenesis of aspirin disease.[4] This hypothesis would explain the complete failure of sodium salicylate to produce symptoms.

CROSS-SENSITIZATION TO DRUGS

Much has been written on the subject of cross-sensitization between chemically related drugs. Cross-sensitization is said to occur when hypersensitivity phenomena induced by one compound are subsequently induced in the same patient by another compound having a similar chemical structure or a similar spatial configuration of the molecule. Much of the information on this subject has been derived from studies on allergic contact dermatitis in animals and is probably not generally applicable to drug reactions in humans mediated by other immunologic mechanisms.[2]

The risk of cross-sensitization to drugs varies so greatly between individuals that it is almost impossible to predict the result of substituting a related drug for one which has previously induced a hypersensitivity reaction. In addition, it is a widely accepted clinical aphorism that individuals who develop hypersensitivity to one class of drugs are more likely to react adversely to other classes of drugs, regardless of chemical structure. Nevertheless, it is worth remembering that certain commonly used drugs have similar chemical structures (see Table 20-6), and whenever possible it is safest to substitute drugs of an entirely different chemical composition once a suspected hypersensitivity reaction has taken place.

TESTS FOR DRUG HYPERSENSITIVITY

Apart from procedures which detect drug-induced sensitization of blood cells, in vitro or in vivo testing for drug hypersensitivity is generally unsatisfactory. Nevertheless, a number of techniques have been suggested as possible methods for distinguishing between allergic and nonallergic drug reactions. Some of these attempts will be reviewed briefly in this section.

SKIN TESTS

Patch testing with suspected cutaneous allergens is often of considerable assistance in the etiologic diagnosis of allergic contact dermatitis or photosensitivity dermatitis (see Chapter 5). Otherwise, skin tests are of very limited value in establishing the cause of suspected hypersensitivity reactions to drugs.

The value and limitations of intradermal testing with penicillin or with penicilloyl-polylysine has already been discussed in this chapter. In addition, there have been isolated case reports of immediate type wheal and flare reactions with low molecular weight drugs such as sulfadiazine, chloramine-T, tannic acid, and phenylmercuric compounds.[10] Similarly, delayed-type reactions have been described in selected patients following the intradermal injection of procaine hydrochloride, benzalkonium chloride, and merthiolate.[11] While there was good correlation between specific symptoms and positive tests in the small number of patients reported, the intradermal method of detecting drug hypersensitivity does not appear to have widespread applicability.

TABLE 20-6. Examples of Drugs Which May Result in Cross-Sensitization*

Drugs	Chemical structure shared by drugs in group
Group 1. Drugs Which Share a "Benzamine" Nucleus	
Procaine and related drugs Para-aminosalicylic acid Sulfanilamide† Sulfadiazine†	 NH_2 group linked to a benzene ring
Group 2. Sulfonamides and Related Compounds	
Sulfonamides (e.g., sulfisoxazole, sulfmethoxy-pyradizine, and related drugs)† Sulfonylurea oral hypoglycemic agents (e.g., chlorpropamide, tolbutamide, and related drugs) Thiazide diuretic agents (e.g., chlorothiazide, chlorthalidone and related drugs) Carbonic anhydrase inhibitors (e.g., acetazolamide and related drugs)	SO_2NH SO_2NH group linked to a benzene ring
Group 3. Penicillin and Related Drugs	
Penicillins (e.g., benzylpenicillin, methicillin, oxacillin, ampicillin, and related drugs) Cephalosporins (e.g., cephaloridine and cephalothin)	$NH-CH \quad CH$ $O=C \quad N$ β-lactam ring
Group 4. Phenothiazine Derivatives	
(e.g., Chlorpromazine, promazine, trifluoperazine, thioridazine and related drugs)	Two benzene rings linked by a sulfur and a nitrogen atom

* The drugs listed within each group may sometimes, but not invariably, cross-react with each other.

† Sulfanilamide and sulfadiazine may cross-react with drugs in both Group 1 and Group 2 as they have both an NH_2 group and SO_2NH group linked to a benzene ring.

BASOPHIL DEGRANULATION TEST

The indirect basophil degranulation test is performed by mixing one drop of the patient's serum, one drop of the suspected drug in saline, and one drop of rabbit buffy coat on a glass slide.[15] Marked degranulation of the basophils as compared to control preparations is considered to constitute a positive test. Despite initial enthusiastic reports, subsequent investigators have failed to confirm the value of this test in the diagnosis of drug allergy.

LYMPHOCYTE TRANSFORMATION

More recently, the in vitro transformation of peripheral blood lymphocytes into blast-like cells in the presence of the suspected drug has been used as a test for drug hypersensitivity. Lymphocyte transformation can also be measured by more sophisticated techniques which utilize the uptake of ^{14}C-thymidine by the lymphocytes as an indication of DNA synthesis and mitotic activity. Preliminary experience with the method would indicate that positive tests are obtained in only 10 per cent of patients with well documented drug hypersensitivity reactions.[13] There appear to be very few false-positive results, but the number of false-negative reactions severely limits the usefulness of the procedure.

SKIN WINDOW TECHNIQUE

In this semi-in vitro procedure, drug allergens are applied to an area of abraded normal skin which is then covered with a glass coverslip. As a result of the inflammatory response induced by the abrasion, cells migrate to the injured area and form a monolayer on the coverslip.[5] In patients with drug hypersensitivity, eosinophil counts ranging between 20 and 95 per cent are observed on the coverslip, whereas the eosinophil counts range between 0 and 7 per cent in control subjects. Like the lymphocyte transformation test, positive results are obtained in only a small proportion of patients, and there is a high incidence of false-negative reactions.

REFERENCES

1. Croft, J. D., Jr., Swisher, S. N., Jr., Gilliland, B. C., Bakemeir, R. F., Leddy, J. P., and Weed, R. I. Coombs'-test positivity induced by drugs. Mechanisms of immunologic reactions and red cell destruction. *Ann. Intern. Med.* 68:176, 1968.

2. Eisen, H. N. "Hypersensitivity to Simple Chemicals," in *Cellular and Humoral Aspects of the Hypersensitive States,* ed. by Lawrence, H. S., New York, Hoeber, 1959, p. 89.

3. Feizi, T., and Woodgate, D. The direct antiglobulin (Coombs') test in hypertensive patients. *Vox Sang. 12*:273, 1967.

3a. Feltkamp, T. E. W., Engelfreit, C. P., and van Loghem, J. J. Autoantibodies and α-methyl dopa. *Lancet 1*:644, 1968.

4. Hawkins, D., Pinkard, R. N., Crawford, I. P., and Farr, R. S. Structural changes in human serum albumin induced by ingestion of acetylsalicylic acid. *J. Clin. Invest. 48*:536, 1969.

5. Larsen, W. G. Drug reactions and the skin window. *A.M.A. Arch. Derm. 95*:422, 1967.

6. Levine, B. B. "Immunochemical Mechanisms of Drug Allergy," in *Textbook of Immunopathology,* ed. by Miescher, P. A., and Müller-Eberhard, H. J., New York, Grune and Stratton, 1968, p. 260.

7. Levine, B. B., and Redmond, A. P. Immunochemical mechanisms of penicillin-induced Coombs' positivity and hemolytic anemia in man. *Int. Arch. Allerg. 31*:594, 1967.

8. Levine, B. B., Redmond, A. P., Fellner, M. J., Voss, H. E., and Levystska, V. Immune responses of man to benzylpenicillin and penicillin allergy. *J. Clin. Invest. 45*:1895, 1966.

9. Levine, B. B., and Zolov, D. M.: Prediction of penicillin allergy by immunological tests. *J. Allerg. 43*:231, 1969.

10. Mathews, K. P. Immediate type hypersensitivity to phenylmercuric compounds. *Amer. J. Med. 44*:310, 1968.

11. Reisman, R. E. Delayed hypersensitivity to merthiolate preservative. *J. Allerg. 43*:245, 1969.

12. Samter, M., and Berryman, G. H. Drug allergy *Ann. Rev. Pharmacol. 4*:265, 1964.

13. Sarkany, I. Clinical and laboratory aspects of drug allergy. *Proc. Roy. Soc. Med. 61*:891, 1968.

14. Scott, G. L., Myles, A. B., and Bacon, P. A. Autoimmune hemolytic anemia and mefenamic acid therapy. *Brit. Med. J. 3*:534, 1968.

15. Shelley, W. B. Indirect basophil degranulation test for allergy to penicillin and other drugs. *J.A.M.A. 184*:171, 1963.

16. Shulman, N. R. "A Mechanism of Blood-Cell Damage by Absorption of Antigen-Antibody Complexes," in *3rd International Symposium on Immunopathology,* ed. by Miescher, P. A., and Grabar, P., Basel, Schwabe, 1963, p. 338.

17. Stewart, G. T. Allergenic residues in penicillins. *Lancet 1*:1177, 1967.

18. Vyas, G. N., Sassetti, R. J., Petz, L. D., and Fudenberg, H. H. Experimental study of Aldomet-induced positive antiglobulin reaction. *Brit. J. Haematol. 16*:137, 1969.

21

Infectious Diseases: Serology, Skin Tests, and Immunization Procedures

SAMUEL O. FREEDMAN

IMMUNITY IN INFECTIOUS DISEASES

The relative importance of humoral and cell-mediated immunity in determining resistance to infectious diseases is probably best illustrated by the congenital or acquired immunologic deficiency states discussed in Chapters 11 and 12. The widely held view that impaired cell-mediated immunity results in repeated and progressive fungal, viral, and granulomatous infections, whereas deficient immunoglobulin synthesis results in increased susceptibility to pyogenic infections caused by staphylococci, pneumonococci, streptococci, or *Hemophilus influenzae* probably represents an oversimplification of a complex situation. Nevertheless, this generalization is useful for clinical purposes in most patients.

Although the role of cell-mediated immunity in infectious diseases has

569

not been as widely investigated as the role of antibodies, opsonins, and other serum factors, there is considerable preliminary data to suggest that it may be of equal or greater significance.[8a] Furthermore, cell-mediated immunity may play a part in the production of tissue damage due to infectious agents. For example, it is likely that the lesions in diseases such as tuberculoid leprosy or cutaneous leishmaniasis, are the direct result of local tissue damage caused by a cell-mediated immune reaction against the organism. On the other hand, many of the clinical manifestations of infectious diseases may be due to the damaging effect of immune-complexes formed in the tissues between the antigens of the invading organisms and humoral antibodies. In all likelihood, both humoral and cell-mediated immunity have an important role in determining the amount of host resistance and the amount of tissue damage in most infectious diseases. In other words, the two processes are not mutually exclusive, but probably act together in influencing the clinical course of the disease.

SEROLOGIC DIAGNOSIS OF INFECTIOUS DISEASES

Serologic tests for infectious diseases are most likely to be developed: (1) whenever precise identification of the causative agent by cultural or other methods is difficult or time consuming; or (2) whenever relative inaccessibility of tissues containing infected material makes it difficult to obtain adequate specimens for laboratory examination.

While it is recognized that serologic methods are often helpful when the etiologic agent cannot be recovered, it should be emphasized that isolation and identification of the organism is always the procedure of choice. The presence of specific antibodies against a given organism in the patient's serum suggests past or present infection, but does not necessarily indicate active disease. Furthermore, cross-reactivity between organisms which are antigenically similar, but pathogenically different, is a fairly common occurrence.

It is for these reasons that serologic tests for the diagnosis of infectious diseases are largely limited to a relatively small number of selected procedures which will be described in the section to follow. (Immunologic techniques for the identification of microorganisms in culture or tissue samples are considered to be beyond the scope of this book.)

BACTERIAL INFECTIONS

Salmonellosis

Serologic testing by the agglutination method is frequently used in the diagnosis of suspected salmonella infections. *Salmonella typhosa* is the cause of typhoid fever in man, whereas *Salmonella paratyphi A* (*Salmonella paratyphi*), *Salmonella paratyphi B* (*Salmonella schottmülleri*), *Salmonella paratyphi C* (*Salmonella hirschfeldii*), and *Salmonella choleraesuis* are causes of milder types of gastrointestinal disturbances, sometimes known as paratyphoid fever.

The salmonella possess three types of antigens which are useful in sero-diagnosis: the H (flagellar) antigens which are associated with the flagellae, the O (somatic) antigens which are associated with the bacterial cell wall, and the Vi (capsular) antigens which are associated with the capsule surrounding the cell.

In the classic form of the Widal reaction, dilutions of the patient's serum are mixed with suspensions of O and H antigens prepared from *S. typhosa, S. paratyphi A,* and *S. paratyphi B.* The highest dilution at which agglutination occurs gives an estimate of the antibody content of the patient's serum. The agglutinating antibodies directed against the O antigen of *S. typhosa* belong predominantly to the IgM immunoglobulin class, but IgG and IgA antibodies may also be detected in lesser amounts.[3]

Although testing is usually carried out with both H and O antigens, the O agglutinins are of more significance since some patients fail to develop H antibodies. Furthermore, H antibodies may persist for years following prophylactic immunization, whereas O antibodies usually disappear within 6 months. It is not necessary to routinely include Vi antigens in the agglutination test for typhoid fever as Vi antibodies rarely occur in the absence of O or H agglutinins. Although the measurement of Vi antibodies may occasionally be of assistance in the detection of typhoid carriers, it should not be relied upon as the sole criteria for diagnosis. In one series of patients, the Vi hemagglutination procedure detected only about 50 per cent of bacteriologically proven typhoid carriers.[25]

Specific agglutinins usually appear in the serum 7 to 10 days after the onset of the acute, febrile illness and reach their peak in 3 to 4 weeks. In general, the demonstration of a rising titer of specific agglutinins is considered as definite evidence of infection with a particular salmonella strain. However, if only a single specimen is available, an O agglutinin titer of more than 1:50 during the first 10 days of illness, or more than 1:500 after 3 or 4 weeks, is considered as presumptive evidence of infection, provided the patient has not been immunized within 2 years. The interpretation of the results of the Widal agglutination reactions in recently immunized individuals is extremely difficult.

The immobilization of Salmonella organisms in the living state by antibodies directed against H antigens has been used extensively in experimental immunology as a sensitive method of detecting antibody formation.

Brucellosis

Human brucellosis is the result of infection with one of three species of *Brucella: B. abortus* (cattle), *B. suis* (hogs), or *B. melitensis* (goats).

Agglutination tests are frequently utilized in the serodiagnosis of suspected brucellosis because of difficulties often encountered in isolating the causative organisms. In the tube agglutination procedure, dilutions of test serum from 1:10 to 1:5120 are mixed with the suspected organism in the smooth phase. A rising titer or a titer of greater than 1:160 is considered presumptive evidence of active disease. The antibodies responsible for the agglutination reaction in human brucellosis belong to the IgM class of immunoglobulins.

In interpreting the results of the agglutination test in brucellosis, it should be remembered that individuals who habitually handle brucella infected animals may show significant titers in the absence of active infection. Furthermore, agglutinins may persist in the serum for years after recovery from brucellosis.

Recently, there has been considerable interest in complement-fixation tests and antiglobulin tests for the serodiagnosis of human brucellosis.[23] Both of these procedures detect predominantly IgG antibodies rather than the IgM antibodies detected by the classic agglutination procedure. A complement-fixation titer greater than 1:10 is usually due to the presence of living bacilli in the tissues, although occasionally it may be the result of repeated occupational contact with brucella organisms. The antiglobulin test would appear to be particularly useful in the diagnosis of chronic brucellosis and in the surveillance of patients following treatment for acute brucellosis.

Syphilis

A wide variety of procedures have been developed over the years in an attempt to provide a reliable and reproducible serologic test for syphilis (STS). In general, these tests may be divided into: (*1*) those which measure Wassermann antibodies (reagins) directed against extracts of normal beef hearts;[34] and (*2*) those which actually measure antibodies against treponemal antigens.[7] The term reagin used in this context must be distinguished from the reagins found in patients with atopic diseases. It has been suggested that the Wassermann antibody is produced as the result of spirochetes combining with the patient's tissue, and that what is measured is an antibody to tissue components rather than to treponemata. Historically, the Wassermann antibody was discovered by chance during the investigation of syphilitic heart disease. The Wassermann antibodies are predominantly IgM, whereas the antibodies directed against treponemal antigens may belong to the IgG, IgA, or IgM classes of immunoglobulins.[5]

Some of the more common serologic tests for syphilis will be described below:

Kahn Test. The Kahn test is a flocculation procedure which employs a crude lipoidal antigen extracted from normal beef heart. In the usual procedure, a constant volume of undiluted serum is mixed with different concentrations of antigen. The size of the floccules formed and the numbers of tubes in which flocculation occurs are used as criteria for a positive reaction. The test measures reagin and has been widely used in the past as a screening procedure. However, this type of test should probably now be abandoned because of the difficulty in standardizing the crude antigen preparation.

VDRL Test. The Venereal Disease Research Laboratory slide test is also a flocculation procedure, but employs a purified cardiolipin-lecithin antigen which can be standardized by chemical and serologic methods. It provides more uniform results than the Kahn test.

Wassermann Test. The Kolmer modification of the Wassermann reaction is a good example of a complement-fixation test using purified cardiolipin-lecithin antigen. The Wassermann reaction and its various modifications are relatively simple to perform and have provided valuable diagnostic information for a period of over 40 years. Nevertheless, these tests measure reagin, and are not quite as specific as the tests which measure treponemal antibodies. It is for this reason that the Wassermann type of complement-fixation test is gradually being replaced with the treponemal tests to be described below.

TPI Test. The Treponema Pallidum Immobilization test utilizes as the antigen live spirochetes (*T. pallidum*, Nichols strain) obtained from rabbit orchitis. The demonstration of antibodies is accomplished by the immobilization of the spirochetes in the presence of the patient's serum and complement. The antibody measured is different from reagin because serum absorbed with cardiolipin antigen will still immobilize spirochetes in undiminished titer.[29] The major problem with the TPI test is related to its technical complexity and the dangers of working with live organisms.

FTA-ABS Test. The Fluorescent Treponemal Antibody Absorption test is based on the immunofluorescent staining of dead spirochetes. In this procedure, the test serum is brought into contact with the organisms which are then exposed to fluorescein labelled antibodies against human γ-globulin.[14] Recent studies would suggest that the FTA-ABS test, as presently performed, is somewhat more sensitive than the TPI test, particularly in late syphilis.[1]

RPCF Test. The Reiter Protein Complement Fixation test is similar to the Kolmer modification of the Wassermann reaction, except that the antigen is extracted from the Reiter spirochete. This organism is a nonpathogenic strain which can be cultured with relative ease. The RPCF appears to be less specific than the FTA-ABS test, but gives better results than the Kolmer modification of the Wassermann reaction. Some authorities now consider the RPCF test to be obsolete.[26]

Serologic tests for syphilis are commonly negative during the first 1 to 3 weeks after the development of the primary lesion. Thereafter, with very few exceptions, patients with the typical clinical manifestations of syphilis have positive serologic tests. In latent syphilis, serologic tests are usually positive, and indeed, the positive test may constitute the only evidence for the diagnosis. Serum antibodies directed against treponemal antigens do not penetrate into the spinal fluid. Therefore, the presence of antibodies in the CSF constitutes strong presumptive evidence in favor of central nervous system involvement. Although there is no definite proof, it must be assumed that at least some of the antibodies found in cerebrospinal fluid are produced locally (see Chapter 18).

The titers of the various serologic tests for syphilis have been used for many years as a guide for evaluating the results of therapy. Following adequate treatment in primary syphilis, the titers will usually become negative after 2 to 3 months. In secondary syphilis, the titers fall more gradually, becoming negative in 12 to 18 months in approximately 80 per cent of patients. In patients treated during the late or latent stages of syphilis, the STS will probably never become negative, although there may be a gradual reduction in titer. There is evidence to show that the more sensitive treponemal tests such as the TPI or FTA-ABS may remain positive for 12 to 15 years or more in presumably adequately treated cases of late syphilis.[1] Thus, a positive STS does not necessarily indicate active disease.

The biologic false-positive (BFP) reactions to serologic tests for syphilis occur in a wide variety of diseases when cardiolipin-lecithin antigens are employed (e.g., the Kahn, VDRL, or Wassermann reactions). False-positive reactions occur most commonly in disease caused by other spirochetes (e.g., yaws, pinta, and relapsing fever), leprosy, collagen-vascular diseases (particularly SLE), Hashimoto's thyroiditis, sarcoidosis, lymphomas, infectious mononucleosis, a wide variety of febrile illnesses, and following immunization to almost any antigen.[16] The treponemal tests are of great assistance in distinguishing biologic false-positive reactions from those of specific diagnostic significance.

In view of the above discussion, the following approach to serologic testing for syphilis appears to be the most satisfactory for clinical purposes:

1. The VDRL test should be performed as the initial screening procedure. If the VDRL is negative and there is no clinical evidence of syphilis, the patient may be considered to be noninfected.

2. The FTA-ABS test should be performed on the sera of patients with a positive VDRL to rule out false-positive reactors. If the FTA-ABS test is positive, the patient may be considered to have previous or active syphilitic infection.

3. The FTA-ABS test is also indicated for patients who have a negative VDRL, but who have clinical signs suggestive of syphilis. About 40 per cent of patients with late syphilis may have a negative VDRL, and thus may be overlooked if only a reagin test is used to exclude the diagnosis.[14]

Gonorrhea

A complement-fixation test is available for the serodiagnosis of gonorrhea, but is not considered to be sufficiently reliable for diagnostic purposes. More recently, a flocculation procedure which utilizes the "B" antigen isolated from *Neisseria gonorrhae* was found to be positive in 85 per cent of women proved by culture to have gonococcal infections.[31] The principal value of this relatively simple test is in screening high-risk patients in less time and at lower cost then is required for culture techniques.

Streptococcal Infections

Several types of hemolysins are associated with streptococci. Of particular interest is streptolysin O which is produced by most strains of β-hemolytic streptococci responsible for human poststreptococcal disease (see Chapters 6 and 7). The antistreptolysin O (ASO) test is based on the observation that the sera of patients who have had recent infections with β-hemolytic streptococci have a transient rise in antibodies directed against streptolysin O. The streptolysin O antigen is capable of lysing human or rabbit erythrocytes. Hence, antistreptolysin O antibody can be demonstrated by its ability to neutralize the lytic action of streptolysin O.

A rising titer, or a titer above 250 Todd units on a single determination is considered presumptive evidence of recent streptococcal infection. The ASO titer may be increased nonspecifically in infectious hepatitis and other forms of liver damage.

C-Reactive Protein (CRP)

C-reactive protein is a serum β-globulin which reacts with the C polysaccharide of the pneumococcus in the presence of calcium ions. Although it is specific for the C polysaccharide, it is not a true antibody and appears nonspecifically in a wide variety of inflammatory, necrotic, and infective conditions (e.g., rheumatoid arthritis, rheumatic fever, myocardial infarction, and extensive neoplasia). The most accurate quantitative method of measuring CRP is by radial immunodiffusion in agar gel against antisera prepared in rabbits.[27]

Tuberculosis

A number of attempts have been made to devise a satisfactory serologic technique for the diagnosis of active pulmonary tuberculosis. These methods have included the measurement of IgG hemagglutinins,[11] precipitins, complement-fixing antibodies, and antibodies that bind radiolabelled antigen. The major disadvantage of all of these methods is that the serologic manifestations of pulmonary tuberculosis may not become apparent until the infection has been present for several months, and the test may remain positive for years after bacteriologic remission.

RICKETTSIAL INFECTIONS

Epidemic (Louse-Borne) Typhus Fever

The etiologic agent responsible for epidemic typhus is *Rickettsia prowazeki*. The serologic diagnosis of this disease can now be established with reasonable certainty by the demonstration of serum antibodies which specifically agglutinate suspensions of *R. prowazeki*. Similar agglutination reactions are available for the detection of specific antibodies in other rickettsial infections such as murine typhus, rocky mountain spotted fever, rickettsialpox, and Q fever.

Previously, the Weil-Felix reaction was used extensively for the diagnosis of suspected typhus and other rickettsial infections. The Weil-Felix test is based on the observation that sera of patients with typhus fever agglutinate suspensions of a strain of *Proteus* known as OX-19, presumably due to cross-reacting antigens shared by both organisms. The test, although nonspecific, is highly reliable. A rising titer from a low level (e.g., 1:20) or a value greater than 1:160 is considered to be diagnostic.

MYCOPLASMA INFECTIONS

Mycoplasma pneumoniae (Eaton Agent)

The diagnosis of pneumonia caused by *Mycoplasma pneumoniae* may be confirmed serologically by a specific immunologic response to the causative organism. Serum antibodies to *M. pneumoniae* may be demonstrated by complement-fixation, hemagglutination, or immunofluorescent techniques. Of these, the complement-fixation test is the simplest and best suited for routine diagnostic purposes, whereas the immunofluorescence test using infected chick-embryo lung sections is probably the most sensitive.

Before specific serologic tests were available, the demonstration of cold agglutinins with an anti-I specificity in the serum (see Chapter 9) constituted a valuable, but nonspecific, diagnostic aid. Cold agglutinins appear in approximately 50 per cent of patients with specific *M. pneumoniae* antibodies demonstrable by the immunofluorescent technique. Occasionally, the cold agglutinins may result in a hemolytic anemia. Nonspecific antibodies which agglutinate streptococcus MG suspensions may be detected with varying frequency during the course of Eaton agent pneumonia. Recent evidence would suggest that *M. pneumoniae* and streptococcus MG share common antigenic components.[22] Neither of these nonspecific serologic tests are of major importance now that more specific tests for the etiologic agent are widely available.

VIRAL INFECTIONS

There is no question that isolation or visualization of the causative agent is the diagnostic procedure of choice in most viral diseases. However, in many instances, virus isolation is not practical as a routine procedure, and, as a result, the treating physician is forced to rely on the indirect evidence provided by serologic tests. The serologic tests for viral diseases are based on the fact that virus proteins are often potent antigens, and usually lead to the formation of specific antibodies in the human host that they infect.

Nevertheless, there are numerous potential pitfalls in the interpretation of serologic tests for viral diseases, and great care must be exercised in applying the results to individual clinical situations. Low residual titers of viral antibodies may persist for years following previous infection or prophylactic immunization. Therefore, at least a fourfold rise in antibody titer in two consecutive blood samples obtained at least 14 days apart is required for a presumptive diagnosis of active viral infection in most instances. Another difficulty frequently encountered in the serologic diagnosis of viral diseases is the number of antigenically different viruses which may cause similar clinical symptoms. Unless one has prior knowledge of the possible etiologic agent, the demonstration of specific viral antibodies is often impractical because of the large numbers of tests required. In addition, extensive antigenic cross-reactivity between certain viruses may make serologic testing impossible because of lack of specificity.

Three types of serologic tests (as well as other types of tests) are commonly employed for the detection of viral antibodies.

Complement-fixation Test.   (See Chapter 22 for a description of the complement-fixation procedure.)

Hemagglutination Inhibition Test.   The fact that a number of viruses (e.g., influenza, parainfluenza, mumps, arboviruses) are capable of inducing non-immunologic agglutination of erythrocytes in vitro forms the basis for this test. Antiserum containing specific viral antibodies will inhibit hemagglutination produced by the virus under investigation.

Virus Neutralization Test.   The virus neutralization test consists of mixing the patient's serum in suitable proportions with the virus under investigation and inoculating the mixture into susceptible laboratory animals, embryonated eggs, or tissue cultures. The presence of specific antibodies leads to protection from the usual pathogenic effects of the virus.

Other Tests.   Double diffusion in agar gel, agglutination, and precipitin reactions are occasionally utilized for the identification of antiviral antibodies.

In most viral diseases, antibodies detected by hemagglutination-inhibition and neutralization appear first and are predominantly IgM immunoglobulins, whereas antibodies detected by complement-fixation appear somewhat later and are predominantly IgG.

Those viral diseases in which serologic methods constitute a useful diagnostic procedure are listed in Table 21-1 together with the tests commonly employed for each disease.

FUNGAL INFECTIONS

Histoplasmosis

Serologic tests are frequently employed in the diagnosis of suspected infection by *Histoplasma capsulatum*.

The complement-fixation test is probably the most reliable and widely used serodiagnostic procedure in histoplasmosis. The test may be performed using either histoplasmin, a broth filtrate of *H. capsulatum* in the mycelial phase, or a suspension of yeast phase cells as the antigen. In acute infections, antibodies detected by the complement-fixation test appear in 4 to 12 weeks and may persist for many months or years. A rising titer or a titer greater than 1:8 on a single determination is strongly suggestive of active infection. There is considerable advantage to determining titers of complement-fixing antibodies to both histoplasmin and the yeast phase antigen because the sera of some patients with culturally proven histoplasmosis will react with one antigen but not with the other.

There is a certain degree of antigenic cross-reactivity between histoplasmin and other fungal extracts as measured by the complement-fixation test. However, the titers are always significantly higher for the etiologic agent proven by cultural isolation.

It should also be noted that skin tests with histoplasmin may result in the production of antibodies which remain present for several weeks. It is therefore essential that blood be drawn for serologic tests before skin tests are performed.

Precipitin tests may be carried out in capillary tubes or in agar, using histoplasmin as the antigen. The precipitin tests become positive in 1 to 3 weeks and disappear in 12 to 16 weeks. A latex fixation test for the detection of agglutinins to *H. capsulatum* is commercially available, but is not as sensitive or as reliable as the complement-fixation procedure. Fluorescent antibody techniques are useful for determining antigenic relationships between *H. capsulatum* and other pathogenic fungi, but their technical complexity limits their applicability as a routine diagnostic test.

Aspergillosis

Positive agar gel precipitin tests with extracts of *Aspergillus fumigatus* are obtained in: (*1*) 80 to 90 per cent of patients with pulmonary eosinophilia due to aspergillosis; and (*2*) almost all patients with pulmonary aspergilloma. The diagnostic and etiologic significance of these reactions is discussed in detail in Chapter 4.

Thermophilic Actinomycetes

The value of serologic tests for antibodies to *Micropolyspora faeni* (*Thermopolyspora polyspora*) and *Micromonospora vulgaris* in the diagnosis of farmer's lung and related diseases is discussed in detail in Chapter 4.

PARASITIC INFESTATIONS

Toxoplasmosis

Human toxoplasmosis is a protozoal disease resulting from infection with *Toxoplasma gondii*. Serologic tests are often used as a diagnostic aid in

TABLE 21-1. Serologic Tests in the Diagnosis of Viral Diseases

Etiologic agents	Common clinical manifestations	Serologic tests commonly used			Remarks
		C.F.*	H.I.†	N.‡	
Respiratory Tract Viruses					
Influenza A, B, and C	Influenza	+	+		Antibodies maximum at 14 days
Parainfluenza	Croup, bronchitis, bronchopneumonia	+	+	+	Especially common in children
Adenoviruses	Upper respiratory symptoms, pharyngitis, conjunctivitis	+		+	Antibodies maximum at 14 to 21 days
Respiratory syncytial virus	Rhinitis, bronchitis, bronchopneumonia, bronchiolitis	+		+	Antibodies less common in infants under 7 months
Enteric Viruses					
Coxsackieviruses	Herpangina, aseptic meningitis, exanthems, rhinitis, pleurodynia, pericarditis, myocarditis of the newborn	+		+	May coexist with poliovirus in patients with paralytic disease
Echoviruses	Aseptic meningitis, paralytic disease, encephalitis, exanthems, myalgias, gastroenteritis, respiratory disease			+	Neutralization tests only practical in epidemics or following virus isolation because of the large number of virus types
CNS Viruses					
Polioviruses	Poliomyelitis, upper respiratory infection, gastroenteritis	+		+	C.F. antibodies may persist for 1 to 5 years, N. antibodies for life
Arboviruses	Eastern equine encephalitis, Western equine encephalitis, Yellow fever, Dengue, St. Louis encephalitis, Japanese encephalitis, tick-borne encephalitis, etc.	+	+	+	Extensive antigenic cross-reactivity between the numerous viruses in this group

Virus	Disease / clinical condition	C.F.*	H.I.†	N.‡	Remarks
Lymphocytic choriomeningitis virus	Aseptic meningitis, respiratory symptoms, exanthems	+			C.F. antibodies appear in 2 weeks, N. antibodies in 6 to 8 weeks
Cytomegalovirus	Brain damage in congenital infections, respiratory symptoms in primary and acquired immunologic deficiency states	+			Indirect immunofluorescence test for cytomegalovirus IgM antibodies positive in 95% of infants with congenital infection
Skin and Mucous Membrane Viruses					
Measles virus	Measles and its complications	+	+	+	Diagnosis usually made on clinical features
Rubella virus	German measles and its complications	+	+	+	N. antibodies may persist for many years
Poxviruses	Smallpox, vaccinia, cowpox and their complications	+	+		H.I. antibodies appear in 4 to 5 days, C.F. antibodies in 8 to 9 days
Varicella–Herpes zoster viruses	Chickenpox, herpes zoster and their complications	+			The viruses that cause chickenpox or herpes zoster are antigenically indistinguishable
Miscellaneous					
Mumps virus	Mumps and its complications	+	+	+	Antibodies appear in 7 to 14 days
Psittacosis–Lymphogranuloma venereum agents	Psittacosis, lymphogranuloma venereum and their complications	+	+		Antibodies maximum in 20 to 30 days. The viruses which cause LGV and psittacosis are antigenically similar

* Complement-fixation.
† Hemagglutination inhibition.
‡ Neutralization.

congenital or acquired toxoplasmosis because of the difficulties frequently encountered in isolating the causative organism.[30a]

The Sabin-Feldman dye fixation test is carried out by exposing *Toxoplasma* organisms obtained from the peritoneal exudates of infected mice to serum antibodies in the presence of methylene blue. If antibodies are present in the patient's serum, the normal staining of the *Toxoplasma* cytoplasm is inhibited. The antibodies detected by the dye test usually appear approximately 1 week after infection, and may persist for many years in low titer (e.g., 1:100). The Sabin-Feldman dye test has been reported to be positive in 20 to 60 per cent of adults in the United States, presumably due to previous asymptomatic infections with *T. gondii*. Therefore, a rising titer in consecutive blood samples or a titer greater than 1:512 in a single determination is usually considered necessary for the confirmation of active infection.

Serum antibodies in toxoplasmosis may also be detected by the complement-fixation reaction.[13] Despite years of experience with complement-fixing antibodies in toxoplasmosis, there is no general agreement on diagnostic titers. However, a rising titer or a titer greater than 1:10 in a single determination is highly suggestive of acute infection. Complement-fixing antibodies tend to appear later (3 to 4 weeks) and disappear more rapidly than antibodies detected by the dye test. Therefore, a strongly positive dye test and a negative complement-fixation test is occasionally found in patients with recent *Toxoplasma* infections.

A direct microagglutination test which utilizes suspensions of dead organisms as the antigen may eventually prove to be of considerable value in the serodiagnosis of toxoplasmosis.[12] Similarly, the indirect fluorescent antibody (IFA) test appears to be a highly sensitive and specific method for the detection of serum antibodies to *T. gondii,* and is now the routine serologic test for *Toxoplasma* antibodies in an increasing number of laboratories.[10]

Because toxoplasmosis may be transmitted in utero, it is of importance to note that maternal antibodies may be transferred to the infant through the placenta. In noninfected infants, the antibodies usually disappear within 6 to 8 months. On the other hand, the detection of a higher antibody titer in the infant's serum than in the maternal serum indicative of infection in the child.

Trichinosis

A variety of serologic tests have been devised for the diagnosis of suspected trichinosis, including the complement-fixation test, precipitin tests, and a fluorescent antibody test.[24]

The complement-fixation test has been used for many years as the principal serodiagnostic procedure in trichinosis. Antibodies detected by this method appear approximately 2 to 3 weeks after infection in 80 to 90 per cent of patients, and may persist for 10 to 12 months. Complement-fixing antibodies against *Trichinella spiralis* are almost never found in normal individuals, so that even low titers (e.g., 1:8) may be of diagnostic significance.

The ring precipitin test is carried out by the overlaying of *Trichinella* antigen on the patient's serum in small test tubes. It is relatively easy to perform, becomes positive at approximately the same time as the complement-fixation test, and may remain positive for periods up to 2 years. Like most precipitin tests, false-positive reactions may occur in patients with hypergammaglobulinemia due to any cause. Recently, there has been considerable interest in an indirect fluorescent antibody procedure which utilizes the washed muscle larvae of *T. spiralis*. This procedure is highly specific, but requires specialized technical skills.

Schistosomiasis (Bilharziasis)

Serologic tests including the complement-fixation reaction, flocculation tests, and an indirect immunofluorescence procedure may be of considerable assistance in the diagnosis of some patients with schistosomiasis.

Pneumocystosis

Recent studies suggest that a complement-fixation test using antigen prepared from pneumocystis-infected human lungs is frequently positive in infants and children infected with this organism.[2]

SKIN TESTS IN THE DIAGNOSIS OF INFECTIOUS DISEASES

Over the years, literally hundreds of skin tests which employ various bacterial, viral, fungal, or parasitic antigens have been developed for the rapid detection of infection with microorganisms. In the section which follows only those tests which are widely used, commonly available, and of proven diagnostic value will be considered in detail. In general, a positive skin test with microbial antigens indicates only that the individual has been infected in the past, and is not a reliable guide to active infection, resistance, immunity, or prognosis.

Because of their complexity, the skin tests for tuberculosis and diphtheria will be discussed in detail, while the remainder will be described in summary form in Table 21-2.

TABLE 21-2. Diagnostic Skin Tests in Infectious Diseases

Disease: organism and (name of test)	Material	Administration	Type, diameter, and description of positive test	Remarks
		Bacterial Infections		
Tuberculosis: *M. tuberculosis* (Mantoux)	Tuberculin purified protein derivative (PPD), 0.05 mg/ml	0.1 ml, intradermal	Delayed, 48–72 hr, induration over 5 mm with or without surrounding erythema	See text
Tuberculosis: *M. tuberculosis* (Tine)	Disc saturated with tuberculin PPD, 2 mg/ml	4 multiple punctures through disc to depth of 1–2 mm with special apparatus	Delayed, 48–72 hr, four or more indurated papules over 1 mm which may coalesce	See text
Diphtheria: *C. diphtheriae* (Schick)	Culture filtrate containing 1/50 MLD of diphtheria toxin per 0.1 ml (control is diphtheria toxoid)	0.1 ml, intradermal, of antigen and control	See text	See text
Leprosy: *M. Leprae* (Lepromin)	Saline suspension of human leprous tissue (Mitsuda) or dried, defatted bacilli (Fernandez)	0.1–0.2 ml, intradermal	1. Delayed, 24–72 hr, 6–20 mm (Fernandez) 2. Granuloma type reaction, 3–4 weeks (Mitsuda)	Neither reaction diagnostic for leprosy, but diagnostic for type of leprosy, both reactions obtained in tuberculoid leprosy, but not in lepromatous leprosy, high incidence of false-positive Mitsuda reactions

Viral Infections

Lymphogranuloma Venereum LGV agent (Frei)	Killed LGV agent from yolk sac of chick embryo (control is normal yolk sac)	0.1 ml, intradermal of antigen and control	Delayed, 48–72 hr, over 6 mm of induration with surrounding erythema, control less than 5 mm	Becomes positive 7–40 days after infection; good reliability
Mumps: mumps virus	Killed mumps virus from allantoic fluid of chick embryo (control is normal allantoic fluid)	0.1 ml, intradermal of antigen and control	Delayed, 48–72 hr, over 15 mm of erythema with or without induration (control less than 10 mm)	Of epidemiologic rather than diagnostic value, positive in 5–10 days, cross-reacts with other viral antigens
Cat scratch disease: unknown organism	Heat treated suspension of infected lymph nodes or pus	0.1 ml, intradermal	Delayed, 48 hr, 5–10 mm of erythema and induration	Surprisingly reliable considering unknown nature of etiologic agent

Fungal Infections

Histoplasmosis: H. capsulatum (Histoplasmin)	1:100 dilution of filtrate from mycelial phase of H. capsulatum	0.1 ml, intradermal	Delayed, 24–72 hr, over 5 mm of erythema and induration	Appears 14 days after infection, cross-reacts slightly with blastomycin and coccidioidin, may induce false-positive serologic tests
Blastomycosis: B. dermatitidis (Blastomycin)	1:100 dilution of filtrate from mycelial phase of B. dermatitidis	0.1 ml, intradermal	Delayed, 24–48 hr, over 5 mm of erythema and induration	Cross-reacts slightly with histoplasmin and coccidioidin
Coccidioidomycosis: C. immitis (Coccidioidin)	1:100 dilution of filtrate from mycelial phase of C. immitis	0.1 ml, intradermal	Delayed, 24–48 hr, over 5 mm of erythema and induration	Cross-reacts slightly with coccidioidin and blastomycin; appears 3–4 weeks after infection
Aspergillosis: A. fumigatus	Protein fraction of aqueous extracts of A. fumigatus, 10 mg/ml	0.025 ml, intradermal	1. Immediate: wheal and erythema over 5 mm, maximal in 15–20 min 2. Arthus: maximal at 7–8 hr	Patient may show immediate reaction only, or a dual reaction consisting of an immediate reaction followed by an Arthus reaction (see Chapter 4)

TABLE 21-2. (*Continued*)

Disease: organism and (name of test)	Material	Administration	Type, diameter, and description of positive test	Remarks
		Parasitic Infections		
Toxoplasmosis: *T. gondii* (Toxoplasmin)	Inactivated peritoneal exudate from infected mice (control is splenic suspension from noninfected mice)	0.1 ml, intradermal, of antigen and control	Delayed, 48–72 hr, over 5 mm of erythema and induration (control negative)	May not become positive for several weeks after infection, used mostly for epidemiologic surveys, large number of reactors in general population, not reliable for diagnosis of acute disease
Trichinosis: *T. spiralis* (Trichinellin)	1:10,000 dilution of dried ground trichinae in saline (control is saline)	0.1 ml, intradermal, of antigen and control	1. Immediate: wheal and erythema over 5 mm, maximal in 15–20 min (control less than 3 mm) 2. Delayed: 24–48 hr, 10–30 mm of induration	1. Appears 2–3 weeks after infection, false-positive and false-negative tests fairly common, standardization of antigen to 0.20 mg antigen N/ml reduces false-positive reactions 2. Occasionally present 3–10 days after infection
Echinococcosis: *E. granulosis* (Casoni)	Inactivated hydatid cyst fluid from humans or animals standardized to contain 0.015 mg of antigen N/ml	0.025 ml, intradermal	1. Immediate: wheal and erythema over 5 mm, maximal in 15–20 min 2. Delayed: 24–48 hr, over 5 mm of erythema and induration	High incidence of false-positive reactions unless cyst fluid is standardized in terms of antigen nitrogen content, may cross-react with *Taenia saginata* and *Schistosoma mansoni*

TUBERCULOSIS

The familiar tuberculin test has been widely utilized for many years, and is recognized universally as the prototype of delayed type hypersensitivity. Despite the vast amount of literature which has accumulated on the subject, the performance and interpretation of tuberculin skin tests is still under active investigation.

The antigens commonly used today are: (1) Old Tuberculin (O.T.) prepared by concentrating the heat-inactivated filtrate of a culture broth in which tubercle bacilli have been grown; or (2) purified protein derivatives of tuberculin (PPD) prepared by ammonium sulphate (PPD-S) or trichloracetic acid precipitation of culture filtrates of *M. tuberculosis*. Because biologic activity varies with different lots, both O.T. and PPD preparations are biologically standardized in guinea pigs or man in terms of International Tuberculin Units (T.U.). The appropriate equivalent "strengths" of commonly used tuberculin preparations are listed in Table 21-3.

TABLE 21-3. Approximate Comparison of Tuberculin Preparations

PPD (mg/dose)	O.T. (dilution)	Tuberculin Units (T.U.)
0.00002 (1st strength)	1:10,000	1
0.0001 (intermediate)	1:2,000	5
0.005 (2nd strength)	1:100	100

For mass surveys, or routine testing in general hospitals, the most satisfactory procedure is probably the intradermal test (Mantoux) with intermediate strength PPD. If active tuberculous disease is suspected, it is customary to start with first strength PPD, and then repeat the test with second strength material if there is no reaction. In this way, unpleasantly severe or necrotic skin reactions can be avoided in individuals expected to be hypersensitive to tuberculin. Old Tuberculin is somewhat less satisfactory as a test material because it contains larger quantities of lipids, polysaccharides, and culture media contaminants than PPD. These nonprotein components or contaminants may provoke false-positive reactions in the 1:100 dilution, or may induce transient febrile episodes in patients with extreme tuberculin hypersensitivity.

Multiple puncture methods such as the tuberculin tine test (TTT) are widely employed for mass surveys because of their economy and convenience. The tine test is as sensitive as the intradermal test, but is slightly less specific and less quantitative when active pulmonary tuberculosis is suspected.[18] At present, neither the scratch test (von Pirquet) nor the patch test (Vollmer) is considered adequate for mass surveys or the routine testing of normal individuals. The criteria for positive reactions with intracutaneous and multiple puncture techniques are documented in Table 21-2.

The tuberculin skin test reaction usually becomes positive within 3 to 4 weeks following infection with *M. tuberculosis* and may persist for many years or for life. False-negative reactions to tuberculin may occur during the course of disseminated tuberculosis, measles, sarcoidosis, lymphoma, or other diseases which produce a generalized depression of cell-mediated hypersensitivity. For reasons which are not well understood, tuberculin sensitivity is also transiently depressed following vaccination with measles, poliomyelitis, or yellow fever vaccine. In addition, the administration of immunosuppressive drugs such as corticosteroids or azathioprine may reduce or abolish the tuberculin skin reaction.

False-positive reactions, on the other hand, are more likely to create difficulties of interpretation than false-negative reactions. Positive reactions to the larger doses of tuberculin (e.g., 50 to 250 T.U.) occur with surprising frequency in certain geographic areas such as the southeastern portion of the United States. Presumably, at least some of these weak reactions may be attributed to infection with "atypical" mycobacteria (e.g., Battey bacillus, photochromogens, scotochromogens, nonchromogens) which cross-react antigenically with *M. tuberculosis.*[6] Scotochromogens and nonchromogens can be readily isolated from the soil in areas where reactions to atypical bacteria are common. Thus, these organisms probably account for a significant proportion of apparently false-positive reactions to the higher concentrations of PPD. However, the importance of "atypical" mycobacteria in the production of positive tuberculin skin reactions cannot be assessed adequately until test antigens for each of these organisms (e.g., PPD-B derived from the Battey bacillus) have been widely available over a period of several years.

The use of intermediate strength PPD also tends to decrease the number of false-positive tuberculin tests. However, it is sufficiently sensitive for most clinical purposes. Individuals who have received BCG vaccination will usually have positive tuberculin skin test reactions for several years afterwards.

As noted previously, a positive skin test to tuberculin is not, in itself, diagnostic of active infection. However, the recent conversion of a previously negative test, or a positive tuberculin test in an infant is highly suggestive of recent infection, and are often regarded as indications for beginning specific chemotherapy.[20] The major value of the tuberculin skin test is to exclude tuberculosis as a diagnostic possibility in patients with pulmonary lesions, or to determine the prevalence of tuberculous infection in epidemiologic studies.

DIPHTHERIA

The Schick test for determining susceptibility to diphtheria is a toxin-antitoxin neutralization test and, as such, is not a true hypersensitivity reaction. The test consists of the injection into the skin of diphtheria toxin in sufficient quantity ($\frac{1}{50}$ M.L.D. per 0.1 ml) to provoke localized erythema and induration (see Table 21-2). However, if sufficient circulating antitoxin is present ($\frac{1}{30}$ to $\frac{1}{100}$ of a unit/ml), the toxin is neutralized, no skin reaction appears, and the patient is considered to be immune to infection with *Corynebacteria diphtheriae*.

Some immune individuals may show delayed type skin hypersensitivity to diphtheria toxin or its contaminants. These allergic reactions may result in false-positive Schick tests, but they are much less common now that highly purified diphtheria toxins are available. Nevertheless, it is usually considered desirable to perform a control test with purified diphtheria toxoid at a concentration of 0.01 Lf/ml in the same diluent as the toxin.

Thus, 4 types of reactions to the Schick test are possible:

1. Positive: An area of redness and induration appears at the site of toxin injection in 12 to 72 hours and reaches a maximum diameter of about 3 cm in approximately 1 week. Necrotic or pigmented areas may appear at the center of the lesion. The control test remains negative. The patient is therefore susceptible to infection with *C. diphtheriae*.

2. Negative: There is no reaction at either the site of toxin injection or the control site. The patient is immune to infection with *C. diphtheriae*.

3. Pseudoreaction: A delayed type cutaneous response appears both at the site of toxin injection and the control site. These reactions reach a maximum in 48 to 72 hours in contrast to a true positive Schick test which persists for a week or more. The patient is thus immune to infection with *C. diphtheriae*, but hypersensitive to diphtheria toxin, diphtheria toxoid, or contaminants contained in both materials.

4. Combined Reaction: Very occasionally, after the pseudoreaction described above has faded, a typically positive Schick test appears at the test site. This type of reaction is often difficult to interpret. It most commonly indicates either hypersensitivity to contaminants in the test preparations, or previous inapparent infection which was sufficient to produce hypersensitivity, but not protective immunity, to diphtheria toxin. In either case, the patient is susceptible to infection with *C. diphtheriae*.

IMMUNIZATION PROCEDURES

Before recommending any immunization procedure, it is necessary to establish that: (1) the disease is of sufficient severity or frequency to justify immunization against it; (2) the proposed immunization procedure is effective; and (3) the risk of the disease is greater than the risk of immunization. Although these are almost self-evident statements, they are not infrequently forgotten in the scientific excitement which follows the discovery of a new vaccine or other immunization procedure.

The types of biologic substances available for passive and active immunization are summarized in Table 21-4. The preferential use of live vaccines

TABLE 21-4. Common Types of Immunization Against Infectious Diseases

Active Immunization	
Bacterial diseases	
Toxoids	Inactivated bacterial toxins (e.g., diphtheria and tetanus toxoids)
Live bacterial vaccines	Organism is modified or attenuated in culture or animals so that it produces a mild or inapparent infection, but still confers immunity against fully virulent organisms (e.g., BCG)
Killed bacterial vaccines	Virulent organisms are killed with minimal change in their antigenic composition (e.g., pertussis and typhoid vaccines)
Viral diseases	
Live viral vaccines	Virus is attenuated so that it produces a mild or inapparent infection, but still confers immunity against fully virulent organisms (e.g., oral poliovirus, measles, and most other viral vaccines)
Killed viral vaccines	Virulent viruses are killed with minimal change in their antigenic composition (inactivated poliovirus vaccine is the only one in this category in common use)
Passive Immunization	
Normal human immunoglobulin	Prepared from large pools of individual plasmas, assumed to contain antibodies against common infectious diseases
Hyperimmune globulin	Prepared against a specific agent from the plasma of hyperimmunized or convalescent individuals (e.g., antitetanus or antivaccinial-immunoglobulins)

is based on the assumption that the living organisms multiply in the individual who receives them, and, thus, stimulate natural antibody formation. In general, live vaccines produce higher antibody titers than killed vaccines, but lower titers than natural infections. The superior protection afforded by live vaccines constitutes their principal advantage as immunizing agents.

The major disadvantage of live vaccines is that it is much more difficult to evaluate their safety than it is with killed vaccines. On the other hand, over-attenuation of live vaccines in an attempt to produce a safer product occasionally results in complete loss of immunogenicity. In addition, it is important to be certain that live virus vaccines do not contain pathogenic passenger viruses as contaminants, and do not produce communicable illnesses in the recipients.

The major indication for passive immunization is a need for rapid protection. Active immunization may result in lifetime immunity, but it may take several days or weeks to achieve protective antibody levels. By contrast, passive immunization may provide protection within minutes or hours, but the protection will last for only a few weeks.

Only those immunization procedures which are in common use, and are of proven value and safety are summarized in the section which follows. (A complete and detailed review of immunization procedures against infectious diseases appears in a recent issue of the *British Medical Bulletin*.[9])

ROUTINE IMMUNIZATION PROCEDURES IN CHILDHOOD

Diphtheria Toxoid, Pertussis Vaccine and Tetanus Toxoid (Combined)

It is a widely accepted procedure in the practice of preventive pediatrics to routinely immunize infants with DPT preparations during the first year of life (see Table 21-5). A single dose of a typical combined preparation contains approximately 40 Lf of diphtheria toxoid, 8 Lf of tetanus toxoid, and 15 billion killed bacilli from strains of *Bordetella pertussis*.

The most desirable age for beginning immunization is 6 months for several reasons: (*1*) before the age of 6 months the infant's antibody response may be reduced by the presence of maternal antibody; (*2*) the infant's own antibody forming mechanism may be immature before 6 months of age; (*3*) adverse reactions to the pertussis component of the triple vaccine are less frequent in infants over 6 months of age; and (*4*) immunization after 6 months of age confers the highest degree of protection during the pre-school years when the exposure to infectious diseases is greater than during infancy.[8]

A possible disadvantage associated with delaying DPT immunization until the age of 6 months is the clinical observation that pertussis is a serious disease only during the first 4 months of life. On the other hand, most adverse reactions to the triple vaccine in childhood can be attributed to its content of killed *B. pertussis* bacilli. Febrile reactions, shock, convulsions, and encephalitis are stated to be more common in infants with a history of frequent convulsions, or convulsions following a previous injection of combined vaccine. These infants should therefore be given a vaccine containing only diphtheria and tetanus toxoids as adverse reactions to these components are uncommon in children. The question of hypersensitivity reactions to diphtheria and tetanus toxoids in adults will be discussed subsequently in the section on Special Immunization Procedures.

TABLE 21-5. Typical Routine Immunization Schedule for Children*

Age	Procedure	Remarks
6–8 months	Diph/pert/tet and oral polio vaccine (1st dose)	Better immunologic response obtained if 1st dose delayed until after 6 months
8–10 months	Diph/pert/tet and oral polio vaccine (2nd dose)	Preferably 6–8 weeks after 1st dose
12–14 months	Diph/pert/tet and oral polio vaccine	Preferably 4–6 months after 2nd dose
2nd year	Measles vaccination	An interval of at least 4 weeks should be allowed between the administration of two live vaccines
2nd year	Smallpox vaccination	Primary vaccination is no longer advised during the 1st year of life
5 years or school entry	Diph/tet/polio vaccine; smallpox revaccination	
15–19 years or school leaving	Tet/polio vaccine; smallpox revaccination	

* Adapted from British Ministry of Health Schedule (1968).

The DPT combination is administered in three doses of 1.0 ml. For maximum antibody response, it is preferable to administer the second dose after an interval of 6 to 8 weeks and the third dose after an interval of 6 months. A booster dose of diphtheria and tetanus toxoids (e.g., 50 Lf of diphtheria toxoid and 10 Lf of tetanus toxoid) may then be given at the age of 5 years or immediately prior to beginning school. Provided the initial three-dose schedule is spaced as outlined above, the booster doses formerly recommended at 2 years and at 8 to 12 years are no longer considered necessary. A booster dose of tetanus toxoid alone (e.g., 10 Lf) may be given at 15 to 19 years of age or following the completion of high school.

The efficacy of the various components of the triple vaccine combination varies somewhat. Available epidemiologic data would suggest that 15 per cent of patients with well documented pertussis had been immunized with pertussis vaccine, whereas the comparable figure for tetanus toxoid is 4 per cent. Immunization with diphtheria toxoid reduces the risk of contracting diphtheria fourfold, and the risk of dying of diphtheria 25-fold. Thus, DPT immunization is an effective procedure.

Poliomyelitis

The most widely used preparation for the prevention of poliomyelitis is oral poliovirus vaccine administered as a suspension of live attenuated types 1, 2, and 3 polioviruses.

In infancy, it is most convenient to give the 0.2 ml dose orally at the same time as the infant receives his diphtheria, pertussis, and tetanus immunization parenterally (see Table 21-5). Three doses of the oral trivalent poliovirus vaccine are considered necessary because the three types of poliovirus sometimes interfere with each other and prevent colonization of the gut by one or more poliovirus types. Furthermore, coexisting enteroviruses may also interfere with multiplication in the gut. It is for this reason that oral vaccine is not entirely suitable for booster doses. It is unlikely that a single booster dose of oral vaccine will invariably increase immunity to all three types of polioviruses.

Therefore, a single injection of 1 ml of combined diphtheria toxoid, tetanus toxoid, and killed poliovirus vaccine constitutes an economical and convenient method of administering the booster doses previously recommended at the time of school entry. Similarly, combined tetanus toxoid and killed poliovirus vaccine is recommended at the time of leaving school.

The immunity conferred by oral poliovirus vaccine is manifest in several ways. There appears to be resistance to a second infection of the alimentary canal, presumably due to the local production of secretory IgA antibodies. In addition, high levels of neutralizing antibodies appear in the circulation shortly after immunization. These circulating antibodies, which are first IgM and then IgG, probably prevent the spread of the virus from the gut to the central nervous system. Detectable circulating antibody responses are found in over 90 per cent of children who receive a full course of oral poliovirus vaccine.

Smallpox

Smallpox vaccine is prepared from the vaccinial lesions of inoculated cows or sheep. The vaccine is available both as a glycerinated vaccine containing live virus or as a lyophilized powder which must be reconstituted in a glycerinated diluent. In infants, smallpox vaccine is applied by rubbing the vaccine into a small scratch on the skin surface, or by the multiple pressure method through a drop of vaccine on the unbroken skin surface.

Despite the widespread use of smallpox vaccine for over 100 years, its efficacy has never been precisely determined in controlled studies. Nevertheless, it is generally agreed that vaccination properly performed with a potent vaccine provides a high degree of immunity for 3 years, and substantial but decreasing protection for 10 years or more.

There is a definite risk of serious complications following primary vaccination.[21a] These complications are twice as common in infants under the age of 1 year and include generalized vaccinia, eczema vaccinatum, post-vaccinial encephalitis, severe febrile reactions, thrombocytopenic purpura, glomerulonephritis, and myocarditis (see Table 21-6). Vaccinia gangrenosum is especially common in infants with immune deficiency syndromes.

TABLE 21-6. Rates of Complications per Million Smallpox Vaccinations*

	Under 1 year	1–2 years	5–14 years
Generalized vaccinia	44.3	14.6	26.5
CNS complications	14.6	3.3	30.3
Eczema vaccinatum	3.0	6.7	7.6

* British Ministry of Health data for England and Wales for 1951–1960.

Because of the increased risk of generalized vaccinia, or eczema vaccinatum, prophylactic smallpox vaccination is contraindicated in infants with: atopic or other forms of generalized dermatitis in either the infant or a family contact, leukemia, lymphoma, immune deficiency syndromes, or in infants receiving corticosteroids, immunosuppressive drugs, or radiotherapy.

Recently it has been demonstrated that the incidence of eczema vaccinatum is significantly reduced in children suffering from atopic dermatitis or other skin disorders by the use of the CVI-78 strain of attenuated live vaccinia virus instead of the standard preparations.[19] It remains to be established whether the CVI-78 strain is sufficiently safe and effective for elective vaccination of children suffering from eczema. Certain thiosemicarbazone derivatives have been reported to show a short-term protective effect against smallpox and a possible therapeutic effect against vaccinal complications.

Because of the risk of adverse reactions and because smallpox is not endemic in many parts of the world, the routine vaccination of infants remains somewhat controversial. There are those who feel that smallpox vaccination should be restricted to children or adults who plan to travel to endemic areas. The risk of serious complications is higher when primary vaccination is carried out in later life, but presumably the total number of individuals subjected to this risk would be significantly lowered if selected vaccination were carried out. On the other hand, recent experience with cases of smallpox imported into the United States, England, and Canada from endemic areas would suggest that inadequate quarantine regulations or failure to diagnose the first case might lead to serious epidemics if routine smallpox vaccination in childhood were abandoned. However, the routine primary vaccination of previously unvaccinated adults living in nonendemic areas is not considered advisable because of the higher risk of complications.

A compromise position which appears to be widely accepted at the present time is to defer primary vaccination until the second year of life in order to reduce the incidence of complications.[28] Waiting until the second year of life also gives the physician the opportunity to recognize possible contraindications to vaccination. Revaccination should then be performed at the same time as the booster doses for diphtheria, tetanus, and poliomyelitis are carried out (i.e., at the age of 5 years and at the time of school leaving).

The primary vaccination should be inspected 6 to 8 days after vaccination. Unless there is a typical vesicle at the site of inoculation, the vaccination should be repeated with another lot of vaccine. On revaccination there are two possible reactions defined by the WHO Expert Committee on Smallpox: (1) A "major reaction" consists of a vesicular or pustular lesion at the inoculation site, and is considered to indicate that the revaccination was successful; (2) any other type of reaction should be regarded as "equivocal" and may result from immunity adequate to suppress virus multiplication, or may represent only an allergic reaction to inactive vaccine. If an "equivocal" reaction is observed, the revaccination should be repeated with another lot of vaccine. The terms "accelerated" and "immune" reactions are no longer in common usage.

Measles

Live attenuated measles virus vaccine prepared from the Schwarz strain is prepared in chick embryo culture, is suitable for administration without human antimeasles immunoglobulin, and is usually given in a dose of 0.5 ml subcutaneously. Immunization with inactivated measles virus vaccine is no longer a recommended procedure.

Measles vaccine produces mild or inapparent, noncommunicable infection in those who receive it. About 15 per cent of infants receiving the Schwarz strain virus experience fever of 103° F or higher beginning about the sixth day after vaccination and persisting for no longer than 5 days.

Live, attenuated measles vaccine is one of the safest immunizing agents presently available. Nevertheless, there are certain precautions and contra-indications associated with its use. Theoretically, infants allergic to egg proteins might develop severe anaphylactic reactions to measles vaccine, but, as yet, no such cases have been reported. More definite contraindica-tions are leukemia, lymphoma, immune deficiency syndromes, and altered resistance following the administration of immunosuppressive drugs or radiation. Severe complications such as a giant cell pneumonia have been reported in children with leukemia who have received measles vaccine.

Immunization with measles vaccine is advocated as a routine procedure because of the relatively high incidence (1:1000) of encephalitis following measles which often causes permanent brain damage or mental retardation. The reported death rate for measles is 1 per 10,000 cases.

It is customary to administer measles vaccine as a single dose during the second year of life because residual maternal antibodies may occasionally persist as long as 12 months. It is generally recommended that there should be an interval of 3 to 4 weeks between giving live measles vaccine and other live virus vaccines (e.g., poliovirus and smallpox). Although there is no definite proof, it is possible that diminished antibody responses might result from the simultaneous administration of two live virus vaccines. Furthermore, the incidence of febrile reactions is undoubtedly increased by the simultaneous administration of two or more antigens.

Over 90 per cent of children who receive measles vaccine develop detect-able antibody titers.

Mumps

Live attenuated mumps virus vaccine is prepared in chick embryo cell culture.[17] It produces an inapparent, noncommunicable infection following administration, but febrile reactions have not been associated with the vac-cine. The recommended dose is two subcutaneous injections of 1.0 ml at an interval of 1 to 4 weeks. The vaccine provides excellent protection and a demonstrable rise in antibody titers for four years after administration. Data concerning its efficacy for longer periods of time is not yet available because mumps vaccine has only recently become available for general distribution.

Mumps is one of the common communicable diseases in children, but is only rarely associated with serious sequelae such as aseptic meningitis or meningoencephalitis. In contrast to measles, the central nervous system manifestations of mumps have a good prognosis. Another potentially serious complication is the occurrence of bilateral mumps orchitis in approximately 5 per cent of males who develop mumps after the onset of puberty.

Thus, there is little indication for the introduction of mumps vaccination as a routine procedure, but its use may be considered in male children approaching puberty who have never had mumps.

SPECIFIC IMMUNIZATION PROCEDURES

Immunization procedures which are recommended for: (1) individuals who have contracted specific infections; (2) individuals exposed to specific infections; (3) individuals traveling to areas where specific diseases are endemic; and (4) individuals in certain occupations are described in the section which follows.

When passive immunization with preparations made by isolating immuno-globulins from pools of normal human plasma is indicated, the term normal human immunoglobulin will be used instead of the older terms gamma globulin, immune serum globulin, or normal gamma globulin. Most of the commercially available immunoglobulin preparations contain 15 to 16 gm of IgG per 100 ml, and negligible quantities of the other immunoglobulins.

Similarly, terms such as human antivaccinial immunoglobulin or human antitetanus immunoglobulin will be used to designate immunoglobulin preparations containing increased amounts of specific antibodies. These names will be used to replace older terms such as hyperimmune gamma globulin or convalescent gamma globulin.

Whenever it is noted that vaccines are prepared from organisms propagated in chick embryos, or the use of horse serum preparations is advocated, it is assumed that precautions regarding possible sensitivity to egg proteins or horse serum will be observed (see Chapter 2).

Tuberculosis

BCG (Bacille Calmette-Guerin) is an attenuated live vaccine derived in 1908 from a strain of *M. tuberculosis var. bovis*. Despite its use for over

50 years as a method of providing protection against tuberculosis, its efficacy remains controversial.[32] The rationale for BCG vaccination is based on the observation that when primary infection with *M. tuberculosis* occurs, most individuals develop an increased resistance to subsequent infection. The mechanism of protection in tuberculosis is believed to be based on cell-mediated immunity rather than humoral antibodies.

Most of the confusion regarding the efficacy of BCG vaccination stems from the fact that preliminary tuberculin testing is an integral part of all clinical trials. Only those patients with negative tuberculin tests are at present considered eligible for vaccination. As noted in the section on tuberculin testing, it has been recognized in recent years that a significant number of individuals in certain geographic areas have weakly positive tuberculin tests due to infection with atypical mycobacteria, and presumably have little or no immunity to *M. tuberculosis*. These individuals are not usually considered eligible for BCG vaccination, and thus the results are less satisfactory in geographic areas where infections with atypical mycobacteria are common.

Currently available data would suggest that a potent BCG vaccine is capable of conferring 80 per cent protection against tuberculosis for a period of up to 10 years.[15] A typical BCG vaccine preparation contains 2 to 8 million viable organisms per milliliter supplied as a freeze-dried preparation. The dose is 0.1 ml by intradermal injection. Undesirable side-effects include occasional discharging ulcers at the injection site and febrile reactions.

Since 1951, the World Health Organization (WHO) and the United Nations Children's Fund (UNICEF) have sponsored BCG vaccination in children on an extensive scale in the developing countries. About 80 per cent of reported cases in the world and approximately 2 to 3 million deaths due to tuberculosis occur each year in these countries.

There is preliminary evidence to suggest that vaccination of tuberculin-positive subjects has no adverse effects. If this observation is confirmed by subsequent studies, mass BCG vaccination in developing countries would be made simpler by eliminating the need for tuberculin testing.

In areas where the prevalence of tuberculosis is low, BCG vaccination should probably be reserved for the following groups of tuberculin-negative individuals in the population: (1) children exposed to household contacts with active tuberculosis; (2) medical students, nurses, and other individuals entering the medical and paramedical professions; (3) individuals planning to take up residence in countries where tuberculosis is prevalent (including armed forces and Peace Corps volunteers); and (4) residents of the economically deprived "inner-core" of large cities.

Tetanus

The most effective protection against tetanus is provided by active immunization with tetanus toxoid. If the basic immunization program has not been carried out in childhood, adults may be immunized with three intramuscular injections of 0.5 ml of adsorbed tetanus toxoid. The first and second injections are given 4 to 6 weeks apart, and the third 6 months later. Once the basic immunization is accomplished, the normal individual probably retains for life the capacity to develop a protective antibody response after a booster dose. However, in the absence of conclusive information on this subject, it is recommended that prophylactic booster doses be administered every 15 to 20 years.

Severe local tenderness and swelling at the site of injections, which begins in 24 to 48 hours and may persist for as long as 10 days, is not uncommon in adults given tetanus toxoid. These reactions occur in about 16 per cent of adults receiving their third dose of tetanus toxoid according to the schedule outlined above, and in approximately 2 per cent of adults given booster doses at the time of injury. Practically all individuals who react to tetanus toxoid in this manner give a typical delayed type skin reaction following the intradermal injection of small quantities of purified tetanus toxoid.

In recent years there has been a tendency to "overimmunize" with tetanus toxoid. Many severe local reactions could be avoided by primary immunization in childhood, and by eliminating the fairly common practice of giving unnecesssarily frequent booster doses to exposed individuals.[30]

Active or passive immunization given at the time of injury is considerably less effective in preventing the clinical manifestations of tetanus. The risk of tetanus is greatest following certain types of injury (e.g., perforating wounds on the limbs, extensive tissue damage, injuries contaminated with soil, and retained foreign bodies) (Fig. 21-1). All such patients should receive thorough surgical debridement of the wound as soon as possible following injury as well as large doses of penicillin (e.g., 1,000,000 units/day) given both parenterally for a period of 5 days and by direct infiltration into the wound. Local infiltration with penicillin is strongly recommended because the blood supply to the wound is often compromised. Despite its demonstrated effect against tetanus organisms, penicillin has no effect against the toxin once it has formed. Therefore, completely vaccinated patients should receive a booster dose of toxoid unless they have had one within the year previous to injury.

Unvaccinated or incompletely vaccinated patients should receive the initial dose of tetanus toxoid at the time of injury, followed by completion of active immunization according to the usual schedule. In addition, human antitetanus immunoglobulin (250 to 500 units) should be administered at the same time as the first dose of toxoid. At present, passive immunization with tetanus antitoxin of equine origin is considered obsolete because of the dangers of allergic reactions, and because its efficacy has never been established with certainty.

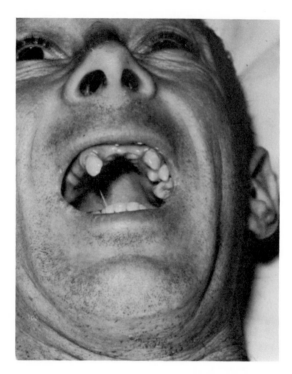

FIG. 21-1. Patient with tetanus showing characteristic spasm of the muscles of mastication and trismus. This patient had not received active immunization against tetanus.

Neonatal tetanus constitutes a major public health problem in rural areas throughout the world, or whenever the umbilical cord becomes contaminated with soil. This disease can be prevented by immunizing the mother during the first 6 weeks of pregnancy with two intramuscular injections of tetanus toxoid.

Diphtheria

Immunization with diphtheria toxoid is rarely recommended for adults or children over the age of 12 years because of the high incidence of severe delayed local reactions. If diphtheria toxoid appears to be indicated for adults, a delayed type response to the Schick test control serves as a reliable guide for predicting hypersensitivity reactions. Such individuals are considered to be immune, and immunization is not recommended.

Treatment of diphtheria with antitoxin of equine origin is still the only available specific treatment. Various types of antitoxin are produced in different parts of the world, but the most commonly used preparation is the pseudoglobulin fraction of horse antitoxin modified by digestion with pepsin. The purification procedures are intended to reduce the antigenicity of the horse serum without destroying the efficacy of the antitoxin.

Therapeutic doses of diphtheria antitoxin range from 20,000 to 100,000 units depending on the severity of the illness. There is no advantage in repeating the treatment once the initial dose has been given. Because of the length of time required for specific antibodies to reach maximum levels in the circulation after intramuscular injection, it is customary to administer $\frac{1}{2}$ the total dose by the intravenous route. The recommended prophylactic dose for diphtheria contacts is 1000 units intramuscularly.

Botulism

Botulism is fortunately not a common disease at the present time. Recently, a new trivalent antitoxin of equine origin (*Clostridium botulinum,* types A, B, and E) has become available for general distribution. This preparation contains 7,500 I.U. type A, 5500 I.U. type B, and 8500 I.U. type E antitoxin per dose. It is recommended that two injections according to the manufacturer's instructions be given as initial therapy, and this dose may be repeated within 2 to 4 hours.[21]

The efficacy of botulinus antitoxin is not clearly established by controlled clinical trials, but its administration would appear to be indicated on the basis of observations that "unfixed" botulinus toxin may remain in the circulation for several days.

Gas Gangrene

In contrast to the toxins of *C. botulinum,* the toxins of the clostridial organisms which cause gas gangrene are rapidly "fixed" to the tissues at the site of entry and cannot be demonstrated in the circulation. Therefore, the prophylactic or therapeutic use of polyvalent gas gangrene antitoxin of equine origin is of questionable value in the management of devitalized wounds or postabortal sepsis.

Influenza

Influenza virus vaccine has a protective effect only when the viruses incorporated into the vaccine are antigenically similar to those causing the epidemic disease. Because there are periodic and largely unpredictable antigenic variations in the prevalent influenza viruses, prevention of influenza in the general population is presently not feasible. Thus, a strain which will protect the patient one year may fail to do so in subsequent years if a new strain appears. Furthermore, most influenza vaccines are only marginally effective, and offer protection for only brief periods of time. Annual immunization with influenza virus vaccine is a commonly recommended procedure for patients who suffer from debilitating diseases, but there is no conclusive proof that influenza vaccine diminishes mortality in the elderly or chronically ill.

Polyvalent or bivalent influenza vaccines are attenuated virus vaccines containing two or more strains of influenza virus propagated in chick embryos. The composition of polyvalent vaccines is changed periodically depending on prevalent strains. Prior to anticipated influenza epidemics due to a known strain, additional immunization with a monovalent vaccine may be necessary if the new strain differs significantly from those contained in the polyvalent vaccines. However, even monovalent vaccines are only about 50 per cent effective in the civilian population.

Only a single booster dose of 1.0 ml of polyvalent or bivalent vaccine is needed in individuals who received one or more doses of monovalent vaccine containing Hong Kong (A_2) strain during the 1968–1969 epidemic. All other individuals should ideally receive two doses at least 2 months apart and the immunization should be scheduled to be completed by early December. The dose varies according to age as follows: adults and children over 10 years old—1.0 ml; children 6 to 10 years old—0.5 ml; children 3 months to 6 years—0.1 to 0.2 ml, 2 weeks apart, followed by a third dose of 0.1 to 0.2 ml, 2 months later. The manufacturer's instructions regarding the administration of monovalent vaccines should be followed when their administration is indicated.

Serious reactions to influenza virus vaccine do not occur. However, local tenderness, febrile reactions, malaise, and exacerbations of pre-existing intrinsic bronchial asthma are not uncommon.

Typhoid

Routine typhoid immunization is not a recommended procedure in North America or Western Europe except under special circumstances: (1) household or institutional exposure to a known typhoid carrier; (2) during a local community or institutional epidemic; and (3) prior to travel to areas where typhoid fever is endemic. There appears to be little evidence to support the rather widely held view that immunization against typhoid fever is necessary for individuals attending summer camps or living in areas where flooding has occurred.

A typical typhoid vaccine preparation contains approximately 1500 million killed *Salmonella typhosa* organisms per milliliter in saline suspension. Recommended dosage schedules are as follows: adults and children over 10 years—0.5 ml subcutaneously on two occasions, separated by 4 or more weeks; children 6 months to 10 years—0.25 ml subcutaneously on two occasions separated by 4 or more weeks. Under conditions of continued exposure, a booster dose of the same quantity of vaccine should be administered every 3 to 5 years. Unpleasant febrile reactions or local tenderness at the injection site are common following typhoid vaccine, but no other side-effects have been reported.

The efficacy of paratyphoid A and paratyphoid B vaccines has never been conclusively established and their administration is not recommended. Similarly, there appears to be no obvious rationale for the routine use of the widely distributed TABT (typhoid-paratyphoid-tetanus) vaccine.

Measles

Because of the high incidence of serious central nervous system complications associated with measles, passive immunization with human antimeasles immunoglobulin is frequently recommended for unvaccinated contacts. Most immunoglobulin preparations are standardized for their content of measles antibodies by tissue culture techniques.

A simplified dosage schedule is now widely accepted: (1) for attenuation, all ages, 250 mg; (2) for prevention, under 1 year, 250 mg; 1 to 2 years, 500 mg; 3 year or more, 750 mg.

Rubella

There is no convincing evidence at present that passive immunization with normal human immunoglobulin is effective in preventing German measles in pregnant women exposed to the disease. Even if a satisfactory method of passive immunization were developed, there is no assurance that the suppression of clinical symptoms in the mother would prevent viremia and fetal damage.

A live attenuated rubella virus vaccine, satisfactory for general distribution, has been developed recently.[33] This vaccine appears to be safe and protective for children, but is not recommended for pregnant women because of an undetermined risk for the fetus. Currently available information would suggest that antibody levels persist for at least 4 years, and probably longer.

Although detailed recommendations concerning immunization practices with rubella virus vaccine have not yet been established, it would seem logical to begin mass vaccination programs with children in elementary schools because they are the major source of virus dissemination in the community. Women of child-bearing age should not be vaccinated unless one can be certain that the patient will not become pregnant in the following 2 months.

Ideally, women in the child-bearing age should be tested for susceptibility to rubella by the hemagglutination inhibition test. If immune, vaccination is unnecessary. If the patient is considered susceptible to rubella, rubella virus vaccine should be administered only if the patient is willing to follow a recognized method of contraception for the ensuing 2 months.

Infectious Hepatitis

The prophylactic use of normal human immunoglobulin is recommended for individuals recently exposed to infectious hepatitis or for persons traveling to endemic areas. Normal human immunoglobulin does not appear to provide complete protection when given in the later stages of the incubation period. Nevertheless, passive immunization of infectious hepatitis contacts is considered a worthwhile procedure because it often reduces the severity of the disease and allows the individual to become actively immunized.

Areas where the risk of infection is significantly greater than it is in North America or Western Europe include India, Asia, Africa, South America, the Pacific Islands, and rural Mexico. A simplified dose schedule for travelers is outlined in Table 21-7. A dose of 0.02 to 0.04 ml/kg of body weight is recommended for the attenuation of infectious hepatitis in household contacts.

Normal human immunoglobulin does not appear to be helpful in the prevention of transfusion hepatitis associated with chronic hemodialysis or open heart surgery.

Varicella

Healthy individuals do not need to be protected against chickenpox. However, there is evidence that normal human immunoglobulin in doses of 0.4 to 0.6 ml/kg will provide amelioration of the disease in newborn infants, patients with immune deficiency syndromes, patients on corticosteroids and immunosuppressive drugs, or other high risk individuals. Recently, it was reported that human antizoster immunoglobulin, in a dose of 2 ml, will

TABLE 21-7. Dose Schedule of Normal Human Immunoglobulin
for Prophylaxis of Infectious Hepatitis in Travelers
to Endemic Areas*

Weight of individual (lbs.)	Dose (ml)	
	Travel for 1–2 months	Travel for 3–6 months
Less than 50	0.5	1.0
50–100	1.0	2.5
More than 100	2.0	5.0

* Recommended by National Communicable Disease Center, U.S.
Public Health Service.

prevent chickenpox in susceptible children if given within 72 hours of
exposure.[4]

Smallpox

Smallpox is still an endemic disease in India, Pakistan, Africa, and South
America. Following routine immunization in childhood as outlined in the
previous section, revaccination in individuals living in nonendemic areas
is desirable at approximately 10-year intervals. However, revaccination at
3-year intervals is recommended for persons in the medical and allied professions and for travelers to endemic areas.

Following exposure to smallpox or suspected smallpox, previously vaccinated individuals should be revaccinated as soon as possible. However,
contacts given smallpox vaccine may not develop antibodies in sufficient
time to protect them from the disease. It is therefore recommended that
human antivaccinial immunoglobulin be administered 12 to 24 hours after
revaccination. The recommended prophylactic dose is 0.3 ml/kg of body
weight, intramuscularly. Antivaccinial immunoglobulin may also be used
in the treatment of eczema vaccinatum (0.6 ml/kg body weight), but is
of no value in the management of postvaccinial encephalitis. Certain
thiosemicarbazone derivatives have recently been reported to show a short-
term protective effect against smallpox and a possible therapeutic effect
against some vaccinial complications.

Vaccinia virus may occasionally cross the placenta during any stage of
pregnancy and infect the fetus. If smallpox vaccination during pregnancy
is indicated for any reason, human antivaccinial immunoglobulin should

be given simultaneously, particularly if the patient is undergoing primary vaccination.

Rabies

A rational approach to the prophylaxis of rabies in individuals bitten or scratched by animals suspected of being rabid is often a perplexing problem for the practicing physician. The prevalence of rabies has decreased markedly in domestic animals over the past 20 years, but has apparently increased in wildlife such as skunks, foxes, and bats. Wild animals constitute the most frequent source of infection for both domestic animals and man in North America at the present time.

Before initiating antirabies prophylaxis, the following factors should be considered: (1) carnivorous animals (e.g., skunks, foxes, coyotes, raccoons, dogs, and cats) and bats are more likely to be infective than other animals; (2) an unprovoked attack is more likely to mean that the animal is rabid; (3) multiple or deep puncture wounds, or any bites on the head, face, or neck are more likely to cause disease than scratches, lacerations, or abrasions on other parts of the body; (4) a properly immunized adult domestic animal has only a minimal chance of transmitting rabies; and (5) the prevalence of rabies in domestic animals in the region may also serve as a guide as to the necessity for administering antirabies vaccine.

The first step in postexposure prophylaxis is thorough cleansing and debridement of the wound. Active immunization against rabies is now almost always carried out with inactivated rabies virus vaccine prepared from duck embryo cultures. A typical dosage schedule consists of 14 to 21 single daily subcutaneous injections of vaccine in the dose recommended by the manufacturer. These should be given in the abdomen, lower back, or lateral aspects of the thigh with frequent rotation of the injection sites. Two booster doses should be given at 10 and 20 days respectively after the completion of the primary course of immunization. The risk of postvaccinial encephalitis (see Chapter 18) with duck embryo vaccine (DEV) is considerably less than with the older vaccines of nervous tissue origin, but rare paralytic reactions do occur. Other adverse reactions to DEV include local pain and tenderness at the site of injection, low-grade fever, and, occasionally, shock during the later stages of the treatment schedule.

The effectiveness of antirabies vaccine has been questioned by some investigators because its value as a prophylactic agent can only be assessed in terms of the number of rabies deaths among unvaccinated persons. Unfortunately, a large percentage of individuals receiving antirabies vaccine probably do not require it on the basis of the criteria outlined above.

Nevertheless, only 7 deaths from rabies occurred in 172,000 individuals treated with DEV in the United States between the years 1957 and 1967. Because of its relative freedom from encephalitogens, it seems reasonable to advocate the use of antirabies vaccine in individuals with a high risk of developing a fatal disease.

Passive immunization with rabies hyperimmune serum of equine origin is recommended for use in conjunction with antirabies vaccine. The usual dose is 1,000 units (1 vial) per 40 lb of body weight. A small portion is used to infiltrate the wound locally, and the remainder is administered as an intramuscular injection.

Pre-exposure immunization has been advocated for persons in high risk occupations (e.g., veterinarians, laboratory workers, and members of the armed forces or other individuals who have frequent contact with wild animals in endemic areas).[31a] The recommended dosage is two 1.0-ml injections of DEV given subcutaneously in the deltoid area 1 month apart, followed by a third dose 6 to 7 months later. Individuals with a continuing risk of exposure should receive 1.0-ml boosters every 3 years. Such individuals should be given a series of five daily boosters after suspected rabies exposure, followed by another booster 20 days later. The efficacy of pre-exposure immunization remains to be established.

Cholera

Cholera occurs in epidemic and endemic form in the continent of India, in Southeast Asia, and in certain areas of the Middle East. Because infection is almost always acquired from food or water, the traveler's best protection in endemic areas is to use standard accommodations and to avoid potentially contaminated food or water.

Nevertheless, primary vaccination or revaccination is generally required for persons traveling to or from countries reporting cholera. A typical cholera vaccine preparation consists of a suspension of 8000 million killed *Vibrios cholerae* organisms of the Inaba and Ogawa strains per milliliter.

Two single injections, 3 to 4 weeks apart, given according to the schedule outlined in Table 21-8 provides immunity for no longer than 6 months. Therefore, booster injections should be given every 6 months as long as the risk of exposure persists. The only known reactions to cholera vaccine are redness and swelling at the injection site, fever, malaise, and headache. Cholera vaccine is essentially unchanged since its development in 1898 and provides protection in less than 50 percent of recipients. However, it is hoped that a new toxoid, currently undergoing clinical trials, will provide a more satisfactory immunologic response.

TABLE 21-8. Recommendations for Cholera Vaccination*

| Age (years) | Primary vaccination (ml) | | Boosters (ml) |
	1st dose	2nd dose	(every 6 months)
Under 5	0.1	0.3	0.3
5–10	0.3	0.5	0.5
Over 10	0.5	1.0	1.0

* National Communicable Disease Center, U.S. Public Health Service.

Yellow Fever

Yellow fever is considered to be endemic today in large areas of continental South America and Africa.

Yellow fever vaccine is a live vaccine prepared from the avirulent 17 D strain propagated in chick embryos. It is one of the safest and most effective vaccines available today, and the only serious complications have been very rare cases of non-fatal encephalitis in children under the age of 1 year. A single subcutaneous injection of 0.5 ml of 17 D vaccine is sufficient to produce immunity in humans for 15–20 years. Hence, vaccination is recommended for all travelers to endemic areas, but should be avoided whenever possible in children under the age of 1 year.

Plague

In some countries of Asia, Africa, and South America, epidemic plague results when the domestic rat population becomes infected. At the time of writing, the area of most intensive epidemic infection is in Viet Nam. In addition, a few sporadic human cases occur each year in the western United States after exposure to infected wild rodents.

Routine vaccination is not necessary for all persons traveling to countries reporting cases. However, selective immunization is recommended for individuals traveling to Viet Nam, Cambodia, and Laos, and for all persons in endemic areas whose work brings them in frequent contact with wild rodents.

Plague vaccine is an inactivated suspension of killed *Pasteurellae pestis* organisms. For primary vaccination, the first two doses should be given 3 to 4 weeks apart followed by a third dose 4 to 12 weeks after the second injection. Suggested doses for adults and children are listed in Table 21-9. Booster injections should be given every 6 to 12 months when the risk of exposure persists. Adverse reactions are mild, and usually consist of discomfort at the site of injection, fever, headache, and malaise.

TABLE 21-9. Recommendations for Plague Vaccination*

| Age (years) | Primary vaccination (ml) | | | Boosters (ml) |
	1st dose	2nd dose	3rd dose	(every 6–12 months)
Under 1	0.1	0.1	0.04	0.04
1–4	0.2	0.2	0.08	0.08
6–10	0.3	0.3	0.12	0.12
Over 10	0.5	0.5	0.2	0.2

*National Communicable Disease Center, U.S. Public Health Service.

The effectiveness of plague vaccine has never been precisely established, but it is widely believed to reduce the prevalence and severity of the disease.

Typhus

Epidemic (louse-borne) typhus is not a serious public health problem for residents of North America or Western Europe who wish to visit other countries. Furthermore, vaccination against typhus is not required by any country as a condition for entry. In fact, there is no risk for the traveler except in cold or mountainous areas where local conditions favor louse infestation. At present, vaccination is recommended only for persons traveling to rural or remote areas of Ethiopia, Rwanda, Burundi, Mexico, Ecuador, Bolivia, or Peru, and the mountainous areas of Asia.

Typhus vaccine is prepared from killed *Rickettsiae prowazekii* organisms propagated in chick embryos. The usual recommended dosage is 1.0 ml subcutaneously at an interval of 3 to 4 weeks, with a single booster injection of 1.0 ml given every 6 to 12 months as long as the risk of exposure continues. Pain and tenderness at the site of injection and an occasional febrile reaction are the only reported adverse effects. Although no controlled studies have been carried out, experience during the North African campaign in World War II has led to the conclusion that the prevalence of the disease is lower in vaccinated individuals. It should be emphasized that vaccination provides protection only against louse-borne (epidemic) typhus, and not against murine or scrub typhus.

REFERENCES

1. Atwood, W. G., Miller, J. L., Stout, G. W., and Norins, L. C. The TPI and FTA-ABS tests in treated late syphilis. *J.A.M.A. 203:*549, 1968.

2. Barta, K. Complement fixation test for pneumocystosis. *Ann. Intern. Med. 70:*235, 1969.

3. Bellanti, J. A., and Jackson, A. L. Characterization of serum immunoglobulins to the somatic antigen of *S. typhosa* in an infant following intrauterine immunization. *J. Pediat. 71:*783, 1968.

4. Brunell, P. A., Ross, A., Miller, L. H., and Kuo, B. Prevention of varicella by zoster immune globulin. *New Eng. J. Med. 280:*119, 1969.

5. Cannefax, G. R., Norins, L. C., and Gillespie, E. J. Immunology of syphilis. *Ann. Rev. Med. 18:*471, 1967.

6. Carpenter, R. L., Patnode, R. A., and Goldsmith, J. B. Comparative study of skin-test reactions to various mycobacterial antigens in Choctaw county, Oklahoma. *Amer. Rev. Resp. Dis. 95:*6, 1967.

7. Deacon, W. E., and Hunter, C. F. Treponemal antigens as related to identification and syphilis serology. *Proc. Soc. Exp. Biol. Med. 110:*352, 1962.

8. Dick, G. Immunization of children against virus diseases. *Brit. J. Hosp. Med. 2:*463, 1969.

8a. Editorial. Cellular immunity in infectious diseases. *Lancet 2:*253, 1969.

9. Evans, D. G. (ed.) Immunization against infectious diseases. *Brit. Med. Bull. 25:*119, 1969.

10. Fletcher, S. Indirect fluorescent antibody technique in the serology of *Toxoplasma gondii. J. Clin. Path. 18:*193, 1965.

11. Freedman, S. O., Dolovich, J., Turcotte, R., and Sault, F. Circulating IgG hemagglutinins to tuberculin in pulmonary tuberculosis. *Amer. Rev. Resp. Dis. 94:*896, 1966.

12. Fulton, J. D. Micro-agglutination test for *Toxoplasma* antibodies. *Immunology 9:*491, 1965.

13. Fulton, J. D., and Fulton, F. Complement fixation tests in toxoplasmosis with purified antigen. *Nature 205:*776, 1965.

14. Harner, R. E., Smith, J. L., and Israel, C. W. The FTA-ABS test in late syphilis. A serological study in 1,985 cases. *J.A.M.A. 203:*545, 1968.

15. Hart, P. D. Efficacy and applicability of mass B.C.G. vaccination in tuberculosis control. *Brit. Med. J. 1:*587, 1967.

16. Harvey, A. M., and Shulman, L. E. Connective-tissue disease and the chronic biologic false positive test for syphilis (BFP reaction). *Med. Clin. N. Amer. 50:*1271, 1966.

17. Hilleman, M. R., Buynak, E. B., Weibel, R. E., Stokes, J. Live, attenuated mumps-virus vaccine. *New Eng. J. Med. 278:*227, 1968.

18. Hull, F. E. Tuberculin tine test. A comparative study with purified protein derivative of tuberculin. *J.A.M.A. 203:*562, 1968.

19. Kempe, C. H., Fulginitti, V., Minamitani, M., and Shinefield, H. Smallpox vaccination of eczema patients with a strain of attenuated live vaccinia (CVI-78). *Pediatrics 42:*980, 1968.

20. Kent, D. C., Reid, D., Sokolowski, J. W., and Houk, V. N. Tuberculin conversion. The iceberg of tuberculous pathogenesis. *Arch. Environ. Health (Chicago) 14:*580, 1967.

21. Koenig, M. C. Trivalent botulinus antitoxin. *Ann. Intern. Med. 70:*643, 1969.

21a. Lane, J. M., Ruben, F. L., Neff, J. M., and Millar, J. D. Complications of smallpox vaccination 1968. National surveillance in the United States. *New Eng. J. Med. 281:*1201, 1969.

22. Lind, K. Immunological relationships between *Mycoplasma pneumoniae* and *Streptococcus* MG. *Acta Path. Microbiol. Scand. 73:*237, 1968.

23. Macdonald, A., and Elmslie, W. H. Serological investigations in suspected brucellosis. *Lancet 1:*380, 1967.

24. Miller, L. H., and Brown, H. W. The serologic diagnosis of parasitic infections in medical practice. *Ann. Intern. Med. 71:*983, 1969.

25. Moss, K. G., Fulmer, H. S., and Deuschle, K. L. The present status of typhoid carriers in Kentucky. *Arch. Environ. Health (Chicago) 14:*407, 1967.

26. Nicholas, L. Serodiagnosis of syphilis. *Arch. Derm. 96:*324, 1967.

27. Nilsson, L. A. Comparative testing of precipitation methods for quantitation of C-reactive protein in blood serum. *Acta Path. Microbiol. Scand. 73:*129, 1968.

28. Neff, J. M., and Lane, J. M. Smallpox vaccination: Before or after one year of age? *Pediatrics 42:*986, 1968.

29. Nelson, R. A., and Mayer, M. M. Immobilization of *Treponema Pallidum* in vitro by antibody produced in syphilitic infection. *J. Exp. Med. 89:*369, 1949.

30. Peebles, T. C., Levine, L., Eldred, M. C., and Esdall, G. Tetanus toxoid emergency boosters: A reappraisal. *New Eng. J. Med. 280:*682, 1969.

30a. Remington, J. S. Toxoplasmosis: Recent developments. *Ann. Rev. Med. 21:*201, 1970.

31. Schmale, J. D. Serologic detection of gonorrhea. *Ann. Intern. Med. 72:*592, 1970.

31a. Sikes, R. K., Rabies immunization. *Ann. Intern. Med. 72:*434, 1970.

32. Smith, D. W. Why not vaccinate against tuberculosis? *Ann. Intern. Med. 72:*419, 1970.

33. Weibel, R. E., Stokes, J., Jr., Buynak, E. B., and Hilleman, M. R. Rubella vaccination in adult females. *New Eng. J. Med. 280:*682, 1969.

34. Wright, D. J. M., Doniach, D., Lessof, M. H., Turk, J. L. Grimble, A. S., and Catterall, R. D. New antibody in early syphilis. *Lancet 1:*740, 1970.

22

Laboratory Tests in Clinical Immunology

SAMUEL O. FREEDMAN

The results of immunologic tests, although rarely diagnostic in themselves, often constitute valuable supportive evidence for the confirmation of suspected immunologic disease. In this chapter, no attempt will be made to describe detailed methodology for the performance of laboratory tests in clinical immunology. Instead, the emphasis will be placed on the indications for, the normal values, and the interpretation of those immunologic tests which appear to be of value in clinical medicine. Before describing specific test procedures, the general methods of measuring antigen-antibody reactions will be outlined in order to facilitate the subsequent discussion of individual diagnostic techniques.

GENERAL METHODS OF MEASURING ANTIGEN-ANTIBODY REACTIONS

According to the unitarian hypothesis of antibody formation, all humoral antibodies were considered to be capable of equal reactivity in all serologic procedures including precipitation, agglutination, complement-fixation, lysis, opsonization, and their various modifications. Although this concept is no longer tenable in all of its aspects, most antibody molecules can take part in a number of in vitro reactions to a greater or lesser extent. In the majority of instances, the name applied to a test for the detection of a specific antigen or antibody does not imply that the antibody which participates in the reaction has exclusive functional properties. Terms such as precipitins, agglutinins, or complement-fixing antibodies are merely semantic conveniences that describe the conditions under which the reaction is performed. For example, a "precipitating antibody" might well demonstrate agglutinating activity if its corresponding soluble antigen is conjugated to erythrocytes, and might well participate in reactions of complement-fixation or lysis if complement is added to the mixture under suitable conditions.

On the other hand, it should be noted that certain types of antibodies in humans, particularly those belonging to the IgE class of immunoglobulins (reagins or homocytotropic antibodies), probably do not participate in conventional serologic reactions such as precipitation, agglutination, or lysis. It is of interest that these reaginic antibodies are chemically and functionally distinguishable from antibodies belonging to other immunoglobulin types (see Chapter 1), although they may have apparently identical specificities for the same antigen. Furthermore, both reaginic and nonreaginic antibodies may be produced at approximately the same time in a single individual following antigenic exposure. The exact relationship between the function of antibodies in vivo and their participation in in vitro reactions will only be established with certainty as more knowledge becomes available concerning the physicochemical properties of antibody molecules.

In considering the general principles of serologic testing, it should be noted that most conventional antibody tests, such as precipitation or complement-fixation, measure the secondary effects of a primary antigen-antibody reaction rather than the capacity of an antiserum to bind antigen. The importance of measuring antigen binding capacity rather than the degree of precipitation is best illustrated by the observation that some populations of antibodies do not precipitate spontaneously even in the presence of optimum concentrations of antigen. Nevertheless, both the *primary* and *secondary* manifestations of antigen-antibody interaction have well established applications in the clinical immunology laboratory (Table 22-1).

PRIMARY MANIFESTATIONS OF ANTIGEN-ANTIBODY REACTIONS

Radioimmunoassay Techniques

Radioimmunoassay methods are particularly useful for the measurement of antigens and antibodies which are of low avidity or exist in low concentrations. One example of this type of technique is the ammonium sulfate method. The procedure is based on the observation that many antigens are not precipitated by ammonium sulfate, whereas ammonium sulfate in suitable concentration will precipitate immunoglobulins semi-quantitatively. Thus, if a radiolabelled antigen is added to its corresponding antiserum and the resultant mixture is treated with half-saturated ammonium sulfate, the precipitate will contain no radioactivity unless an antigen-antibody reaction has occurred. The amount of radiolabelled antigen bound by the antigen-antibody complex can be used to determine, in quantitative terms, the amount of antibody present. Several sophisticated variations of this very sensitive method have been developed for the quantitative measurement of either antigen or antibody.

TABLE 22-1. General Methods of Measuring
Antigen-Antibody Reactions

Primary Manifestations
    Radioimmunoassay techniques
    Immunofluorescence techniques
Secondary Manifestations
    Precipitation in solution
    Precipitation in gel
    Radial precipitation (radial immunodiffusion)
    Immunoelectrophoresis
    Direct agglutination tests
    Passive agglutination tests
    The Coombs' (antiglobulin) test
    Complement-fixation tests
    Tests of immune cytolysis
    Tests of opsonization and phagocytosis
    Tests for reagins

Other immunoassay techniques depend upon the competition for antibody between unlabelled antigen in the patient's serum and radiolabelled antigen which is added to the reaction mixture in predetermined amounts. The unbound radiolabelled antigen and the antigen-antibody complex may then be separated by physical methods, such as centrifugation or electrophoresis, and the amount of radioactivity can be used to calculate the quantity of antigen in the test sample.

Immunofluorescence Techniques

Antibodies can be made fluorescent without altering their immunologic properties or specificity by attaching them to a dye such as fluorescein isothiocyanate, or Lissamine-Rhodamine. The fluorescent antibodies can then be used to demonstrate both antigens and antibodies in tissue sections or cell smears when these preparations are examined microscopically under ultraviolet light.

Intrinsic tissue antigens such as nuclear antigens or immune reactants (e.g., immunoglobulins or complement) deposited in tissues can be demonstrated in tissue sections by the *direct* application of specific fluorescent antibodies. In the *indirect* immunofluorescence technique, an antiserum containing unlabelled antibodies is applied to the section which is then treated with a fluorescent anti-γ-globulin antiserum of the appropriate species specificity. The advantage of the indirect technique is that it is necessary to prepare only a single fluorescent antiserum for a variety of tests. Furthermore, the sensitivity of the test is increased considerably because more labelled antibody becomes attached to the section than in the direct technique.

Another application of the indirect immunofluorescence technique is the detection in human sera of antibodies directed against tissue antigens. A section of normal tissue (not necessarily of human origin) is first treated with the serum under investigation. If antitissue antibodies present in the serum become attached to the tissue antigens, the subsequent application of a fluorescent antihuman immunoglobulin antiserum will reveal a typical pattern of fluorescence.

SECONDARY MANIFESTATIONS OF ANTIGEN-ANTIBODY REACTIONS

Precipitation in Solution

The mechanism of the precipitation reaction in vitro constitutes the basis for most theories of antigen-antibody interaction, and thus it is of theoretic as well as practical significance. If increasing amounts of a soluble antigen are added to a constant amount of antiserum, a typical precipitation curve is formed (Fig. 22-1). The antigen-antibody precipitate first appears in the zone of antibody excess, reaches its maximum in the equivalence zone, and then decreases again in the zone of antigen excess. This phenomenon is best explained by the framework or lattice theory which postulates that the participating antigen and antibody molecules have more than one combining site. The hypothetical structures of immune precipitates and soluble complexes according to the lattice theory are illustrated schematically in Figure 22-2.

Precipitation in Gel

At the present time, one of the several available gel diffusion techniques is the most common method of demonstrating precipitin reactions between soluble antigens and their corresponding antibodies. In the double diffusion plate test described by Ouchterlony, buffered agar is poured into a Petri dish or on a glass slide, allowed to harden, and two or more wells are then cut in the gel. (Gelatin, agarose, silica gel, cellulose acetate, acrylamides, and other substances have also been used as the supporting medium, but agar is used most frequently in clinical laboratories.) The antigen and antiserum are placed in separate wells, allowed to diffuse through the agar, and a visible band of precipitation occurs where the antigen and antibody meet in optimal proportions.

Increasing amounts of antigen added
to constant amount of antiserum

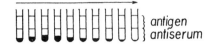

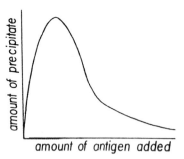

FIG. 22-1. Schematic representation of a typical precipitin curve. (From Sehon, A. H. in Harris, M. C., and Shure, N., *Sensitivity Chest Diseases,* Philadelphia, Davis, 1964.)

Because different antigens migrate through the agar at different rates depending on their equivalence zones, the number of separate bands observed when an antigen mixture reacts with an antiserum directed against all of its components provides an approximate indication of the number of antigenic constituents in the mixture. If two antigen mixtures are diffused simultaneously against the same antiserum, precipitin bands due to a common antigenic component fuse to form a continuous line (reaction of identity), whereas bands due to different antigenic components cross each other (reaction of nonidentity) (see Fig. 22-3). Additional advantages of this procedure are that equivalence is automatic, and that it requires relatively small amounts of antigen and antisera.

Radial Precipitation (Radial Immunodiffusion)

Radial immunodiffusion tests have proved to be extremely useful in clinical immunology laboratories for the measurement of various plasma protein constituents with reasonable accuracy, simplicity, and economy of reagents. In the method most commonly employed, a small amount of antiserum is incorporated in agar on a glass slide or plate and the antigen is placed in a well cut in the agar. The concentration of antigen can then be calculated from the radius of the precipitin ring surrounding the antigen well.

PRECIPITIN REACTION IN LIQUID MEDIA

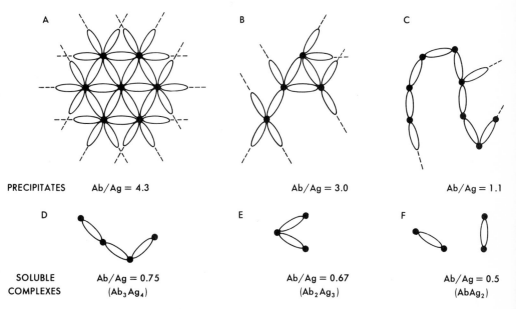

FIG. 22-2. Schematic representation of the lattice theory. **Black circles** represent antigen molecules; **Open elipses** represent antibody molecules; **numbers** refer to mole ratios of antibody (Ab) to antigen (Ag). **Dotted lines** indicate that precipitates may continue to extend. Precipitates correspond to those found in the antibody excess zone (A), the equivalence zone (B), and the antigen excess zone (C). Soluble complexes correspond to those found in supernatants in moderate (D), far (E), or extreme (F) antigen excess. (From Davis, B. D., Dulbecco, R., Eisen, H. N., Ginsburg, H., and Wood, W. B. Microbiology, New York, Hoeber Medical Division, Harper & Row, 1967.)

Immunoelectrophoresis

The process of immunoelectrophoresis entails a combination of the methods of precipitation in gel and electrophoresis. Its major application in clinical immunology is for the identification of normal and abnormal serum proteins, although it may be used for other purposes. The serum, or a serum fraction, is placed in a well on a slide coated with agar, and an electric current is applied across the slide in order to cause a separation of protein components. After the slide is removed from the electrophoresis aparatus, antihuman immunoglobulin or antiwhole human serum antiserum is placed in a longitudinal trough and allowed to diffuse against the separated protein constituents. The various protein constituents of the serum appear as overlapping areas of antigen-antibody precipitate which can be identified by their shape and position on the slide (Fig. 22-4).

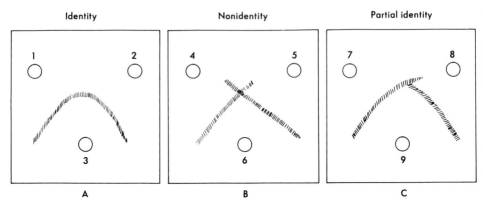

FIG. 22-3. Precipitation in gel showing reactions of identity (*A*), nonidentity (*B*), and partial identity (*C*). (From Davis, B. D., Dulbecco, R., Eisen, H. N., Ginsburg, H., and Wood, W. B. *Microbiology,* New York, Hoeber Medical Division, Harper & Row, 1967.)

Direct Agglutination Tests

The direct agglutination technique is used in clinical immunology for the detection of antigens located on the surfaces of formed blood elements or on microorganisms. The test is most commonly performed by mixing dilutions of antiserum with a suspension of the particulate material containing surface antigens. The reaction between antigen and antibody is manifested by agglutination or aggregation of particles in a test tube, in wells, or on a slide. The mechanism of the agglutination reaction is considered to be similar to that of the precipitin reaction. It is postulated that multivalent antibodies combine with surface antigen and the particles become cross-linked to form three dimensional visible clumps. In general, agglutination procedures in which antigen molecules are fixed to cell surfaces are far more sensitive than precipitation procedures in which the antigen mole-

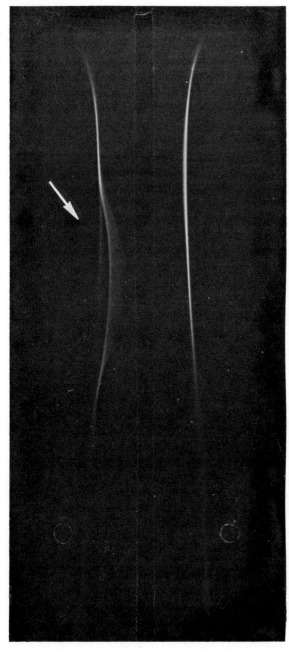

FIG. 22-4. Example of immunoelectrophoresis of human myeloma serum (*upper well*) and human normal serum (*lower well*) against antihuman IgG antiserum in the trough. The additional and abnormally shaped band in the upper portion is due to an IgG myeloma protein.

cules are free in solution. The reason for the higher sensitivity of the agglutination reaction is that the bulk of the combining mass is provided by the cells or microorganisms which contain the surface antigens.

Passive Agglutination Tests

The specific agglutination of red cells, collodion, latex, or bentonite particles passively coated with soluble antigen constitutes a highly sensitive method for the detection of antibodies present in extremely low concentrations. Protein antigens may be nonspecifically adsorbed to the red cell surface by treatment with tannic acid or they may be covalently linked to the red cell by the use of reagents such as bis-diazotized benzidine (BDB), carbodiimide, or toluene-2,4-diisocyanate. The latter methods tend to be more sensitive since the antigen is firmly linked to the red cell. Otherwise, antigen which separates from the red cells may inhibit the hemagglutination reaction. Many polysaccharide antigens will link nonspecifically to red cells and no special treatment is required.

Neutral carriers such as bentonite or latex particles adsorb antigens nonspecifically. The reactions obtained with these carrier materials may be observed as agglutination in tubes or as flocculation on slides depending on the antigen, the carrier, and the conditions of the test.

The Coombs' (Antiglobulin) Test

The direct and indirect Coombs' tests are sophisticated variations of the agglutination procedure, and are most commonly employed to detect antigen-antibody reactions between anti-Rh antibodies and Rh blood group antigens. The Coombs' test is described in detail in Chapter 9.

Complement-Fixation Tests

The hemolytic complement-fixation test is based on the principle that a standard amount of complement added to a mixture of antigen and its corresponding antibody is fixed by the antigen-antibody complex which is formed. The reaction mixture of complement, antigen, and antibody is then tested for the presence of free complement in the second stage of the procedure by adding a mixture of erythrocytes and anti-erythrocyte antibodies. If the erythrocytes are not lysed by their specific antibodies, it means that complement was utilized by an antigen-antibody reaction which occurred in the first stage of the test. One of the advantages of the complement-fixation procedure is that it can be utilized with both soluble and particulate antigens and it is not dependent on the chemical nature of the antigenic determinants.

Tests of Immune Cytolysis

The mechanism of destruction of cells in vitro through the combined action of complement and their specific antibodies is discussed in detail in Chapters 1 and 9.

Tests of Opsonization and Phagocytosis

The principles underlying the commonly used tests for the assessment of opsonization and phagocytosis are discussed in Chapter 11.

Tests for Reagins

Direct skin testing for reaginic antibodies, the Prausnitz-Küstner reaction, and those in vitro tests for reagins which have potential clinical applications are discussed in Chapters 1 and 3.

SPECIFIC TESTS IN CLINICAL IMMUNOLOGY

The number and variety of tests performed in clinical immunology laboratories obviously differs widely between institutions. In this section, a brief description of those procedures which are carried out in the Clinical Immunology Laboratory of The Montreal General Hospital will be presented together with comments regarding their significance and interpretation. Most of the tests to be discussed are listed in the requisition form in use at The Montreal General Hospital which is reproduced in Figure 22-5. Many variations of these procedures exist, are carried out in other laboratories, and are equally useful in clinical immunology. However, a detailed description of all available methods is beyond the scope of this book.

IMMUNOGLOBULIN PROFILE

In the Clinical Immunology Laboratory of The Montreal General Hospital, a routine "Immunoglobulin Profile" consists of the following determinations: (*1*) total serum proteins determined by conventional biochemical methods; (*2*) cellulose acetate electrophoresis; (*3*) quantitative immunoglobulins; (*4*) immunoelectrophoresis when indicated; and (*5*) analytic ultracentrifugation when indicated. The information derived from the first three determinations is essential for a preliminary assessment of the immunoglobulin status of a given patient, and the last two are very helpful in selected problems to be discussed later in this section.

MR ☐
MRS ☐
MISS ☐

SURNAME _____

GIVEN NAMES _____

UNIT NO. _____ ROOM NO. _____

ADDRESS _____
(If Out Patient)

ATTENDING PHYSICIAN _____
(If Private Patient)

DATE ORDERED _____

ORDERED BY _____

DIAGNOSIS

RELEVANT LABORATORY AND PHYSICAL FINDINGS

FOR BLOOD TESTS SEND 20ml CLOTTED BLOOD
Tests marked with an asterisk * available on consultation only on ward patients, and by special request (Local 740) on private and semi-private patients.

☐ IMMUNOGLOBULIN PROFILE	NORMAL	RESULTS
QUANTITATIVE IMMUNOGLOBULINS		
IgG mg/100 ml	600-1500	
IgA mg/ 100 ml	19-495	
IgM mg/100 ml	57-200	
Total proteins _____ gm/100ml		
☐ ULTRACENTRIFUGATION*		

AUTOIMMUNE PROFILE
☐ R.A. TEST
☐ ANTI–DNA
☐ ANTI–THYROID
☐ ANTI–MUSCLE
☐ COMPLEMENT (C'3)
☐ DNA BINDING*

IMMUNO– FLUORESCENCE
☐ KIDNEY *
☐ ANTI– NUCLEAR*
☐ THYROID*
☐ ADRENAL*
☐ GASTRIC*
☐ MUSCLE*

☐ LIGHT CHAINS (SERUM)
☐ LIGHT CHAINS (URINE)
☐ PLASMA VISCOSITY (HEPARINIZED)
☐ CRYOGLOBULINS DELIVER IMMEDIATLY
☐ SELECTIVE PROTEIN CLEARANCE
☐ IMMUNE DEFICIENCY PROFILE*
☐ LYMPHOCYTE * TRANSFORMATION
☐ OTHER TESTS (SPECIFY)

CELLULOSE ACETATE ELECTROPHORESIS

IMMUNOELECTROPHORESIS

REPORT:

FIG. 22-5. Requisition form in use for the Clinical Immunology Laboratory of The Montreal General Hospital.

Cellulose Acetate Electrophoresis

Immunoglobulins, like other serum proteins, can be separated electrophoretically according to their electrical charge and molecular size. In the cellulose acetate methods, a linear application of serum is made towards one end of a strip of cellulose acetate, an electric current is applied across the strip for 45 to 60 minutes, and the separated proteins are then stained to make them visible. The amount of protein which migrates in the albumin, $\alpha 1$, $\alpha 2$, β, and γ-globulin regions can then be determined quantitatively through the use of a scanning densitometer and integrator (Fig. 22-6). Normal values obtained by this method are listed in Table 22-2.

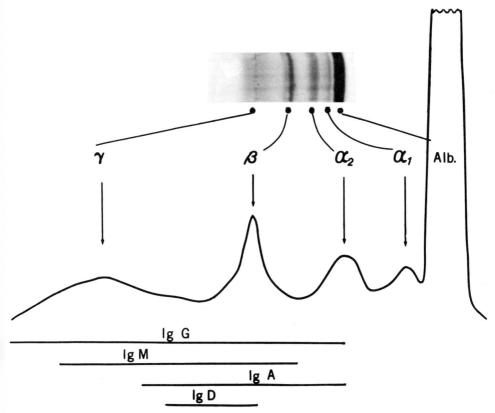

FIG. 22-6. Schematic representation of the pattern obtained on scanning a cellulose acetate electrophoretic strip of normal human serum.

The results of cellulose actate electrophoresis when considered together with the total protein values are extremely useful in making the diagnosis

TABLE 22-2. Normal Adult Values for Electro-phoretic Fractionation of Serum Proteins by the Cellulose Acetate Method

	Gm/100 ml
Total proteins	6.5–8.2
Albumin	3.3–5.0
α1-globulin	0.2–0.4
α2-globulin	0.6–0.8
β2-globulin	0.6–1.1
γ-globulin	0.9–1.9

TABLE 22-3. Immunologic Deficiency Disorders Which May Be Associated with Hypogammaglobulinemia

Primary Disorders (see Chapter 11)
1. X-linked thymic alymphoplasia with agammaglobulinemia
2. Autosomal recessive alymphocytic agammaglobulinemia (Swiss-type agamma-globulinemia)
3. Lymphopenia-agammaglobulinemia with agranulocytosis
4. Primary agammaglobulinemia
5. Transient hypogammaglobulinemia of infancy
6. The dysgammaglobulinemias
7. Wiskott-Aldrich syndrome
8. Ataxia telangiectasia

Secondary Disorders
1. Chronic lymphocytic leukemia
2. Lymphosarcoma
3. Reticulum cell sarcoma
4. Giant follicular lymphoma
5. Plasma cell disorders (some cases—see Chapter 10 for explanation)
6. Administration of corticosteroids, immunosuppressive agents, and cancer chemotherapeutic drugs
7. Nephrotic syndrome
8. Protein losing gastroenteropathy
9. Thymoma
10. Myotonic dystrophy
11. Congenital rubella syndrome

of hypergammaglobulinemia, hypogammaglobulinemia, or hypoalbuminemia. In addition, the shape of the electrophoretic scan produced by the densitometer is essential for the detection of and distinction between polyclonal and monoclonal gammopathies (see Figs. 10-2 and 10-4).

The diseases associated with polyclonal hypergammaglobulinemia are listed in Table 10-1; the diseases associated with monoclonal hypergammaglobulinemia are listed in Table 10-2; and the disorders associated with hypogammaglobulinemia are listed in Table 22-3.

Quantitative Immunoglobulin Determination

The serum levels of individual immunoglobulin classes can be determined with a high degree of sensitivity and reproducibility by the technique of radial immunodiffusion previously described. The measurement of individual immunoglobulin values, as opposed to the total electrophoretic γ-globulin values, is particularly useful as a screening procedure in the detection of certain immunologic deficiency states, the dysgammaglobulinemias, multiple myeloma, Waldenstrom's macroglobulinemia, and the various causes of hypergammaglobulinemia. Normal serum immunoglobulin values for children and adults are presented in Table 22-4.

TABLE 22-4. Range of Immunoglobulin Levels in the Sera of Normal Subjects at Various Ages

Age	IgG (mg/100 ml)	IgM (mg/100 ml)	IgA (mg/100 ml)
Newborn	750–1650	2–30	0–10
1–3 months	275–750	10–70	5–60
4–6 months	200–1150	10–80	10–90
7–24 months	250–1500	20–150	15–125
2–3 years	400–1500	20–150	20–250
3–8 years	550–1500	20–150	20–300
9–16 years	600–1600	35–150	20–400
Adults	600–1600	60–200	20–500

The correlation between serum immunoglobulin abnormalities and clinical disease is illustrated by the data obtained from 1000 consecutive patients referred for investigation to the Division of Clinical Immunology of The Montreal General Hospital. The referrals were obtained from all departments in the hospital, but the majority originated from the general medical

TABLE 22-5. Common Causes of Immunoglobulin Abnormalities Not Associated with a Monoclonal Peak

Diagnosis	Number of patients	Patients with abnormal findings	Electrophoresis γ-globulins ↑	→	IgA ↑	IgG ↑	→	IgM ↑	↓	IgA and IgG ↑	IgA and IgM ↑	IgG and IgM ↑	→	IgA, IgG, and IgM ↑	↑IgG and ↓IgM	↑IgG, ↑IgA, and ↓IgM
Liver disease																
Cirrhosis	19	19	8		4	1		4	2	4		4				
Chronic active hepatitis	4	4	2					1				1			1	1
Collagen-vascular disease																
Rheumatoid arthritis	151	68	6	7	9	8		27	10	4		4	1	4		
Systemic lupus erythematosus	11	9	4	2		1	2			2						
Sjögren's syndrome	2	2	2					2			1	2		1		
Temporal arteritis	2	1						1								
Polymyositis	5	2	2			1				1						
Pulmonary fibrosis	4	3			2			1								
Leukemia																
Chronic myelogenous	3	3	2			1		1						1		
Chronic lymphatic	5	3		2				1	1				1			
Plasma cell	1	1	1													
Hodgkin's disease	11	9		5		1			4			1	3	1		
Chronic infections	4	4			1	1		1		1						
TOTALS	222	128	27	16	16	14	2	39	17	12	1	12	5	7	1	1

wards or from the specialty services of clinical immunology, rheumatology, hematology, and dermatology. Thus, the patients studied were drawn from a highly selected group of adults who were expected to show some form of immunoglobulin abnormality. Nevertheless, the results are of interest because they serve to illustrate both the value and the limitations of immunoglobulin studies as a diagnostic technique.

Of the 1000 patients studied, 128 showed immunoglobulin abnormalities not associated with a monoclonal peak on cellulose acetate electrophoresis (see Table 22-5), and 25 showed immunoglobulin abnormalities associated with a monoclonal peak (see Table 22-6). Examination of the tables reveals that polyclonal hypergammaglobulinemias were detected most frequently in patients with Laennec's cirrhosis, chronic active hepatitis, a variety of collagen-vascular diseases, and chronic infections. Monoclonal gammopathies occurred most commonly in patients with multiple myeloma, but were also detected in Waldenstrom's macroglobulinemia, lymphosarcoma, Sjögren's syndrome, and infectious hepatitis. Hypogammaglobulinemia, on the other hand, was most frequently associated with rheumatoid arthritis (perhaps due to chronic steroid therapy), Hodgkin's disease, chronic lymphatic leukemia, multiple myeloma, and the nephrotic syndrome of systemic lupus erythematosus.

TABLE 22-6. Monoclonal Gammopathies (M Proteins)

Diagnosis	Number of patients	Immunoglobulin class of monoclonal peak		
		IgG	IgA	IgM
Multiple myeloma	17	9	8	—
Waldenstrom's macroglobulinemia	2	—	—	2
Lymphosarcoma	2	1	—	1
Sjögren's syndrome	2	1	—	—
Chronic active hepatitis	1	1	—	—
Idiopathic	1	1	—	—
Total	25	13	8	3

Immunoelectrophoresis

Immunoelectrophoresis of the patient's serum against antiwhole serum, anti-total immunoglobulin, anti-IgG, anti-IgM, and anti-IgA antisera is indicated whenever there is a monoclonal or polyclonal peak in the electrophoretic scan, or whenever there is a significant increase or decrease in one of the immunoglobulin fractions. This procedure is particularly useful for the detection and identification of the abnormal immunoglobulins such as those which occur in multiple myeloma and related disorders (Fig. 22-4). In addition, immunoelectrophoresis against antilambda chain or antikappa chain antiserum can be employed for the detection and identification of free light chains in the patient's serum or concentrated urine.

Analytic Ultracentrifugation

In patients with macroglobulinemia, the demonstration of 19S components in the ultracentrifuge may provide confirmation of the findings obtained by electrophoresis, quantitative immunoglobulin determinations, and immunoelectrophoresis. It should be remembered that the quantitative determination of immunoglobulins by radial immunodiffusion is dependent on the antigenic properties of the immunoglobulin molecule, rather than its structural properties. Thus, if a patient's serum demonstrates a monoclonal peak composed of monomer IgM, instead of the more common pentamer IgM (see Chapter 1), the serum IgM level will be increased, but there will be no abnormal macromolecular component detected on ultracentrifugation. The presence of monomer IgM can be confirmed more positively by techniques involving the use of column chromatography.

OTHER TESTS OF VALUE IN THE STUDY OF IMMUNOGLOBULIN ABNORMALITIES

Plasma Viscosity

In patients with large amounts of IgM or other macromolecules in their serum, the plasma viscosity may be increased and may result in the hyperviscosity syndrome described in Chapter 10. The plasma viscosity is most conveniently measured in a semi-micro-dilution viscometer, and is usually expressed as the relative viscosity compared to water. The average normal value is 1.65 times that of water, but clinical symptoms associated with hyperviscosity rarely appear until the relative viscosity levels are in the range of 5 to 6.

Cryoglobulins

The types of cryoglobulins which may occur in human disease states, as well as their clinical significance, is discussed in detail in Chapter 10. If cryoglobulinemia is suspected, a fresh sample of nonheparinized blood is drawn into a syringe, and allowed to clot and separate at 37° C. The serum is then stored at 4° C for 48 hours and examined for precipitation or gel formation. If a cryoprecipitate is formed, an attempt should be made to determine its nature by double diffusion in agar gel against anti-human IgG, IgM, IgA, and C3 antisera.

IMMUNE DEFICIENCY PROFILE

The investigation of a patient with a possible primary or secondary immunologic deficiency state will, of course, vary depending on the suspected underlying disorder, and the age of the patient. The procedures which are most frequently utilized for this purpose are listed in Table 22-7 and their clinical significance is discussed in detail in Chapter 11.

TABLE 22-7. Immune Deficiency Profile*

Tests of Phagocytic Function
1. White blood cell count for polymorphonuclear leukocytes
2. Bone marrow smear for polymorphonuclear leukocytes and their precursors
3. Scanning of liver and spleen with radioactive colloid
4. Nitroblue tetrazolium test (see Chapter 11)
5. Bactericidal assay

Tests of Lymphocyte Function (Cell-Mediated Immunity)
1. White blood cell count for lymphocytes
2. Response of lymphocytes to phytohemagglutinin (see Chapter 1)
3. Biopsy of regional lymph node 4 days after booster dose of DPT (see Chapter 21), or 10 days after primary immunization
4. Tests of delayed hypersensitivity
   a. Induction of delayed hypersensitivity to dinitrochlorobenzene (DNCB)
   b. Skin response to monilia, trichophyton, and streptodornase
   c. Skin response to tuberculin PPD in individuals previously immunized with BCG
   d. Allograft rejection time

Tests of Plasma Cell Function (Humoral Immunity)
1. Determination of serum immunoglobulin levels by quantitative gel diffusion
2. Determination of serum isohemagglutinin titers
3. Determination of primary antibody response by measuring H and O agglutinins following a single dose of typhoid vaccine
4. Determination of secondary antibody response by measuring diphtheria and tetanus antitoxin levels following a booster dose
5. Demonstration of plasma cells in a lymph node biopsy obtained after a secondary antigenic response

* Adapted from Janeway, C. A. *J. Pediat.* 72:885, 1968.

In the most commonly used test of deficient cell mediated immunity, a sensitizing dose of 0.1 ml of a 2% solution of 2,4 dinitrochlorobenzene (DNCB) in acetone is applied topically to the skin of the patient's forearm. After 10 to 14 days have elapsed, a challenging dose of 0.1 ml of a 0.1% solution of DNCB is applied to the opposite forearm. Under these circumstances, approximately 90 per cent of individuals with normal cell-mediated immunity will develop allergic contact dermatitis (see Chapter 5) at the site of challenge.

AUTOIMMUNE PROFILE

A number of laboratory procedures may be utilized to detect the presence of serum autoantibodies. Because multiple autoantibodies are often detected in patients with autoimmune syndromes (see Table 9-4), it should be remembered that autoantibodies do not always have organ-specific pathogenetic significance. Nevertheless, their presence may be of considerable assistance in confirming the diagnosis of autoimmune diseases which are suspected on clinical grounds or on the basis of other laboratory findings.

Rheumatoid Factors (R.A. Test)

Although a number of test procedures have been devised for the detection of rheumatoid factor, the sensitized sheep cell agglutination test is probably the most sensitive and most reliable method for routine clinical purposes. A commonly used modification of the test consists of a passive agglutination procedure in which the patient's serum is allowed to react with sheep erythrocytes which have been coated with pooled human normal γ-globulin (Cohn Fraction II) by the tanned cell method. An agglutination titer of 1:500 or greater is considered to constitute a positive test. The nature and properties of rheumatoid factor are discussed in Chapter 8, and the diseases which may be associated with rheumatoid factor activity are listed in Table 8-2.

Antinuclear Antibodies

As is the case with rheumatoid factor, numerous tests exist for the detection of antinuclear antibodies in the serum. In the Clinical Immunology Laboratory of The Montreal General Hospital, an indirect immunofluorescence technique for the detection of antinuclear antibodies is carried out by applying a 1:5 dilution of the patient's serum to a section of rat liver. Staining of the nuclei by antinuclear antibodies in the patient's serum is subsequently detected in the treated section by the addition of fluorescein labelled goat antihuman IgG, IgA, and IgM antisera. The correlation between a positive immunofluorescence test and disorders known to be associated with antinuclear antibodies (see Table 8-1) is excellent. The relationship between the LE cell phenomenon and antinuclear antibodies, and the significance the various patterns of nuclear staining is discussed in detail in Chapter 8.

Tests for Free DNA

As noted in Chapter 8, free DNA may appear in the sera of some patients in the absence of detectable antinuclear antibodies. The presence of free DNA is best detected by a modification of the ammonium sulfate method for the demonstration of primary antigen-antibody binding.

Antithyroid Antibodies

The types of thyroid antibodies which can occur in association with thyroid disorders are described fully in Chapter 15 (see Table 15-1). For clinical purposes, the most satisfactory procedures for the detection of thyroid antibodies in human sera are: (1) a passive agglutination procedure in which human group O, Rh+ erythrocytes are coated with a crude extract of normal human thyroid tissue by the tanned cell method; and (2) an indirect immunofluorescence test involving the use of the patient's serum, human thyroid tissue and fluorescein labelled goat antihuman IgG, IgM, and IgA antisera. A tanned cell hemagglutination titer greater than 1:25 is considered to constitute a positive test.

The incidence of thyroid antibodies in human thyroid disease is listed in Table 15-2 and the incidence of thyroid antibodies in other disease states is listed in Table 9-4.

Antiskeletal Muscle Antibodies

The presence of antiskeletal muscle antibodies in human sera can be detected: (1) by a passive hemagglutination test in which group O, Rh+ erythrocytes are coated with a crude extract of normal human skeletal muscle by the tanned cell method; and (2) by an indirect immunofluorescence technique involving the use of rat skeletal muscle, the patient's serum, and fluorescein labelled goat antihuman IgG, IgM, and IgA antisera. A tanned cell hemagglutination titer of 1:40 or greater is considered to constitute a positive test, and the significance of the pattern of immunofluorescent staining of striated muscle in myasthenia gravis is fully discussed in Chapter 19.

In myasthenia gravis, antiskeletal muscle antibodies can be detected by the tanned cell method in approximately 40 per cent of patients, and by the immunofluorescence technique in approximately 20 per cent of patients. However, when myasthenia gravis is associated with a thymoma, antiskeletal muscle antibodies are almost universally present.

Anti-Adrenal Antibodies

The presence of anti-adrenal antibodies in human sera is best demonstrated by an indirect immunofluorescence technique involving the use of normal human adrenal tissue, the patient's serum, and fluorescein labelled anti-human IgG, IgM, and IgA antisera. The incidence of anti-adrenal antibodies in patients with idiopathic adrenal atrophy (Addison's disease) is approximately 66 per cent for females and 33 per cent for males (see Chapter 15). In addition, anti-adrenal antibodies may be found in certain other human disease processes with immunologic features, and these are summarized in Table 9-4.

Antigastric Antibodies

Antigastric antibodies may be demonstrated in human sera by an indirect immunofluorescence technique involving the use of rat or human gastric tissue, the patient's serum, and fluorescein labelled goat antihuman IgG, IgM, or IgA antisera. The incidence of antigastric (parietal cell) antibodies in pernicious anemia, and in other diseases with immunologic features is summarized in Table 9-4.

Antibodies in Renal Disease

The direct immunofluorescent staining of renal biopsies with antihuman IgG, IgM, IgA, and C3 antisera constitutes an extremely valuable procedure in the differential diagnosis of immunologic renal disease. The significance of the "anti-GBM" and the "immune-complex" patterns of immunofluorescent staining is discussed in detail in Chapter 6, summarized in Tables 6-1 and 6-2, and illustrated in Figure 6-1.

Antibodies in Cutaneous Disease

Using an indirect immunofluorescence technique, it has been shown that the sera of approximately 65 per cent of patients with pemphigus vulgaris contain an antibody which localizes in the intercellular areas of stratified squamous epithelium. On the other hand, the antibodies are localized in the epithelial basement membrane in approximately 65 per cent of patients with bullous pemphigoid, and no antibodies are found in the sera of patients with dermatitis herpetiformis, erythema multiforme, or other bullous skin diseases. (See Table 5-5.) The indirect immunofluorescence technique employed in the differential diagnosis of bullous skin diseases involves the use of sections of stratified squamous epithelium obtained from the upper one-third of the rat esophagus, the patient's serum, and fluorescein labelled goat antihuman IgG, IgM, or IgA antisera (see Chapter 5).

In addition, the direct immunofluorescent staining of skin biopsies with antihuman IgG, IgM, IgA, and C3 antisera may provide confirmatory evidence for the existence of a cutaneous vasculitis of immunologic etiology.

Antibodies in Liver Disease

By means of indirect immunofluorescence techniques, it has been shown that the sera of some patients with chronic active hepatitis, primary biliary cirrhosis, or cryptogenic cirrhosis contain antibodies against smooth muscle, bile cannaliculi, on glomerular cytoplasmic (mitochondria constituents. The immunofluorescence technique involves the use of sections of rat uterus (smooth muscle), rat liver (bile cannaliculi), or rat kidney (cytoplasmic), the patient's serum, and goat antihuman immunoglobulin antisera. The incidence of various autoantibodies in several forms of chronic liver disease is presented in Table 16-1.

COMPLEMENT

There are at least three methods of studying complement in human disease: (1) the measurement of serum levels of C3 by quantitative gel diffusion (normal values 120 to 175 mg/100 ml); (2) the measurement of serum levels of complement by determining the degree of lysis by human complement of sheep erythrocytes sensitized with rabbit antibody as compared to a standard guinea pig complement preparation; and (3) the immunofluorescent demonstration of complement deposition in tissue sections using antisera directed against C3 (see Chapters 6, 7, and 8). The quantitative gel diffusion test, although relatively simple to perform, measures only a single complement component and does not discriminate between active and inactive C3. The hemolytic complement test, on the other hand, provides an indication of the functional activity of all the complement components, but does not detect minor variations in single complement components. The causes of decreased and increased serum complement levels are listed in Table 11-5.

SUGGESTED READING

1. Cohen, A. S. (ed.). *Laboratory Diagnostic Procedures in The Rheumatic Diseases,* Boston, Little, Brown, 1967.

2. Davis, B. D., Dulbecco, R., Eisen, H. N., Ginsberg, H. S., Wood, B. D., Jr. "Antibody-Antigen Interactions," in *Microbiology,* New York, Hoeber, 1967.

3. Kabat, E. A., and Mayer, M. M. *Experimental Immunochemistry,* Ed. 2, Springfield, Ill., Thomas, 1961.

4. Miescher, P. A., and Müller-Eberhard, H. J. (eds.) *Textbook of Immunopathology,* Vols. I and II, New York, Grune and Stratton, 1968.

5. Nairn, R. C. (ed.) *Fluorescent Tracing,* Ed. 2, Edinburgh, Livingstone, 1964.

6. Weir, D. M. (ed.) *Handbook of Experimental Immunology,* Philadelphia, Davis, 1967.

7. Williams, C. A., and Chase, M. W. (eds.) *Methods in Immunology and Immunochemistry,* Vols. I and II, New York, Academic Press, 1968.

Index

71 72 73 74 75 76   10 9 8 7 6 5 4 3 2 1